Ophthalmology - Current Clinical and Research Updates
http://dx.doi.org/10.5772/57076
Edited by Pinakin Gunvant Davey

Contributors

Pinakin Gunvant Davey, Makoto Ishikawa, Takeshi Yoshitomi, Yukitoshi Izumi, De-Quan Li, Cintia de Paiva, Stephen Pflugfelder, Balwant Singh Gendeh, Vikas Tah, James Myerscough, Kamran Saha, Stephen Tuft, Muhamad Ahad, Jason Ho, Bennett McAllister, Rebecca Kammer Od, Jie Shen, Elliot Marc Kirstein, Hezheng Zhou, Artashes Arto Zilfyan, Arto Zilfyan, Aaron Seitz, Jenni Deveau, Gary Lovcik, Felicia M. Ferreri, Italo Giuffre', Ipek Midi, Magdalena Zdybel, Barbara Pilawa, Umit Yolcu, Omer Faruk Sahin, Fatih Cakir Gundogan, Roshini Sanders, Hannah Timlin, Peizeng Yang, Patricio Pacheco

Published by InTech

Janeza Trdine 9, 51000 Rijeka, Croatia

Publishing Process Manager Iva Lipovic

Technical Editor InTech DTP team

Cover InTech Design team

First published September, 2014

Printed in Croatia

Additional hard copies can be obtained from orders@intechopen.com

Ophthalmology - Current Clinical and Research Updates, Edited by Pinakin Gunvant Davey

p. cm.

ISBN 978-953-51-1721-6

OPHTHALMOLOGY - CURRENT CLINICAL AND RESEARCH UPDATES

Edited by **Pinakin Gunvant Davey**

For EU product safety concerns:
IN TECH d.o.o., Prolaz Marije Krucifikse Kozulić 3, 51000 Rijeka, Croatia, info@intechopen.com or visit our website at intechopen.com.

Meet the editor

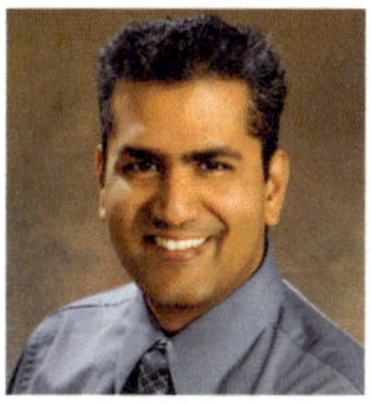

Dr. Pinakin Gunvant Davey is a tenured Professor at Western University of Health Sciences, College of Optometry. He holds Doctor of Optometry degree from Southern College of Optometry and a Ph.D. from Anglia Ruskin University in Cambridge, England, in the area of glaucoma. His post-doctoral research fellowship at University of Louisville was focused on improving imaging techniques in glaucoma. He has authored over 40 international publications, and has given over 100 conference and invited presentations both nationally and internationally. Dr. Davey research area is focused on retinal and optic nerve physiology and researches methods of improving vision in glaucoma and macular degeneration. Dr. Davey is on editorial board of 10 journals in the fields of ophthalmology, optometry and biomedical sciences.

Contents

Preface

In an era of information overload, boundaries that restrict information access must be demolished. To this, the Open Access books and journals are truly serving the purpose of not only breaking the barriers and but also abolishing in part "information poverty". The pioneering and up-to-date information in this book will be freely available without delay and restrictions. A great applaud is due to all the clinicians and researchers who authored chapters in this book; who believe in the Open Access model and have devoted their precious resources to publish in this book. Of course, a lot more needs to be done to eradicate the *information poverty* and we are indeed in the right direction with Open Access and we can dream of a day that "knowledge and information will be free flowing to all world, both developed and developing.

This book brings together both a review and updates in clinical and research areas of ophthalmology, optometry and vision science. The chapters will be of interest to a wide audience. On one hand, the review and update of clinical practices will interest students and residents, on the other, cutting edge research chapters will be of interest to the researchers in the field.

The book is divided into four parts: 1) Review and Updates in Diagnostic Testing, 2) Updates in Anterior Segment Diseases, 3) Updates in Posterior Segment Diseases, and 4) Updates in Research in Ophthalmology, Optometry and Vision Science. The chapters are written by experts and individuals with special interests in topics with a focus on clinical application and translational benefit to eye care.

This book was a significant undertaking and has come to fruition with assistance from numerous individuals that need to be thanked. I am grateful to Drs. Donald Egan and Raymond Maeda for their role of reviewers of book chapters. I am grateful to Miss Iva Lipović for all her help as a managing editor throughout the book project.

A special thanks to my family, my parents Gunvant and Minaben Davey for their support, my brother and sister Karthik Davey and Darshna Vyas whose strength I have always depended on. I am in debt to my wife Payal and my loving children Ved and Jash who allowed me to steal the time from them, to complete the book project, so I could see my dream come true. Thank you!

Dr. Pinakin Gunvant Davey
College of Optometry
Western University of Health Sciences
Pomona, California, USA

Section 1

Review and Updates in Diagnostic Testing

Chapter 1

Imaging in Ophthalmology

Umit Yolcu, Omer Faruk Sahin and
Fatih C. Gundogan

Additional information is available at the end of the chapter

http://dx.doi.org/10.5772/58314

1. Introduction

The imaging systems have a unique role in the ophthalmologic routine practice. While imaging has an auxiliary role in other branches of medicine, it is the most essential part of the ophthalmic examination. In other words, it can be said that ophthalmic examination is almost impossible without imaging. In this chapter, a basic review of the essentials of imaging techniques in ophthalmology will be presented.

2. Anterior segment imaging systems

2.1. Slit-lamp biomicroscopy

The slit lamp biomicroscopy is an important tool in ophthalmic practice. It is basically designed for examination of anterior segment but with the appropriate attachments, all ocular structures can be viewed. Most important advantage of biomicroscopy in examining the eye structures is stereopsis, in other words ophthalmologist can examine eye structures in three dimensions. It is a routine examination tool of most practitioners. In order to use all benefits of this tool, clinician should understand the basic imaging principle of the instrument.

Modern slit-lamp biomicroscopes have two major parts; observation and illumination systems. The illumination system of slit lamp projects bright slit light onto the focus plane. Illumination part delivers very sharp, thin and undistorted slit light in order to view true representation of the ocular structures. Blue and green filters are available in most slit-lamps to visualize fluorescein stain, micro-aneurysms and nerve fiber layer. In recent years LED illuminated slit lamps are also available. LED illuminated systems provides sharpest, brightest and most homogeneous slit beam. The other advantages LED systems on halogen lamps are last 100 times longer, have special light spectrum and they consume less energy.

Observation part comprises many optical lenses in order to deliver magnified view of ocular structures. Its magnification range differs between 5x to 40x depending on the manufacturer (Figure 1 A-F). It can enable magnification by flip-type, Galilean rotating barrel and continuous zoom methods [1]. High magnified view may be desirable for many clinicians however image quality compromises with high magnification. Therefore least required magnification should be used for the examination to achieve the best possible resolution. Resolution of a slit-lamp is depends on the wavelength of light used, the refractive index between the eye and objective, the working distance, and the diameter of the objective lens. Most biomicroscope oculars have 10 to 15 degree convergence angle to minimize convergence need of the examiner during the examination.

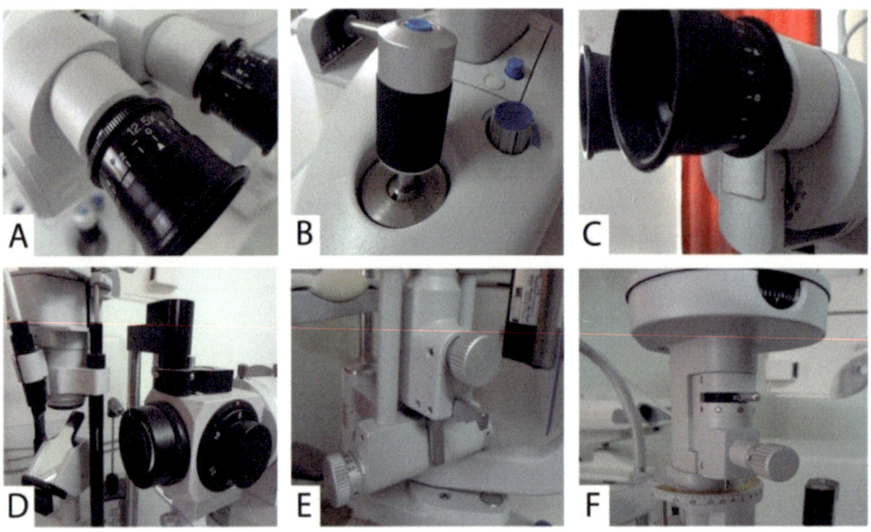

Figure 1. A. Binocular eyepieces provide stereoscopic vision and can be adjusted for examiners refraction. B. Joystick allows focusing with movement to forward, backward, laterally and diagonally. It can be rotated to lower or elevate the light beam. C. Eyepieces can be adjusted for Interpupillar distance of examiner D. Magnification can be changed with between 6x to 40 x. E. Releasing the knob allows separation of illumination and observation point. F. Slit height, color and angle can be adjusted with knurled knob.

In normal usage illumination system and observation system are coupled on a common focal plane and point. Both moves around a common focus point. It can horizontally uncoupled by releasing a knob. It is recommended that before using the slit lamp, distance between eyepieces should be adjusted for inter pupillary distance of the practitioner and focused by the help of a rod for his or her refraction. This procedure helps comfortable binocular viewing. Examination also should be conducted in semi-dark light conditions.

http://dx.doi.org/10.5772/58314

2.1.1. Examination techniques

2.1.1.1. Diffuse illumination

Diffuse illumination is a simple illumination method for examining the eye and surrounding structures. Slit width should be set to maximum, magnification to low and light at approximately 45-degree (Figure 2). Details cannot be viewed by this method; it just gives overview of eye and adnexia. High magnification should not be used with this method. Corneal scars, foreign bodies, pigmentary changes should be noted by this gross inspection method [2]. Findings obtained by the diffuse illumination should be investigated by other illumination techniques.

Cobalt blue filter and red free (green) filter can be used with this method. After instillation of fluorescein stain corneal epithelial defects, tear break up time and contact lens positioning can be viewed under cobalt blue light. With the green filter, bulbar conjunctival vessels and small hemorrhages and aneurysms can be viewed.

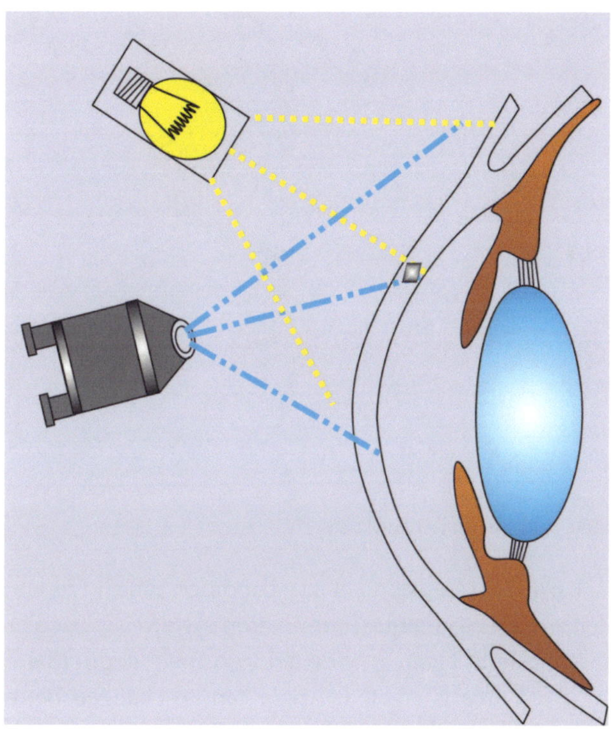

Figure 2. Diffuse illumination

a. Direct Illumination

Direct focal illumination is the most commonly used method. Observer focuses on the area directly illuminated by the slit light. Magnification can be increased to maximum if needed. Direct illumination can be used with different type of light beams.

Optic section of the cornea, anterior chamber and lens can be examined with optic section technique. Depth of any foreign body, stromal thinning, epithelial edema, layers of cornea, anterior chamber depth and different layers of lens can be determined. In this technique, illumination system is placed on the side of cornea or lens (i.e. temporal) and is set at angle between 30-60 degrees. Light beam is narrowed to minimum, light intensity is adjusted to maximum. Then examiner should focus on the middle point of horizontal corneal or lens section. Middle or maximum magnification can be used (Figure 3) [2].

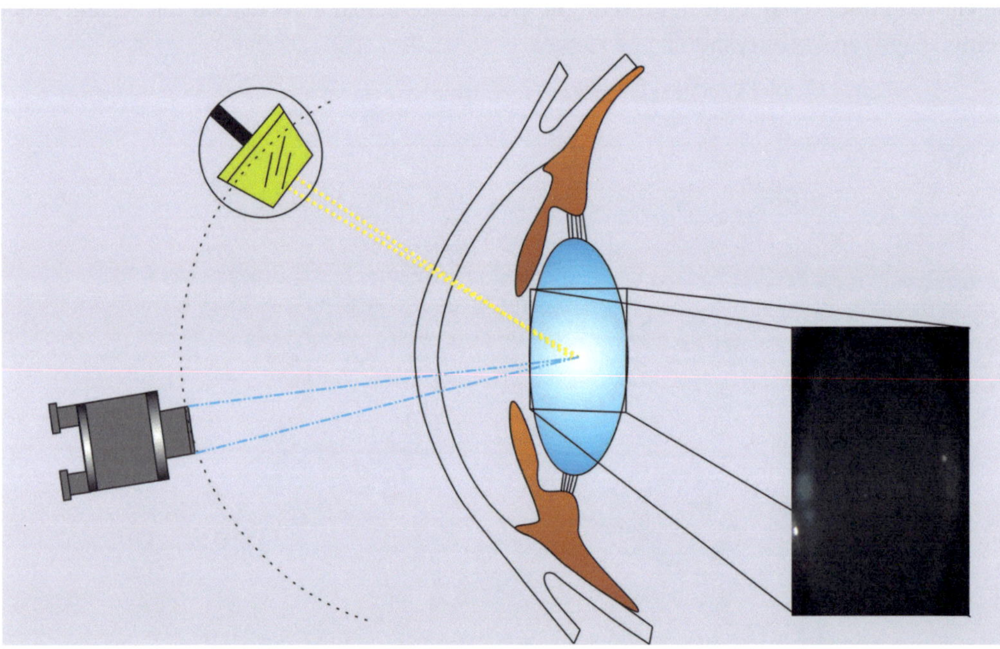

Figure 3. Direct illumination, optic section technique.

Parallelepiped technique provides detection of any condition which obscures corneal transparency or crystalline lens. In this technique illumination system is placed on the side of cornea or lens (i.e. temporal) and light beam is widened to corneal depth (3-4 mm). By this way a parallelepiped illuminated area is created. Angle can be changed between 30-60 degrees. Magnification may vary between 10x-40x (Figure 4). By focusing on the anterior side of the parallelepiped light, corneal epithelial alterations and protein deposits and debris in a contact lens wearer can be viewed. Endetolial pigment changes, keratic precipitates, other deposits and striations on the endotelium can be viewed by using parallelepiped technique [2].

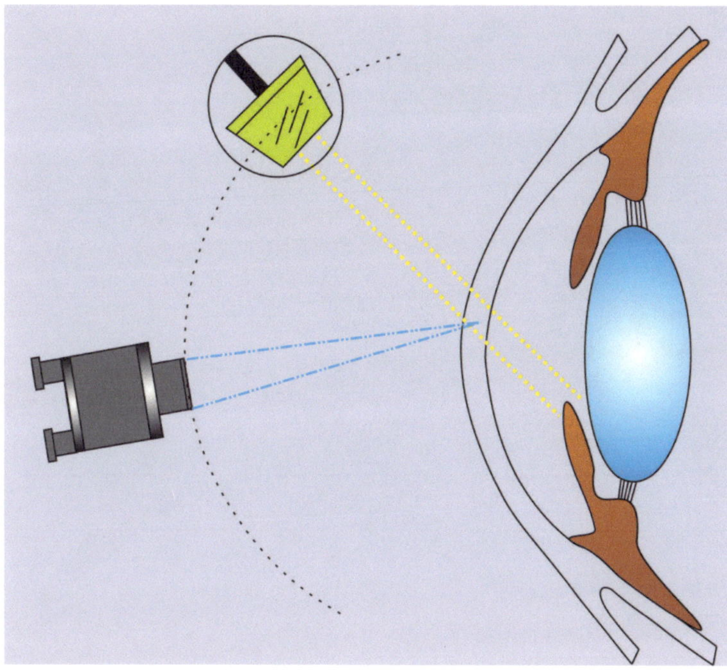

Figure 4. Direct illumination, parallelepiped technique

Crystalline lens transparency and opacities can be evaluated by using with a 0.5 to 2 mm wide beam. Different from the corneal examination illumination, system should be set to a smaller angle, 10 to 45 degree. Detailed examination can be performed by directing the light towards the pupil area and focusing different layers of the lens [2].

Wide beam illumination is useful for the inspection of contact lens surface. By this method, protein deposits, mucus secretion, corneal nerve fibers, infiltrative keratitis, corneal opacities, iris and lens surface can be viewed. Setup of the method is similar to parallelepiped method except slit width is wider then corneal depth. Light intensity should get reduced and angle of the illumination adjusted depending on the surface of under inspection, generally more than 45 degrees [2].

Conical beam illumination is useful in viewing the inflammatory cells and proteins in the anterior chamber. In this method width and height of the slit light beam is reduced until obtaining a point light. Height is reduced to 1-2 mm. Light intensity is set to maximum. Examination should be done in dark conditions (Figure 5) [2]. The number of cells in the anterior chamber is assessed from side to side of the anterior chamber in medium magnification and high-angle illumination.

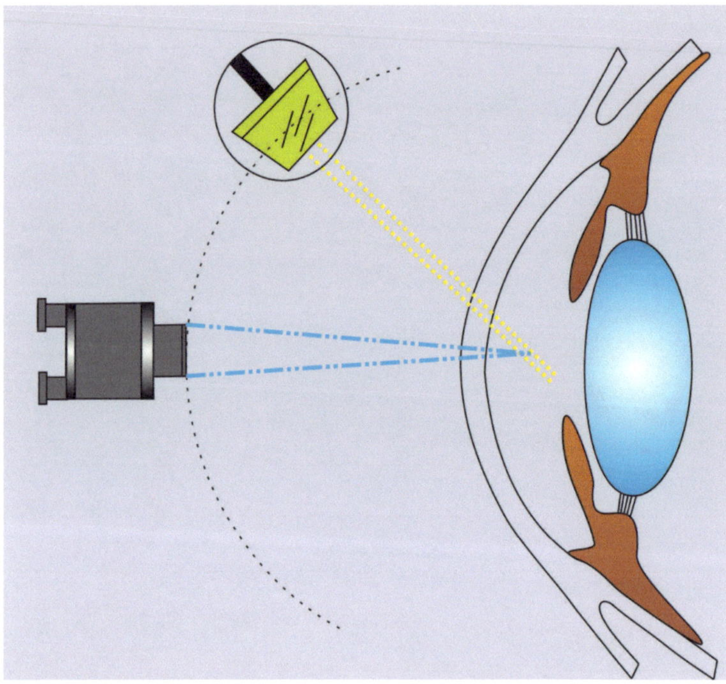

Figure 5. Conical beam illumination

b. Indirect illumination

In this technique light beam is projected to a different area other than the focal point of the observation system. Illumination system is get moved off from its click position by releasing a knob (Figure 6). Therefore two systems do not coincide at same point. Procedure is similar to parallelepiped illumination technique exceptionally, in this method, observed area is not directly the illuminated area but just beside the anterior border of parallelepiped area. With this method, transparency loss or loose contrast differences in transparent structures can be viewed such as subtle corneal opacities, bulbar conjunctival vessels and lens opacities [2].

Scleral scatter is used for especially small changes in large transparent areas. Central corneal clouding, bullous keratopathy, corneal scars, contact lens edges can be examined with this method. In this method, parallelepiped beam focused on central cornea then after releasing the knob illumination system moved out its click position and beam can be projected to nasal or temporal limbus (Figure 7). With correct positioning of the illumination system, a halo of scatter light around the cornea can be viewed [2]. Any condition which alters corneal transparency obstructs the internal reflecting light and becomes visible as a whitish color over pupil background.

http://dx.doi.org/10.5772/58314

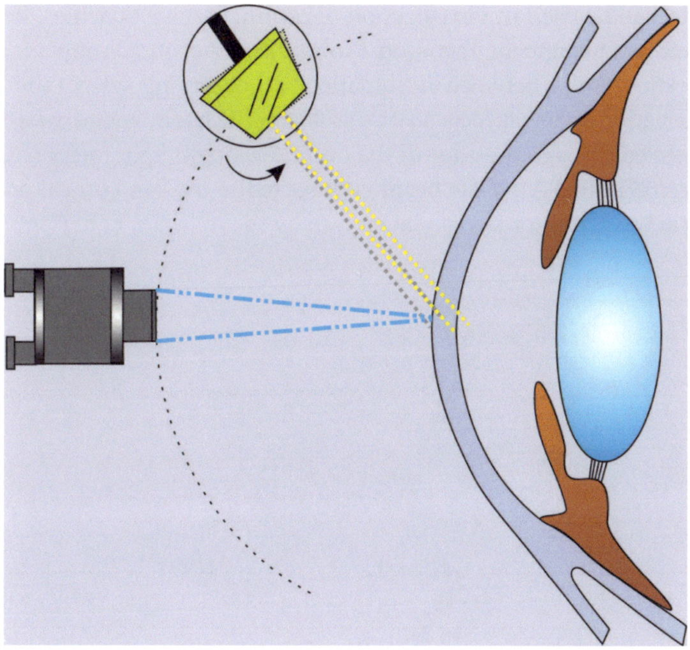

Figure 6. Indirect illumination

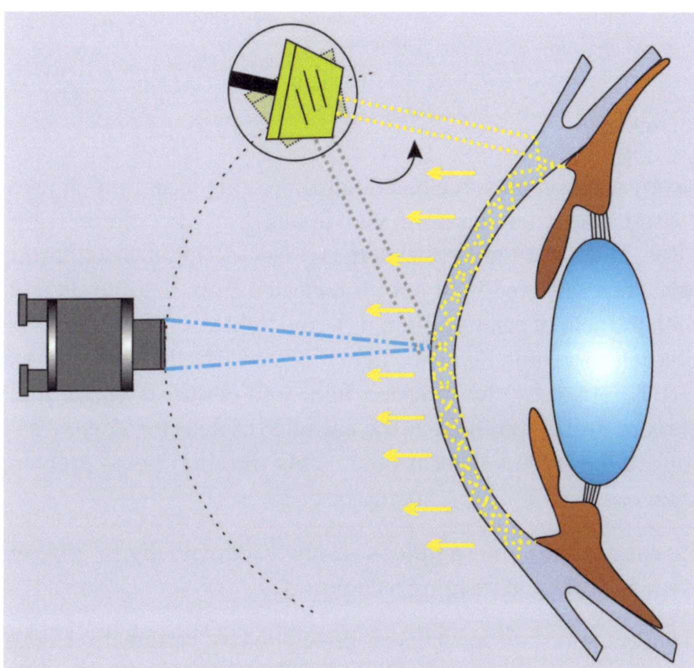

Figure 7. Indirect illumination, scleral scatter technique

Retro illumination can be used in visualization of central corneal opacities, lens and vitreous opacities, iris defects and pigment liberation. Procedure of the retro illumination is started with releasing of the knob. Angle between illumination and observing system should be set about zero. Then illumination system is focused on the object which is intended to be observed. When the beam is projected through the edge of the pupil, the bright light reflex returning from the retina can be seen (Figure 8A). If the beam is projected to the iris, corneal opacities and any vascularisation in the cornea or iris can be viewed by the reflected light (Figure 8 B) [2].

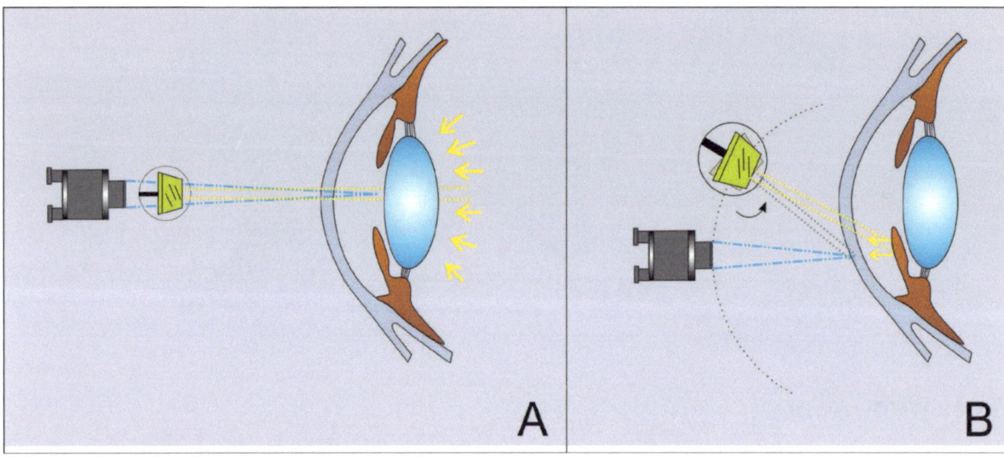

Figure 8. A. Fundus retro illumination. B. Iris retro illumination

2.2. Confocal microscopy

Confocal microscopy is a non-invasive histological imaging technique. It uses reflected light from the living tissue. Therefore, it is an in vivo imaging method of the living cornea. It uses focused light or laser beam. A bright light beam is projected and focused through an objective lens to the cornea. Then reflected light spot is collected from the illuminated tissue area by objective lens. With the help of beam splitter, reflected light is separated from the light mixture and directed to the detection unit. Reflected light reaches to the detection apparatus by passing a pin-hole. Detector transcodes the reflected light into electrical signal and records to the storage media (Figure 9). The pin-hole at the entrance of detector apparatus filters the light coming from outside the intended focal point. This filtration helps grabbing sharper and clearer images than conventional light microscopy [3].

For two-dimensional imaging, the sample is scanned sequentially in different focal planes. There are three types of confocal imaging techniques.

a. *Tandemn scanning confocal microscopy* was developed by Petran and Hadravsky [4]. Basic part of the system is the real time point illumination and point detection. It was developed by Nipkow in 1884 [5]. System provides real-time images at true color and marginal image quality based on the low intensity of reflected light [6]. Future development in tandemn

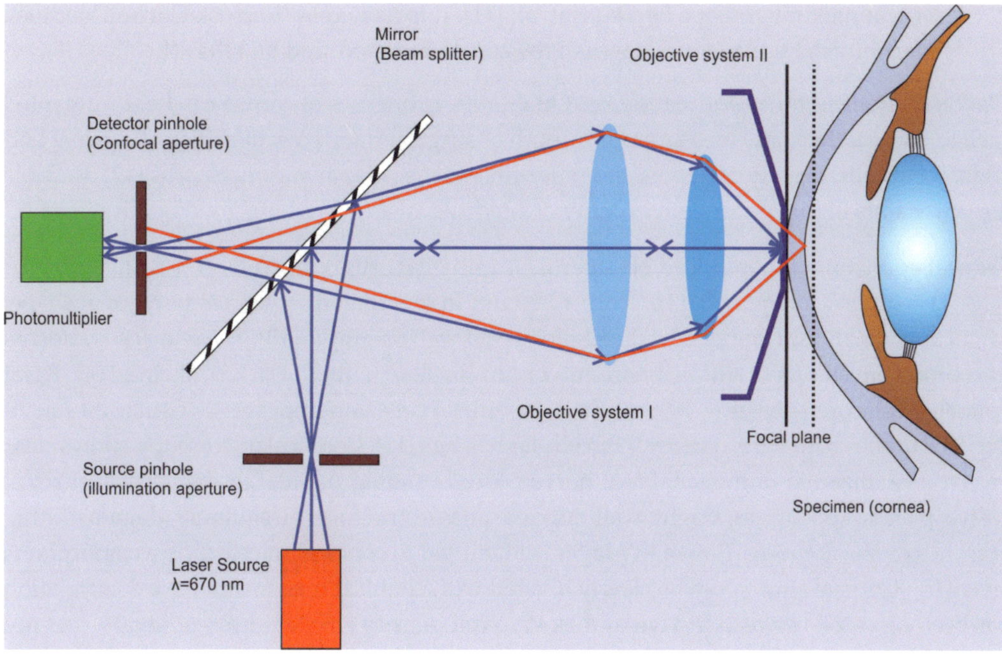

Figure 9. Working principle of confocal microscopy.

scanning was done by Xiao et al [7]. They used set of pin-holes on the same side of Nipkow disk for illumination and detection. The pinholes need to be as small as possible to eliminate the scattered light [4]. Design was simple but it has disadvantage of low intensity of illumination for image formation. Clinical version was produced but no longer in production [3].

b. *Scanning slit confocal microscopy* is an alternative scanning method to point scanning which uses a slit illumination. It scans over the back focal plane of the microscope. Advantage of slit scanning is that many points on the axis of the slit are scanned at the same time and therefore scanning time is markedly decreased. Scanning slit systems also have superior light brightness compared to point scanning. In comparison to pin-hole systems, slit scanning systems have lower axial and transverse resolution. Slit height, width and amount of light can be adjusted in slit scanning systems. By this way, visualization quality and optic section area can be modified based on the specimen i.e. transparent or opaque specimens.

c. *Laser scanning confocal microscopy* was developed by Webb in 1987 [8-10]. A coherent laser beam is used as a light source and specimen scanned by laser beam with the help of galvanometer scanning mirrors which provides fast scanning. Reflected light is refocused and projected to the photomultiplier through the pin-hole aperture. Heidelberg Retinal Tomograph is an example of in vivo confocal imaging systems. It uses 670 nm diode laser as a light source to acquire and analyze the optic nerve for glaucomatous damage. With the help of detachable optical attachment, HRT II was modified to high resolution confocal laser scanning microscope by Stave et. al. [11]. It is named as 'Rostock Cornea Module'. High-contrast, high quality images of the cornea are produced by HRT III.

Clinical applications of confocal microscopy: Qualitative properties of cornea can be documented such as corneal thickness measurement, depth of surgical interfaces, densities of stromal and endothelial cells, density or nerves and reflectance and scatter at various depths [12]. Reliable measurements highly depend on experienced technician and grabbing good quality images.

Corneal epithelium is comprised of superficial epithelial cells, wing cells and basal epithelial cells. The superficial epithelial cells are 40-50 μm in length and appear as polygonal shape, bright nucleus and surrounded by dark halo in confocal imaging [5, 13]. The wing cells appears in confocal images as bright cell borders, bright nucleus without dark oval ring [14]. Basal epithelial cells are smaller (8-10 μm) than superficial cells and appears as regular mosaic of dark cell bodies with light, narrow intercellular borders [13]. Confocal microscopy allows clear in vivo visualization of the sub-basal nerve plexus running parallel to the corneal surface. Nerve plexus appears as bright well-defined linear structures, frequently demonstrating branches or anastomoses. Bowman's layer is identified in confocal microscopy as amorphous layer [15]. Corneal stroma can be clearly imaged with confocal imaging and good correlation has been reported between in vivo and ex vivo cell density [16, 17]. Stromal keratocytes are identified as hyperreflective cell nuclei with poorly visualized cell processes. Cell process may become more visible in corneal edema or trauma [15, 18]. Descement membrane appears as an acellular layer between posterior stroma and endothelium [15]. Confocal microscopy provides clear images of the corneal endothelium despite of moderate corneal edema [19]. Endothelial cells appear in confocal imaging as hexagonal shape cells with a honeycomb order [15].

The introduction of confocal microscopy into the research and clinical practice, represented a revolutionary approach to the inherited corneal diseases. It allowed the clinician in vivo microscopic analysis of affected corneas and screening of unaffected family members [20]. Besides the inherited corneal diseases, confocal microscopy can be used in determining the acanthamoeba keratitis, fungal keratitis, bacterial and viral keratitis [3, 21, 22]. Wound healing response can be analyzed after refractive surgery with confocal microscopy [3].

2.3. Scheimpflug imaging

The Scheimpflug principle, first described by Theodor Scheimpflug, a cartographer of the Austrian navy [23]. According to him, obliquely tilted object can be documented with maximal possible depth of focus and minimal image distortion. In a normal imaging camera, all planes are parallel to each other. But in a Scheimpflug imaging principle, all planes cuts each other in an intersection point (Figure 10). Scheimpflug principle was first introduced in ophthalmology by Drews, Niesel, Brown, Dragomirescu and Hockwin [24-27]. Scheimpflug imaging technique provides high resolution and wide depth-of-focused sharp images from anterior corneal surface to the posterior crystalline lens capsule. In this technique camera rotates along with a monochromatic slit light source around the optical axis of the eye to obtain slit images. This system scans the cornea from zero to 180° and each one of the photographs belongs to the

http://dx.doi.org/10.5772/58314

specific angle of corneal section (Figure 11). During the scanning process, a center placed static camera detects pupil contours and controls fixation.

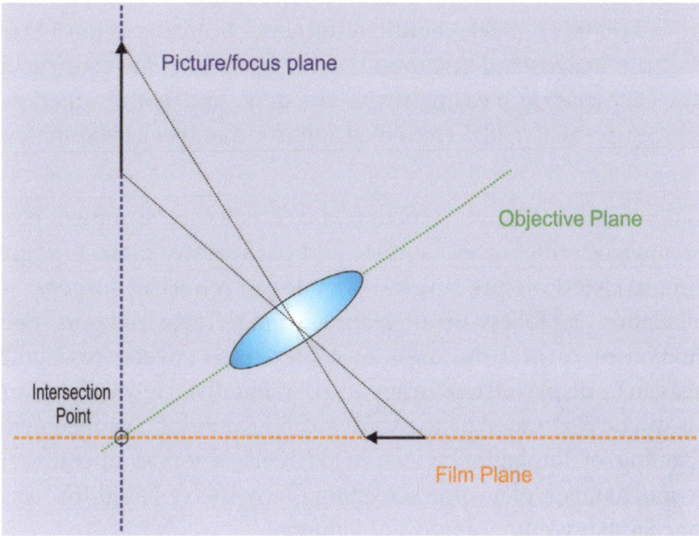

Figure 10. Scheimpflug principle imaging

Reconstruction of anterior and posterior corneal surface topography is done by analyzing of multiple photographs taken from specific angle. Corneal pachymetry, wavefront aberrations, densitometry of crystalline lens and anterior chamber calculations and measurements are provided by bundled software. Pentacam is a Scheimpflug imaging device available in market. There are three different model Pentacam versions available in the markets which are basic, classic and HR (high resolution). Differences between models are mostly in software but resolution upgrade is available in HR model [28].

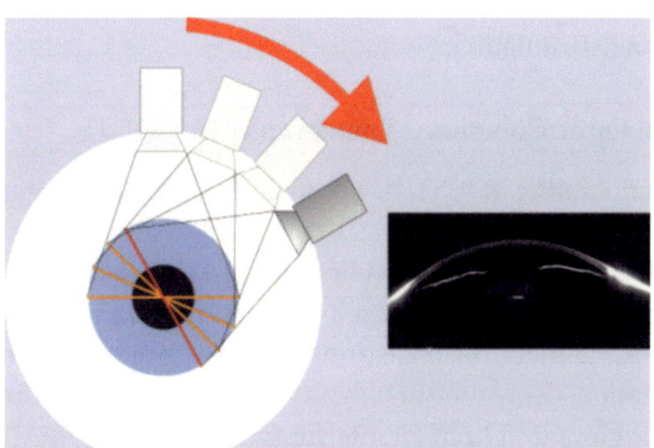

Figure 11. Scheimpflug photography technique

The other one is Galilei dual Scheimpflug analyzer which integrates a placido disc with a dual rotating Scheimpflug system [29]. Both systems acquire images simultaneously to obtain information on the curvature and elevation of the cornea. After scanning the anterior chamber, Scheimpflug images are transferred to PC to get analyzed and used to construct 3-D model of the anterior segment of the eye by the bundled software. Accuracy of the 3-D model increases with the count of the images and resolution of the camera. After constructing 3-D model, topographic and pachymetric measurements are done and entire anterior and posterior surfaces of the cornea are analyzed. Remodeled anterior chamber can be analyzed and viewed in any direction.

Basic software allows qualitative assessment of the cornea such as topography and elevation data of anterior and posterior corneal surface and pachymetry map. Topography maps are used for keratoconus detection, pre-surgical planning of refractive surgery, intra ocular lens (IOL) power calculation and follow-up after corneal and refractive surgery. Pachymetry maps allow representation of corneal thickness in color which covers from limbus to limbus. Measured values can be displayed and represented manually at any point. Corneal wavefront Zernike analysis can be performed by the software. 3-D anterior chamber analysis is used for pre-surgical planning of implantation of phakic IOLs, pre-post operative comparison of changes in anterior chamber, glaucoma screening, pachymetry-based IOP correction, assessment of anterior chamber volume, angle and volume.

Optional software modules such as Holladay Report, Holladay EKR Detail Report, Belin/ Ambrosio Enhanced Ectasia Display, Contact Lens Fitting, 3D Posterior chamber IOL Simulation Software and 3D cataract analysis can be installed. The Holladay Report was developed by Jack T. Holladay, M.D [30]. It calculates the real relationship of the posterior corneal surface to the anterior corneal surface and provides data for calculating the optimal IOL refractive power for patients who have undergone refractive corneal surgeries. The Belin/Ambrosio display is the first keratoconus screening tool. It provides height data of the anterior and posterior corneal surface in combination with a progression analysis of the corneal thickness. It was developed by Michael W. Belin, M.D. and Renato Ambrosio Jr., M.D [31]. This module is used to early detection of keratoconus. Contact Lens Fitting module allows automatic display of all necessary measurement data for fitting contact lenses, automatic suggestions for contact lenses and realistic image simulation.

2.4. Anterior Segment Optic Coherence Tomography (AS-OCT)

Optical coherence tomography (OCT) is a non-contact imaging method which provides detailed cross-sectional images of biological tissues. It works with similar principle with ultrasound imaging. Delay time of reflected light is measured and used to visualize the target tissue in depth. A beam of infrared light is used instead of sound wave. Light travels extremely faster than sound wave and therefore measuring the delay time of infrared light is impossible. To overcome this limitation, delay time of light is measured by comparing the sample reflected light with a reference reflected light in an interferometer.

Resolution of OCT depends on the coherence length of the light and ranges from 2 μm to 20μm. High resolution capability and transparent structure of the anterior segment makes OCT an ideal imaging technology. High frequency ultrasound of anterior segment and confocal microscopy also can reach similar resolution but OCT is more practical, non-contact, and faster.

OCT was invented by David Huang and colleagues in 1991 [32]. Joseph Izatt described anterior segment OCT in 1994 [32, 33]. First anterior segment OCT was based on time domain technique and used 1310 nm wavelength infrared light. Time domain technique requires mechanical movement of a mirror to estimate the latency of every axial scan (A scan) in the projecting light. Wavelength of light that is used in this technique limits the resolution to 18 μm and the mechanical part limits the speed of A-scans performed by the device to 2000 scan/sec [34].

With the invention of spectral domain OCT (SD-OCT), axial resolution is increased to 5μm and the A-scan speed to about 26000 – 40000 (depends upon manufacturer) per second with the 840 nm light and without a movable mechanical part. In SD-OCT, reference mirror is fixed and A-scan is produced by Fourier transformation of spectral interference patterns between the sample and reference reflections. SD-OCT can visualize bowman layer as a parallel line, thickness profile of epithelial and stromal layer separately. However, time-domain OCT cannot easily visualize epithelial layer and stromal layer separately. Time-domain OCT still has advantage of visualizing deep tissue structures and anterior chamber biometry [34].

Newest technology for AS-OCT is Swept-Source OCT (SS-OCT). It uses 1310 nm infrared light source and categorized as fourier-domain OCT. SS-OCT makes possible to reconstruct the three dimensional images of the anterior segment of the eye more accurately [35]. SS-OCT has 10μm vertical resolution and capable to make 300.000 A-scan in one second for 16 mm section. Scan width of SS-OCT is higher than SD-OCT (16mm versus us 6 mm) [34]. It is quite simple and less expensive than SD-OCT. SS-OCT based OCT device has been announced in the market recently.

AS-OCT enables objective evaluation of anterior chamber. It provides comparable data of anterior chamber depth and irido-corneal angle dimensions with ultra sound biomicroscopy (UBM) [36]. Specific dimensions of the iris and chamber angle provided by AS-OCT can be used in predicting the development of angle-closure glaucoma [37]. AS-OCT is also useful in evaluating anterior chamber anatomy and positioning filtering devices after glaucoma surgery [37]. Anterior chamber measurements provided by AS-OCT are also useful in pre-operative evaluation of keratorefractive surgery. Measurement of chamber depth is useful in sizing and predicting the postoperative position of phakic intraocular lenses to the corneal endothelium [38, 39]. AS-OCT produced pachymetry map helps preoperative prediction of keratoconus and postoperative evaluation of ectasia and corneal thinning [40]. It is also useful in analysis of corneal wound structure after refractive surgery. AS-OCT is also useful in placement of intracorneal ring segments. It can identify incision depth and intrastromal position of the ring segments precisely. Assessment of segment position may help physician to avoid depth related complications [41].

AS-OCT can provide useful information before and after corneal surgery including corneal transplants. In preoperative setting, it is useful for evaluation of graft donor tissue for thickness and structural preservation [42]. After descement stripping endothelial keratoplasty, it detects posterior lamellar dislocation, primary graft failure and anterior chamber crowding with consequent chamber angle encroachment, possible descement membrane detachment and pupillary block [43]. It can successfully detect descement membrane detachment in case of corneal edema after corneal transplant or cataract extraction [44].

Beyond the surgeries, AS-OCT is a valuable tool in determining the hereditary or infective corneal pathologies. AS-OCT can visualize the full-thickness intrastromal deposits, and confirm the pattern and the depth of these intrastromal infiltrates in granular corneal dystrophy Type 2 [45]. It is ideal for evaluating the depth of injury due to a foreign body, laceration or ocular burn [46]. In microbial keratitis, AS-OCT can illustrate corneal infiltrates as hyper-reflective areas [47].

2.5. Ultrasound biomicroscopy (UBM)

Ultrasound biomicroscopy allows in vivo detailed assessment of anterior segment structures even if an optical opacity is presented. UBM was developed by Pavlin, Sherar and Foster [48]. It is based on 50-100 MHz transducers which are incorporated into a B mode clinical scanner [48-50]. Similar with other imaging techniques, penetration decreases but, resolution increases with the increasing frequency. It requires supine positioning of the patient and ocular contact with a coupling gel or fluid bath. One percent methyl cellulose is used for fluid bath but saline can also be used. During the examination, transducer moves continuously. Careful attention must be paid not to contact the transducer with the eye during the examination, otherwise corneal abrasion may occur. Most of the commercially available devices provide 25μm axial resolution and 50μm lateral resolution. Tissue penetrations of these devices are approximately 4-5 mm [51]. Scanning procedure can be viewed in real time and recorded on media. Qualitative measurements can be done with using electronic calipers of bundled software. UBM device can record the B-mode images to the media and software can reconstruct 3D anatomy model of the scanned area. The images can be viewed in any direction after examination. UBM also can be used for ocular biometry to calculate IOL power but popularity has reduced due to be a invasive technique and commercialization of partial coherent interferometry technique which is non-invasive.

UBM systems are also suitable for imaging other parts of the eye. With the eye movement, conjunctiva, underlying sclera and even peripheral retina can be examined. It can provide diagnostic images for corneal diseases, glaucoma, cysts, tumors and lens implants. Anterior chamber depth can easily be measured with UBM. Corneal layers can be identified in cross section. The first highly reflective layer is corneal epithelium. Under the epithelium, bowman layer also can be differentiated as a highly reflective layer. Corneal stroma reveals low reflectivity under the bowman layer. Endothelium cannot be differentiated from descement membrane by UBM, but both can be seen as a highly reflective layer at the posterior corneal margin [52]. Corneoscleral junction and scleral spur can be distinguished. Trabecular meshwork cannot be visualized with UBM but identification of scleral spur locates its posterior extent. Iris epithelium forms as highly reflective layer on the posterior iris surface. This layer is useful in determining the interaction of intra-irideal lesions from lesions behind the iris [52].

UBM provides valuable information about anterior segment related diseases. It allows classification of angle closure glaucoma based on their anatomic differences [53]. It can help to understand the mechanisms of angle closure glaucoma, pigmentary glaucoma, malignant glaucoma and other glaucoma types [53-55]. It can also help defining the mechanisms and results of various types of glaucoma surgery [56]. UBM appearance of filtration bleb is characterized by a fluid tract from the anterior chamber through the internal ostium, beneath the scleral flap and into the subconjunctival space. Low internal reflectivity is a sign of better IOP control. Location of accurate obstruction site of fluid flow can be determined by UBM imaging [51].

UBM can visualize patients with opaque corneas before making decision for corneal transplantation [57]. Depth of anterior chamber, state of the angle presence of synechiae and position of intraocular lens can be determined before surgery [52]. UBM is also useful in scleral diseases. It can differentiate extra-scleral and intra-scleral diseases and degree of scleral thinning [58].

In case of traumatic hypotony, UBM can detect cyclodialysis cleft even in the presence of anterior chamber swallowing [59]. After trauma, other causes of hypotony such as occult wound leakage, ciliary body membranes can also be detected. UBM can show the anterior chamber traumatic opacities and can detect small foreign bodies [60, 61]. UBM can provide valuable information in the management of anterior segment tumors [62].

3. Posterior segment and orbital imaging system

3.1. Fundus camera

Fundus camera is a specially designed low power microscope. It can take photo from surface to the posterior pole of the eye with an attached camera. It is used for imaging the eye, monitoring progression of a disease and screening purposes. With the retinal angiograph attachment, it can be used for diagnostic purposes. Most of the commercially available fundus cameras have 30-50 degrees view angle with magnification of 2.5x. Most of them have some modifications which allow visualizing 5x magnified view of 15 degree central retinal area. With the wide angle lenses, 140 degree retinal area can be visualized which minifies the image by half.

Fundus camera uses flash bulb as a light source. The light follows different paths in both observation and illumination systems. Observation light is focused via a series of lenses through a doughnut shaped aperture. When passing distance between the camera objective and corneal surface, it forms an annulus through central aperture. Reflected light coming back from the retina passes through the unilluminated hole in the doughnut formation [63]. Independent light travelling system minimizes the reflections of light source in the captured image. Retinal image projected through a low powered telescopic eye-piece allows selecting and focusing the retinal image. When the capture button is pressed, a mirror interrupts the illumination system and allows flash bulb light. Simultaneously, another mirror falls in front of the observation system which redirects the retinal image to the CCD camera. New devices use infrared light instead of a visible light to observe the retina to improve patient comfort, minimize reflections and to take undilated fundus images. Once the images have been captured, they are transferred to a connected PC for observation and analysis.

Bundled software's are capable of creating panoramic images of retina with processing multiple images taken from different areas of retina. Most of the fundus cameras have internal fixation point or external fixation point for taking images from different regions of retina and patient cooperation.

Digital SLR (single-lens-reflex) cameras provide superior image quality. They also require less illumination to capture photographs. This means less flash light requirement and better patient comfort. Recent devices combine digital SLR devices with fundus cameras to take digitally editable, high quality images. Capability of fundus camera instruments varies by model and manufacturer. They can perform color fundus photography, stereo fundus photography, red-free imaging, autoflourescence imaging and angiography of retina. Stereo fundus photography permits clinician to view the patient's fundus pathology in three dimensional from the print-out or computer screen.

In Recent years, usage of scanning laser technology in imaging of the posterior segment also allowed fast and wide field retinal image capturing. For example P200 (Optos PLC, Dunferline, Scotland) ultra-wide field non-contact retinal imaging camera uses red and green laser to scan the retina. It can produce up to 200 degree of high resolution retinal images in a single capture. It can also capture autofluorescence and fluorescein angiography images with additional modules [64].

Fundus photographs are visual records of the current opthalmoscopic appearance of a patient's retina. They allow the physician to identify retinal changes on follow-up or share the patient's condition with colleagues. It is mostly used for follow-up of glaucoma and diabetic retinopathy. Glaucoma is a condition which damages optic nerve over time. Physician can identify subtle changes in the optic nerve with serial fundus photographs and can recommend appropriate therapy to the patient.

It can document macular edema, newly occurred micro aneurysms and neovascularisation clearly. Detecting the macular edema may be easier with stereo fundus photographs..

3.2. Fundus Fluorescein Angiography (FFA)

FFA changed the diagnosis of macular and choroidal pathologic lesions in a revolutionary way. Although retina can be examined by slit lamp biomicroscopy, FFA provides valuable additive information to the practitioner. Fluorescein dye was first synthesized by Adolf von Baeryer in 1871 [65]. However, it was used as a diagnostic tool in 1960s by MacLean and Maumenee [66]. Modernization of fundus camera features, invention of special camera filters, improved optics, high resolution digital cameras and better understanding of biologic properties of fluorescein have changed FFA to a sophisticated valuable diagnostic tool in ophthalmology.

Fluorescein is used in ophthalmology as hydrocarbon salt of sodium with molecular formula $C_{20}H_{10}O_5Na_2$ (Figure 12) [67]. Molecular weight of fluorescein is 376.67 daltons and it is highly water soluble. Fluorescein has the ability to give off longer wavelength light after being exposed to a specific wavelength light. Excitation wavelength is 465 to 490 nm and fluorescence wavelength is 520-530 nm [68].

http://dx.doi.org/10.5772/58314

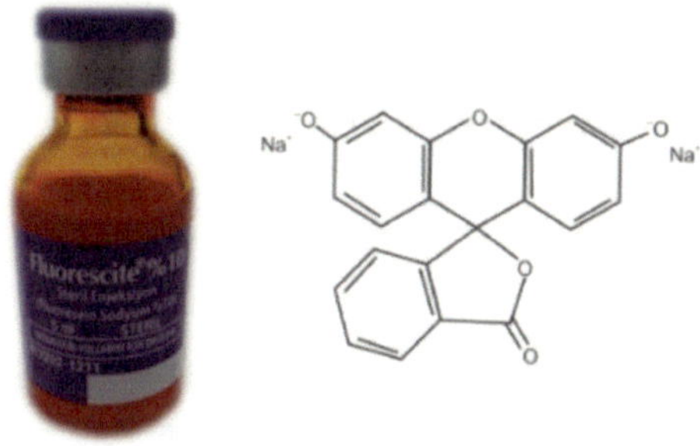

Figure 12. Marked form and chemical structure of sodium fluorescein.

Molecular weight is too large to pass through the RPE cells to pass through the RPE cells (Outer blood-retina barrier) and large choroidal vessels. But it is small enough to diffuse easily through the capillaries except central nervous system and retina (inner blood retina barrier) and these features makes it ideal for visualizing vessels [69]. Special feature for diagnostic purposes in ophthalmology is able to leak from disrupted blood-retina barrier areas. After injecting the fluorescein from antecubital vein, 80-85% of fluorescein binds to plasma proteins especially albumin [67, 69]. Unlike bound fluorescein, free fluorescein is able to absorb and emit light. Fluorescein is eliminated by glomerular filtration in the kidney and metabolized by liver [70].

The risks of angiography have been well described in literature [70, 71]. Mild reactions due to fluorescein angiograph are nausea, emesis, pruritus and vasovagal symptoms. The incidence of these reactions can be as low as 0,6% or as high as 15% [67, 69]. Most of the adverse effects are rapidly onset after injection and normally resolves approximately in 1,5 hours [71]. Severe reactions such as laryngeal edema, broncho spasm, anaphylaxis, shock, myocardial infarction, cardiac arrest and convulsion can be seen [72]. These reactions may even be fatal (1 in 222,000) [73]. Absolute contraindications include first trimester of pregnancy [74]. Relative contraindications are second and third trimesters of pregnancy, congestive cardiac, renal and hepatic failures [69].

After administration of fluorescein several phases can be seen in retinal circulation. Understanding the normal phases is essential for correct interpretation of FFA. These phases of FFA are shown in Figure 13. After administration of dye, fluorescence can be visualized in optic nerve and choroid within 10-15 seconds. But this interval can be changed by many factors such as injection site and circulation speed [75].

After initial appearance of dye in the choroid, arterial filling occurs 1-3 seconds later. Complete filling of arteries should finish less than 1 second. Venous filling phase occurs slower than arterial phase. Laminar filling of veins with dye can be seen in all individuals 2-3 seconds after completion of arterial filling (arterio-venous phase). It is named as also laminar venous filling. Venous filling should be completed in 11 seconds after first appearing the dye in arteries (Venous phase). Recirculation phase starts at 30th second after injection of dye and lasts approximately 2 minutes. In this phase, vessels are filled for the second cycle. With the elimination of dye through the glomerular filtration, concentration of the dye in the blood stream declines during the recirculation phase. In the late phase of angiogram, no dye should be detected in the vessels. Fluorescence can be detected in the vessels in case of vascular leakage secondary to inflammation [75].

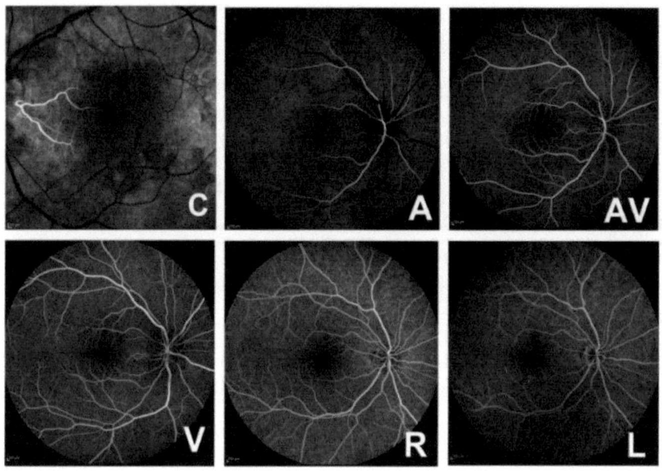

Figure 13. Phases of fluorescence angiography. C. Choroidal, A. Arterial, AV.Arteriovenous, V.Venous, R. Recirculation, L. Late phase.

Hypofluoresence can be detected in the FFA secondary to filling defects or blockage of fluorescence by an opaque medium. Filling defects can be seen by occlusion of small vessels in diabetes, radiation retinopathy, sickle cell disease or talc retinopathy. Capillary filling defects can be seen in diabetes and retinal vein and artery occlusion and Behcet's disease. Retinal arterial occlusion is observed as hypofluoresence in the retinal area distal to the site of the occlusion (Figure 15, A-B) [75].

Hyperfluorescence can be observed in 4 circumstances; leakage, staining, pooling and window defect. Window defect implies partial or total loss of blocking effect of RPE. It can be seen in geographic atrophy in macular degeneration and tear of the RPE. Neovascularisation in diabetic retinopathy, sickle cell retinopathy and choroidal neovascular membrane in AMD or myopic degeneration leads to leaking appearance. Microaneurysms in diabetes, Irvine-Gass syndrome, uveitis induced macular edema and arterial macroaneurysms are example of leakage due to the permeability loss of vessels [75]. Pooling means accumulation of the dye in fluid filled spaces. Examples of pooling appearance are central serous chorioretinopathy, pigment epithelial tear in AMD and intra ocular tumors. Staining is increased intensity of hyperfluorescence in a lesion. Examples of staining are disciform scars, regressed neovascular tissue, myopic degeneration and gyrate atrophy (Figure 14, C-F).

http://dx.doi.org/10.5772/58314

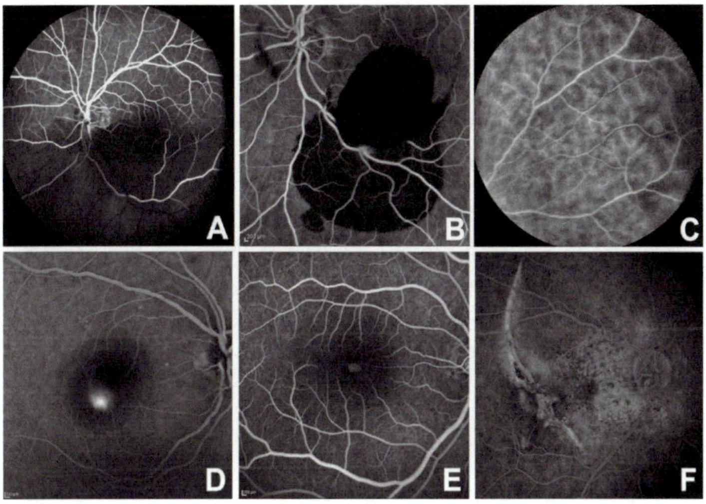

Figure 14. Sample FFA images A. Filling defect due to the occlusion of major artery, B. Blockage of fluorescence in intravitreal hemorrhage C. Leakage in behcet uveitis. D. Pooling in SSR, E. Window defect in macular hole, F. Late staining in choroidal scar.

3.3. Indocyanine green angiography

Investigations for visualizing the choroidal vasculature introduced the indocyanine green (ICG) angiography into the ophthalmology. It was first introduced into medicine in 1957 for measuring the cardiac output [76, 77]. In 1986 Hayashi et. al improved new filter combinations with sufficient sensitivity [78]. Indocyanine green is a water soluble dye and molecular weight is 775 daltons. Molecular formula is C43H47N2NaO6S2 [79] (Figure 15). It absorbs near-infrared light the range of 790-805 nm. Emission spectrum is in the range of 770-880 nm, peak at 835 nm. Indocyanine green bounds to plasma proteins with 98% but unlike fluorescein, 80% of indocyanine green bounds to the globulins such as A1-lipoprotein [79]. Therefore indocyanine dye cannot escape from choroidal vasculature and allows visualizing of the choroidal vasculature. ICG diffuses through the choroidal stroma slowly and stains in the choroid during the 12 minutes after injection.

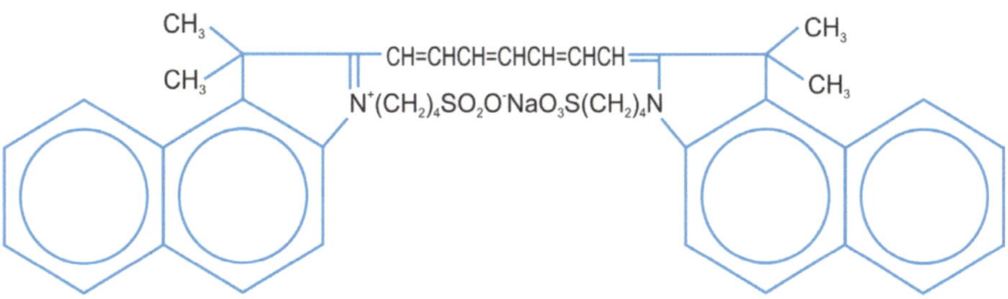

Figure 15. Molecular structure of indocyanine green

Standard dosage of ICG is 25 mg which is dissolved in 5 ml solvent. It should be injected rapidly through the antecubital vein. It is taken up by liver and secreted into the bile without metabolic alteration. It is a safer dye than fluorescein. Adverse reactions are rare. Nausea, vomiting and pruritus can be seen in 0.15% of patients. Isolated vasovagal type reactions and anaphylactic shock have been reported in the literature [80-82].

Image acquisition from ICG done by the near infrared laser or light through the excitation filter. Excited ICG molecules emits slightly different wavelength of light. Before being captured by the camera, emitted light passes the barrier filter which blocks the light with a shorter wavelength than 825 nm. Therefore, the camera captures only the light which is emitted by ICG, not the projected light near infrared spectrum [79].

Digital image capturing and processing systems made it easy to capture, view and store the acquired images. The Charge coupled device captures the ICG angiography images and converts to digital data. SLO systems provide high capturing sensitivity and allow simultaneous capturing with fluorescein angiography and ICG angiography. SLO systems use infrared diode laser (795 nm) to excite the ICG. The use of wide angle lenses allows instantaneous imaging of large fundus areas.

ICG angiography is widely used in the detection and follow-up of AMD related lesions. Serous pigment epithelial detachment is an ovoid or circular detachment of retina pigment epithelium and seen as blockage of normal choroidal vessels in ICG. Choroidal neovascularization (CNV) is a choroidal capillary proliferation through a break in the bruch membrane. Classic CNV can be detected as an area of bright hyperfluorescence but it can be better delineated by fluorescence angiography. Occult CNV without serous pigment epithelial detachment can be seen as early vascular hyperfluorescence and late staining of abnormal vessels. Occult CNV with serous pigment epithelial detachment reveals as early vascular hyperfluoresence and late staining of the CNV [83, 84]. Hot spot or focal CNV is seen as well delineated and no more than one disc diameter in size with ICG angiography.

Polipoidal choroidal vasculopathy is an abnormality of the choroidal circulation. it is seen as distinct network of vessels in choroid at the early phases. Retinal angiomatous proliferation is characterized by dilated retinal vessels, retinal hemorrhages and exudates. In ICG, it reveals as focal areas of intense hyperfluorescence (hot spot) and late extension of leakage which corresponds to intraretinal neovascularization. Central serous chorioretinopathy is a collection of fluid under the retina and makes visual distortion. It is detected in ICG angiography as multifocal areas of hyperfluorescence in early and late phases. ICG angiography is a valuable diagnostic tool in the evaluation of intraocular tumors. Pigmented choroidal melanomas absorb and block ICG fluorescence. It can be used for differentiation of choroidal melanomas from non-pigmented intra ocular tumors [79].

ICG angiography also can provide valuable information about intraocular inflammatory conditions.

http://dx.doi.org/10.5772/58314

3.4. Scanning Laser Ophthalmoscope (SLO)

SLO is a tool which can be used for FFA, ICG angiography, autoflourescence detection and acquiring OCT images with modification. Combination of low powered laser illumination and confocal imaging technique provides high contrast and detailed images. Using very narrow and exact wavelength laser allows more efficient excitation than filtered flash illumination of the fundus camera. Due to the monochromatic laser, captured images are in gray scale.

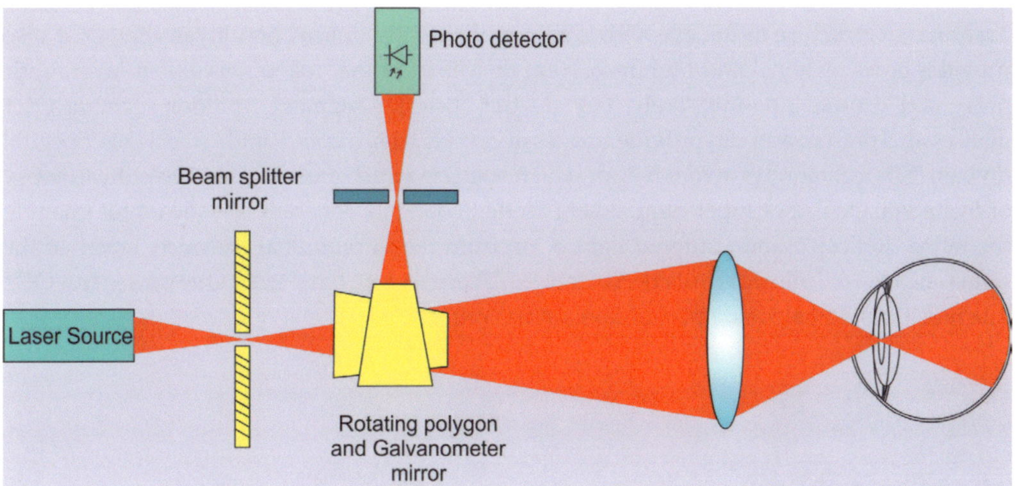

Figure 16. Working scheme of scanning laser opthalmoscope

SLO imaging principle basically starts with the pre-shaped laser beam which is focused to the retina. Pre-shaped laser beam passes through the 2mm aperture of a beam splitter mirror. Beam is deflected horizontally by a rotating polygon mirror to form a line scan. Galvanometric mirror is deflected vertically to form a two dimensional raster. Two dimensional raster laser beams are focused to a single point at the patient's lens which refocuses it onto the retina. The light reflected from the retina travels the same path and rescanned by two scanning mirrors. Beam separator collects the reflected light and focuses it onto the photo detector (Figure 16). Photo detector converts the reflected light to the images and transmits to the computer for processing and recording. Advantage of SLO is reduced scattered light in the reflected light. Reduced scattered light results with improved image contrast.

There are two types of SLO-based device available in the market. These are Heidelberg Retinal Tomography (HRT) and Heidelberg Retinal Angiography (HRA). HRT is designed to acquire images from especially optic nerve and macula. It provides quantitative three dimensional imaging of the posterior segment. HRA uses 670nm laser diode and confocal aperture to acquire images. HRT II has 15-degree scan area. Image resolution is 384x384 pixels. Scan depth ranges between 1 to 4 mm. Sixteen images are captured at each 1 mm. After acquiring images, bundled software allows the analysis of retinal thickness and optic nerve topography [85].

HRA is a confocal SLO designed for simultaneous FA, ICG angiography and autoflourescence imaging. Blue laser (488nm) is used for exciting fluorescein and near infrared laser (795nm) is used for exciting indocyanine green dye. Barriers for acquiring emitted light are 500nm for FA and 810nm for ICG angiography. The field of range starts from 10°x10° to as much as 150°x 150° with the contact lens attachment [86]. Another firm 'Optos' also combined the scanning laser ophthalmoscope with OCT [87].

3.5. Optical Coherence Tomography (OCT)

Transparent structure of the eye allows us visualizing the fundus non-invasively. OCT also provides cross sectional and high resolution images of retina, retina nerve fiber layer, optic nerve and choroid non-invasively. Beyond the posterior segment, anterior segment OCT devices also present and can provide images of cornea, lens, iris and angle structures. Spectral domain (SD) technique provides 5-7μm axial resolution which means an in-vivo optical biopsy of the retina. OCT uses super luminescent diode to obtain a coherent laser beam for imaging the retina. Reflected and scattered light beam from the vitreoretinal interface, layers of the retina and choroid allows acquisition of images. There are two basic technique present for OCT imaging; time-domain and spectral domain techniques.

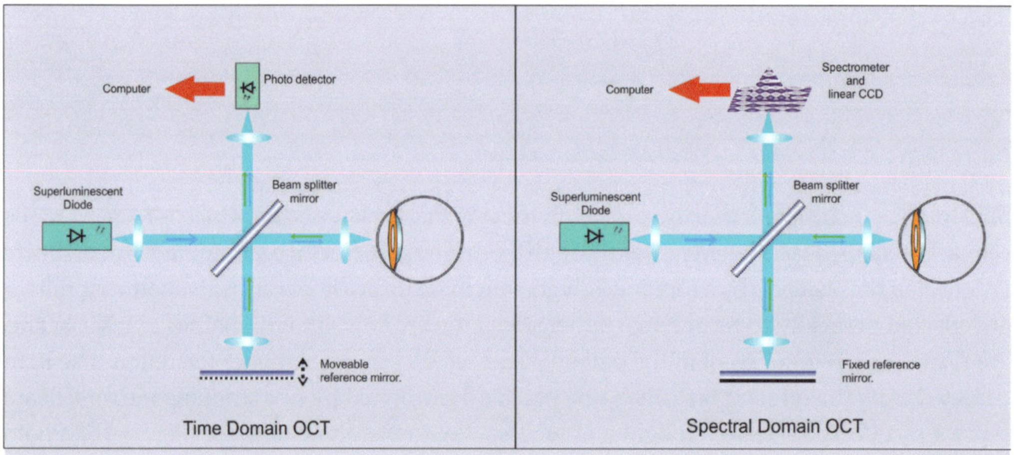

Figure 17. Comparison of time domain and spectral domain OCT working principle

Time-domain technique emits laser beam by super luminescent diode. The beam is splitted into two different paths by a beam splitter. First beam is sent to ocular media, other beam is sent to the movable mirror. Reflected light from the ocular media and movable mirror are combined on the same path and a partial interference is created. Photo detector and the computer measure the interference amplitude and calculate the depth information for each A-scan. To create a B scan image, A-scan sequences are repeated for different directions. Obtained image quality depends on the count of A-scan in each direction (Vertical, horizontal, oblique) and absorption rate of the projected light by tissue. Time-domain devices can provide 400 A scans per second with a maximal axial resolution of 8-10μm (Figure 17). High quality images require longer time to create. Therefore time is the major limitation of this technique. Time-domain technique cannot visualize deeper layers such as choroid due to the light scattering feature of the RPE and low signal-noise ratio [88](Figure 18 A).

In SD-technique, the light source is the same as in time-domain technique. There is also a reference mirror, but it is fixed unlike time-domain technique. This technique uses spectrometer and linear CCD for analyzing interferences between sample beam and reference beam. Fourier transform equation is used for calculating interference information. Absence of movable mirror speeds up the image acquisition up to 50 times. This technique enables to obtain large numbers of A-scans that allows creating high resolution images. SD devices can provide 20.000-52.000 A-scan per second with a 5-7μm resolution [89](Figure 18 B). Such a speed reduces the eye movement artifacts. Obtaining large numbers of images in a short period of time allows 3D reconstruction of the examined area.

One of the newer techniques in OCT imaging modalities is swept-source OCT (SS-OCT). It uses a different form of fourier analysis and employs tunable frequency swept laser source. Unlike spectral OCT measurements, interference is detected with photo detectors instead of spectrometer. Axial scan rate of SS-OCT is 100.000 to 236.000 per second with 11μm tissue resolution [90-92]. Prototype OCT systems using longer wavelength light are also present. Using longer wavelength light provides better penetration of deep tissues and allows visualizing of the choroid and opaque media in better detail [93]. Another new technology is Doppler OCT which detects the precise location of vascular abnormalities using cross sectional imaging. It can evaluate blood flow and volume of retinal and choroidal vasculature [94].

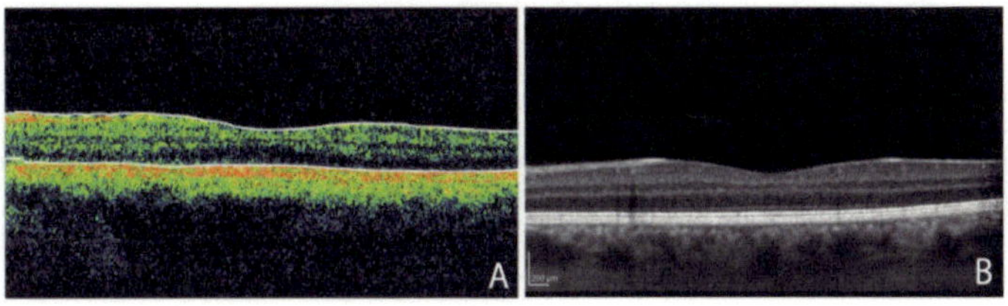

Figure 18. A. Macular cross-section acquired by time domain OCT, B. Macular cross-section image acquired by spectral-domain OCT

Automated retinal thickness measurements calculated by OCT devices are used for monitoring disease progression and response to therapies such as AMD, diabetic macular edema and vein occlusions. Accurate measurement of the retinal thickness helps physician for clinical decision regarding treatment in these conditions. Determining the retinal nerve fiber layer profile with OCT provides valuable information in detecting and management of glaucoma patients. OCT helps in diagnosing and classification of the macular holes. The determined size and configuration by OCT helps predicting the surgery outcomes [95, 96]. It allows evaluation of the vitreoretinal interface in epiretinal membrane and vitreoretinal traction [97]. OCT contributed to better understanding the AMD and helped monitoring the progression and therapeutic response to the intravitreal injections [98]. It is a valuable tool for early diagnosis, analysis and monitoring of diabetic retinopathy with high repeatability and resolution [99]. OCT provides quantitative assessment of retinal thickness in diabetic retinopathy [100].

3.6. Ocular ultrasonography

Ultrasound is a safe, non-invasive, widely used diagnostic tool in medical imaging. It has an important role in ophthalmological diagnosis. Ultrasound produces two-dimensional cross-sectional views of the eye and orbit. It has especially important role for imaging intraocular lesions in the presence of anterior segment opacities. Ultrasound devices produce acoustic sound waves above the audible range of 20KHz to visualize ocular and orbital tissues. Acoustic sound is created by a piezoelectric crystal which is a transducer for converting electric energy into the ultrasound. A short acoustic wave generated by a piezoelectric crystal is sent to the examining tissue. Some of the ultrasound waves are reflected back to the probe. Probe converts returned echoes into electrical signal and image of the tissue is created with processing and combining every electrical signal (Figure 19).

Currently ophthalmic ultrasound devices use 8-100 MHz frequency echoes. In other fields 2-6 MHz frequency is mostly used. Higher frequencies provide increased resolution but decreased pentrance. Eye is a superficially located tissue and has low absorptive properties which make the use of high frequencies practical.

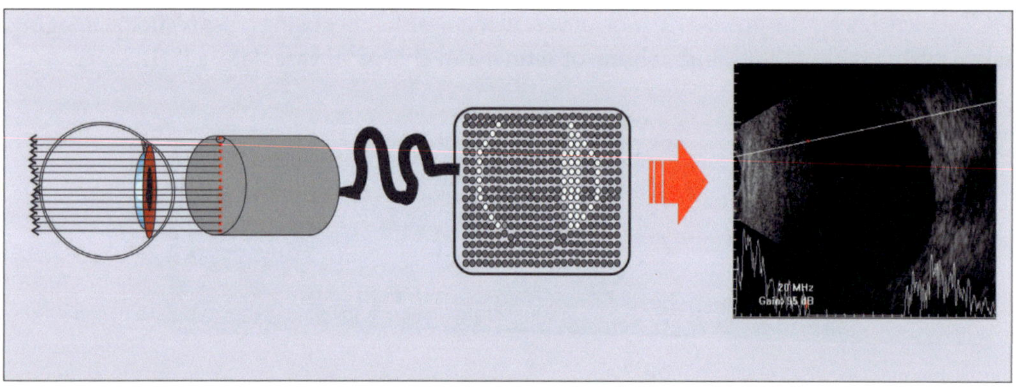

Figure 19. Working principle of ultrasonography

First report of ultrasound applied in ophthalmology belongs to Munth and Hughes who reported A-scan ultrasonography of intraocular tumors in 1956 [101]. B-scan images of the specific ocular diseases and tumors has been described two year later after the initial publication [102]. Most frequently used ultrasound imaging modes are A-scan, B-scan, ultrasound biomicroscopy, color doppler ultrasonography and three dimensional ultrasonography. Ultrasound biomicroscopy has been discussed in detail above.

Ocular ultrasonography is frequently used for evaluating intra ocular tissue integrity, searching and diagnosing intraocular foreign bodies, assessment of intraocular or peri-ocular lesions and examining trauma patients. It is frequently used in the presence of opaque media such as cataract, corneal pathologies, etc. It can be used for determining intralesional characteristics or ecographic nature of a visible mass or foreign body.

A-scan imaging is a one dimensional display of echo strength over time. Vertical height corresponds to echo intensity. There are two types of A-scan present in opthalmological use; biometric A-scan and standardized diagnostic A-scan. Biometric A-scan is used for axial length measurement and corneal pachymetry in evaluation of ocular hypertension and calculation of intraocular lens power [103]. It uses 10-12 MHz frequency and has linear amplification curve. Standardized A-scan is used with 8MHz probe. It is used to determine and differentiate abnormal intraocular tissues. Retina consists highly dense ocular structures such as sclera and choroid which produces 100% echo spikes.

B-scan is the two dimensional view of the combined multiple A-scan echoes. Unlike A-scan, every spike is encoded as a bright dot and every dot brightness changes with the strength of the echo. B-scan images are highly accurate representations of ocular structures and provide shape, location and extensive information. Most of the ophthalmic ultrasound devices use 10MHz frequency for B-scan imaging. The evaluation and differentiation of intraocular lesions are one of the primary indications for ultrasonography. Combined use of B-scan and A-scan provides more reliable information for evaluating ocular lesions. Simultaneously viewing kinetic properties of echo amplitudes (A scan) with B-scan provides more accurate evaluation of intraocular lesions such as choroidal melanomas [104].

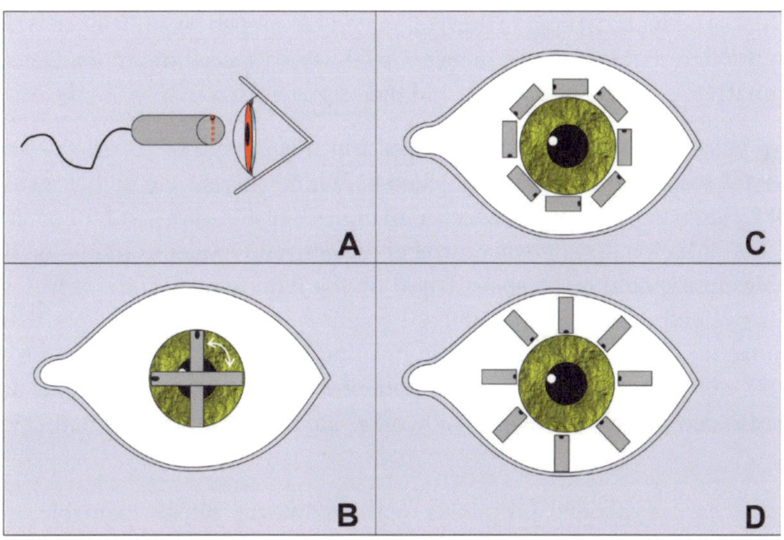

Figure 20. B-scan orientations A. External view of axial scan probe orientation B. Axial scan orientation, C. Transverse scan orientation, D. Longitudinal scan orientation

B-scan probe can be applied to the eye in axial, transverse and longitudinal orientation. Axial scan can be obtained by placing the probe across the visual axis through the cornea and lens. It is the easiest and mostly used orientation but sound attenuates due to the lens. This limits

its diagnostic use (Figure 20). Longitudinal scan can be obtained by placing the probe on sclera to visualize the specific clock hour anterior-posterior cross section. Transverse B-scan also can be obtained by placing the probe on the sclera parallel to the limbus. It provides antero-posterior dimension of the lesion. These two methods is not affected by the attenuation effect of the lens. It provides lateral dimension of the lesion.

Color-doppler ultrasonography allows evaluating B-scan image of the eye and blood flow simultaneously. If the flow moves toward the transducer it is coded with red color. The blood flow that moves away from the transducer is coded with blue color. It provides valuable information about vasculature of orbital tumors, carotid disease, central retinal artery and vein occlusions and non-arteritic ischemic optic neuropathy [105-107].

Ophthalmic 3D ultrasonography uses multiple consecutive two-dimensional B-scan images to create three-dimensional blocks with the help of bundled software. Specially designed transducer probe rapidly scans the eye in trans-scleral orientation and software creates the 3D image. It is useful for calculating the volume of the intraocular lesions [108].

3.7. Computerized Tomography (CT)

Computed tomography is a useful imaging tool in the evaluation of most orbital and ocular lesions. It allows us to detect location, extent and configuration of the lesion. It also provides tissue mass composition and helps planning of an appropriate surgical approach to minimize morbidity. Computed tomography works slightly different than conventional X-ray imaging methods. CT uses x-rays but it emits a thin collimated fan shaped beam. The beam is attenuated as it passes through the tissues and detected by array of special detectors. Detectors create electrical signals from attenuated X-rays and then signals are converted to the images.

CT provides images from thin slices of tissues and it is devoid of superimposition. Spatial resolution of CT scan depends on slice thickness. Thinner slices have higher resolution. Slice thickness of CT imaging can vary between 1-10 mm. Thin slices are good for ocular use but it requires higher radiation dose, greater number of slices and longer examination time. Therefore, slice thickness should be balanced based on the requirement of the case. Optimal slice thickness for eye and orbit is 2 mm [109]. CT requires less time and cheaper than magnetic resonance imaging (MRI). CT is superior in imaging bony structures and in the presence of blood. Therefore, it is excellent in trauma patients. Iodinated contrast agents are used for enhancement to detect intracranial extension of orbital tumors and to evaluate optic chiasmal lesions.

CT is indicated in unexplained propitosis, opthalmoplegia, pitosis, palpable orbital mass, preseptal cellulites, orbital trauma and orbital signs of paranasal sinus diseases. One should request CT imaging only when absolutely indicated because of X-ray exposure.

3.8. Magnetic Resonance Imaging (MRI)

MRI has complex working principle but it has one of the largest diagnostic potential in medicine. It is especially used for imaging neural tissue visualization and has substantial advantage to other imaging methods. MRI creates images with the help of magnetic field and radio waves. It is based on the ability of a small number of protons within the body to absorb and emit radio wave energy when the body or tissue is exposed to strong magnetic field. Soft tissue contrast ratios of MRI are superior to other imaging modalities. Differences in the density of protons in different tissues are provides discriminating one from other. Different tissues absorb and release radio wave energy at different characteristic rates.

Various pulse sequence techniques are used in MRI imaging but most popular ones are T1 and T2-weighted images. T1 images measures ability of protons in a tissue to exchange energy with the surrounding environment or how fast the tissue is magnetized. T2 images measures how quickly the tissue loses its magnetization. In T1 images, fat appears as bright and water appears dark. Reverse view is present in T2 images. T1 images are used especially for viewing anatomy. T2 images are more valuable for detecting pathology. Contrast materials enhance recognition of primary pathology by demonstrating areas of breakdown of the blood-brain barrier.

MRI uses non-ionizing radiation. It can generate images through the entire body. It can visualize the tissue in sagittal, coronal and axial planes. It can visualize vascular tissues with or without contrast material. Beyond the advantages, it is relatively expensive and not widely available. Claustrophobia may be a problem for some patients. Cardiac pacemakers or implanted ferromagnetic foreign bodies are contraindications for MRI.

3.9. Angiography

There are three type of angiography imaging techniques. These are digital subtraction angiography, CT-angiography and MR-angiography. Digital subtraction angiography uses X-rays and iodine based intra-arterial contrast material. It subtracts the structures other than the vascular system, such as bone and muscles. It is still the gold standard method for imaging intra- and extra-cranial vasculature and in the diagnosis of cerebral aneurysms.

CT-angiography uses X rays and iodine based contrast agent. After bolus injection of the contrast agent from antecubital vein, high speed CT scan is performed. It provides images of three dimensional view of surface anatomy with color and blood vessel anatomy without color. It needs shorter examination times that MR-angiography and superior image resolution. Implanted magnetic foreign body is not a contraindication. It is safer and faster than digital subtraction angiography. It can outline surgical anatomy finer than MR-angiography.

No requirement of ionizing radiation and iodinated contrast agent are the main advantages of MR angiography over CT scan.

4. Conclusion

Imaging modalities has changed greatly in recent years. Especially newest OCT technologies promise better understanding and diagnosing of the disease. Advances in laser technologies and optical systems also have enhanced image quality and resolution in most of the imaging techniques. Newest digital technologies enable more easily reproducible information and facilities telemedicine applications. Examination in Ophthalmology starts with imaging the eye either with inspection or a sophisticated tool. Caution should be taken no to skip the basic techniques and principles while evaluating the patients. Otherwise we can spend valuable time and money with sophisticated tests unnecessarily.

Author details

Umit Yolcu[1*], Omer Faruk Sahin[2] and Fatih C. Gundogan[3]

*Address all correspondence to: umit_yolcu@hotmail.com

1 Siirt Military Hospital, Ophthalmology, Siirt, Turkey

2 Etimesgut Military Hospital, Ophthalmology, Ankara, Turkey

3 GATA Medical School, Ophthalmology, Ankara, Turkey

References

[1] Nema HV, Nema N. Diagnostic Procedures in Ophthalmology. New Delhi2009.

[2] González J, Benavides C. Atlas of Slit Lamp: (ocular Biomicroscopy): Imagen y Comunicación Multimedia; 2004.

[3] Guthoff RF, Zhivov A, Stachs O. In vivo confocal microscopy, an inner vision of the cornea - a major review. Clinical & experimental ophthalmology. 2009;37(1):100-17.

[4] Petran M, Hadravsky M. Tandem scanning microscope--a new tool for three-dimensional microanatomy. Progress in clinical and biological research. 1989;295:551-8.

[5] Bohnke M, Masters BR. Confocal microscopy of the cornea. Progress in retinal and eye research. 1999;18(5):553-628.

[6] Bohnke M, Masters BR. Long-term contact lens wear induces a corneal degeneration with microdot deposits in the corneal stroma. Ophthalmology. 1997;104(11):1887-96.

[7] Xiao GQ CT, Kino GS. Real-time confocal scanning optical microscope. Applied Physics Letters. 1988;53(8):716–18.

[8] Davidovits P, Egger MD. Scanning laser microscope. Nature. 1969;223(5208):831.

[9] Davidovits P, Egger MD. Scanning laser microscope for biological investigations. Applied optics. 1971;10(7):1615-9.

[10] Webb RH, Hughes GW, Delori FC. Confocal scanning laser ophthalmoscope. Applied optics. 1987;26(8):1492-9.

[11] Stave J, Zinser G, Grummer G, Guthoff R. [Modified Heidelberg Retinal Tomograph HRT. Initial results of in vivo presentation of corneal structures]. Der Ophthalmologe : Zeitschrift der Deutschen Ophthalmologischen Gesellschaft. 2002;99(4):276-80.

[12] Erie JC, McLaren JW, Patel SV. Confocal microscopy in ophthalmology. American journal of ophthalmology. 2009;148(5):639-46.

[13] Jalbert I, Stapleton F, Papas E, Sweeney DF, Coroneo M. In vivo confocal microscopy of the human cornea. The British journal of ophthalmology. 2003;87(2):225-36.

[14] Masters BR, Thaer AA. In vivo human corneal confocal microscopy of identical fields of subepithelial nerve plexus, basal epithelial, and wing cells at different times. Microscopy research and technique. 1994;29(5):350-6.

[15] Mustonen RK, McDonald MB, Srivannaboon S, Tan AL, Doubrava MW, Kim CK. Normal human corneal cell populations evaluated by in vivo scanning slit confocal microscopy. Cornea. 1998;17(5):485-92.

[16] Patel S, McLaren J, Hodge D, Bourne W. Normal human keratocyte density and corneal thickness measurement by using confocal microscopy in vivo. Investigative ophthalmology & visual science. 2001;42(2):333-9.

[17] Patel SV, McLaren JW, Camp JJ, Nelson LR, Bourne WM. Automated quantification of keratocyte density by using confocal microscopy in vivo. Investigative ophthalmology & visual science. 1999;40(2):320-6.

[18] Vanathi M, Tandon R, Sharma N, Titiyal JS, Pandey RM, Vajpayee RB. In-vivo slit scanning confocal microscopy of normal corneas in Indian eyes. Indian journal of ophthalmology. 2003;51(3):225-30.

[19] Hara M, Morishige N, Chikama T, Nishida T. Comparison of confocal biomicroscopy and noncontact specular microscopy for evaluation of the corneal endothelium. Cornea. 2003;22(6):512-5.

[20] Vincent AL, Patel DV, McGhee CN. Inherited corneal disease: the evolving molecular, genetic and imaging revolution. Clinical & experimental ophthalmology. 2005;33(3):303-16.

[21] Zhivov A, Stachs O, Kraak R, Stave J, Guthoff RF. In vivo confocal microscopy of the ocular surface. The ocular surface. 2006;4(2):81-93.

[22] Knappe S, Stave J, Guthoff RF. [Epidemic keratoconjunctivitis. In vivo images of corneal structures with the confocal Rostocker laser scanning microscope (RLSM)]. Der Ophthalmologe : Zeitschrift der Deutschen Ophthalmologischen Gesellschaft. 2005;102(8):798-801.

[23] Scheimpflug T. Der photoperspektrograph und seine anwendung. Photogr Korr. 1906;43:516–31.

[24] Drews RC. Depth of Field in Slit Lamp Photography. An Optical Solution Using the Scheimpflug Principle. Ophthalmologica Journal international d'ophtalmologie International journal of ophthalmology Zeitschrift fur Augenheilkunde. 1964;148:143-50.

[25] Niesel P. [Slit-lamp photography of lens for measurement purposes]. Ophthalmologica Journal international d'ophtalmologie International journal of ophthalmology Zeitschrift fur Augenheilkunde. 1966;152(5):387-95.

[26] Brown N. Slit-image photography. Transactions of the ophthalmological societies of the United Kingdom. 1970;89:397-408.

[27] Brown N. Quantitative slit-image photography of the lens. Transactions of the ophthalmological societies of the United Kingdom. 1972;92:303-7.

[28] OCULUS, Optikgeräte, G.m.b.H. http://www.pentacam.com/sites/index.php (accessed in 29 august 2013).

[29] Ziemer, Ophthalmic, Systems, AG. http://galilei.ziemergroup.com/key-features-g4.html (accesed in 29 august 2013).

[30] Holladay JT. Corneal topography using the Holladay Diagnostic Summary. Journal of cataract and refractive surgery. 1997;23(2):209-21.

[31] Belin MW, Ambrosio R, Jr. Corneal ectasia risk score: statistical validity and clinical relevance. Journal of refractive surgery. 2010;26(4):238-40.

[32] Huang D, Swanson EA, Lin CP, Schuman JS, Stinson WG, Chang W, et al. Optical coherence tomography. Science. 1991;254(5035):1178-81.

[33] Izatt JA, Hee MR, Swanson EA, Lin CP, Huang D, Schuman JS, et al. Micrometer-scale resolution imaging of the anterior eye in vivo with optical coherence tomography. Archives of ophthalmology. 1994;112(12):1584-9.

[34] Maeda N. Optical coherence tomography for corneal diseases. Eye & contact lens. 2010;36(5):254-9.

[35] Yasuno Y, Madjarova VD, Makita S, Akiba M, Morosawa A, Chong C, et al. Three-dimensional and high-speed swept-source optical coherence tomography for in vivo investigation of human anterior eye segments. Optics express. 2005;13(26):10652-64.

[36] Dada T, Sihota R, Gadia R, Aggarwal A, Mandal S, Gupta V. Comparison of anterior segment optical coherence tomography and ultrasound biomicroscopy for assessment of the anterior segment. Journal of cataract and refractive surgery. 2007;33(5): 837-40.

[37] Jancevski M, Foster CS. Anterior segment optical coherence tomography. Seminars in ophthalmology. 2010;25(5-6):317-23.

[38] Goldsmith JA, Li Y, Chalita MR, Westphal V, Patil CA, Rollins AM, et al. Anterior chamber width measurement by high-speed optical coherence tomography. Ophthalmology. 2005;112(2):238-44.

[39] Doors M, Cals DW, Berendschot TT, de Brabander J, Hendrikse F, Webers CA, et al. Influence of anterior chamber morphometrics on endothelial cell changes after phakic intraocular lens implantation. Journal of cataract and refractive surgery. 2008;34(12):2110-8.

[40] Mohamed S, Lee GK, Rao SK, Wong AL, Cheng AC, Li EY, et al. Repeatability and reproducibility of pachymetric mapping with Visante anterior segment-optical coherence tomography. Investigative ophthalmology & visual science. 2007;48(12): 5499-504.

[41] Lai MM, Tang M, Andrade EM, Li Y, Khurana RN, Song JC, et al. Optical coherence tomography to assess intrastromal corneal ring segment depth in keratoconic eyes. Journal of cataract and refractive surgery. 2006;32(11):1860-5.

[42] Choi CY, Youm DJ, Kim MJ, Tchah H. Changes in central corneal thickness of preserved corneas over time measured using anterior segment optical coherence tomography. Cornea. 2009;28(5):536-40.

[43] Lim LS, Aung HT, Aung T, Tan DT. Corneal imaging with anterior segment optical coherence tomography for lamellar keratoplasty procedures. American journal of ophthalmology. 2008;145(1):81-90.

[44] Wylegala E, Nowinska A. Usefulness of anterior segment optical coherence tomography in Descemet membrane detachment. European journal of ophthalmology. 2009;19(5):723-8.

[45] Hong JP, Kim TI, Chung JL, Huang D, Cho HS, Kim EK. Analysis of deposit depth and morphology in granular corneal dystrophy type 2 using fourier domain optical coherence tomography. Cornea. 2011;30(7):729-38.

[46] Wylegala E, Dobrowolski D, Nowinska A, Tarnawska D. Anterior segment optical coherence tomography in eye injuries. Graefe's archive for clinical and experimental ophthalmology = Albrecht von Graefes Archiv fur klinische und experimentelle Ophthalmologie. 2009;247(4):451-5.

[47] Konstantopoulos A, Kuo J, Anderson D, Hossain P. Assessment of the use of anterior segment optical coherence tomography in microbial keratitis. American journal of ophthalmology. 2008;146(4):534-42.

[48] Pavlin CJ, Harasiewicz K, Sherar MD, Foster FS. Clinical use of ultrasound biomicroscopy. Ophthalmology. 1991;98(3):287-95.

[49] Pavlin CJ, Harasiewicz K, Foster FS. Ultrasound biomicroscopy of anterior segment structures in normal and glaucomatous eyes. American journal of ophthalmology. 1992;113(4):381-9.

[50] Pavlin CJ, Sherar MD, Foster FS. Subsurface ultrasound microscopic imaging of the intact eye. Ophthalmology. 1990;97(2):244-50.

[51] Dada T, Gadia R, Sharma A, Ichhpujani P, Bali SJ, Bhartiya S, et al. Ultrasound biomicroscopy in glaucoma. Survey of ophthalmology. 2011;56(5):433-50.

[52] Arun D, Hayden BC, Pavlin CJ. Ophthalmologic Ultrasound, An Issue of Ultrasound Clinics, 1e (The Clinics: Radiology): Saunders; 2008.

[53] Pavlin CJ, Foster FS. Ultrasound biomicroscopy in glaucoma. Acta ophthalmologica Supplement. 1992(204):7-9.

[54] Potash SD, Tello C, Liebmann J, Ritch R. Ultrasound biomicroscopy in pigment dispersion syndrome. Ophthalmology. 1994;101(2):332-9.

[55] Pavlin CJ, Easterbrook M, Harasiewicz K, Foster FS. An ultrasound biomicroscopic analysis of angle-closure glaucoma secondary to ciliochoroidal effusion in IgA nephropathy. American journal of ophthalmology. 1993;116(3):341-5.

[56] Yamamoto T, Sakuma T, Kitazawa Y. An ultrasound biomicroscopic study of filtering blebs after mitomycin C trabeculectomy. Ophthalmology. 1995;102(12):1770-6.

[57] Milner MS, Liebmann JM, Tello C, Speaker MG, Ritch R. High-resolution ultrasound biomicroscopy of the anterior segment in patients with dense corneal scars. Ophthalmic surgery. 1994;25(5):284-7.

[58] Pavlin CJ, Easterbrook M, Hurwitz JJ, Harasiewicz K, Eng P, Foster FS. Ultrasound biomicroscopy in the assessment of anterior scleral disease. American journal of ophthalmology. 1993;116(5):628-35.

[59] Gentile RC, Pavlin CJ, Liebmann JM, Easterbrook M, Tello C, Foster FS, et al. Diagnosis of traumatic cyclodialysis by ultrasound biomicroscopy. Ophthalmic surgery and lasers. 1996;27(2):97-105.

[60] Berinstein DM, Gentile RC, Sidoti PA, Stegman Z, Tello C, Liebmann JM, et al. Ultrasound biomicroscopy in anterior ocular trauma. Ophthalmic surgery and lasers. 1997;28(3):201-7.

[61] Deramo VA, Shah GK, Baumal CR, Fineman MS, Correa ZM, Benson WE, et al. Ultrasound biomicroscopy as a tool for detecting and localizing occult foreign bodies after ocular trauma. Ophthalmology. 1999;106(2):301-5.

[62] Pavlin CJ, McWhae JA, McGowan HD, Foster FS. Ultrasound biomicroscopy of anterior segment tumors. Ophthalmology. 1992;99(8):1220-8.

[63] THE, OPHTHALMIC, PHOTOGRAPHERS', SOCIETY, INC. Fundus Photography Overview. Available from: http://www.opsweb.org/?page=fundusphotography (accesed in 29.08.2013).

[64] Optos PLC D, Scotland KY11 8GR UK. Available from: http://www.optos.com/en/Products/Retinal-imaging-products/Ultra-widefield-imaging/ (accesed in 31.12.2013).

[65] Baeryer Av. Uber ein neue Klasse van farbstoffen. Der Deutschen Chem Ges. 1871(4): 555.

[66] Maclean AL, Maumenee AE. Hemangioma of the Choroid. Transactions of the American Ophthalmological Society. 1959;57:171-94.

[67] Anand R. Fluorescein angiography. Part 1: Technique and normal study. Journal of ophthalmic nursing & technology. 1989;8(2):48-52.

[68] Brancato R, Trabucchi G. Fluorescein and indocyanine green angiography in vascular chorioretinal diseases. Seminars in ophthalmology. 1998;13(4):189-98.

[69] Cavallerano AA. Ophthalmic fluorescein angiography. Optometry clinics : the official publication of the Prentice Society. 1996;5(1):1-23.

[70] Bloome MA. Fluorescein angiography: risks. Vision research. 1980;20(12):1083-97.

[71] Jennings BJ, Mathews DE. Adverse reactions during retinal fluorescein angiography. Journal of the American Optometric Association. 1994;65(7):465-71.

[72] Kelley JS. Fluorescein angiography: techniques and toxicity. International ophthalmology clinics. 1977;17(2):25-33.

[73] Yannuzzi LA, Rohrer KT, Tindel LJ, Sobel RS, Costanza MA, Shields W, et al. Fluorescein angiography complication survey. Ophthalmology. 1986;93(5):611-7.

[74] Halperin LS, Olk RJ, Soubrane G, Coscas G. Safety of fluorescein angiography during pregnancy. American journal of ophthalmology. 1990;109(5):563-6.

[75] J. Fernando Arevalo. Fluorescein Angiography: General Principles and Interpretation. Retinal Angiography and Optical Coherence Tomography: Springer; 2009.

[76] Ó. G. Björnsson RM, and V. S. Chadwick. Physicochemical studies of indocyanine green (ICG): absorbance/concentration relationship, pH tolerance and assay precision in various solvents. Experientia. 1982;38(12):1441–2.

[77] Engel E, Schraml R, Maisch T, Kobuch K, Konig B, Szeimies RM, et al. Light-induced decomposition of indocyanine green. Investigative ophthalmology & visual science. 2008;49(5):1777-83.

[78] Hayashi K, Hasegawa Y, Tokoro T. Indocyanine green angiography of central serous chorioretinopathy. International ophthalmology. 1986;9(1):37-41.

[79] Klais CM, Ober MD, Yannuzzi LA. Indocyanine Green Angiography: General Aspects and Interpretation. In: Arevalo JF, editor. Retinal Angiography and Optical Coherence Tomography: Springer; 2009.

[80] Benya R, Quintana J, Brundage B. Adverse reactions to indocyanine green: a case report and a review of the literature. Catheterization and cardiovascular diagnosis. 1989;17(4):231-3.

[81] Gilmore DM, Khullar OV, Jaklitsch MT, Chirieac LR, Frangioni JV, Colson YL. Identification of metastatic nodal disease in a phase 1 dose-escalation trial of intraoperative sentinel lymph node mapping in non-small cell lung cancer using near-infrared imaging. The Journal of thoracic and cardiovascular surgery. 2013;146(3):562-70.

[82] Wolf S, Arend O, Schulte K, Reim M. Severe anaphylactic reaction after indocyanine green fluorescence angiography. American journal of ophthalmology. 1992;114(5): 638-9.

[83] Orth DH, Patz A, Flower RW. Potential clinical applications of indocyanine green choroidal angiography--preliminary report. Eye, ear, nose & throat monthly. 1976;55(1):15-28, 58.

[84] Bischoff PM, Flower RW. Ten years experience with choroidal angiography using indocyanine green dye: a new routine examination or an epilogue? Documenta ophthalmologica Advances in ophthalmology. 1985;60(3):235-91.

[85] Heidelberg, Engineering, Inc. http://www.heidelbergengineering.com/us/products/hrt-glaucoma-module/hrt-product-specifications/ (accesed in 29.08.2013).

[86] Heidelberg, Engineering, Inc. http://www.heidelbergengineering.com/us/wp-content/uploads/2106_Product%20Lit_HRA%20wBluePeak_Product%20Sheet_v2.pdf (accesed in 29.08.2013).

[87] Optos. plc. http://www.optos.com/en-US/Products/Retinal-imaging-products/OCT-imaging/ (accesed in 31.12. 2013).

[88] Adhi M, Duker JS. Optical coherence tomography--current and future applications. Curr Opin Ophthalmol. 2013;24(3):213-21.

[89] Leitgeb R, Hitzenberger C, Fercher A. Performance of fourier domain vs. time domain optical coherence tomography. Optics express. 2003;11(8):889-94.

[90] Grulkowski I, Liu JJ, Potsaid B, Jayaraman V, Lu CD, Jiang J, et al. Retinal, anterior segment and full eye imaging using ultrahigh speed swept source OCT with vertical-cavity surface emitting lasers. Biomedical optics express. 2012;3(11):2733-51.

[91] Srinivasan VJ, Huber R, Gorczynska I, Fujimoto JG, Jiang JY, Reisen P, et al. High-speed, high-resolution optical coherence tomography retinal imaging with a frequency-swept laser at 850 nm. Optics letters. 2007;32(4):361-3.

[92] Huber R, Adler DC, Srinivasan VJ, Fujimoto JG. Fourier domain mode locking at 1050 nm for ultra-high-speed optical coherence tomography of the human retina at 236,000 axial scans per second. Optics letters. 2007;32(14):2049-51.

[93] Povazay B, Bizheva K, Hermann B, Unterhuber A, Sattmann H, Fercher A, et al. Enhanced visualization of choroidal vessels using ultrahigh resolution ophthalmic OCT at 1050 nm. Optics express. 2003;11(17):1980-6.

[94] Wang Y, Lu A, Gil-Flamer J, Tan O, Izatt JA, Huang D. Measurement of total blood flow in the normal human retina using Doppler Fourier-domain optical coherence tomography. The British journal of ophthalmology. 2009;93(5):634-7.

[95] Haouchine B, Massin P, Tadayoni R, Erginay A, Gaudric A. Diagnosis of macular pseudoholes and lamellar macular holes by optical coherence tomography. American journal of ophthalmology. 2004;138(5):732-9.

[96] Hillenkamp J, Kraus J, Framme C, Jackson TL, Roider J, Gabel VP, et al. Retreatment of full-thickness macular hole: predictive value of optical coherence tomography. The British journal of ophthalmology. 2007;91(11):1445-9.

[97] Barak Y, Ihnen MA, Schaal S. Spectral domain optical coherence tomography in the diagnosis and management of vitreoretinal interface pathologies. Journal of ophthalmology. 2012;2012:876472.

[98] Fung AE, Lalwani GA, Rosenfeld PJ, Dubovy SR, Michels S, Feuer WJ, et al. An optical coherence tomography-guided, variable dosing regimen with intravitreal ranibizumab (Lucentis) for neovascular age-related macular degeneration. American journal of ophthalmology. 2007;143(4):566-83.

[99] Goebel W, Kretzchmar-Gross T. Retinal thickness in diabetic retinopathy: a study using optical coherence tomography (OCT). Retina. 2002;22(6):759-67.

[100] Sanchez-Tocino H, Alvarez-Vidal A, Maldonado MJ, Moreno-Montanes J, Garcia-Layana A. Retinal thickness study with optical coherence tomography in patients with diabetes. Investigative ophthalmology & visual science. 2002;43(5):1588-94.

[101] Mundt GH, Jr., Hughes WF, Jr. Ultrasonics in ocular diagnosis. American journal of ophthalmology. 1956;41(3):488-98.

[102] Baum G, Greenwood I. The application of ultrasonics locating techniques to ophthalmology; theoretic considerations and acoustic properties of ocular media. I. Reflective properties. American journal of ophthalmology. 1958;46(5 Part 2):319-29.

[103] Şahin ÖG. Central corneal thickness, axial length, intraocular pressure and visual field indices in patients with ocular hypertension. Gulhane Medical Journal. 2010;52(4):266-9.

[104] Ossoinig KC. Ruling out posterior segment lesions with echography. International ophthalmology clinics. 1978;18(2):117-20.

[105] Lieb WE, Cohen SM, Merton DA, Shields JA, Mitchell DG, Goldberg BB. Color Doppler imaging of the eye and orbit. Technique and normal vascular anatomy. Archives of ophthalmology. 1991;109(4):527-31.

[106] Lieb WE, Shields JA, Cohen SM, Merton DA, Mitchell DG, Shields CL, et al. Color Doppler imaging in the management of intraocular tumors. Ophthalmology. 1990;97(12):1660-4.

[107] Baxter GM, Williamson TH. Color Doppler flow imaging in central retinal vein occlusion: a new diagnostic technique? Radiology. 1993;187(3):847-50.

[108] Romero JM, Finger PT, Rosen RB, Iezzi R. Three-dimensional ultrasound for the measurement of choroidal melanomas. Archives of ophthalmology. 2001;119(9): 1275-82.

[109] Naik MN, Tourani KL, Sekhar GC, Honavar SG. Interpretation of computed tomography imaging of the eye and orbit. A systematic approach. Indian journal of ophthalmology. 2002;50(4):339-53.

Chapter 2

Imaging Devices and Glaucoma Management

Pinakin Gunvant Davey

Additional information is available at the end of the chapter

http://dx.doi.org/10.5772/58568

1. Introduction

The definition of glaucoma varies depending upon the source or criteria of the randomized controlled trial evaluated. Thus the diagnosis of glaucoma can be enigmatic due to lack of universally accepted definition of glaucoma that covers all facets of glaucoma pathogenesis. The classic definition of having the triad of visual field damage, nerve head damage and elevated intraocular pressure is no longer valid. Although intraocular pressure remains arguably the most important risk factor its absolute value may be elevated or remain within the statistical limits of normality depending upon the type of glaucoma. Issues related to glaucoma management are anything but cookbook type Therefore glaucoma remains interesting for clinicians that manage patients with glaucoma and researchers that study its pathogenesis.

The patients at risk of glaucoma undergo cellular level damage that is manifests as both structural damage at posterior pole of the eye and damage to functional vision. The major goals of glaucoma management are quite clear; to halt the progressive damage of the disease and maintain functional vision with least disruption to quality of life. As we know now that structure damage (optic nerve or retinal nerve fiber layer) often precede functional damage, however this is not universal as imaging devices many not be sensitive enough to pick up subtle damages.[1] Given that scenario it is the recommendation of both and American Optometric association and American Academy of Ophthalmology to record both structure and visual function in patients at risk of glaucomatous optic neuropathy.[2 3]

Obtaining objective data on the morphology and the structure of optic nerve and nerve fiber layer is of great advantage particularly if it is repeatable and reproducible because there is great amount of intra and inter observer variability amongst clinicians. To this accord the computerized imaging technologies can obtain automated evaluation of structural damage in eyes at risk of glaucoma particularly because imaging is less influenced by disease severity and has low long term variability. [4] This article will cover: 1) the technology behind each imaging device, 2) understand parts of the output that is important parameters that have shown to be clinically useful, having diagnostic or prognostic ability. This article will also evaluate: 3) the output of imaging devices to evaluate progressive damage in individuals at risk of glaucoma. Further this article will also discuss the common imaging artifacts that can influence the outcome of the imaging tests.

Most experts in the field will agree to the fact that stereo optic disc imaging is perhaps the gold standard of all techniques of optic disc evaluation.[3 5 6] Fundus cameras can generate a stereo disc images by either displacing the camera system thus creating an offset and obtain two pictures sequentially. The disadvantage of such a technique is that the amount of displacement can differ from one visit to another that can lead to erroneous judgment. Ideally stereo optic disc pictures should be captured by simultaneously this can be achieved by having a dual camera system that captures two images simultaneously. Also until recent years automated analysis of the optic disc morphology was not readily available and investigators of various studies performed planimetry to evaluate disc morphology.[5 6] With the advances in automated analysis this technique may see a revival and increased use in clinical care.

The computerized imaging devices are fundamentally Scanning Laser Ophthalmoscope, Scanning Laser Polarimeter or Optical Coherence Tomograph. These technologies may provide similar information but there are fundamental differences between devices that makes the measurements obtained from each non-interchangeable. Furthermore there is benefit to be gained by performing multiple imaging on the same patient as it may yield additional clinical details.

2. Scanning laser ophthalmoscope

Heidelberg Engineering manufactures Heidelberg Retina Tomograph III (HRT which is the current generation scanning laser ophthalmoscope that provides topographical data of the optic nerve and peri-papillary retina. Using high speed raster scanning technique and diode laser for illumination HRT obtains two-dimensional images of retina and optic nerve. The depth of focal plane is automatically adjusted to obtain multiple two-dimensional images. The HRT III acquires 16 to 64 2-dimentional images to a maximum depth of 4 mm that starts at vitreo-retinal interface to beyond the bottom of the optic disc cupping. The number of optic section varies in different eyes. The eye with deep cupping has an increase in number of sections (two-dimensional images). The optic sections are combined to produce a three-dimensional topography of the optic disc surface. This is repeated up to six time and the best three are selected and averaged to obtain the final output.

2.1. Interpretation of a HRT III output

There are various reports with different level of information that is produced by the device. The author believes that the OU report (Figure 1) is an excellent output of various parameters that are clinically useful in making judgment and patient education. The quality of the scan is judged on the value of standard deviation; the lower the value of standard deviation the better is the quality of the scan (see section A Figure 1). The HRT III provides useful information on

http://dx.doi.org/10.5772/58568

optic disc size. The device software classifies the optic disc, average or large once the user has outlined the optic disc margin (see section A Figure 1). Overall HRT's optic disc analysis provides details of cup information, neuro-retinal rim information and retinal nerve fiber layer (RNFL) information. The right eye of the patient is compared to the left eye and the between eyes asymmetry is also provided. All parameters provided are also compared to the normative database to evaluate if parameters are within statistical limits of normality, borderline or outside normal limits.

A color coded figure provides the cupping information (section B Figure 1). The cupping is represented by the red color where as the neuro retinal rim is represented by blue and green with blue being sloping rim and the green the stable rim. The cup volume is provided as one of the parameters and in eyes suspicious of glaucoma or progressive loss of neuro-retinal rim we can see an increase in cup volume. The cup shape measure is an overall value of three-dimensional representation of cupping and the values are negative in an ocular healthy eye and more positive in an eye suspicious of glaucoma.

The rim details provided are rim area and rim volume both will see a decline with progression of glaucomatous optic neuropathy (see Section C Figure 1). Additionally once the outline of optic disc is marked the device automatically generates Moorfields Regression Analysis. This is arguably the single most important parameter and is discussed in greater detail below. HRT also provides RNFL which is measured 360 degrees just outside the disc margin (see Section D Figure 1). This location of measurement differs from the location of measurement of both the Scanning Laser Polarimeter-GDx-Pro and Optical Coherence Tomograph. Thus the RNFL measured using one technology will not match the values obtained by other and should not be used interchangeably.

All HRT parameters are given symbols of green check mark, yellow exclamation point, or red X which represents statistical limits of normality that is within normal limits, borderline or outside normal limits respectively.

2.2. Moorefield's regression analysis

The Moorfields Regression Analysis was developed by Dr. David Garway-Heath and colleagues [7 8] at the Moorfields hospital, London England. The Moorfields Regression Analysis (MRA) provides an ability to perform cross-sectional analysis, thus classifying an eye as at risk or within normal limits. The analysis exploits prior knowledge that the neuro retinal rim area is positively correlated with the disc size that is the larger the disc size greater is the rim area[9 10] and additionally the rim area narrows in eyes with glaucomatous optic neuropathy[11 12]. The MRA provides information if the rim area of an eye is within 95%, 99% or 99.9% of population. The optic nerve is divided into six sectors, superior 90 degrees is divided into superior nasal and superior temporal, similarly inferior 90 degrees are divided into inferior nasal and inferior temporal. The nasal and temporal 90 degrees form the remaining two sectors. If a rim area falls between 95 to 99% or greater than 99% of predicted population interval it is labeled as borderline or outside normal limits respectively. If any sector falls in either of these two categories the MRA is classified as Outside Normal Limits.

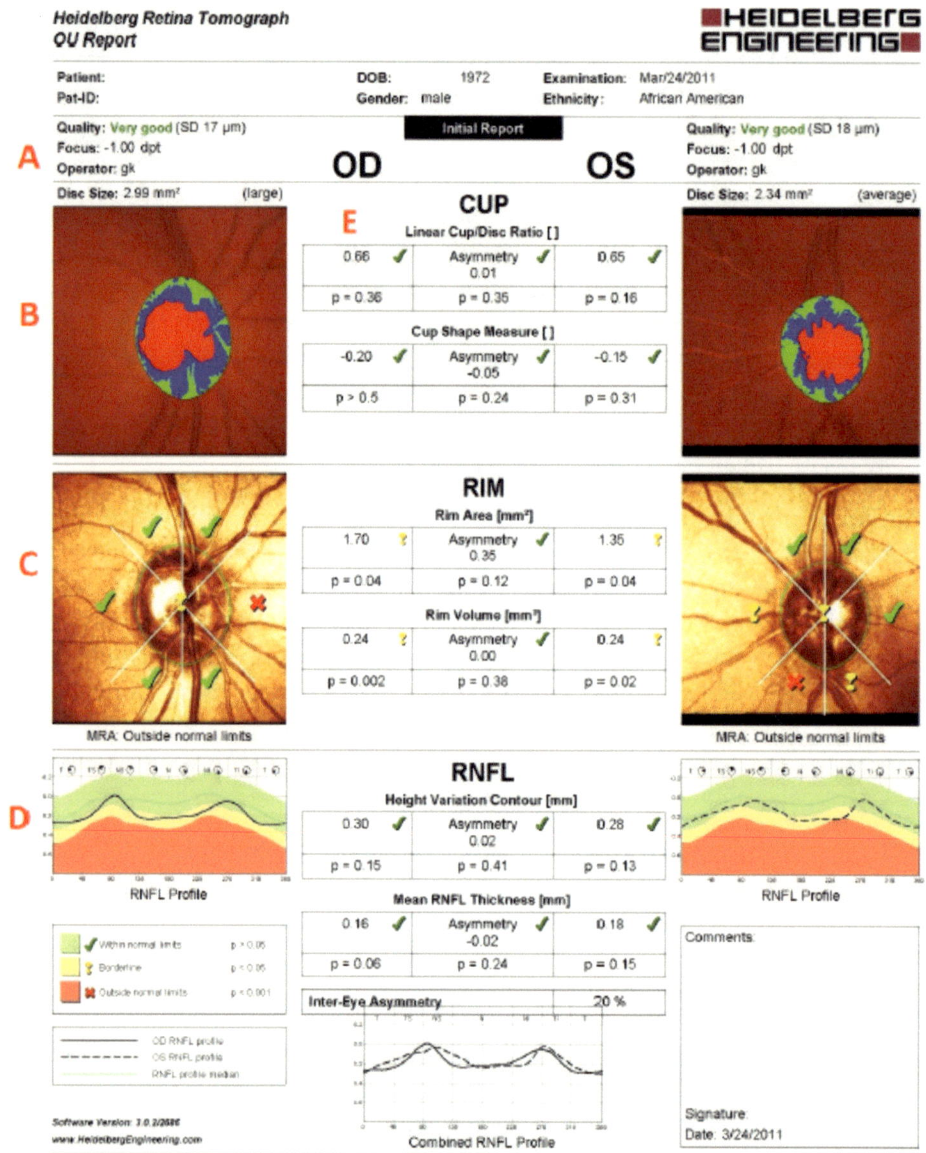

Figure 1. An OU report obtained using HRT III. Section A shows that reliability of the scan and the size of the disc which is obtained once the operator outlines the disc margin. Section B is a courtesy pseudo-isochromatic fundus image that shows the rim and cupping. Red color represents the cupping whereas the blue and the green are rim tissue. Section C shows the Moorfields regression analysis of various sectors of optic disc and section D shows RNFL in the TSNIT region. The section E provides the right eye and left eye information of various parameters measured and its asymmetry analysis along with statistical significance

This parameter was investigated in an Ancillary Study to Ocular Hypertension Treatment Study and was found to be a significant predictor of future development of glaucomatous optic neuropathy in a group of ocular hypertensive eyes.[13] Additionally a more recent report from

http://dx.doi.org/10.5772/58568

the same study indicates that these parameters are as effective as stereo photographs at estimating risk of development of primary open angle glaucoma in a group of ocular hypertensive eyes. [14]

3. Scanning laser polarimetry

Carl Zeiss Meditec manufactures the GDx-Pro which is the current generation scanning laser polarimeter. The scanning laser polarimeter uses near infrared laser (780 nm) in a raster pattern to image both the macula and peripapillary region. Details about the working principles can be found in detail elsewhere. [15] Birefringence is optical property that split a light wave by a polar material into two components. These components travel at different velocities which creates a relative phase shift. The phase shift is termed retardation. A few ocular structures, cornea, lens and retinal nerve fiber layer that are highly organized and parallel structures are birefringent. The scanning laser polarimeter is a confocal scanning laser ophthalmoscope that is capable of measuring retardation. It is shown that the RNFL retardation measured using the scanning laser polarimeter correlates well with the retinal RNFL determined by histology. [16 17]

3.1. Measurement and Interpretation of GDx — Pro output

The scanning laser polarimeter as a first step calculates anterior segment birefringence. This procedure is needed only once when examining the patient for the first time as anterior segment birefringence remains similar throughout life If there is a significant change in anterior segment like refractive or cataract surgery it is recommended to re-calculate the anterior segment birefringence. [18-20] Second part of the test is to obtain the brirefringence of the peripapillary retina. Clinicians can choose to scan the eye once or thrice. Obtaining more than one scan during the visit and averaging the scans decreases the variability in measurements obtained.

The output of optic nerve head and peripapillary images are divided into three parts the fundus image, retinal nerve fiber layer map and deviation map (see Figure 2 section A, B and C respectively). The fundus image (Figure 2 section A) in a GDx-Pro printout is a misnomer because the device uses a monochromatic light to capture the image. This image is only utilized to evaluate the focus, centration of scan and to be certain that the scan is evenly illuminated. The retinal nerve fiber layer map provides information about the thickness of retinal nerve fiber layer in a 20-degree image with the optic nerve in the center (Figure 2 section B). It is expected that in healthy eyes inferior and superior retinal nerve fiber layer is thick and represented with bright red and yellow where as the nasal and temporal regions are thinner and is represented with cooler colors like blue. The deviation map provides information if the retinal nerve fiber layer thickness points on the 20 degree image is within statistical limits of normality or has a less than 5%, 2%, 1% or 0.5% chance of being normal (Figure 2 section C).

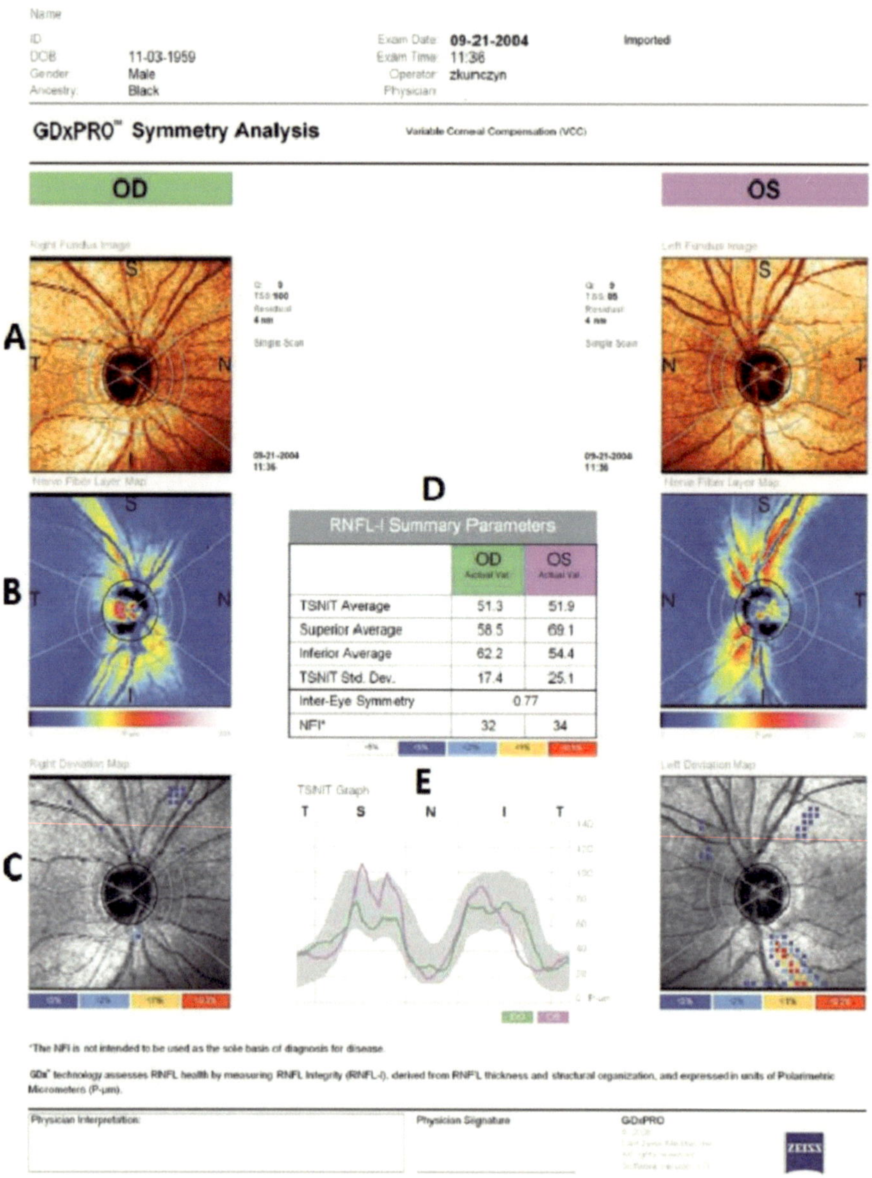

Figure 2. An output obtained using the GDX-Pro scanning laser polarimeter. Section A, B and C represents the courtesy pseudo-isochromatic fundus image, RNFL thickness plot and the deviation plot respectively. The Section C left eye shows a cluster of superpixels in the inferior temporal region that possibly indicates early damage. Section D and E provide the various parameters and TSNIT RNFL plot that can be used diagnostically. Image Courtesy Dr. Joseph Sowka OD, Professor, Nova Southeastern University, College of Optometry.

The two white rings shown on the three image maps is the region where the RNFL is measured to provide the various parameters (figure 2 D) and the thickness profile of the retinal nerve fiber layer in the temporal, superior, nasal, inferior and temporal (TSNIT) region in the

http://dx.doi.org/10.5772/58568

peripapillary retina of both eyes (Figure 2 E). The more similar the profiles are the less likely they are glaucomatous, however one has to remember the two eyes of an individual although similar most definitely will have differences.

There are various thickness parameters like TSNIT average, inferior average, superior average are provided along with color coding to indicate if they are within statistical limits of normality. The GDx-Pro also provides with a classifier the Nerve Fiber Indicator (NFI) that ranges 0 to 100 and a higher number is likely suggestive of damage. The manufacturers recommend that a NFI value of less than 30 has a low likelihood of glaucoma, a value between 30 and 50 should be considered a suspect and a value greater than 50 has a high likelihood of glaucoma. Numerous studies have shown that the NFI is the best GDx parameter at differentiating ocular healthy and glaucoma eyes. [21-24]

4. Optical coherence tomography

It is indeed an understatement to say that optical coherence tomography (OCT) has revolutionized clinical imaging in eye care. It was one of the fastest accepted technologies in eye care which is capable of obtaining micron resolution cross-sectional or tomographic scans of biological tissue in vivo. The principles of OCT are similar to ultrasound devices. The OCT uses light instead of sound thus providing excellent resolution (5-10 microns and 15 microns transverse). The echo time delay (that is the delay in time from when the ray of light leaves the device till the reflected light is received back) is calculated thus measuring distance that is an axial scan (A-scan). This is done at about 400 times per second. The axial scans are added to obtain the B-scan of the location being measured. The OCT principles described above is a "Time-domain (TD) OCT". The TD OCT devices are manufactured by Carl Zeiss Meditec. Although a phenomenal breakthrough in itself it was limited by number of scans it was capable of measuring. The scan regions measured were small and time taken was much larger. This was remedied by the "Fourier-Domain" technology. The Fourier domain technology uses a broader band width light source than the time domain OCT with a spectrometer to obtain the spectral interferogram that when analyzed using Fast-Fourier Transformation obtains the A-scan. The A-scans are obtained at a rate of 26,000 to 40,000 per second. Thus large amounts of data can be obtained in a short duration which was not possible accurately using the Time-domain OCT.

Numerous companies' manufacture the Fourier-domain OCT. This article will discuss general parameters output by all OCTs. Furthermore the OCT is capable of measuring both anterior segment and posterior segment. This article is going to restrict to analyzing output of posterior segment scan.

The OCT outputs the retinal nerve fiber layer thickness map and a deviation map (Figure 3 sections A and B). The RNFL thickness map (Figure 3 section A) is similar in interpretation as GDx-Pro which is color coded and it is expected that the inferior and superior region will show thicker RNFL compared to nasal and temporal regions in healthy eyes. The deviation map (Figure 3 section B) provides information if the given region is within statistical limits of normality. It also doubles as a fundus image; a careful look at this region is a must, to evaluate centration, focus and identify any errors in imaging (see next section for further details). The section B, similar to other devices and should not be utilized as a substitute to fundus photography.

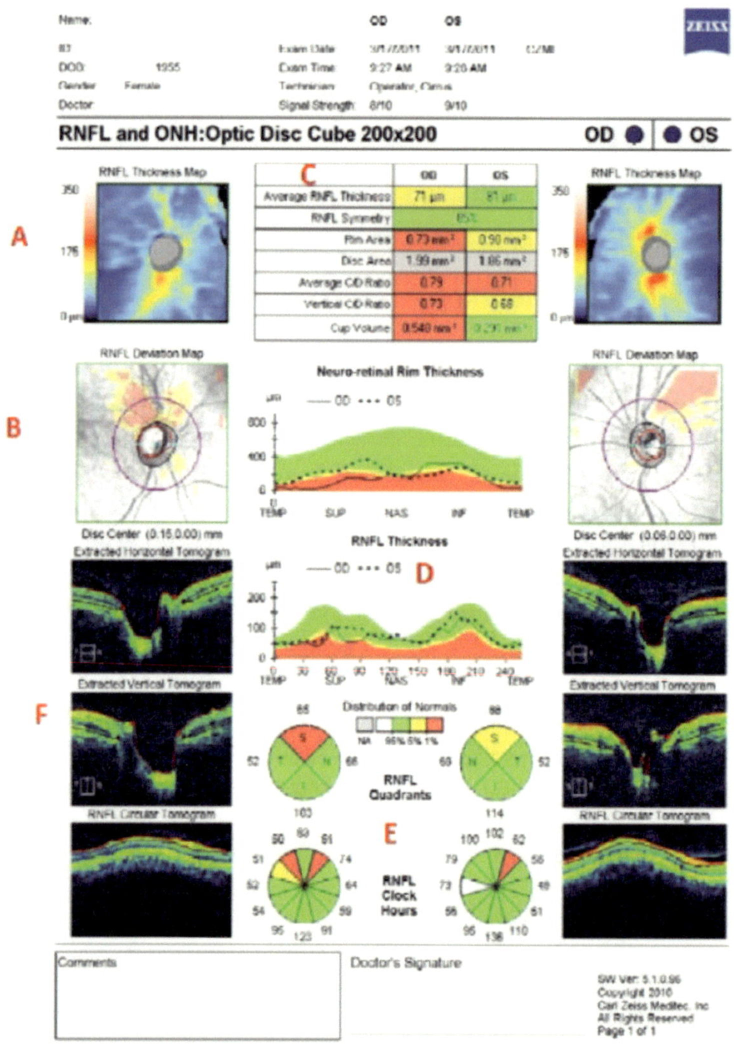

Figure 3. An output of RNFL analysis of Cirrus OCT. Section A shows the thickness map and section B shows the fundus image and highlights regions that are not within statistical limits of normality. Section C provides with the table of various parameters. Section D provides the TSNIT RNFL thickness profile and Section E provides thickness in various sectors and clock hours respectively. The section B,C, D and E are color coded to give an idea if the thickness measurement region or a parameter are within statistical limits of normality or outside normal limits. Section F provides with the vertical and horizontal tomogram obtained at the 12 and 6 O'clock & 3 and 9 O'clock of disc and peripapillary retina providing layer by layer thickness profile of retina and optic disc. The Circular tomogram in Section F is the cross-sectional thickness profile taken on the region of purple ring in section B.

The purple ring in Figure 3 Section B denotes the region where the RNFL is measured on the Temporal Superior, Nasal, Inferior and Temporal (TSNIT) region. This is utilized to calculate the RNFL parameters like the Average RNFL thickness and symmetry provided in the table (Figure3 Section C). The RNFL thickness profile obtained from the purple ring around the optic nerve is plotted graphically for both eyes to obtain symmetry information (Figure 3 section D). The graph has three color coded regions: 1) green represents 95% of normal distribution. 2) The yellow in RNFL plot represents the population that has less than 5% but greater than 1% chance of being normal and is also called the "borderline" category, whereas, 3) the red in the RNFL plot represents <1% chance of being normal; the "outside normal limits" category. The OCT also provides disc parameters in the table of parameters that includes cup to disc ratio cup volume, disc area and rim area (Figure 3 section C). The OCT also provides the RNFL values in each quadrant and each clock hour (Figure 3 Section E). The analysis reports of Optovue OCT Heidelberg and Engineering Spectralis is very similar to that of explained of Cirrus OCT (See Figure 4 and 5).

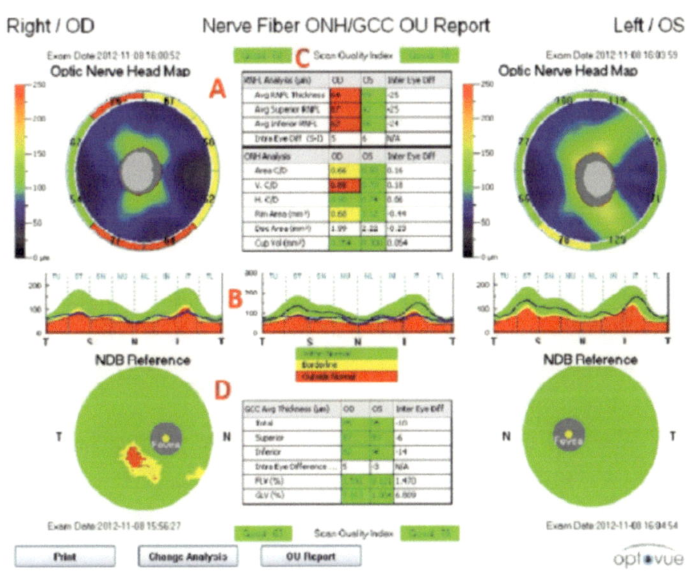

Figure 4. A combined output of retinal nerve fiber layer and ganglion cell complex map obtained by Optovue iVue OCT. The section A provides thickness information around the disc, section B the RNFL thickness in TSNIT region and section C provides the various parameters. The section D provides the ganglion cell complex parameters and the map. The right eye data shows that the infero temporal macula region shows damage that is statistically significant. All sections are color coded to provide information on statistical significance. Image courtesy Dr. Qienyuan Zhou PhD Optovue Inc.

Because OCTs are relatively new technology, automated machine learning algorithms similar to NFI of GDx-Pro and Moorfields regression analysis of HRT III are not available in OCT. It is seen that inferior average consistently shows up as the best parameter in differentiating early glaucoma from ocular healthy eyes.[5 25-32]

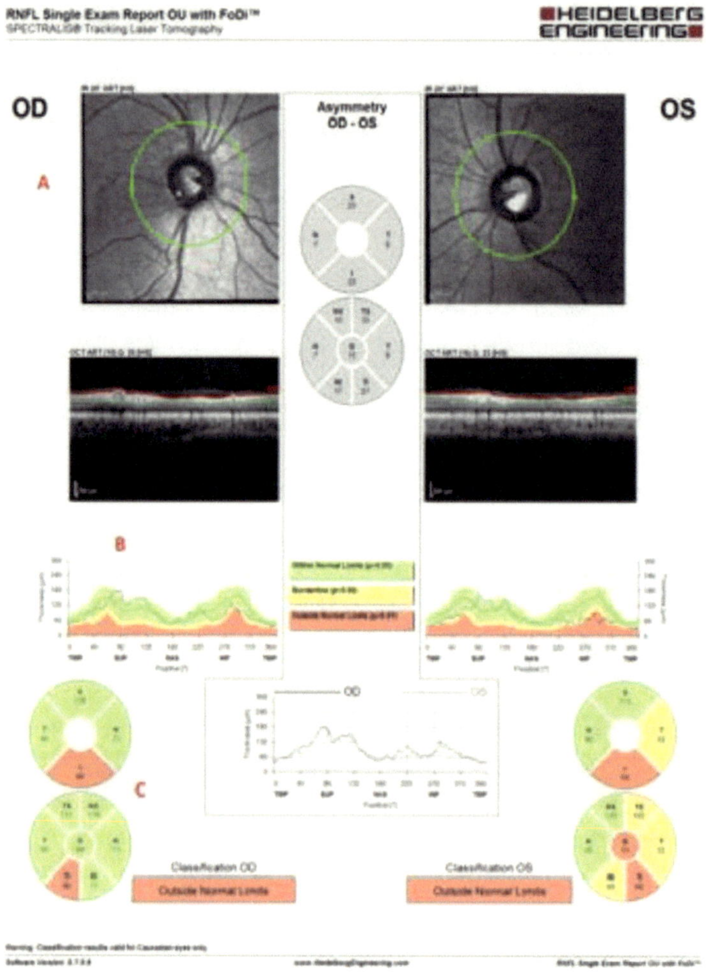

Figure 5. An OU report of RNFL with section A, B and C showing fundus image, RNFL thickness profile in TSNIT region and RNFL thickness in various quadrants respectively. Both the section B and C are color coded to provide information on statistical significance. Image courtesy Mr. Ali Tafreshi of Heidelberg Engineering.

4.1. Macula analysis in glaucoma

A new macula analysis is proposed to evaluate patients at risk of glaucoma. This analysis was proposed by Dr. Sanjay Asrani MD as additional data that might help managing glaucoma patients.[33 34] A separate scanning of the macula region is needed to obtain ganglion cell analysis. Different manufactures perform the analysis with slight variation. The Optovue manufactures of RTvue and iVue OCT call it the Ganglion Cell Complex that includes the nerve fiber layer, ganglion cell layer and the inner plexiform layer (Figure 4 section D). Carl Zeiss Meditec the manufacturers of Cirrus OCT calls it the Ganglion Cell Analysis that includes the

http://dx.doi.org/10.5772/58568

Ganglion cell layer and inner plexiform layer. There is no agreement if one analysis yields better results than the other. Further there is some conflicting reports about the diagnostic accuracy of the macular parameters in glaucoma however they tend to perform at par with other parameters generated by Fourier domain OCT (See review article by Wong et al., [35].)

5. Imaging artifacts

Although invaluable in clinical practice imaging devices like other clinical diagnostic techniques are susceptible to artifacts. Some which can be controlled and some that are not possible to control. When there is reduced signal strength which could possibly be due to image focusing issues, eye movement, tear film issues, or optical quality lowered due to presence of media opacity there is degradation in image quality which leads to errors in measured parameters and diagnostic ability of the devices.

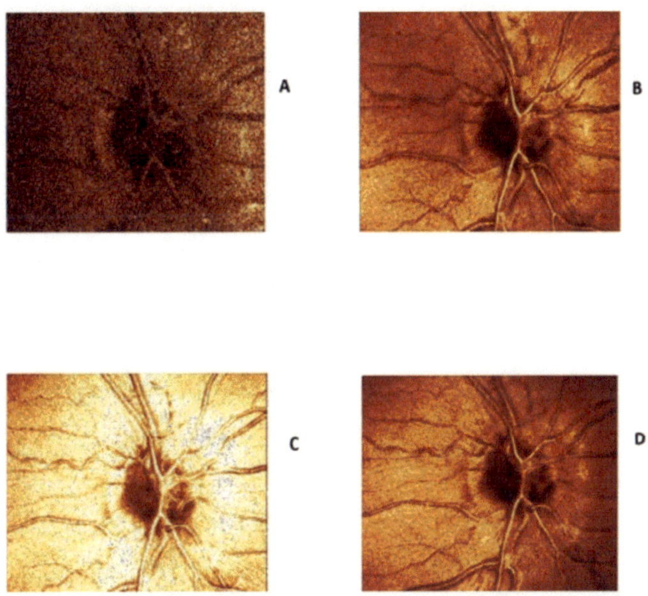

Figure 6. Common errors in imaging, these decrease the signal strength and image quality which in turn decreases the accuracy of parameters obtained. Section A shows an image of a severe dry eye patient that improved upon instillation of artificial tears (Section B). Section C shows the same patient with 2 diopter myopic defocus. As seen the image is over exposed with imaging artifacts visible. Section D shows the same patient with appropriate focus set.

All imaging devices outcomes would be affected if the image is defocused or if there was image quality degradation. Studies have looked at the effect of dryness and tear film issues that influence the outcome of the imaging. [36-38] It is advisable that patient's blink regularly between scans or artificial tears/lubricants be utilized to form a uniform regular optical surface. It is also be ideal if procedures that require ocular contact be avoided and performed after imaging is complete. Similarly reduced pupil size and optic media can have effect on imaging because the amount of light reaching retina will be decreased thus signal received from the eye will be of decreased leading to missing details.[36] This causes erroneous estimation of parameters measured and also to excessive false positive diagnosis. See figure 6 A-D for error in imaging due to dry eye or defocus and improvement in images when appropriate corrective methods were used.

Involuntary eye movement often leads to measurements obtained not at the intended region. [39] This leads to major errors in imaging. Some of these errors may be obvious to detect however some so subtle and leaving no obvious artifacts (See figure 7A B C and D "eye movement artifacts"). The eye movement artifacts are particularly a serious issue in the case of time domain OCTs slow scans or any scan that takes longer time. The errors in imaging due to eye movements can be avoided in the image acquisition phase as done by re-scanning as done in Spectralis OCT or done post acquisition (post image capture) processing as done in Optovue's OCTs.

The device may also fail in identifying appropriate layers of retinal and thus leading to segmentation errors. The scans should be viewed carefully and imaging performed again if such errors are observed. These errors are becoming less common with advanced instrumentation and algorithms that are in development to provide image registration.

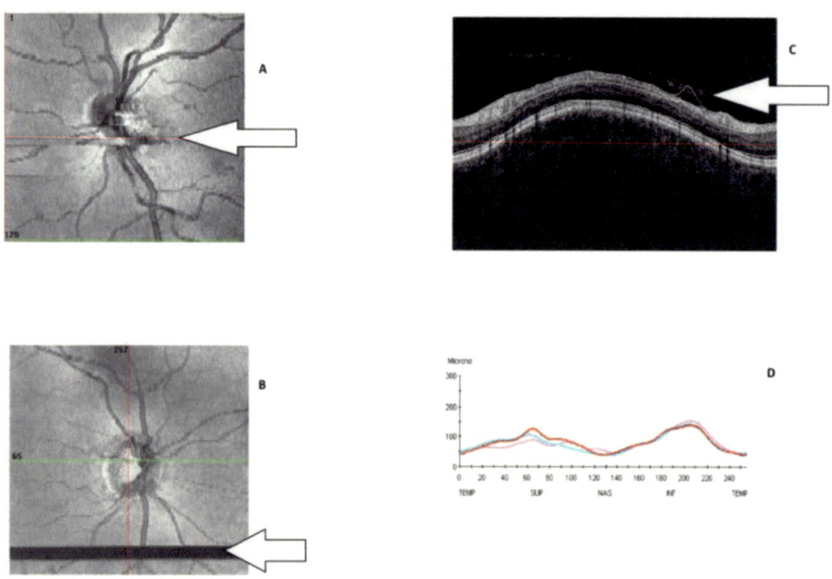

Figure 7. Various errors in imaging marked by an arrow in individual images. Section A shows an eye movement artifact that and is seen as non continuous blood vessels and optic disc. Section B shows blink artifact that is seen as a black band of missing data. Section C shows a segmentation error of RNFL which the machine algorithm has outlined incorrect upper lower layer of RNFL erroneously including the vitreo-retinal interface. Section D shows three consecutive scans obtained using Time domain OCT that were obtained 1-minute apart in a patient moving his eye. Images A,B, C courtesy Miss Kelly Soules Optovue Inc.

Atypical Birefringence pattern is an imaging artifact that affects images obtained in eyes with poor choroidal pigmentation also called "blonde fundus" and influenced results obtained using the prior generation polarimetry device GDx-Variable Corneal Compensator (VCC). These patterns were prevalent in 10-15% of the population when examined with GDx-VCC. [22 40] The images tended to not follow the normal physiological pattern of nerve fiber layer and the RNFL map shows "bicycle spoke like pattern" or "tie dye pattern" (See figure 8). These eyes were deemed not appropriate for imaging using GDx-VCC. With the new generation polarimetr GDx-Pro (Enhanced Corneal Compensator) has dramatically decreased the prevalence of these atypical patterns and long term measurement variability.[41]

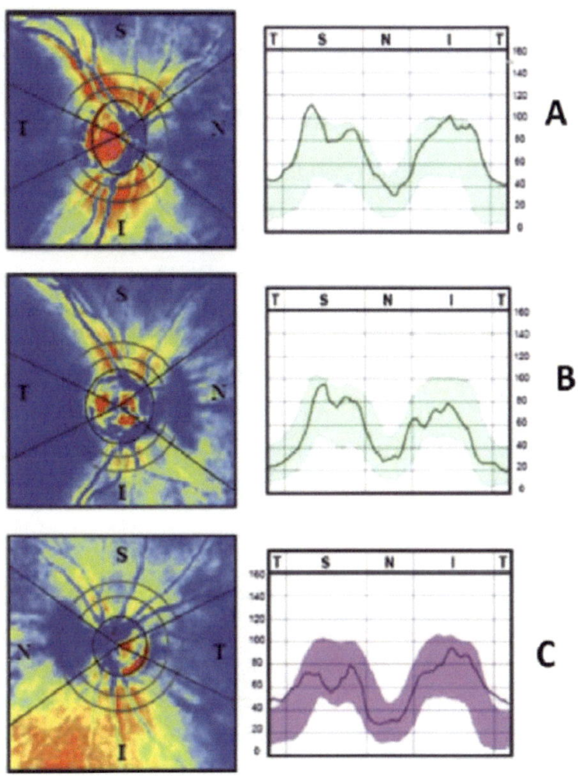

Figure 8. Three eyes with Atypical Retardation Pattern also known as "tie-dye" pattern in RNFL thickness profile map. These are an outcome of poor signal to noise ratio due to poor choroidal pigmentation. These scans are an outcome of an artifact and should not be utilized in managing patients.

6. Diagnostic accuracy and comparison of individual devices

Overall the principles behind the confocal scanning laser ophthalmoscope HRT-I, HRT-II and HRT-III manufactured by Heidelberg engineering are very similar that the data can be transferred from one generation to another. The agreement in stereometric parameters obtained by HRT-I is very similar to HRT-II.[42] Thus as expected the diagnostic accuracy of these different generation devices should be similar.

Whereas where GDx is concerned each generation of technology has fixed an error or problem in the imaging. For example the initial generation device: GDx-Fixed Corneal Compensator (GDx-FCC) used a standard correction factor to correct for anterior segment birefringence. The anterior segment birefringence varies in population thus the technology was changed to GDx Variable Corneal Compensator (GDx-VCC). [43 44] Recently the new generation GDx-Pro was introduced to improve upon the GDx-VCC. It is shown that the GDx-Enhanced Corneal Compensator (ECC now called GDx-Pro) better characterized the RNFL, decreased the number of atypical retardation pattern found in the study population.[45] It is shown by Mai and co-workers that the GDX-Pro has better repeatability, diagnostic ability, and a better structure and function relationship than GDx-VCC.[46-48] Thus it has to be remembered that where polarimetry is concerned newer devices are better than older generation devices.

Similarly the Fourier domain OCT compared to the older generation "time-domain" TD-OCT shows a marked improvement as it tried to address issues related to improved resolution, faster scanning speed. Where glaucoma is concerned the diagnostic accuracy of the TD OCT is similar to FD OCT [49 50], also the population mean RNFL values may not vary significantly however it has to be remembered the RNFL measurements are not comparable and cannot be used interchangeably.[51] The TD OCT RNFL tends to be thicker than FD OCT except for advanced glaucoma.[51] Unlike GDx-Pro and HRT III there are various manufacturers that make the Fourier Domain OCT. Overall comparing various Fourier domain OCT techniques the diagnostic accuracy in identifying individuals with glaucomatous optic neuropathy is very similar in these devices despite having difference in resolution and scanning speed.[52]

7. Comparison of diagnostic accuracy of various devices

Diagnostic accuracy of the imaging devices varies as a function of disease severity.[28 53-57] As the severity of glaucoma increases devices accuracy to detect glaucoma accurately also increases. For various reasons it is difficult to compare all imaging devices and its ability to diagnose glaucoma as there is no large scale population based study that have compared the latest technology that is available. Additionally there are inherent differences in the design and population of the cross-sectional studies that will influence the outcome of the study. For example the nerve fiber layer analysis may better suit than disc topography in evaluating myopes at risk of glaucoma. [58] These factors need to be kept in mind when comparing diagnostic accuracy of various imaging devices.

Studies have compared diagnostic capacity of GDx, OCT and HRT and although slight differences exist in identification of true-positive overall the ROC area which is a function of sensitivity and specificity (true positive and true negative) is similar in all the devices.[32 59] Because both the OCT and GDx provide RNFL data and numerous studies have evaluated its ability in identifying individuals with glaucoma.[5 32 59-62]. Over all these studies report that the diagnostic accuracy of GDx is very similar to OCT in identifying glaucoma eyes from a group of ocular healthy eyes. So in summary it is safe to conclude that although there are differences in diagnostic accuracy of various imaging devices overall they tends to perform quite similar.

8. Progression and imaging

Detecting progression or change over time in eyes at risk of glaucoma or with glaucoma is probably one of the most difficult tasks clinically. Progression in an optic nerve due to open angle glaucoma is subtle, slow and can easily be missed in casual observation. Thus the objectivity and reproducibility of the imaging devices can be of great benefit. All imaging devices have parameters that can be followed over time to monitor progression. These algorithms are overall based on simple regression analysis that is analyzing change in parameters with follow-up over time. This analysis identifies if there is a trend of values lowering or increasing over time was statistically significant also known as trend analysis.

Heidelberg retina tomography has topographical change analysis (TCA). The TCA is a statistical method that compares topographic values in small discrete regions of 4x4 pixels called superpixels. This method is distinctly different than trend analysis as the analysis is performed on raw topography values. The figure 9 shows an optic nerve head with progressive damage compared to the baseline scans. Studies have shown that this may be useful in identifying progressive damage in glaucoma.[63 64]

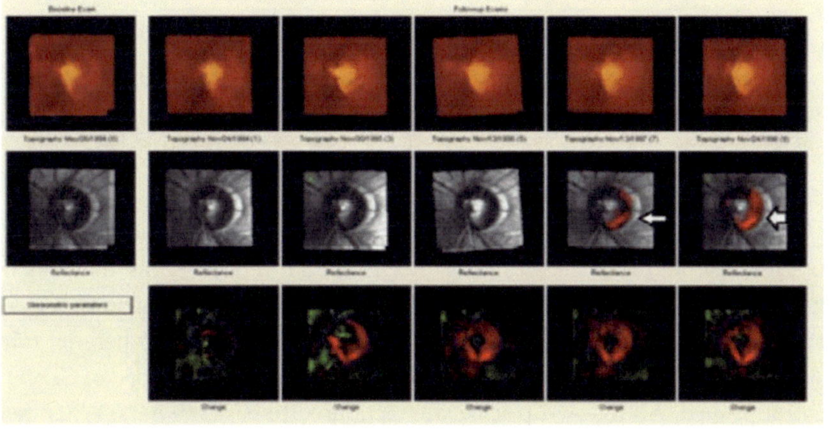

Figure 9. A Topographical Change Analysis output obtained using the HRT. The arrows indicate region of change in thickness particularly thinning in rim area. Image courtesy Mr. Ali Tafreshi of Heidelberg Engineering.

The scanning laser polarimetry GDx-VCC has advanced serial analysis that outputs trend over time in diagnosing progressive change in glaucoma (Figure 10). More recently an advanced

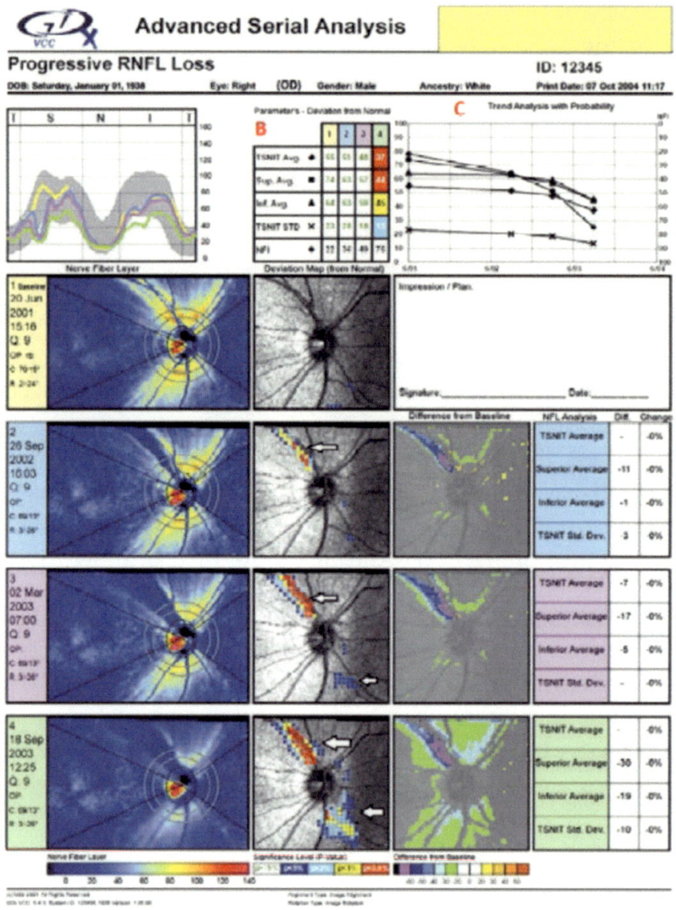

Figure 10. An advanced serial analysis of GDx. The deviation map shows an increase in number of superpixels (see arrow) that are statistically significant showing progressive thinning of retinal nerve fiber layer. The various parameters shown in section B and trend over time shown in section C show progressive decline. Image Courtesy Carl Zeiss Meditec.

"Guided Progression Analysis" that investigates changes in overall 20 degree area of the scan, TSNIT RNFL graph and the thickness parameters. Initial reports show that this may be of advantage in identifying progressive damage. [65-67] This software is however not cleared FDA approval and is not available for sale in USA. The Cirrus optical coherence tomography has a Guided Progression Analysis (figure 11) very similar to that described of GDx is available and is FDA approved. All follow-up scans are compared to baseline data. When two consecutive examinations show loss data the scans are flagged to be "possible loss" and "Likely loss" when three consecutive examinations show damage.

Glaucoma imaging devices have made a long journey from devices of interest in research arena to clinically useful technology. Its place in clinic and its usefulness in managing patients with glaucoma cannot be dismissed. With newer and improved techniques there is also an im-

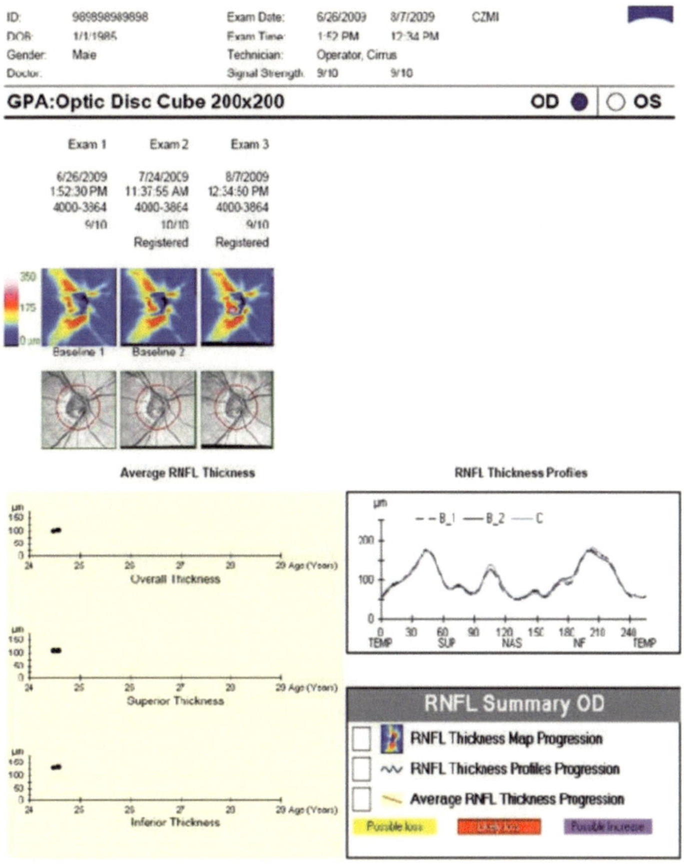

Figure 11. A Guided Progression Analysis (GPA) of Cirrus OCT that is obtained on an ocular hypertensive patient. The scans show no progressive damage in the short duration of follow-up with both RNFL thickness profile and RNFL summary.

provement in correlation of structure-functional loss in eyes with glaucoma.[68-73] This can improve overall diagnostic and prognostic ability in managing patients with glaucoma. With further advance in adaptive optics and improvement in transverse resolution has given us ability to image cones astrocytes, ganglion cells and its dendrites. [74] This should be able to bring the next wave in improvement of patient care and improve understanding of glaucoma pathogenesis.

Author details

Pinakin Gunvant Davey

Western University of Health Sciences, College of Optometry, Pomona CA, USA

References

[1] Gordon MO, Beiser JA, Brandt JD, et al. The Ocular Hypertension Treatment Study: baseline factors that predict the onset of primary open-angle glaucoma. Archives of ophthalmology 2002;120(6):714-20; discussion 829-30

[2] Fingeret M, Mancil L, Bailey IL, et al. Optometric Clinical Practice Guideline: Care of the Patient with Open Angle Glaucoma. Secondary Optometric Clinical Practice Guideline: Care of the Patient with Open Angle Glaucoma 2011.

[3] Prum B, Friedman D, Gedde S, et al. Primary Open Angle Glaucoma. Secondary Primary Open Angle Glaucoma 2010.

[4] Leung CK, Cheung CY, Lin D, et al. Longitudinal variability of optic disc and retinal nerve fiber layer measurements. Investigative ophthalmology & visual science 2008;49(11):4886-92 doi: 10.1167/iovs.07-1187[published Online First: Epub Date]|.

[5] Greaney MJ, Hoffman DC, Garway-Heath DF, et al. Comparison of optic nerve imaging methods to distinguish normal eyes from those with glaucoma. Investigative ophthalmology & visual science 2002;43(1):140-5

[6] Jonas JB, Budde WM, Panda-Jonas S. Ophthalmoscopic evaluation of the optic nerve head. Survey of ophthalmology 1999;43(4):293-320

[7] Garway-Heath DF, Wollstein G, Hitchings RA. Aging changes of the optic nerve head in relation to open angle glaucoma. The British journal of ophthalmology 1997;81(10):840-5

[8] Wollstein G, Garway-Heath DF, Hitchings RA. Identification of early glaucoma cases with the scanning laser ophthalmoscope. Ophthalmology 1998;105(8):1557-63 doi: 10.1016/s0161-6420(98)98047-2[published Online First: Epub Date]|.

[9] Betz P, Camps F, Collignon-Brach C, et al. [Stereophotography and photogrammetry of the physiological cup of the disc (author's transl)]. Journal francais d'ophtalmologie 1981;4(3):193-203

[10] Jonas JB, Gusek GC, Naumann GO. Optic disc, cup and neuroretinal rim size, configuration and correlations in normal eyes. Investigative ophthalmology & visual science 1988;29(7):1151-8

[11] Read RM, Spaeth GL. The practical clinical appraisal of the optic disc in glaucoma: the natural history of cup progression and some specific disc-field correlations. Transactions-American Academy of Ophthalmology and Otolaryngology. American Academy of Ophthalmology and Otolaryngology 1974;78(2):OP255-74

[12] Tuulonen A, Airaksinen PJ. Initial glaucomatous optic disk and retinal nerve fiber layer abnormalities and their progression. American journal of ophthalmology 1991;111(4):485-90

[13] Zangwill LM, Weinreb RN, Beiser JA, et al. Baseline topographic optic disc measurements are associated with the development of primary open-angle glaucoma: the Confocal Scanning Laser Ophthalmoscopy Ancillary Study to the Ocular Hypertension Treatment Study. Archives of ophthalmology 2005;123(9):1188-97 doi: 10.1001/archopht.123.9.1188[published Online First: Epub Date]|.

[14] Weinreb RN, Zangwill LM, Jain S, et al. Predicting the onset of glaucoma: the confocal scanning laser ophthalmoscopy ancillary study to theOcular Hypertension Treatment Study. Ophthalmology 2010;117(9):1674-83 doi: 10.1016/j.ophtha.2010.03.044[published Online First: Epub Date]|.

[15] RNFL analysis with GDx VCC: A primer and a clinical guide. http://www.meditec.zeiss.com/C125679E00525939/EmbedTitelIntern/GDxPrimerChapter2/$File/GDx_Primer_Chapter2.pdf%5Ct_blank, 2004.

[16] Morgan JE, Waldock A, Jeffery G, et al. Retinal nerve fibre layer polarimetry: histological and clinical comparison. The British journal of ophthalmology 1998;82(6):684-90

[17] Weinreb RN, Dreher AW, Coleman A, et al. Histopathologic validation of Fourier-ellipsometry measurements of retinal nerve fiber layer thickness. Archives of ophthalmology 1990;108(4):557-60

[18] Dada T, Behera G, Agarwal A, et al. Effect of cataract surgery on retinal nerve fiber layer thickness parameters using scanning laser polarimetry (GDxVCC). Indian journal of ophthalmology 2010;58(5):389-94 doi: 10.4103/0301-4738.67048[published Online First: Epub Date]|.

[19] Sanchez-Cano A, Pablo LE, Larrosa JM, et al. The effect of phacoemulsification cataract surgery on polarimetry and tomography measurements for glaucoma diagnosis. Journal of glaucoma 2010;19(7):468-74 doi: 10.1097/IJG.0b013e3181c4aed8[published Online First: Epub Date]|.

[20] Zangwill LM, Abunto T, Bowd C, et al. Scanning laser polarimetry retinal nerve fiber layer thickness measurements after LASIK. Ophthalmology 2005;112(2):200-7 doi: 10.1016/j.ophtha.2004.08.019[published Online First: Epub Date]|.

[21] Da Pozzo S, Iacono P, Marchesan R, et al. Scanning laser polarimetry with variable corneal compensation and detection of glaucomatous optic neuropathy. Graefe's archive for clinical and experimental ophthalmology=Albrecht von Graefes Archiv fur klinische und experimentelle Ophthalmologie 2005;243(8):774-9 doi: 10.1007/s00417-004-1118-1[published Online First: Epub Date]|.

[22] Gunvant P, Zheng Y, Toth M, et al. Atypical retardation pattern: can performance of classification be improved? Optometry and vision science : official publication of the American Academy of Optometry 2008;85(6):482-8 doi: 10.1097/OPX.0b013e3181783aa2[published Online First: Epub Date]|.

[23] Iester M, Perdicchi A, De Feo F, et al. Comparison between GDx VCC parameter and achromatic perimetry in glaucoma patients. Journal of glaucoma 2006;15(4):281-5 doi: 10.1097/01.ijg.0000212235.88416.bd[published Online First: Epub Date]|.

[24] Reus NJ, Lemij HG. Diagnostic accuracy of the GDx VCC for glaucoma. Ophthalmology 2004;111(10):1860-5 doi: 10.1016/j.ophtha.2004.04.024[published Online First: Epub Date]|.

[25] Bowd C, Zangwill LM, Berry CC, et al. Detecting early glaucoma by assessment of retinal nerve fiber layer thickness and visual function. Investigative ophthalmology & visual science 2001;42(9):1993-2003

[26] Budenz DL, Michael A, Chang RT, et al. Sensitivity and specificity of the StratusOCT for perimetric glaucoma. Ophthalmology 2005;112(1):3-9 doi: 10.1016/j.ophtha. 2004.06.039[published Online First: Epub Date]|.

[27] Chen HY, Huang ML. Discrimination between normal and glaucomatous eyes using Stratus optical coherence tomography in Taiwan Chinese subjects. Graefe's archive for clinical and experimental ophthalmology=Albrecht von Graefes Archiv fur klinische und experimentelle Ophthalmologie 2005;243(9):894-902 doi: 10.1007/ s00417-005-1140-y[published Online First: Epub Date]|.

[28] Gunvant P, Zheng Y, Essock EA, et al. Application of shape-based analysis methods to OCT retinal nerve fiber layer data in glaucoma. Journal of glaucoma 2007;16(6): 543-8 doi: 10.1097/IJG.0b013e318050ab65[published Online First: Epub Date]|.

[29] Kanamori A, Nakamura M, Escano MF, et al. Evaluation of the glaucomatous damage on retinal nerve fiber layer thickness measured by optical coherence tomography. American journal of ophthalmology 2003;135(4):513-20

[30] Lu AT, Wang M, Varma R, et al. Combining nerve fiber layer parameters to optimize glaucoma diagnosis with optical coherence tomography. Ophthalmology 2008;115(8): 1352-7, 57 e1-2 doi: 10.1016/j.ophtha.2008.01.011[published Online First: Epub Date]|.

[31] Medeiros FA, Zangwill LM, Bowd C, et al. Evaluation of retinal nerve fiber layer, optic nerve head, and macular thickness measurements for glaucoma detection using optical coherence tomography. American journal of ophthalmology 2005;139(1):44-55 doi: 10.1016/j.ajo.2004.08.069[published Online First: Epub Date]|.

[32] Zangwill LM, Bowd C, Berry CC, et al. Discriminating between normal and glaucomatous eyes using the Heidelberg Retina Tomograph, GDx Nerve Fiber Analyzer, and Optical Coherence Tomograph. Archives of ophthalmology 2001;119(7):985-93

[33] Asrani S, Zeimer R, Jampel H, et al. Macular symmetry testing for glaucoma detection. Journal of glaucoma 2006;15(2):182; author reply 82

[34] Mathers K, Rosdahl JA, Asrani S. Correlation of Macular Thickness With Visual Fields in Glaucoma Patients and Suspects. Journal of glaucoma 2013 doi: 10.1097/IJG. 0b013e31829539c3[published Online First: Epub Date]|.

[35] Wong JJ, Chen TC, Shen LQ, et al. Macular imaging for glaucoma using spectral-domain optical coherence tomography: a review. Seminars in ophthalmology 2012;27(5-6):160-6 doi: 10.3109/08820538.2012.712734[published Online First: Epub Date]|.

[36] Asrani S, Edghill B, Gupta Y, et al. Optical coherence tomography errors in glaucoma. Journal of glaucoma 2010;19(4):237-42 doi: 10.1097/IJG.0b013e3181b21f99[published Online First: Epub Date]|.

[37] Hoh ST, Greenfield DS, Liebmann JM, et al. Factors affecting image acquisition during scanning laser polarimetry. Ophthalmic surgery and lasers 1998;29(7):545-51

[38] Stein DM, Wollstein G, Ishikawa H, et al. Effect of corneal drying on optical coherence tomography. Ophthalmology 2006;113(6):985-91 doi: 10.1016/j.ophtha.2006.02.018[published Online First: Epub Date]|.

[39] Koozekanani D, Boyer KL, Roberts C. Tracking the optic nervehead in OCT video using dual eigenspaces and an adaptive vascular distribution model. IEEE transactions on medical imaging 2003;22(12):1519-36 doi: 10.1109/tmi.2003.817753[published Online First: Epub Date]|.

[40] Toth M, Hollo G. Enhanced corneal compensation for scanning laser polarimetry on eyes with atypical polarisation pattern. The British journal of ophthalmology 2005;89(9):1139-42 doi: 10.1136/bjo.2005.070011[published Online First: Epub Date]|.

[41] Grewal DS, Sehi M, Cook RJ, et al. The impact of retardance pattern variability on nerve fiber layer measurements over time using GDx with variable and enhanced corneal compensation. Investigative ophthalmology & visual science 2011;52(7):4516-24 doi: 10.1167/iovs.10-5969[published Online First: Epub Date]|.

[42] Balasubramanian M, Bowd C, Weinreb RN, et al. Agreement between the Heidelberg Retina Tomograph (HRT) stereometric parameters estimated using HRT-I and HRT-II. Optometry and vision science : official publication of the American Academy of Optometry 2011;88(1):140-9 doi: 10.1097/OPX.0b013e3181fc3467[published Online First: Epub Date]|.

[43] Choplin NT, Zhou Q, Knighton RW. Effect of individualized compensation for anterior segment birefringence on retinal nerve fiber layer assessments as determined by scanning laser polarimetry. Ophthalmology 2003;110(4):719-25 doi: 10.1016/s0161-6420(02)01899-7[published Online First: Epub Date]|.

[44] Zhou Q, Weinreb RN. Individualized compensation of anterior segment birefringence during scanning laser polarimetry. Investigative ophthalmology & visual science 2002;43(7):2221-8

[45] Reus NJ, Zhou Q, Lemij HG. Enhanced imaging algorithm for scanning laser polarimetry with variable corneal compensation. Investigative ophthalmology & visual

science 2006;47(9):3870-7 doi: 10.1167/iovs.05-0067[published Online First: Epub Date]|.

[46] Mai TA, Reus NJ, Lemij HG. Structure-function relationship is stronger with enhanced corneal compensation than with variable corneal compensation in scanning laser polarimetry. Investigative ophthalmology & visual science 2007;48(4):1651-8 doi: 10.1167/iovs.06-1003[published Online First: Epub Date]|.

[47] Mai TA, Reus NJ, Lemij HG. Diagnostic accuracy of scanning laser polarimetry with enhanced versus variable corneal compensation. Ophthalmology 2007;114(11): 1988-93 doi: 10.1016/j.ophtha.2007.01.022[published Online First: Epub Date]|.

[48] Mai TA, Reus NJ, Lemij HG. Retinal nerve fiber layer measurement repeatability in scanning laser polarimetry with enhanced corneal compensation. Journal of glaucoma 2008;17(4):269-74 doi: 10.1097/IJG.0b013e31815c3a6b[published Online First: Epub Date]|.

[49] Chang RT, Knight OJ, Feuer WJ, et al. Sensitivity and specificity of time-domain versus spectral-domain optical coherence tomography in diagnosing early to moderate glaucoma. Ophthalmology 2009;116(12):2294-9 doi: 10.1016/j.ophtha.2009.06.012[published Online First: Epub Date]|.

[50] Chen HY, Chang YC, Wang IJ, et al. Comparison of Glaucoma Diagnoses Using Stratus and Cirrus Optical Coherence Tomography in Different Glaucoma Types in a Chinese Population. Journal of glaucoma 2012 doi: 10.1097/IJG. 0b013e3182594f42[published Online First: Epub Date]|.

[51] Knight OJ, Chang RT, Feuer WJ, et al. Comparison of retinal nerve fiber layer measurements using time domain and spectral domain optical coherent tomography. Ophthalmology 2009;116(7):1271-7 doi: 10.1016/j.ophtha.2008.12.032[published Online First: Epub Date]|.

[52] Leite MT, Rao HL, Zangwill LM, et al. Comparison of the diagnostic accuracies of the Spectralis, Cirrus, and RTVue optical coherence tomography devices in glaucoma. Ophthalmology 2011;118(7):1334-9 doi: 10.1016/j.ophtha.2010.11.029[published Online First: Epub Date]|.

[53] Essock EA, Zheng Y, Gunvant P. Analysis of GDx-VCC polarimetry data by Wavelet-Fourier analysis across glaucoma stages. Investigative ophthalmology & visual science 2005;46(8):2838-47 doi: 10.1167/iovs.04-1156[published Online First: Epub Date]|.

[54] Girkin CA, Liebmann J, Fingeret M, et al. The effects of race, optic disc area, age, and disease severity on the diagnostic performance of spectral-domain optical coherence tomography. Investigative ophthalmology & visual science 2011;52(9):6148-53 doi: 10.1167/iovs.10-6698[published Online First: Epub Date]|.

[55] Leite MT, Zangwill LM, Weinreb RN, et al. Effect of disease severity on the performance of Cirrus spectral-domain OCT for glaucoma diagnosis. Investigative ophthal-

mology & visual science 2010;51(8):4104-9 doi: 10.1167/iovs.09-4716[published Online First: Epub Date]|.

[56] Rao HL, Leite MT, Weinreb RN, et al. Effect of disease severity and optic disc size on diagnostic accuracy of RTVue spectral domain optical coherence tomograph in glaucoma. Investigative ophthalmology & visual science 2011;52(3):1290-6 doi: 10.1167/iovs.10-5546[published Online First: Epub Date]|.

[57] Reddy S, Xing D, Arthur SN, et al. HRT III glaucoma probability score and Moorfields regression across the glaucoma spectrum. Journal of glaucoma 2009;18(5):368-72 doi: 10.1097/IJG.0b013e31818c6edd[published Online First: Epub Date]|.

[58] Leung CK, Medeiros FA, Zangwill LM, et al. American Chinese glaucoma imaging study: a comparison of the optic disc and retinal nerve fiber layer in detecting glaucomatous damage. Investigative ophthalmology & visual science 2007;48(6):2644-52 doi: 10.1167/iovs.06-1332[published Online First: Epub Date]|.

[59] Medeiros FA, Zangwill LM, Bowd C, et al. Comparison of the GDx VCC scanning laser polarimeter, HRT II confocal scanning laser ophthalmoscope, and stratus OCT optical coherence tomograph for the detection of glaucoma. Archives of ophthalmology 2004;122(6):827-37 doi: 10.1001/archopht.122.6.827[published Online First: Epub Date]|.

[60] Gunvant P, Zheng Y, Essock EA, et al. Comparison of shape-based analysis of retinal nerve fiber layer data obtained From OCT and GDx-VCC. Journal of glaucoma 2009;18(6):464-71 doi: 10.1097/IJG.0b013e31818c6f2b[published Online First: Epub Date]|.

[61] Kanamori A, Nagai-Kusuhara A, Escano MF, et al. Comparison of confocal scanning laser ophthalmoscopy, scanning laser polarimetry and optical coherence tomography to discriminate ocular hypertension and glaucoma at an early stage. Graefe's archive for clinical and experimental ophthalmology=Albrecht von Graefes Archiv fur klinische und experimentelle Ophthalmologie 2006;244(1):58-68 doi: 10.1007/s00417-005-0029-0[published Online First: Epub Date]|.

[62] Leung CK, Chan WM, Chong KK, et al. Comparative study of retinal nerve fiber layer measurement by StratusOCT and GDx VCC, I: correlation analysis in glaucoma. Investigative ophthalmology & visual science 2005;46(9):3214-20 doi: 10.1167/iovs.05-0294[published Online First: Epub Date]|.

[63] Bowd C, Balasubramanian M, Weinreb RN, et al. Performance of confocal scanning laser tomograph Topographic Change Analysis (TCA) for assessing glaucomatous progression. Investigative ophthalmology & visual science 2009;50(2):691-701 doi: 10.1167/iovs.08-2136[published Online First: Epub Date]|.

[64] Chauhan BC, McCormick TA, Nicolela MT, et al. Optic disc and visual field changes in a prospective longitudinal study of patients with glaucoma: comparison of scan-

ning laser tomography with conventional perimetry and optic disc photography. Archives of ophthalmology 2001;119(10):1492-9

[65] Alencar LM, Zangwill LM, Weinreb RN, et al. Agreement for detecting glaucoma progression with the GDx guided progression analysis, automated perimetry, and optic disc photography. Ophthalmology 2010;117(3):462-70 doi: 10.1016/j.ophtha.2009.08.012[published Online First: Epub Date]|.

[66] Grewal DS, Sehi M, Greenfield DS. Detecting glaucomatous progression using GDx with variable and enhanced corneal compensation using Guided Progression Analysis. The British journal of ophthalmology 2011;95(4):502-8 doi: 10.1136/bjo.2010.180810[published Online First: Epub Date]|.

[67] Kjaergaard SM, Alencar LM, Nguyen B, et al. Detection of retinal nerve fibre layer progression: comparison of the fast and extended modes of GDx guided progression analysis. The British journal of ophthalmology 2011;95(12):1707-12 doi: 10.1136/bjophthalmol-2011-300354[published Online First: Epub Date]|.

[68] Kanamori A, Nakamura M, Tomioka M, et al. Structure-function relationship among three types of spectral-domain optical coherent tomography instruments in measuring parapapillary retinal nerve fibre layer thickness. Acta ophthalmologica 2013;91(3):e196-202 doi: 10.1111/aos.12028[published Online First: Epub Date]|.

[69] 69. Lamparter J, Russell RA, Schulze A, et al. Structure-function relationship between FDF, FDT, SAP, and scanning laser ophthalmoscopy in glaucoma patients. Investigative ophthalmology & visual science 2012;53(12):7553-9 doi: 10.1167/iovs.12-10892[published Online First: Epub Date]|.

[70] 70. Medeiros FA, Zangwill LM, Bowd C, et al. The structure and function relationship in glaucoma: implications for detection of progression and measurement of rates of change. Investigative ophthalmology & visual science 2012;53(11):6939-46 doi: 10.1167/iovs.12-10345[published Online First: Epub Date]|.

[71] Naghizadeh F, Garas A, Vargha P, et al. Structure-Function Relationship Between the Octopus Perimeter Cluster Mean Sensitivity and Sector Retinal Nerve Fiber Layer Thickness Measured With the RTVue Optical Coherence Tomography and Scanning Laser Polarimetry. Journal of glaucoma 2012 doi: 10.1097/IJG.0b013e318264cda2[published Online First: Epub Date]|.

[72] Park HY, Park CK. Structure-function relationship and diagnostic value of RNFL Area Index compared with circumpapillary RNFL thickness by spectral-domain OCT. Journal of glaucoma 2013;22(2):88-97 doi: 10.1097/IJG.0b013e318231202f[published Online First: Epub Date]|.

[73] Sato S, Hirooka K, Baba T, et al. Correlation Between the Ganglion Cell-Inner Plexiform Layer Thickness Measured With Cirrus HD-OCT and Macular Visual Field Sensitivity Measured With Microperimetry. Investigative ophthalmology & visual

science 2013;54(4):3046-51 doi: 10.1167/iovs.12-11173[published Online First: Epub Date]|.

[74] Werkmeister RM, Cherecheanu AP, Garhofer G, et al. Imaging of retinal ganglion cells in glaucoma: pitfalls and challenges. Cell and tissue research 2013 doi: 10.1007/s00441-013-1600-3[published Online First: Epub Date]|.

Chapter 3

Application of Electron Paramagnetic Resonance Spectroscopy in Ophthalmology

Magdalena Zdybel and Barbara Pilawa

Additional information is available at the end of the chapter

http://dx.doi.org/10.5772/58313

1. Introduction

Electron paramagnetic resonance (EPR) spectroscopy is the method of examination of free radicals and the others paramagnetic centers [1-22]. EPR measurements reveal applications in medicine [8-11, 23-34], biology [8-11], pharmacy [35-48], cosmetology [49, 50], biotechnology [51-54]. EPR method is useful to examination of tissues, cells, biopolimers, drugs, cosmetic substances, herbs, and biomaterials [8-11, 23-34]. Free radicals in such mentioned samples may be characterized by EPR spectra, and the influence of physical and chemical factors on them may be tested. The important information about light, oxygen, temperature, gamma irradiation on the biological or pharmacological objects may be obtain from analysis of their absorption signals [8-11, 23-54]. Free radical properties and concentration are determined by the use of electron paramagnetic resonance [1-8]. Applications of EPR method to determine the optimal conditions of photodynamic therapy [24-26], the best conditions of sterilization of drugs [35-48], herbs [22] and cosmetic substances [49, 50], was proposed.

1.1. Aim

The aim of this work is to present usefulness of EPR analysis in ophthalmology. EPR studies of free radicals and their interactions with tissues structures are described. Melanins, which contain o-semiquinone free radicals (S=1/2) and biradicals (S=1) exist in the eye. EPR studies of paramagnetic centers in melanin biopolymers are presented. The effect of light irradiation and temperature on free radicals in melanin biopolymer is shown. The effect of dia- and paramagnetic metal ions on free radicals in melanins is discussed. The effect of drugs on free radicals in melanins tested by EPR is presented. Different types of free radicals, their chemical and thermodynamic stability are compared. Free radicals and reactive oxygen species in ophthalmology are presented.

The effect of electron paramagnetic resonance as the absorption of electromagnetic waves by the sample located in magnetic field and the EPR spectrometer are described. The positive aspects of the EPR analysis in the technical meaning such are bring to light. EPR measurements are not destructive to the samples and only the low amount of the sample is needed. The types of EPR spectrometers and microwave frequencies are presented. EPR spectra of tissues may be multi-component and the frequency of microwaves influences the resolution of detection of EPR lines of different types of free radicals. The parameters of the EPR spectra: amplitudes, integral intensities, linewidths, g-factors, and both physical and practical meaning of them are shown. Amplitudes and integral intensities increase with increasing of free radical concentration in the sample [1-8]. Linewidth depends on molecular structure of the samples and magnetic interactions in the chemical units [1-6]. g-Values let us to determine the type of free radicals [1-3]. Free radical concentration determination and the references for these measurements are shown. The concentration is proportional to the area under the absorption lines [1-8]. The spin probes in EPR investigation to ophthalmology are presented. The professional spectroscopic programs are characterized.

Sample preparation to EPR measurements are presented. The measurements in the wide range of temperatures and microwave powers relative to their usefulness in ophthalmologic samples are discussed. The methods of differentiation of free radicals and biradicals in melanin biopolimers are presented.

2. Paramagnetic centers

2.1. Types of paramagnetic centers

Paramagnetic centers are the molecular units with unpaired electrons and they have characteristic behavior in magnetic field applied in EPR spectroscopy [1-8]. Paramagnetic centers are formed during photolysis, thermolysis, radiolysis, electrolysis, and the others chemical reactions [11]. Oxygen is very active in generation of paramagnetic centers [1, 11, 55]. The most known paramagnetic centers are free radicals, biradicals, paramagnetic metal ions, oxygen O_2 molecules in triplet ground state and paramagnetic conducting species [l, 5, 11]. Paramagnetic centers differ in spins and in stability. Free radicals have spin with the value of 1/2, biradicals and O_2 spins are equal of 1, paramagnetic ions mainly reveal spin of 1/2, delocalized electrons in conducting materials have spins of 1/2. Magnetic moments of paramagnetic centers result from their spins, and they are responsible for the orientations in magnetic field during their EPR detection.

Paramagnetic centers differ in lifetime [8, 11]. Stability of paramagnetic centers is connected with their chemical building and the external conditions in the environment. There is known stabile organic free radicals and labile reactive oxygen species. Samples in vacuum have usually free radicals for the longer times than the samples in air, where oxygen molecules O_2 in paramagnetic triplet states with spin S=1 exist [1, 11]. The reactions with oxygen is stronger in the higher temperatures [11]. The intensive reactions between paramagnetic centers become in the structures with the large amount of unpaired electrons.

2.2. Stable free radicals

Stabile free radicals with different localization of unpaired electrons exist in organic molecular units [10, 11, 55]. Thermodynamic stability of free radicals depend on their chemical structure [55]. The lifetime is longer for free radicals in aromatic units than in aliphatic units. The major types of free radicals exist in cells and tissues, because of differentiation on their building and composition. o-Semiquinone free radicals are the aromatic free radicals [55]. There is known the chain the aliphatic free radicals [55]. The exemplary popular free radicals in living organism are peroxyl radicals (ROO•) and alkoxyl radicals (RO•).

2.3. Reactive oxygen species

The group of reactive oxygen species consists of both paramagnetic free radicals and diamagnetic non-radical compounds [11, 55]. The reactive oxygen species are not stabile, they have the short lifetimes often lower than one second, and they easy react with others molecules. The exemplary paramagnetic reactive oxygen species are hydroxyl radical (•OH), hydroperoxyl radical (HO_2•), superoxide radical anion (O_2•), and nitric dioxide (NO_2•) [11]. Reactive oxygen species appear in inflammatory states in human organism [10, 11], irradiated tissues, in thermally [35-43] and gamma [44-48] sterilized drugs.

2.4. Paramagnetic centers in eye

Paramagnetic centers in eye exist mainly in melanin biopolymer [56]. Melanin is a natural pigment that is found in most organisms. In humans, melanin is found in skin, eyes, hair, leucocytes, *Substantia nigra, Locus coerules* and inner ear [31, 32, 57-60]. Through a process called melanogenesis, melanin is produced by melanocytes [32, 58].

There are three basic types of melanin: eumelanin, which is a brown and black, pheomelanin, which is red or yellow, and neuromelanin, which is present in the brain [33, 59].

Chemically, melanins are amorphous biopolymers consisting of various monomer units i.a. 5, 6-dihydroxy indole-2-carboxylic acid and 5, 6-dihydroxy indole [59, 60]. Chemical structures of eu-and pheomelanins are compared in Figure 1 [59]. Eumelanin contains carbon (C), oxygen (O), and nitrogen (N) atoms. Besides C, O, and N, sulphur (S) exists in pheomelanin [59, 60].

Melanins are found in the eye in higher concentrations than anywhere else in the human body [61]. In the eye, melanin content in the iris, ciliary body, choroid and retinal pigment epithelium (RPE) [60]. Cornea and lens don't have the pigment [60, 62].

Content of melanin differs in various ocular tissues [60, 62]. In humans, scleral melanin levels are higher than retina and central choroid-RPE. Besides, it is also different distribution of melanin in human eyes. The peripheral tissue pigment levels are generally higher compared to the central regions [60]. The melanin content of human RPE decreases with age [56, 62].

Differences in iris color are caused by three factors: the concentration of pigment within stromal melanocytes, light scattering and absorptive properties of extracellular components, and the pigment granules in the iris pigment epithelium (IPE) (located on the back of the iris) [63].

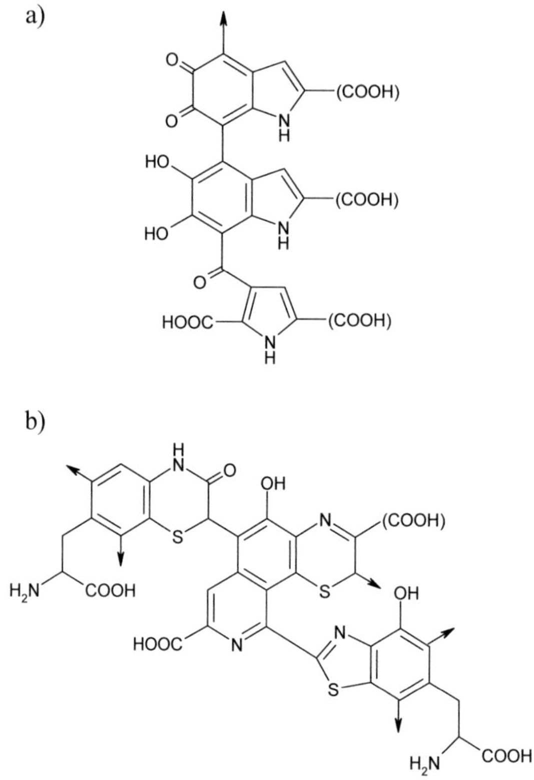

Figure 1. Chemical structure of eumelanin (a) and pheomelanin (b) [59].

Melanin from the IPE is essentially eumelanin, while melanin from IPE-scraped iris (consisting mainly of stroma plus anterior IPE) exhibiting content of both eumelanin and pheomelanin [63].

It is shown that the green iris appear to be more pheomelanic, whereas blue-green iris appear to be more eumelanic [63]. Blue eyes contain little of either pigment, while green-brown and brown irides feature a mixed pigment content [63].

Many drugs and metal ions bind to melanin [32, 52, 64-68]. The binding of drug to melanin is the result of physicochemical properties of the pigment [61]. Melanin protects the pigmented tissues through the absorption of many drugs and chemicals. On the other hand, this may lead to toxic accumulation of these substances in melanin, and consequently to the degradation of pigmented tissues [69, 70]. Differences in melanin content in ocular tissues might contribute to differences in drug binding and toxicity [60].

Melanin in the eyes helps protect them from ultraviolet and high-frequency visible light [34, 61, 70]. Besides, ocular melanin may also play a protective role against free radicals [61].

http://dx.doi.org/10.5772/58313

The main paramagnetic centers in melanin are the o-semiquinone free radicals with spin of 1/2 and with unpaired electrons localized on oxygen atoms [64-68]. Additionally it was spectroscopically proved that biradicals with spin of 1 also exist in melanins [71, 72]. o-Semiquinone free radicals and biradicals were also found in melanin complexes with copper(II) ions and drugs, as kanamycin [71] and netilmicin [72]. So far in eye melanin only o-semiquinone free radicals were studied [56].

3. The effect of electron paramagnetic resonance – Basic theory

Electron paramagnetic resonance (EPR) is the effect which appears in the paramagnetic samples exposed to microwaves in magnetic field [1-3]. Magnetic field causes Zeeman splitting of energy levels. After splitting the energy levels of unpaired electrons in magnetic field relate to different orientation of their magnetic moments, i.e. parallel and non parallel to the magnetic induction vector B. Both the magnetic moments in magnetic field and the magnetic spin quantum number M_S have 2S+1 values [1, 5, 8]. The energy level of unpaired electron with the magnetic spin quantum number M_S in magnetic field is splitted into 2S+1 levels. The unpaired electron may be excited by microwaves and it comes to the higher energy levels, when the frequency and the energy of microwaves are equal as is given in the resonance condition formula [1]:

$$h\nu = E_2 - E_1 = g\mu_B B_r \tag{1}$$

where h – Planck constant, ν – microwave frequency, g – spectroscopic factor, μ_B – Bohr magneton, B_r – resonance induction of magnetic field, E_2 – energy of the excited level of unpaired electron, E_1 – energy of the ground level of unpaired electron.

The energy E of unpaired electron with the magnetic spin number M_S in magnetic field with induction **B** is given as [1, 4]:

$$E(M_S) = M_S g\mu_B B_r \tag{2}$$

The electron paramagnetic resonance (EPR) effect is also called electron spin resonance (ESR), because unpaired electrons in the paramagnetic samples have unpaired spins [1-8]. The described above effect is the basis of EPR (ESR) spectroscopy, which is the experimental method of examination of paramagnetic species. Paramagnetic samples are located in magnetic field and they absorb microwaves with energies fulfill the resonance conditions (1) [1-8]. EPR spectroscopy use to analysis the absorption and the first derivative lines. The first derivative curves are very important for the samples with complex paramagnetic center system, when the several types of paramagnetic species exist [1]. The resolution of the multicomponent EPR spectra to the component lines is easier for the first derivatives than for the absorption curves.

For paramagnetic samples with free radicals, when the spin is S=1/2 the Zeeman splitting of the individual energy level in magnetic field causes the appearance of two levels [1, 3, 5]. The Zeeman splitting for free radicals in magnetic field is shown in Figure 2 [3]. Free radicals mainly exist in eye, so this example is the most important for ophthalmology. In the Figure 2 the energy levels of unpaired electrons of free radicals outside and in magnetic field are presented, and the absorption and the first derivative lines are shown.

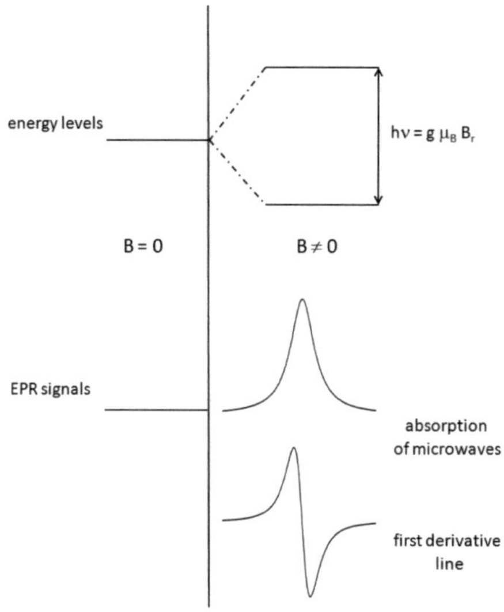

Figure 2. The Zeeman effect in magnetic field for free radicals with spin S=1/2. The absorption and the first absorption EPR curves are presented. B – induction of magnetic field, B_r – magnetic resonance induction, h – Planck constant, ν – microwave frequency, g – spectroscopic factor, μ_B – Bohr magneton, the resonance formula: $h\nu = g\mu_B B_r$. The scheme was prepared by the use of work [3].

4. EPR spectrometers useful in ophthalmology

4.1. The electronic blocks of the continuous microwave (CW) spectrometer

Electron paramagnetic spectrometer with continuous microwaves (CW-EPR) is the most useful apparatus for ophthalmology. For such type of the spectrometer samples are located in magnetic field and the microwaves are continuously send to the tested object [1, 3]. Unpaired electrons of the paramagnetic sample is continuously excited by microwaves and the spin-spin and spin-lattice relaxation processes occur [l, 3, 5, 8]. This spectrometer consists of microwave bridge, waveguides, resonance cavity, electromagnet, the modulation block, detector, and the amplifier. The source of microwaves and attenuator exist in microwave bridge. The attenuator is applied to change microwave power in the experiment. The popular source of microwaves is klystron. The microwave changes with attenuation according to the formula [4]:

$$attenuation\left[dB\right] = 10lg\left(M_0 / M\right) \quad (3)$$

where M_0 – the total microwave power produced by klystron, M – microwave power used during the measurement of EPR spectra.

The EPR spectra should be detect with low microwave power without the saturation effect to obtain the proper amounts of paramagnetic centers in the tested samples [1, 3]. The changes of microwave power and detection of EPR lines is used to characterize magnetic interactions in the samples.

Electromagnetic waves are send from microwave bridge via attenuator by waveguides to the resonance cavity [1-8]. The paramagnetic sample is located in the resonance cavity in the magnetic field produced by electromagnet. The absorption of the microwaves took place in the resonance cavity. Modulation of magnetic field is done by modulator and the signal is measured by detector. The receiver gain is used during the detection. Numerical detection of the EPR lines is done. Magnetic field is measured by NMR detector. Microwave frequency is usually measured, but sometimes the references are used. The measurement of the microwave frequency is necessary to accurately determine g-factor, which is important to study the type of paramagnetic centers in the samples.

The classic CW-EPR spectrometer of Bruker BioSpin GmbH is shown in Figure 3. The exemplary resonance cavity of Bruker BioSpin GmbH is presented in Figure 4. Electromagnet – the source of magnetic field is presented in Figure 5.

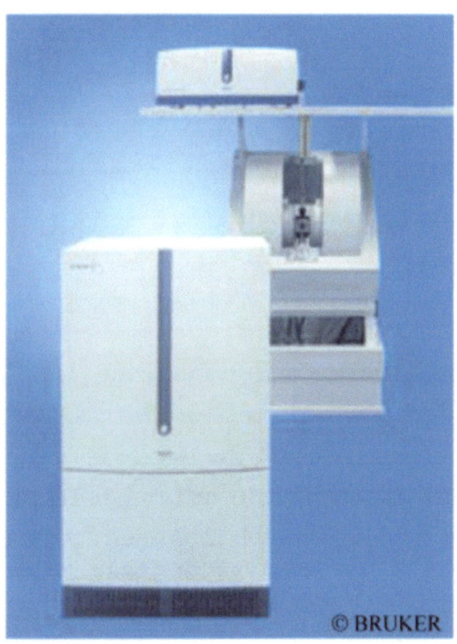

Figure 3. Continuous microwave EPR spectrometer EMXplus produced by Bruker BioSpin GmbH.

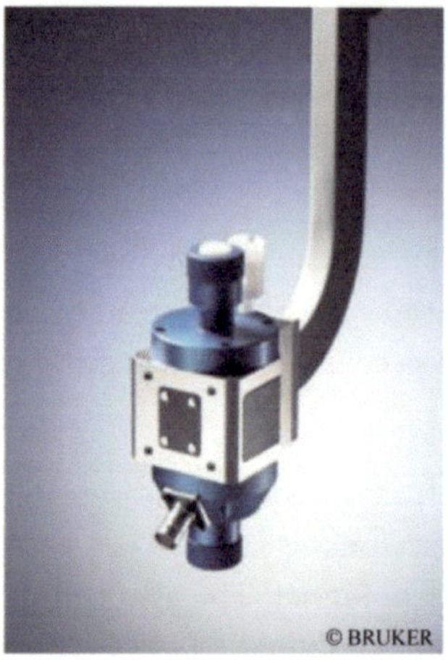

Figure 4. The resonance cavity of CW-EPR spectrometer of Bruker BioSpin GmbH.

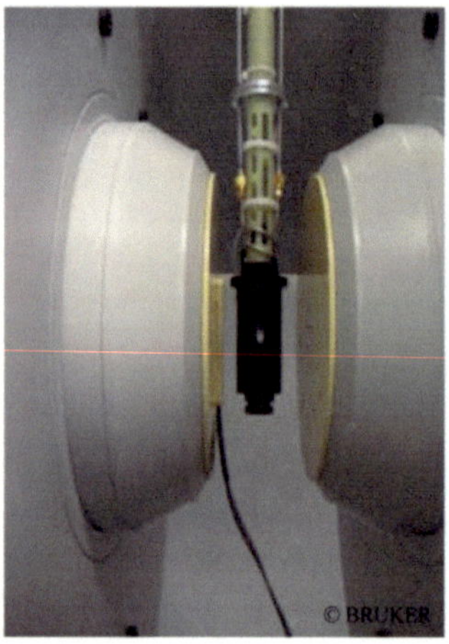

Figure 5. Electromagnet and the resonance cavity of CW-EPR spectrometer produced by Bruker BioSpin GmbH.

The pulsed EPR spectrometers are also used in medicine [1, 8]. These types of spectrometers are useful in examination of kinetics of processes. Microwaves are sent to the paramagnetic sample between poles of electromagnet and the decrease of the absorbed signal is detected. The pulsed EPR spectrometers are applied to test magnetic interactions in the samples [1]. Time of spin-lattice relaxation processes may be obtained by the pulsed method [1, 3, 5, 8]. The different spin-lattice relaxation times of unpaired electrons of major paramagnetic centers brings to light the component signals of them. It is used to determine the number of different types of paramagnetic centers in the samples. Determination of the number of component lines in the CW-EPR spectra is performed by fitting the resultant spectra by superposition of Gauss and Lorentz lines [1, 4].

http://dx.doi.org/10.5772/58313

4.2. Types of microwave bands in EPR spectrometers

Different microwave frequencies are used in the EPR spectrometers [1, 2]. The most popular is the frequency about 9.3 GHz (X-band). The typical microwave bands and corresponding frequencies of electromagnetic waves are presented in Table 1 [1, 2].

Microwave band	Microwave frequency [GHz]
L	1.5
S	3.0
C	6.0
X	**9.3**
K	23
Q	36
V	50
W	95

Table 1. Microwave bands used in EPR spectroscopy [1, 2].

5. EPR spectra

5.1. The parameters of EPR spectra and their practical meaning in studies of eye free radicals

The basic parameters of the first derivative EPR spectra give important information about type of paramagnetic centers in the sample, their amounts, and magnetic interactions which reflect chemical structure of the tested object [1-8]. The following parameters of EPR spectra: amplitudes (A), integral intensities (I), linewidths (ΔB_{pp}), and g-factors are usually analyzed. The parameters for the model eumelanin – DOPA-melanin (from SIGMA-ALDRICH) are shown in Figure 6. The first derivative EPR spectrum of DOPA-melanin is presented, because of the eumelanin mainly exists in eye.

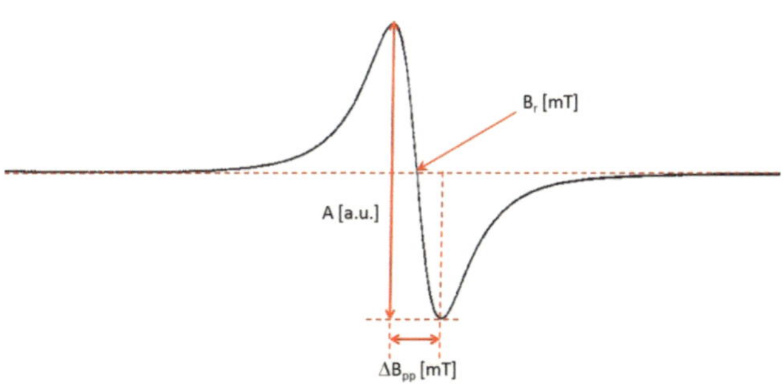

Figure 6. The first derivative EPR spectrum of the model eumelanin – DOPA-melanin and the basic parameters: amplitude (A), linewidth (ΔB_{pp}), and the resonance magnetic induction (B_r).

Amplitudes (A) and integral intensities (I) increase with the increasing of free radical concentration in the samples [1, 8]. The comparison of amplitudes (A) of EPR spectra of different samples from eye give information about the relative contents of free radicals in them. But the free radical concentration in the individual biological sample is determined by integral intensity (I), and it is proportional to the value of this parameter (I). Integral intensity (I) of the EPR spectra is the area under the absorption line, so for the first derivative EPR curve double integrations should be done. Linewidth (ΔB_{pp}) increases for the stronger dipolar interactions of free radicals in the samples [1, 8]. Dipolar interactions increases for decrease distances between free radicals [1, 8].

g-Values are calculated from the resonance condition according to the formula [1]:

$$g = h\nu / \mu_B B_r \tag{4}$$

where h – Planck constant, ν – microwave frequency, μ_B – Bohr magneton, B_r – induction of resonance magnetic field.

Determination of g-value is possible for known microwave frequency (ν) and resonance induction (B_r). Microwave frequency is detected by the recorder, and resonance induction is obtained from the EPR spectrum (Figure 6). g-Values characterize type of free radicals existing in the samples [1, 5]. The individual free radicals have EPR lines in the correspond to their chemical structures magnetic field. The resonance magnetic induction effect on the g-factor of free radicals (formula 4). g-Values are used in EPR spectroscopy to identification of the species which causes paramagnetic character of the sample.

5.2. EPR spectra of complex biological samples

Free radical system in biological samples, for example for species obtained from eye, is usually complex. In cells or tissues several groups of free radicals may exist [8]. The EPR spectra are then multi-component as the superposition of the lines of all the groups of free radicals. The information about the each group of free radicals is obtain by numerical fitting of the shape of the resultant EPR spectrum of the sample by sum of theoretical lines. The shape of the component lines is gaussian or lorentzian [1-4]. The percentage fraction of the individual component lines in the total EPR spectrum means the percentage fraction of their concentration in the sample [1]. Such numerical fitting were done for example for model neuromelanins [29, 30].

The analysis of shape of the EPR spectra and determination of their parameters are performed by spectroscopic programs. The known modern program to spectral analysis is WINEPR of Bruker, ORIGIN 6.0 of Microcal Software, LabVIEW 8.5 by National Instruments (Austin, Texas) or programs of JAGMAR (Kraków, Poland) and EPRAD (Poznań, Poland).

6. Application of EPR spectroscopy in ophthalmology

6.1. Sample preparation to the examination

EPR spectra can be measure for solid state, liquid and gaseous samples [1, 4, 8]. Solid state samples, for example melanin from eye, are examined in glass or quartz tubes with the diameters higher than for liquid samples. The mass of the solid samples located in the tubes should be determined to obtain the content of free radicals in one gram of the probe. The melanin in the glass tubes for spectroscopic studies is shown in Figure 7. The external diameter of the thin walled tube is 3 mm. The materials used in tubes should not reveal EPR signals for the measurement parameters used in the experiment. The EPR spectrum of DOPA-melanin is presented in Figure 8.

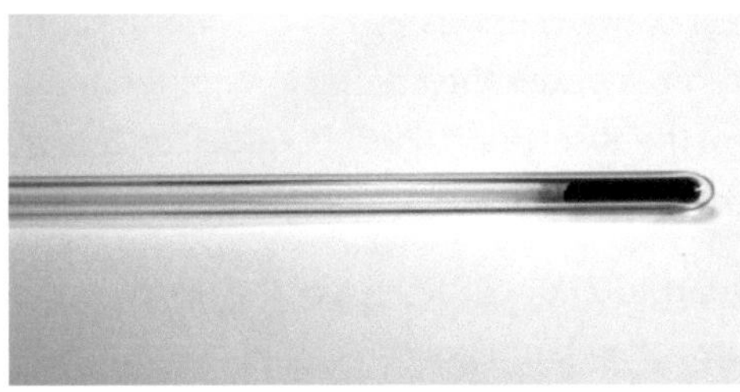

Figure 7. The model eumelanin – DOPA-melanin in the glass tube with diameter of 3 mm for EPR measurements.

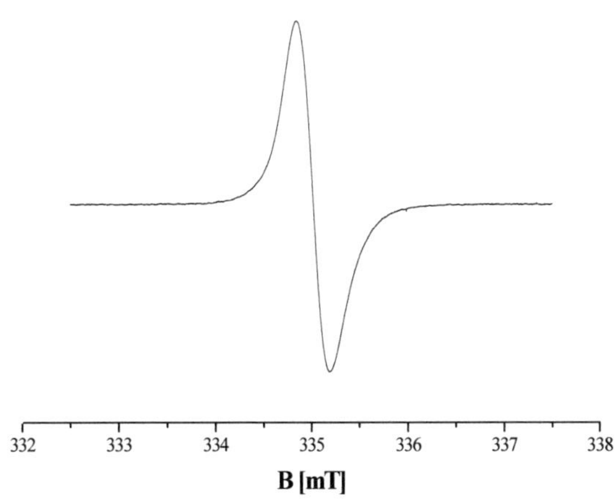

Figure 8. The EPR spectrum of model eumelanin – DOPA-melanin recorded at room temperature with low microwave power of 2.2 mW. B is the induction of magnetic field.

Liquid samples should be measure in the thin glass or quartz tubes with diameter below 1 mm. The special flat cells are also used. Water in the sample quenches EPR signals, so the large dimensions of wet samples are practically not used.

Paramagnetic gases in the environment usually decrease EPR lines of the paramagnetic samples. Such effects were observed for example for melanins [73, 74]. The samples susceptible to oxygen may be evacuated before the EPR measurements.

6.2. Determination of free radical concentration in the samples in ophthalmology

6.2.1. The measurement of the concentration

Free radicals concentrations in the samples are determined by the use of integral intensities of their EPR spectra and the spectra of the reference with the known amounts of paramagnetic centers [1, 3, 8]. Free radical concentrations (N) in the samples are determined as the value which is proportional to the area under the absorption curves and the integral intensity (I) [1, 3, 8]. Integral intensities (I) of the absorption line is obtained by integration of this curve. Double integration of the first-derivative EPR spectra give us the value of integral intensity (I).

To obtain free radical concentration the EPR lines of the tested samples and the references are measured. In our EPR studies of melanin polymers two references were used: ultramarine and the ruby crystal. Amplitudes of the EPR lines of the ruby crystal (A) located with the analyzed sample and ultramarine (A_u) in the resonance cavity were determined. The integral intensities (I) of the EPR spectra of the tested melanin samples and the reference-ultramarine (I_u) were compared.

The concentration of the free radicals (N) in the melanins was calculated as [3]:

$$N = N_u\left[\left(W_u A_u\right)/I_u\right]\left[I/\left(WAm\right)\right] \tag{5}$$

where N_u – the number of paramagnetic center in the ultramarine reference; W, W_u – the receiver gains for sample and the ultramarine; A, A_u – the amplitudes of ruby signal for the sample and the ultramarine; I, I_u – the integral intensities for the sample and ultramarine, m – the mass of the sample.

6.2.2. The paramagnetic references and their properties

The paramagnetic references should contain high amounts of stabile paramagnetic centers [1-8]. In our studies of melanin biopolymer from eye [56], others melanins [64-68, 71-78], cells [24-26, 68], drugs [35-48], ultramarine was used as the reference. In Figure 9 ultramarine in the glass tube is shown. The broad EPR line of ultramarine with paramagnetic centers with unpaired electrons located on sulfur atoms is presented in Figure 10.

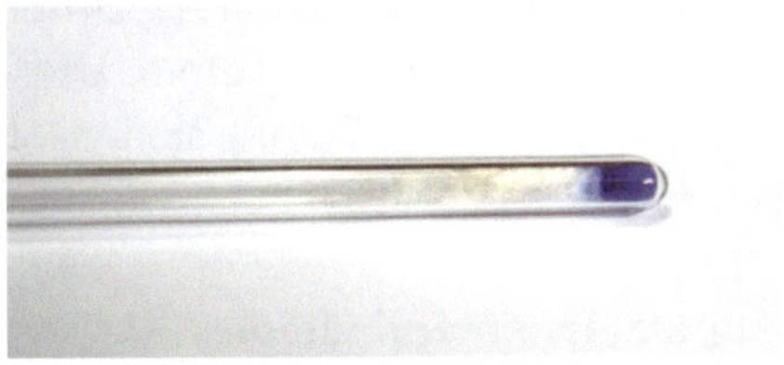

Figure 9. Ultramarine in the glass tube to EPR measurements.

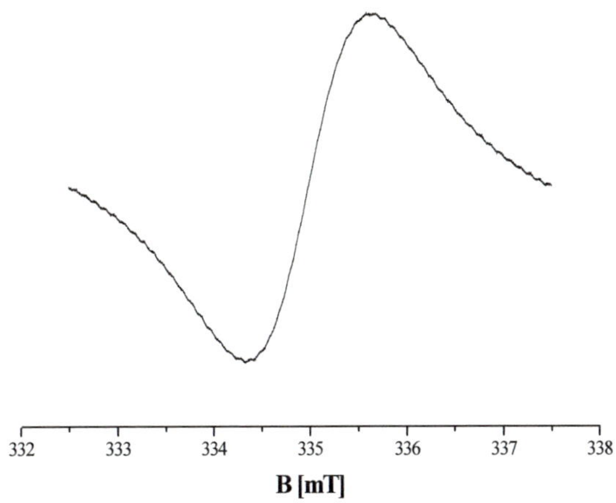

Figure 10. EPR spectrum of ultramarine – the reference for free radical concentration recorded with low microwave power of 2.2 mW. B is the induction of magnetic field.

The second reference – a ruby crystal (Al_2O_3: Cr^3) was permanently placed in a resonance cavity. For tested sample and for ultramarine the EPR line of a ruby crystal are measured. The ruby crystal is shown in Figure 11.

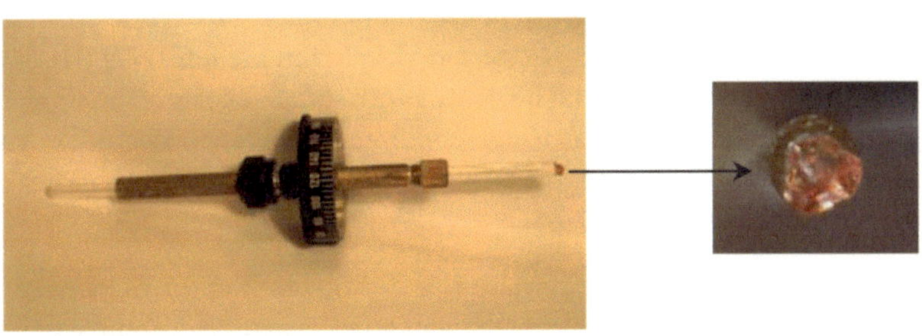

Figure 11. A ruby crystal.

The other reference for free radical concentration is DPPH (2, 2-diphenyl-1-picrylhydrazyl) [4]. Unpaired electron in DPPH is localized on nitrogen atom. DPPH is not so stabile such as ultramarine, because it is susceptible for oxygen. During storage of DPPH in air its free radical concentration decreases, so it should be evacuated.

6.3. Magnetic interactions in ophthalmological samples

Information about magnetic interactions between unpaired electrons in paramagnetic samples gives linewidth and changes of the spectra with microwave power [1-3]. The influence of microwave power (M) on the EPR spectra of the melanin samples from eye [56] and the others melanins [64-68] were examined. The changes of amplitudes (A) and linewidths (ΔB_{pp}) of EPR spectra with increasing of microwave power were analysed to determine type of broadening of EPR lines. The influence of microwave power (M) on amplitudes (A) and linewidths (ΔB_{pp}) of the EPR spectra depend on free radicals distribution (homogeneous or inhomogeneous) in the samples. For homogeneous broadened EPR lines the amplitude (A) increases with increasing of microwave power (M) and for the higher microwave powers it value decreases [1]. The increase of linewidth (ΔB_{pp}) with increasing of microwave power (M) is characteristic for the homogeneously broadened EPR lines [1]. For inhomogeneous broadening of spectral lines the amplitude (A) increases with increasing of microwave power (M) and for the higher microwave powers it value does not change [1]. Linewidth (ΔB_{pp}) of the inhomogeneously broadened EPR lines is unchanged with increasing of microwave power (M) [1].

Spin-lattice interactions in the samples may be characterized by observation of changes of amplitudes (A) of EPR lines with increasing of microwave power [1-3]. The slow and fast spin-lattice relaxation processes in the samples differ in microwave saturation of EPR lines [1-3]. The higher power of microwave saturation of EPR lines reveal the samples with the fast spin-lattice relaxation processes than the samples with the slow spin-lattice relaxation processes [1-4].

6.4. EPR investigation of melanin biopolymer in eye

6.4.1. Free radicals and biradicals in melanin biopolymer

The important paramagnetic structures existing in eye are melanin biopolymers [56, 60-63]. EPR examination of melanins from low temperature of liquid nitrogen to room temperature proved that two types of paramagnetic centers are located in them [71, 72]. The characteristic for both free radicals with spin S=1/2 and biradicals with spin S=1 correlations between integral intensities (I) of EPR lines and the measuring temperature (T) were observed. IT value for free radicals was constant independent on temperature, and the IT values for biradicals depended on the measuring temperature.

Free radicals and biradicals play an important role during binding drugs to melanins [71, 72]. The amounts of these paramagnetic centers changes after formation of complex melanin-drug. Such effects were observed for example for kanamycin [71] and netilmicin [72]. Paramagnetic copper(II) ions influence on free radicals and biradicals in melanin complexes with kanamycin and netlimicin was observed. It is expected that drugs applied in ophthalmology change free radicals and biradicals concentrations in melanin biopolymers in eye. So electron paramagnetic resonance spectroscopy seems to be very useful in examination of interactions of drugs with melanin in eye.

6.4.2. EPR results for melanin in eye

Electron paramagnetic resonance spectroscopy was used to examine free radicals in RPE melanosomes from different aged donors [56]. o-Semiquinone free radicals were identified in RPE melanosomes with the characteristic g-values and single broad EPR lines. Concentrations of free radicals in RPE melanosomes depend on the age of donors. The higher free radicals concentrations were obtained for donors aged > 45 years, than for donors aged < 22 years [56]. Free radicals concentrations in RPE melanosomes (~10^{17} spin/g) [56] were lower than the concentrations in model eumelanin – DOPA-melanin [56], A-375 melanoma cells [68], *Cladosporium cladosporioides* mycelium [52], and *Cladosporium herbarum* mycelium [53]. Free radical concentration in melanin changed after irradiation of eumelanin by visible light [34].

EPR spectra of RPE melanosomes were similar to those observed for DOPA-melanin (Figure 8), which is the synthetic model eumelanin. The unresolved hyperfine structure characteristic for pheomelanins was not observed for melanin of RPE. The exemplary complex shape of EPR spectra with signals of pheomelanin is shown in Figure 12 [52].

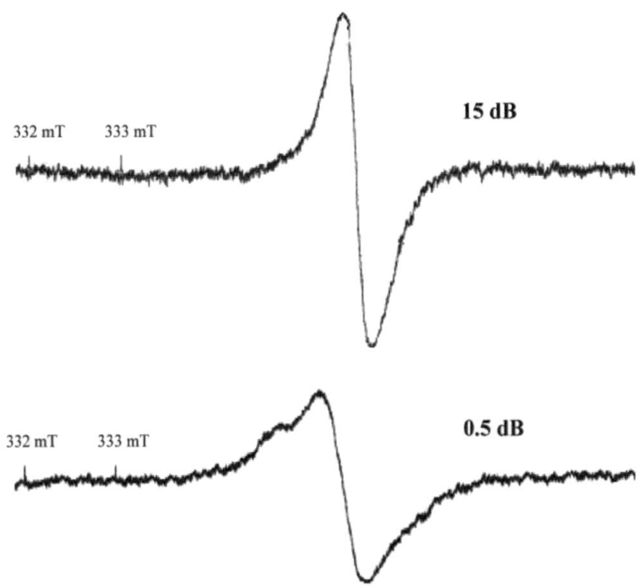

Figure 12. EPR spectra with signals of pheomelanin in *Cladosporium cladosporioides* recorded with different microwaves. The melanin samples were studied in paper [52].

Melanin in *Cladosporium cladosporioides* mycelium is the mixture of eu-and pheomelanin [52, 75-77]. The signal of pheomelanin is clearly visible in the EPR spectrum recorded with 0.5 dB attenuation, while it was not observed in the EPR spectrum measured with attenuation of 15 dB (Figure 12). It is proposed that the lower attenuation and higher microwave powers should be used to search pheomelanin in the biological samples.

6.4.3. EPR method proposed to examine free radicals in drugs in ophthalmology

EPR may be applied to examine of free radicals formed in ophthalmological drugs in process of their sterilization. Drugs used in ophthalmology should not contain microorganisms, and the sterilization is performed to remove or killed them [35-48]. Sterilization methods are gamma irradiation or thermal treatment of drugs [35-48]. Radiative and thermal sterilization should not produce free radicals in drugs, because changes of their interactions on eye as the result of modification of their chemical structure. Free radicals in sterilized optalmological drugs may be responsible for toxic effects during therapy.

Electron paramagnetic resonance spectroscopy was used to optimize sterilization procedure and conditions of antibiotics and the other drugs [35-48]. The methods of sterilization and temperatures for which the low amounts of free radicals are produced in drugs were searched. Similar examination of drugs may be proposed in ophthalmology.

6.4.4. EPR studies of antioxidant properties of drugs in ophthalmology

Electron paramagnetic resonance spectroscopy may be used in ophthalmology to examine antioxidant properties of drugs. The interactions of drugs with free radicals are tested with DPPH as the reference [79-81]. Chemical structure of DPPH is shown in Figure 13 [4]. DPPH is the model source of free radicals in this study. The EPR spectrum of DPPH is presented in Figure 14.

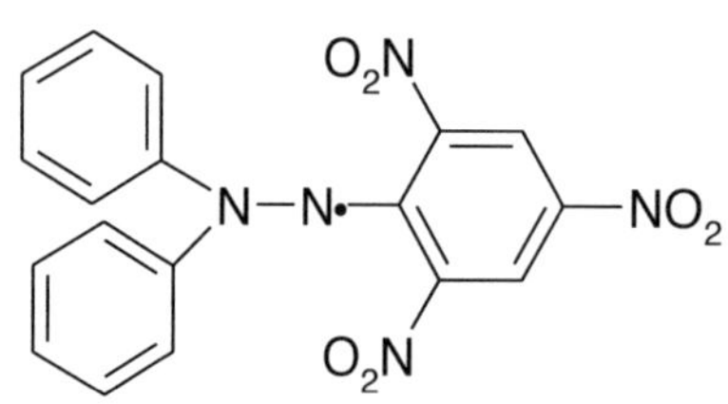

Figure 13. Chemical structure of DPPH [4].

The antioxidant properties of drugs reflects the decrease of amplitudes of the EPR line of DPPH after adding the tested samples to the solution [79-81]. The changes of integral intensities are also observed.

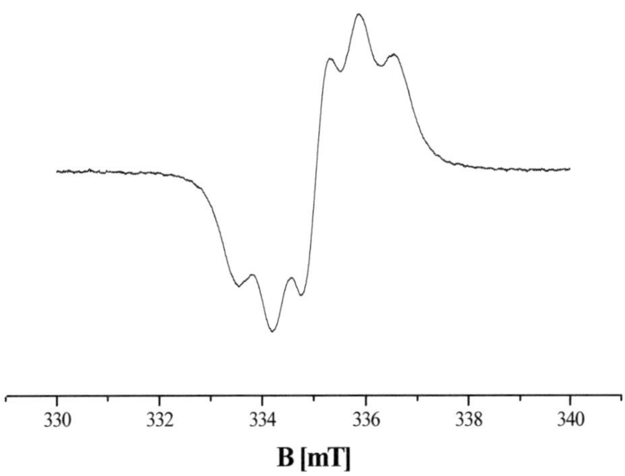

Figure 14. EPR spectrum of DPPH recorded with low microwave power of 2.2 mW. B is the induction of magnetic field.

7. Conclusions – Advantages of EPR measurements in ophthalmology

Electron paramagnetic resonance spectroscopy is the useful method to examine free radicals in eye, drugs and their interactions with free radicals (Table 2). Microbiological tests may be accompanied by EPR analysis to obtain the best conditions of sterilization process. Antioxidant properties of drugs may be determined by EPR measurements.

EPR IN OPHTHALMOLOGY	
Application	**Characteristics**
determination of free radical properties and concentrations in eye structures	type and chemical structure of free radicals, localization of unpaired electrons in free radicals, light and temperature effect on free radicals, oxygen molecules effect on free radicals, para- and diamagnetic metal ions effect on free radicals, changes in free radicals of eye melanin biopolymers after drug binding, spin-spin and spin-lattice interactions depend on chemical structures in eye
examination of biradicals in melanin biopolymers in eye	chemical structure and amounts of biradicals, effect of drugs and physical conditions on biradicals
studies of free radical interactions in eye	kinetics and products of free radicals

EPR IN OPHTHALMOLOGY	
Application	**Characteristics**
determination of antioxidants influence on free radicals in eye	decrease of the amount of free radicals in eye structures after interactions with antioxidant drugs and substances
use of spin-labels to examine biochemical units in eye	numerical analysis of shape of EPR lines of spin-labels to obtain information about chemical units in eyes
determination of antioxidant and free radical properties of ophthalmological drugs	analysis of quenching of free radicals by individual drugs, and study free radicals contents in pharmacological substances
optimization of thermal and radiative sterilization processes of ophthalmological drugs	searching temperatures or doses of irradiation, which do not produce high amounts of free radicals in drugs during heating or gamma irradiation
optimization of storage conditions of ophthalmological drugs	searching effects of light, temperature, and oxygen on free radical formation in drugs; the best conditions of drugs storage do not produce high amounts of free radicals in the samples

Table 2. Application of electron paramagnetic resonance (EPR) spectroscopy in ophthalmology [1-4, 11, 24-48, 52-56, 64-68, 70-81].

The most important advantages of EPR analysis in ophthalmology are the low amount of the samples necessary to test, the non destructive type of this analysis, the major information about free radicals. EPR spectra bring to light type and concentration of free radicals in eye, melanin biopolymer, and drugs.

Acknowledgements

The CW-EPR spectrometer (Figure 3), the resonance cavity (Figure 4), and electromagnet (Figure 5) are presented by courtesy of Bruker BioSpin GmbH. The cited EPR studies in medicine and pharmacy in Department of Biophysics are financially supported by Medical University of Silesia in Katowice (in 2013 grant number KNW-1-137/K/3/0).

Author details

Magdalena Zdybel* and Barbara Pilawa

*Address all correspondence to: mzdybel@sum.edu.pl

Medical University of Silesia in Katowice, School of Pharmacy with the Division of Laboratory Medicine, Department of Biophysics, Sosnowiec, Poland

References

[1] Wertz JE, Bolton JR. Electron Spin Resonance: Elementary Theory and Practical Applications. London: Chapman and Hall; 1986.

[2] Weil JA, Bolton JR. Electron Paramagnetic Resonance: Elementary Theory and Practical Applications. 2nd Edition. New York: John Wiley & Sons; 2007.

[3] Stankowski J, Hilczer W. Wstęp do spektroskopii rezonansów magnetycznych. Warszawa: PWN; 2005.

[4] Kęcki Z. Podstawy spektroskopii molekularnej. Warszawa: PWN; 1999.

[5] Morrish AH. Fizyczne podstawy magnetyzmu. Warszawa: PWN; 1970.

[6] Symons M. Spektroskopia EPR w chemii i biochemii. Warszawa: PWN; 1987.

[7] Kirmse R, Stach J. Spektroskopia EPR. Zastosowania w chemii. Kraków: Uniwersytet Jagielloński; 1994.

[8] Eaton GR, Eaton SS, Salikhov KM., eds. Foundations of Modern EPR. Singapore: World Scientific; 1998.

[9] Pryor W., editor. Free radicals in biology. New York: Acadmeic Press; 1976.

[10] Jaroszyk F., editor. Biofizyka. Warszawa: PZWL; 2008.

[11] Bartosz G. Druga twarz tlenu. Wolne rodniki w przyrodzie. Warszawa: PWN; 2006.

[12] Domagała W, Pilawa B, Lapkowski M. Quantitative in-situ EPR spectroelectrochemical studies of doping processes in poly(3, 4-alkylenedioxythiophene)s: Part 1: PEDOT. Electrochimica Acta 2008;53(13): 4580-4590.

[13] Zykwinska A, Domagala W, Czardybon A, Pilawa B, Lapkowski M. In situ EPR spectroelectrochemical studies of paramagnetic centres in poly(3, 4 ethylenedioxythiophene) (PEDOT) and poly(3, 4-butylenedioxythiophene) (PBuDOT) films. Chemical Physics 2003;292(1): 31-45.

[14] Moskwa T, Domagala W, Czardybon A, Pilawa B, Lapkowski M. ESR spectroelectrochemistry of functionalised long side chain derivatives of poly(3, 4-ethylenedioxythiophene). Synthetic Metals 2005;152(1-3): 189-192.

[15] Pilawa B, Więckowski AB, Trzebicka B. Numerical analysis of EPR spectra of coal, macerals and extraction products. Radiation Physics and Chemistry 1995;45(6): 899-908.

[16] Pilawa B, Więckowski AB. Comparative e. p. r. analysis of interactions between macerals and atmospheric oxygen. Fuel 1997;76(12): 1173-1177.

[17] Pilawa B, Więckowski AB, Pietrzak R, Wachowska H. Microwave saturation of EPR spectra of oxidised coal. Central European Journal of Chemistry 2007;5(1): 330-340.

[18] Pilawa B, Więckowski AB. Groups of paramagnetic center in coal samples with different carbon contents. Research on Chemical Intermediates 2007;33(8-9): 825-839.

[19] Pilawa B, Więckowski AB, Wachowska H, Kozłowski M. Effect of reduction and butylation on coal. Application of saturation of two-component EPR spectra. Applied Magnetic Resonance 2003;24: 73-83.

[20] Więckowski AB, Pilawa B, Lewandowski M, Wojtowicz W, Słowik G. Paramagnetic Centres in Exinite, Vitrinite and Inertinite. Applied Magnetic Resonance 1998;15(3-4): 489-501.

[21] Weszka J, Hajduk B, Zdybel M, Pilawa B. Dependence of EPR spectra on conditions of PPI thin films deposition. Paper presented at: Polymer on the Odra River; 6-7.07.2011; Opole.

[22] Pawłowska-Góral K, Ramos P, Pilawa B, Kurzeja E. Application of EPR spectroscopy to examination of the effect of sterilization process on free radicals in different herbs. Food Biophysics 2013;8(1): 60-68.

[23] Pawłowska-Góral K, Pilawa B. Detection of free radicals formed by in vitro metabolism of fluoride using EPR spectroscopy. Toxicology in Vitro 2011;25(7): 1269-1273.

[24] Pilawa B, Latocha M, Kościelniak M, Pietrzak R, Wachowska H. Oxygen effects in tumor cells during photodynamic therapy. Polish Journal of Environmental Studies 2006;15: 160-162.

[25] Latocha M, Pilawa B, Dudek J, Biniszkiewicz T, Kozdrowska L, Sieroń A, Wilczok T. Free radicals in melanotic human melanoma and human colon adenocarcinoma cells after photodynamic therapy. Physica Medica 2004;20(1): 61-63.

[26] Latocha M, Pilawa B, Zdybel M, Wilczok T. Effect of laser radiation on free radicals in human cancer G361 cells. Acta Physica Polonica A 2005;108(2): 409-412.

[27] Krzywda A, Petelenz E, Michalczyk D, Płonka PM. Sclerotia of the acellular (true) slime mould *Fuligo septica* as a model to study melanization and anabiosis. Cellular & Molecular Biology Letters 2008;13: 130-143.

[28] Okazaki M, Kuwata K, Miki Y, Shiga S, Shiga T. Electron spin relaxation of synthetic melanin and melanin-containing human tissues as studied by electron spin echo and electron spin resonance. Archives of Biochemistry and Biophysics 1985;242: 197-205.

[29] Zecca L, Costi P, Mecacci C, Ito S, Terreni M, Sonnino S. Interaction of human substantia nigra neuromelanin with lipids and peptides. Journal of Neurochemistry 2000;74: 1758-1765.

[30] Zucca FA, Giaveri G, Gallorini M, Albertini A, Toscani M, Pezzoli G, Lucius R, Wilms H, Sulzer D, Ito S, Wakamatsu K, Zecca L. The neuromelanin of human substantia nigra: physiological and pathogenic aspects. Pigment Cell Research 2004;17: 610-617.

[31] Plonka PM, Michalczyk D, Popik M, Handjiski B, Slominski A, Paus R. Splenic eumelanin differs from hair eumelanin in C57BL/6 mice. Acta Biochimica Polonica 2005;52: 433-441.

[32] Sarna T. Badanie struktury i właściwości centrów aktywnych melanin. Zagadnienia Biofizyki Współczesnej 1981;6: 201-219.

[33] Sealy RC, Hyde JS, Felix CC, Menon IA, Prota G. Eumelanins and pheomelanins: characterization by electron spin resonance spectroscopy. Science 1982;217: 545-547.

[34] Jung K, Seifert M, Herrling T, Fuchs J. UV-generated free radicals (FR) in skin: their prevention by sunscreens and their induction by self-tanning agents. Spectrochim Acta A 2008;69(5): 1423-1428.

[35] Zdybel M, Pilawa B, Kościelniak-Ziemniak M, Czyżyk D, Adamczyk J. Application of EPR spectroscopy to examination of free radicals in thermally sterilized chlortalidone. Farmaceutyczny Przegląd Naukowy 2010;7(2): 21-25.

[36] Ramos P, Pilawa B, Stroka E. EPR studies of free radicals in thermally sterilized famotidine. Nukleonika 2013;58(3): 413-418.

[37] Ramos P, Pilawa B, Wilczyński S, Czyż K, Adamczyk J. Effect of heating at 180°C on paramagnetic properties of diclofenac-EPR study. Engineering of Biomaterials 2009;12(87): 7-12.

[38] Skowrońska A, Wojciechowski M, Ramos P, Pilawa B, Kruk D. ESR studies of paramagnetic centers in pharmaceutical materials-Cefaclor and Clarithromycin as an example. Acta Physica Polonica A 2012;121(2): 514-517.

[39] Kościelniak-Ziemniak M, Pilawa B. Application of EPR Spectroscopy for Examination of Free Radical Formation in Thermally Sterilized Betamethasone, Clobetasol, and Dexamethasone. Applied Magnetic Resonance 2012;42(4): 519-530.

[40] Ramos P, Pepliński P, Pilawa B. Free radicals in thermally sterilized verapamil. Engineering of Biomaterials 2009;12(89-91): 162-164.

[41] Krztoń A, Liszka B, Ramos P, Pilawa B. FT-IR and EPR studies of changes of chemical structure of ampicyline during thermal sterilization. Engineering of Biomaterials 2009;12(89-91): 153-156.

[42] Ramos P, Pilawa B, Krztoń A, Liszka B. Free radicals in the thermally sterilized aminoglycoside antibiotics. Pharmaceutica Analytica Acta 2012;3(9): 1-13.

[43] Ramos P, Pilawa P. Effect of temperature and time of thermal sterilization on formation of free radicals in isosorbide. Farmaceutyczny Przegląd Naukowy 2010;7(5): 28-33.

[44] Wilczyński S, Lekki J, Kwiatek W, Chodurek E, Pilawa B. Formation of paramagnetic centers in sterilized gentamicin and neomycin irradiated by protons. Polish Journal of Environmental Studies 2006;15(4): 216-218.

[45] Wilczyński S, Pilawa B, Koprowski R, Wróbel Z, Ptaszkiewicz M, Swakoń J, Olko P. EPR studies of free radical decay and survival in gamma irradiated aminoglycoside antibiotics: sisomicin, tobramycin and paromomycin. European Journal of Pharmaceutical Sciences 2012;45: 251-262.

[46] Wilczyński S, Ptaszkiewicz M, Pierzchała E, Pilawa B, Swakoń J, Olko P. Electron paramagnetic resonance studies of gamma irradiated azithromycin. Current Topics in Biophysics 2008;31: 1-4.

[47] Wilczyński S, Ramos P, Pilawa B, Ptaszkiewicz M, Swakoń J, Olko P. Comparison of free radicals properties in radiosterilized and thermally sterilized streptomycin. Engineering of Biomaterials 2009;12(89-91): 170-172.

[48] Wilczyński S, Pilawa B, Ptaszkiewicz M, Swakoń J, Olko P. Free radicals properties of gamma irradiated solid forms of drugs. Engineering of Biomaterials 2008;11(81-84): 52-54.

[49] Deda A, Wilczyński S, Zdybel M, Pierzchała E, Pilawa B. Zastosowanie spektroskopii elektronowego rezonansu paramagnetycznego (EPR) w kosmetologii. Dermatologia Estetyczna 2010;12(4): 220-225.

[50] Deda A, Pierzchała E, Wilczyński S, Zdybel M, Pilawa B. Badania wolnych rodników w kosmetologii metodą elektronowego rezonansu paramagnetycznego (EPR). Zeszyty Naukowe Wyższej Szkoły Nauk Społecznych z siedzibą w Lublinie – Kosmetologia 2010;1: 11-22.

[51] Pilawa B, Pietrzak R, Wachowska H, Babeł K. EPR studies of carbonized cellulose – oxygen interactions. Acta Physica Polonica A 2005;108(2): 151-154.

[52] Pilawa B, Zdybel M, Buszman E, Witoszyńska T, Cieśla H. Effect of flucytosine on paramagnetic properties of Cladosporium cladosporioides. Engineering of Biomaterials 2009;12(89-91): 167-169.

[53] Zdybel M, Pilawa B, Buszman E, Witoszyńska T, Brotoń B. Paramagnetism of pigmented soil fungi of Cladosporium herbarum. Engineering of Biomaterials 2009;12(89-91): 172-174.

[54] Pawłowska-Góral K, Kurzeja E, Pilawa B, Ramos P. EPR studies of Rhizoma calami. Engineering of Biomaterials 2009;12(89-91): 159-161.

[55] Rozancew EG, Szolle WD. Chemia organiczna wolnych rodników. Warszawa: PWN; 1985.

[56] Bilińska B, Pilawa B, Zawada Z, Wylegala E, Wilczok T, Dontsov AE, Sakina NL, Ostrovsky MA, Ilyasova VB. Electron spin resonance investigations of human retinal pigment epithelium melanosomes from young and old donors. Spectrochimica Acta Part A 2002;58: 2257-2264.

[57] Tran ML, Powell BJ, Meredith P. Chemical and structural disorder in eumelanins: a possible explanation for broadband absorbance. Biophysical Journal 2006;90: 743-752.

[58] Ito S, Wakamatsu K, Ozeki H. Chemical analysis of melanins and its application to the study of regulation of melanogenesis. Pigment Cell Research 2000;13: 103-109.

[59] Wakamatsu K, Ito S. Advanced chemical methods in melanin determination. Pigment Cell Research 2002;15: 174-183.

[60] Durairaj C, Chastain JE, Kompella UB. Intraocular distribution of melanin in human, monkey, rabbit, minipig and dog eyes. Experimental Eye Research 2012;98: 23-27.

[61] Leblanc B, Jezequel S, Davies T, Hanton G, Taradach C. Binding of drugs to eye melanin is not predictive of ocular toxicity. Regulatory Toxicology and Pharmacology 1998;28(2): 124-132.

[62] Schmidt SY, Peisch RD. Melanin concentration in normal human retinal pigment epithelium. Regional variation and age-related reduction. Investigative Ophthalmology & Visual Science 1986;27(7): 1063-1067.

[63] Prota G, Hu DN, Vincensi MR, McCormick SA, Napolitano A. Characterization of melanins in human irides and cultured uveal melanocytes from eyes of different colors. Experimental Eye Research 1998;67(3): 293-299.

[64] Pilawa B, Chodurek E, Wilczok T. Types of paramagnetic centres in Cu^{2+}complexes with model neuromelanins. Applied Magnetic Resonance 2003;24: 417-422.

[65] Beberok A, Buszman E, Zdybel M, Pilawa B, Wrześniok D. EPR examination of free radical properties of DOPA-melanin complexes with ciprofloxacin, lomefloxacin, norfloxacin and sparfloxacin. Chemical Physics Letters 2010;497(1-3): 115-122.

[66] Najder-Kozdrowska L, Pilawa B, Więckowski AB, Buszman E, Wrześniok D. Influence of copper(II) ions on radicals in DOPA-melanin. Applied Magnetic Resonance 2009;36(1): 81-88.

[67] Buszman E, Pilawa B, Zdybel M, Wrześniok D, Grzegorczyk A, Wilczok T. EPR examination of $Zn^{2+}$and Cu^{2+}effect on free radicals in DOPA-melanin-netilmicin complexes. Chemical Physics Letters 2005;403(1-3): 22-28.

[68] Chodurek E, Zdybel M, Pilawa B, Dzierżewicz Z. Examination by EPR spectroscopy of free radicals in melanins isolated from A-375 cells exposed on valproic acid and cisplatin. Acta Poloniae Pharmaceutica – Drug Research 2012;69: 1334-1341.

[69] Hu DN, Savage HE, Roberts JE. Uveal melanocytes, ocular pigment epithelium, and Müller cells in culture: in vitro toxicology. International Journal of Toxicology 2002;21: 465-472.

[70] Sarna T. Properties and function of the ocular melanin-A photobiophysical view. Journal of Photochemistry and Photobiology B: Biology 1992;12: 215-258.

[71] Najder-Kozdrowska L, Pilawa B, Buszman E, Więckowski AB, Świątkowska L, Wrześniok D, Wojtowicz W. Triplet states in DOPA-melanin and in its complexes with kanamycin and copper Cu(II) ions. Acta Physica Polonica A 2010;118(4): 613-618.

[72] Zdybel M. Multi-component system of paramagnetic centers in DOPA-melanin complexes with netilmicin, zinc(II) and copper(II) ions. PhD thesis. Medical University of Silesia in Katowice; 2008.

[73] Zdybel M, Pilawa B, Buszman E, Wrześniok D. Effect of oxygen on free radicals in DOPA-melanin complexes with netilmicin, diamagnetic Zn(II), and paramagnetic Cu(II). Chemical Physics Letters 2013;556: 278-286.

[74] Pilawa B, Latocha M, Buszman E, Wilczok T. Effect of oxygen on spin-spin and spin-lattice relaxation in DOPA-melanin. Complexes with chloroquine and metal ions. Applied Magnetic Resonance 2003;25: 105-111.

[75] Zdybel M, Pilawa B, Buszman E, Witoszyńska T. EPR studies Cladosporium cladosporioides complexes with amphotericin B. Nukleonika 2013;58(3): 401-405.

[76] Matuszczyk M, Buszman E, Pilawa B, Witoszyńska T, Wilczok T. Cd^{2+}effect on free radicals in Cladosporium cladosporioides-melanin tested by EPR spectroscopy. Chemical Physics Letters 2004;394(4-6): 366-371.

[77] Pilawa B, Buszman E, Gondzik A, Wilczyński S, Zdybel M, Witoszyńska T, Wilczok T. Effect of pH on paramagnetic centers in Cladosporium cladosporioides. Acta Physica Polonica A 2005;108(1): 147-150.

[78] Buszman E, Pilawa B, Latocha M, Wilczok T, Tyrawska-Spychałowa D, Bajan C, Bijak A, Bilińska B. Spectroscopic studies of melanins isolated from pigmented soil fungi of the Karkonosze Mountains. Current Topics in Biophysics 1998;22: 21-24.

[79] Kurzeja E, Stec M, Ramos P, Pilawa B, Pawłowska-Góral K. The influence of sterilization on free-radical generation, discoloration and the antioxidant properties of certain spice herbs. Italian Journal of Food Science 2012;24(3): 254-261.

[80] Kurzeja E, Stec M, Ramos P, Pilawa B, Pawłowska-Góral K. Antioxidant properties of water extracts of sterilized and unsterilized Morus Alba L. leaves. International Journal of Food Properties 2013;16(4): 723-737.

[81] Rzepecka-Stojko A, Pilawa B, Ramos P, Stojko J. Antioxidative properties of bee pollen extracts examined by EPR spectroscopy. Journal of Apicultural Science 2012;56(1): 23-31.

Chapter 4

Tonometry

Felicia Ferreri, Rosa Minniti, Alessandra Polimeni,
Lucia Zavettieri, Giuseppina Ferreri,
Paolo Ferreri and Pasquale Aragona

Additional information is available at the end of the chapter

http://dx.doi.org/10.5772/58690

1. Introduction

Tonometry is a diagnostic method which, through the use of different tools, allows the evaluation of the pressure existing inside the human eye.

An elevated intraocular pressure (IOP) is the main risk factor for the development of glaucoma, an ocular disease, that if not properly treated, causes irreversible damage to the optic nerve, leading to blindness.

The aim of tonometry is to detect the IOP that is measured in millimeters of mercury (mmHg); it is performed through the interaction with the ocular structures and in particular with the cornea. The human cornea is a curved structure with an increasing thickness from the center to the periphery and with different radius of curvature in the anterior and posterior faces. From the histological point of view, the cornea has five layers, which, from inside out are:

1. Endothelium: the inner layer made from a layer of hexagonal cells that act as a barrier modulating the penetration of substances within the corneal structure from the aqueous humor;

2. Descemet's membrane: made by collagen;

3. Stroma: it is characterized by particular cells, keratocytes, and by collagen lamellae, arranged in parallel and covered with a mucopolysaccharide substance;

4. Bowman layer: a dense acellular cluster;

5. Epithelium: the outer layer made from non-keratinized cells.

Recently, it has been identified with the electron microscope, another layer, the layer of Dua, localized in the posterior stroma, close to the Descemet's membrane. [1] The cornea, is wetted in the most external part by the tear film that consists of two layers: the mucous-aqueous and the lipid layers. Cornea and tear film play a key-role in assessing the IOP; in fact, all the clinical instruments used to measure the IOP interact with these structures, being the value of IOP obtained studing the corneal deformation resultant from the strength applied on the anterior part of the eye. Therefore tonometry is based on the biomechanical characteristics of cornea, namely the elastic and viscoelastic characteristics, and thus IOP and corneal properties are closely interdependent [2].The ease of corneal deformability is called corneal hysteresis (CH), which is calculated as the difference in air pressures between force-in applanation (P1) and force-out applanation (P2), or (P1 – P2). Studies have shown that CH is altered in various disease.

Measurement of CH also provides a more complete characterization of the contribution of corneal resistance to intraocular pressure measurements than central corneal thickness (CCT) alone [3]. However, corneal hysteresis values can be produced by various combinations of corneal thickness, rigidity, intraocular pressure, and hydration. All these factor interfere with the evaluation of the IOP.

2. Tonometry

The history of the tonometry begins in 1622, when, for the first time, Richard Banister estimated the increase of intraocular pressure (IOP) by finger pressure on the bulb (digital eye pressure) and, for several centuries, this remained the only common and simple method to evaluate IOP.

In fact, in several studies, the digital eye pressure is described as a method to assess the IOP in uncooperative patients.

Nowadays, there is a rating scale for the digital eye pressure

Nt	Normal Tension
T+	Increased Tension
T+1	Appreciable tension
T+2	Manifests tension
T+3	Hardness wooden
T-	Hypotonia
T-1	Appreciable hypotonia
T-2	Manifested hypotonia
T-3	Bulb very soft

Afterwards, several instruments were created to obtain an IOP value, in terms of pressure brought to the cornea needed to achieve the applanation of its curvature.

The tonometry can be distinguished in base at the type of corneal deformation obtained in:

http://dx.doi.org/10.5772/58690

- Schiötz tonometry of known weight
- Applanation tonometry to force variable
- Applanation tonometry to force constant

2.1. Schiötz tonometry of known weight

It was the first tonometer able to give reproducible results, simple and inexpensive to be used in clinical practice,being invented in 1905 by the Norwegian ophthalmologist Hjalmar Schiötz. Schiötz tonometry studies lOP by measuring the indentation of the cornea produced by a known weight applied on the corneal surface. It also measures the facility of aqueous outflow calculating the rate at which the pressure declines with time, being this related to the ease with which the aqueous leaves the eye. The decline in lOP over time can be used to determine outflow facility in micronL/min/mmHg through a series of mathematical calculations.

The Schiötz tonometer (Fig.1) is constituted by a piston, applied directly to the cornea, that moves vertically within a scale. The test is performed with the patient in the supine position. Although the test can be performed in an examination chair that reclines. The right position of the base of the scale applied on the cornea allows, to the piston and the weights fitted, to slide, until the intraocular pressure opposes to the applied force; this is indicated on the linear scale on the instrument and the resulting value is converted to millimeters of mercury by a table called "nomogram of Friedenwald" (Fig.2). Each unit of the scale indicates 1/20 mm of the cornea and evaluate the extent of the corneal deformation caused by a weighted force applied from the outside [4].The Schiötz tonometer does not require the use of the slit lamp, it is simple to use, but the IOP value obtained can be biased since repeated measurements may reduce the IOP value while the supine position is known to increase IOP [5].

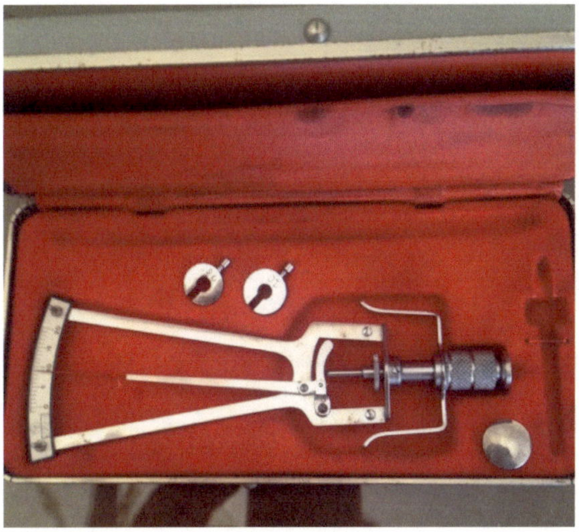

Figure 1. Schiötz tonometer of known weight

The values of IOP obtained with this tool depend on several factors: the elastic properties of the eye, aqueous humor formation and removal, scleral rigidity [6],, high myopia and ocular blood volume changes. Others factors may cause an erroneous result: calibration problems, patient position, squeezing of the eyelids during the measurement, just to name a few although these errors affect the outcome of other tonometers also to some extent. These problems reduce the accuracy and reproducibility of the Schiötz tonometry for an individual patient [7]. In general, Schiötz tonometer finds its best use as a research tool for the investigation of pharmacokinetics and is rarely used clinically.

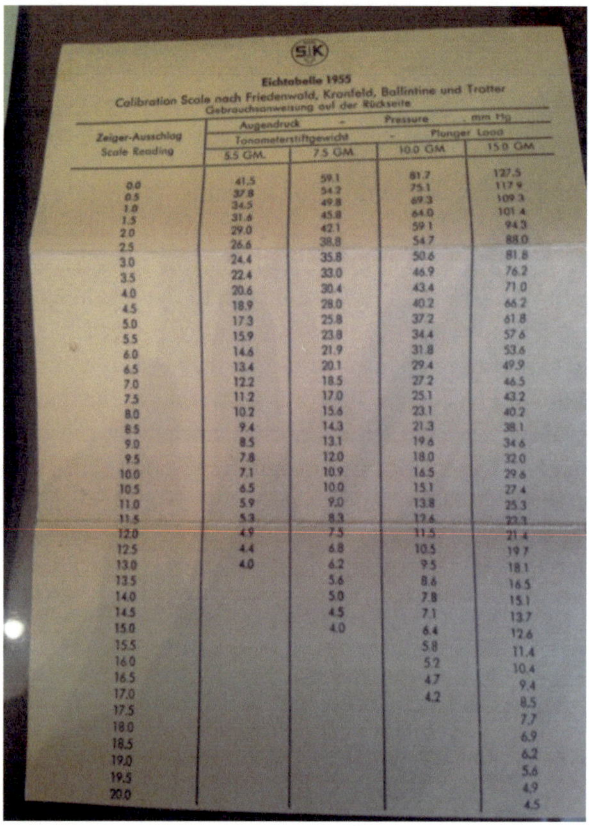

SK

Eichtabelle 1955

Calibration Scale nach Friedenwald, Kronfeld, Ballintine und Trotter

Gebrauchsanweisung auf der Rückseite

Zeiger-Ausschlag Scale Reading	Augendruck - Pressure - mm Hg			
	Tonometerstiftgewicht - Plunger Load			
	5.5 GM.	7.5 GM	10.0 GM	15.0 GM
0.0	41.5	59.1	81.7	127.5
0.5	37.8	54.2	75.1	117.9
1.0	34.5	49.8	69.3	109.3
1.5	31.6	45.8	64.0	101.4
2.0	29.0	42.1	59.1	94.3
2.5	26.6	38.8	54.7	88.0
3.0	24.4	35.8	50.6	81.8
3.5	22.4	33.0	46.9	76.2
4.0	20.6	30.4	43.4	71.0
4.5	18.9	28.0	40.2	66.2
5.0	17.3	25.8	37.2	61.8
5.5	15.9	23.8	34.4	57.6
6.0	14.6	21.9	31.8	53.6
6.5	13.4	20.1	29.4	49.9
7.0	12.2	18.5	27.2	46.5
7.5	11.2	17.0	25.1	43.2
8.0	10.2	15.6	23.1	40.2
8.5	9.4	14.3	21.3	38.1
9.0	8.5	13.1	19.6	34.6
9.5	7.8	12.0	18.0	32.0
10.0	7.1	10.9	16.5	29.6
10.5	6.5	10.0	15.1	27.4
11.0	5.9	9.0	13.8	25.3
11.5	5.3	8.3	12.6	23.3
12.0	4.9	7.5	11.5	21.4
12.5	4.4	6.8	10.5	19.7
13.0	4.0	6.2	9.5	18.1
13.5		5.6	8.6	16.5
14.0		5.0	7.8	15.1
14.5		4.5	7.1	13.7
15.0		4.0	6.4	12.6
15.5			5.8	11.4
16.0			5.2	10.4
16.5			4.7	9.4
17.0			4.2	8.5
17.5				7.7
18.0				6.9
18.5				6.2
19.0				5.6
19.5				4.9
20.0				4.5

Figure 2. Nomogram of Friedenwald

2.2. Applanation tonometry to force variable

There are different type of Applanation tonometry to force variable

- Goldmann Tonometer
- Perkins Tonometer
- Draeger Tonometer

http://dx.doi.org/10.5772/58690

- Mackay-Marg Tonometer
- Tonopen
- Pneumatic applanation tonometer.

2.3. Goldmann applanation tonometer (GAT) (Fig.3)

This instrument is based on an interesting physical principle: the "Imbert –Flick principle", which states that the pressure inside an ideal, dry, infinitely thin, and a perfect sphere is equal to that applied to obtain the applanation of its surface. However, the human eye is not an ideal sphere, since it is not thin-walled and dry, and this produces two confounding forces:

- a force produced by the corneal rigidity (because the cornea is not infinitely thin and is usually toriodal),which is directed towards the outside of the globe;
- a force produced by the surface tension of the tear film (because the eye is not dry), which is directed towards the globe.

Goldmann estimated that a circular area of flattening, of the size of 3.06 mm of diameter applied on the cornea, is sufficient to avoid the influence of sclera and corneal rigidity and surface tension, allowing a realistic measurement of the IOP. The applanating force required to flatten this area, is directly proportional to the intraocular pressure. Specifically, the force (measured in dynes) multiplied by 10 is equal to the intraocular pressure (measured in millimeters of mercury).

The GAT is mounted on the slit lamp to produce a magnified image, and when it touches the tear film and the cornea, a circle appears as to the observer. Staining the ocular surface with fluorescein and using a cobalt blue light in the slit lamp allow obtaining a better observation of the tear film(Fig.4). The final image looks like two semicircles of exactly 3.06 mm in diameter, displaced by the presence of a prism in the head of the instrument, giving the applanation pressure when the half circles just overlap at the central end. The semicircles move with the ocular pulse, and the endpoint is reached when the inner edges of the semicircles touch each other at the midpoint of their excursion(Fig.5). At this point, the IOP value is reported, in millimeters of mercury, on the instrument dial used to modulate the pressure. This measurement is safe, easy to use and relatively accurate in most clinical situations [8].

The GAT remains the gold-standard to assess the IOP, because it is relatively unaffected by ocular rigidity.

An excessive amount of fluorescein results in wide mires and an inaccurately high reading, whereas an inadequate amount of fluorescein leads to artificially low readings.

Marked corneal astigmatism causes an elliptical fluorescein pattern, and the clinician should rotate the prism to obtain an accurate reading [9].

The accuracy of GAT is reduced in certain situations

- Corneal edema: the increased corneal thickness gives falsely high values.

- Soft corneal lens: give falsely low values.
- Scleral rigidity modifications: in the scleral buckling procedures the IOP may appear inappropriately low [10].
- The central corneal thickness (CCT): The IOP value is most accurate with a CCT of 520 micron [11].

Applanation tonometry measurements are not accurate, if CCT is increased or decreased compared to the reference values. Increased CCT may give an artificially high IOP measurement; decreased CCT, an artificially low reading [12].

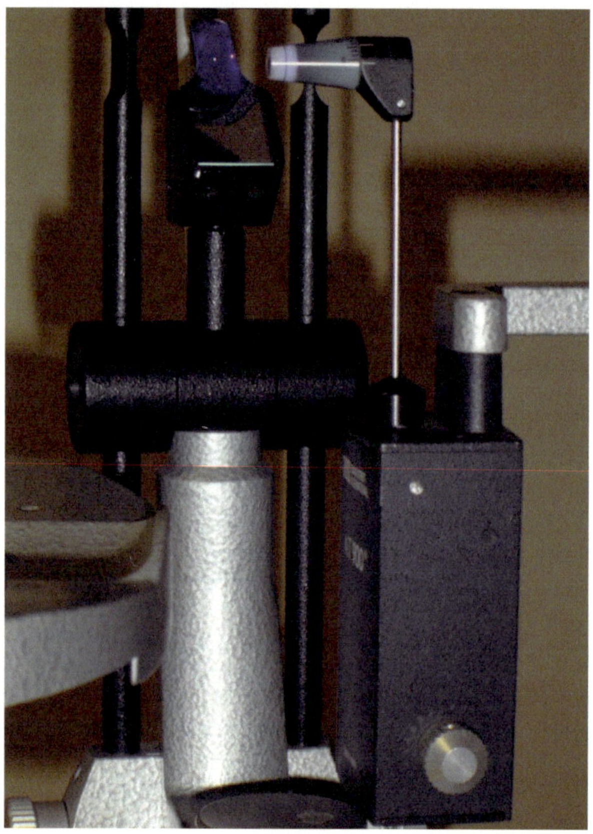

Figure 3. GAT

However, because the relationship of measured IOP and CCT is not linear, it is important to remember that the biomechanical properties of an individual cornea may vary, resulting in changes of the relative stiffness or rigidity of the cornea and altering the measurement. Currently, there is no validated correction factor for the effect of CCT on the GAT [13].

The GAT has some disadvantages [14]:

http://dx.doi.org/10.5772/58690

- The IOP assessment is subjective
- It 's always required the sitting position of the patient
- It is possible to transmit infections if the prism head is not disinfected before each measurement
- The pulsations of the eye can lead to excessive movements of the semicircles
- The amplitude of the semicircles, after application of fluorescein, can influence the readings of IOP
- Repeated or prolonged contact between the cornea and the tonometer may damage the corneal epithelium, resulting in a not reliable assessment of IOP
- The characteristics of the cornea (thickness, astigmatism, corneal surface regularity, viscoelastic properties) may make it difficult or incorrect the reading of the IOP values
- Excessive pressure on the eye, caused by squeezing of the eyes of the patient or by the force applied by the operator on the lid to keep the eyelids open, may induce incorrect readings
- Possible incorrect results due to an altered calibration of the tonometer

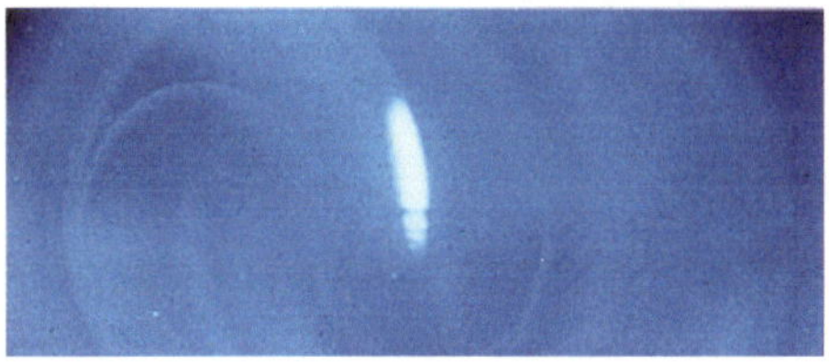

Figure 4. Semicircles

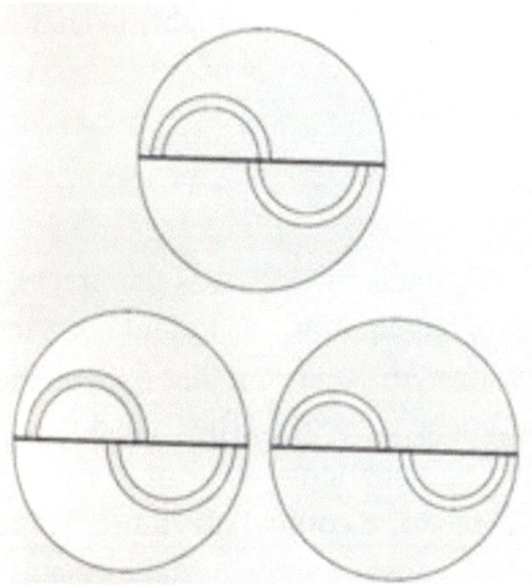

Figure 5. Semicircles readings

2.4. Perkins tonometer

The Perkins tonometer (Fig. 6) is a counterbalanced applanation tonometer that is portable and can be used with the patient either upright or supine [15].

It is similar to the GAT in using a split-image device and fluorescein stained ocular surface. However, the values of IOP are not well correlated with that obtained by Goldmann tonometer [16].

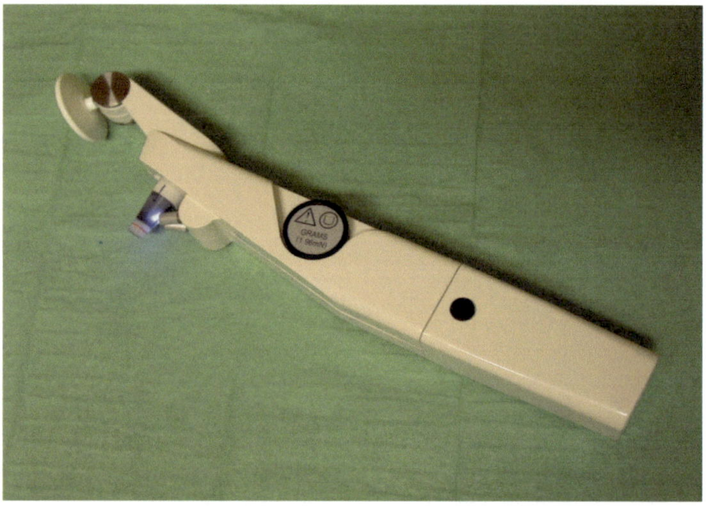

Figure 6. Perkins tonometer

2.5. Draeger tonometer

Portable version, supplied with an electric motor, able to change the applied force.

Less common and more difficult to use

2.6. Mackay-Marg tonometer

The Mackay-Marg model(Fig.7), made in 1959, was the first electronic tonometer and can be said to combine the principles of applanation and indentation. It uses a free-floating transducer to detect the transmitted pressure. An outer ring that flattens the adjacent cornea, reducing its influence on the IOP measurement, surrounds the transducer. The mobile tip that protrudes from a probe has a diameter of applanation of 1.5 mm on the corneal surface and, therefore, it is less affected by corneal thickness and corneal curvature. This device can be used in children and non-cooperative patients because of their portability and ease of use, in irregular and edematous corneas, even in the presence of LAC [17]; it gives values slightly higher compared to those obtained with the GAT [18].

http://dx.doi.org/10.5772/58690

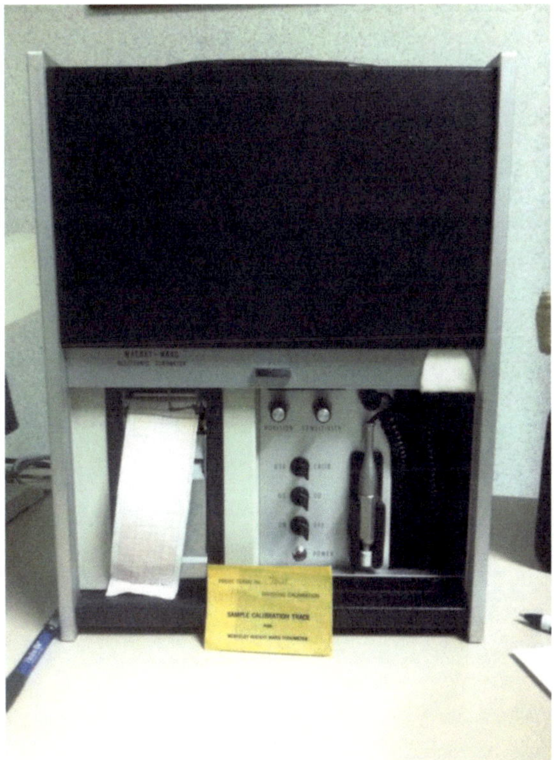

Figure 7. MACKAY-MARG TONOMETER

3. Tonopen (Fig.:8)

It is based on the principle of the MACKAY-MARG tonometer. The values of IOP are converted into an electronic signal that is processed by a microprocessor. The area of applanation is smaller than that of GAT [19].

The instrument performs 4-10 measurements and calculates the average value, giving even higher percentages of reliability for values of 24 mmHg or higher, with a good correlation with the GAT [20].

The values below to 24 mm Hg are overestimated of about 2 mmHg compared to those of GAT.

The advantages of Tonopen are:

- It can be used in irregular corneas
- it allows to perform tonometry on patients in any position
- Easy to use

The disadvantages are that in presence of important corneal irregularities it gives unreliable results.

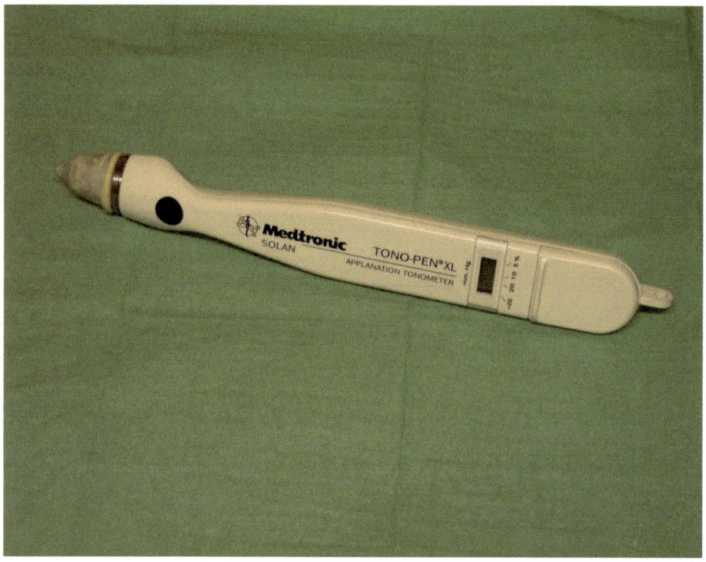

Figure 8. Tonopen

4. Pneumatic applanation tonometer (Fig.9)

The pneumatic tonometer, or pneumotonometer, has a pressure-sensing device that consists of a gas-filled chamber covered by a Silastic diaphragm. The gas in the chamber escapes through an exhaust vent.

As the diaphragm touches the cornea, the gas vent decreases in size and the pressure in the chamber rises.

Because this instrument perform an applanation on only a small area of the cornea, it is especially useful in the presence of corneal scars or edema [21].

The Ocular Blood Flow Analyzer (BFA) is a particular pneumotonometer. It performs the measurements of the IOP, 200 times per second and it records, with great precision, the amplitude of the eye pulse. It is based on the combination of a pneumatic system and an electronic system. A piston is moved by an air-flow until arriving in contact with the cornea, the force required to obtain the cornea applanation is given by the compressed air.

The air can freely exit the tool when far away from the cornea while when the probe is placed on the eye the airflow will be hampered to exit, so creating a proportional pressure. The IOP value is given as the force necessary to obtain the cornea applanation; the values are higher than that obtained by the GAT [22]. Furthermore it is known that its values are influenced by physiological variations in central corneal thickness ([23] and corneal curvature [24] and the values are also not reliable if the cornea is significantly pathological

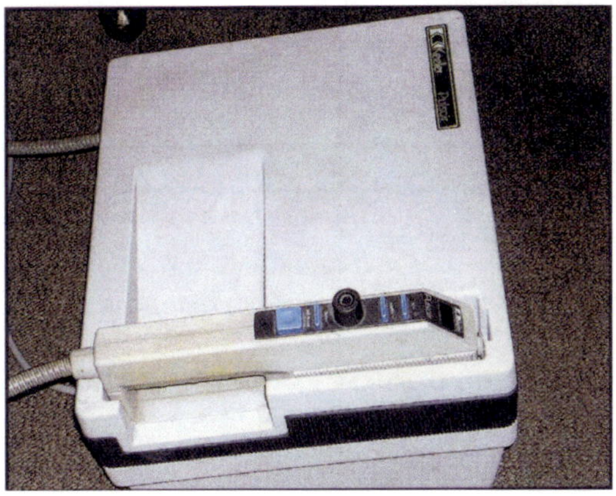

Figure 9. Pneumatic Applanation Tonometer.

5. Applanation tonometry to force variable

5.1. The Non-Contact Tonometries (NCT)

These instruments are based on two processes:

The applanation is obtained by a jet of compressed air that it is properly positioned on the cornea and checked optically ;

The applanation time is assessed by the maximum reflection of a beam incident at an angle of 45° and the speed with which it is obtained corresponds to the IOP.

The influence of corneal thickness is variable. There would be an overestimation for hypotension and underestimation for hypertension [25]

The instruments are often used in large-scale glaucoma-screening programs or by nonmedical health care providers.

5.2. Pascal dynamic contour tonometer (PDCT) (Fig. 10)

This tool entered the market recently and is based on the method of dynamic tonometry. While for the static tonometry, the tool deforms the corneal surface, and this deformation is correlated with the IOP, the dynamic tonometry is based not on the deformation itself, but on the fact that the instrument puts the applanation force on the cornea with a well-defined speed. The relationship between the time and the speed with which the deformation is achieved correlates with the value of IOP. The static IOP assessment is replaced by the concept of dynamic corneal deformation speed and inertial mass. The profiled tip of the tonometer, called SensorTip, has a radius of curvature of 10.5 mm and the contact surface has a diameter of 7.5 mm which determines a line profile with the corneal surface and the tear film. The tip is mounted on a movable arm (cantilever) which is placed on the cornea giving a force equivalent to a gram and constantly kept by a spring mechanism.

A piezo-electric tip with a diameter of 1.2 mm is placed on the center of the contact surface, generates an electrical signal proportional to the IOP.

In conclusion, the PDCT eliminates most of the systematic errors due to individual changes of corneal characteristics, which, instead, influence all types of applanation tonometers. The advantage of measuring the real pressure in combination with the ability to record the dynamic fluctuations of the pressure gives the opportunity to diagnose and classify different types of glaucoma [26]

Indeed, it is important to underline that with the PDCT tonometer is possible to obtain an accurate definition of the pressure fluctuation due to the heartbeat (ocular pulse amplitude-OPA)

In fact, the PDCT seems to be the most accurate method for measuring the ocular pulse amplitude.

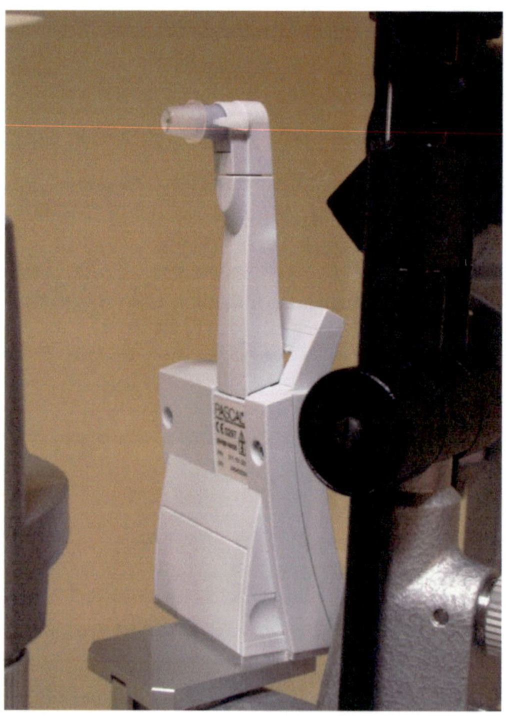

Figure 10. PDCT

http://dx.doi.org/10.5772/58690

5.3. Icare rebound tonometers (Fig.11)

The rebound technology is based on the rebound measuring principle, in which a very light-weight probe is used to make a momentary contact with the cornea.

In the rebound technology, motion parameters of the probe are recorded during the measurement. An induction based coil system is used for measuring the motion parameters. An advanced algorithm, combined with the state of the art software, analyzes deceleration and the contact time of the probe while it touches the cornea. Deceleration and the contact time of the probe change as a function of IOP. In simple terms, the higher the IOP, the faster the probe decelerates and the shorter the contact time.

The Icare rebound tonometer does not require any maintenance calibration, the anaesthesia is not needed since the touch of the probe is so gentle that the measurement is barely noticed by the patient [27].

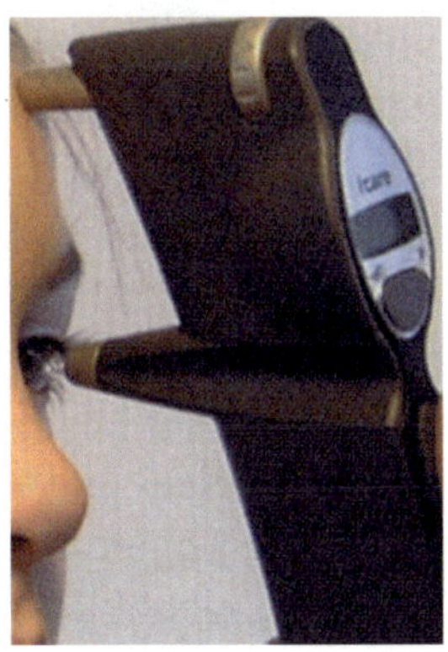

Figure 11. Icare

5.4. The self-tonometers (Fig.13)

The Proview phosphene tonometer is based on an entoptic phenomenon called phosphene (flash of light); that is a feeling of light obtained from the retina by non-luminous stimuli. It looks like a pen, but inside it is present in a small, flat probe, an internal spring and a graduated scale for the values of IOP.

The patient can measure the IOP several times a day, with a device safe, easy to use and inexpensive. The measurement is carried out through the upper lid, does not require either anesthesia or fluorescein stain, it is portable, does not require batteries or electrical outlets.

The patient puts the instrument on the upper eyelid, at the root of the nose, and he presses until he sees a phosphene, and the IOP is recorded.

There is not a corneal applanation, and then tonometry can be performed on the abnormal corneas or after ocular surgery [28].

The Proview may be useful for perform a self-tonometry, but it needs to be calibrated with the GAT to have a good correlation between the values obtained by the two instruments [29]

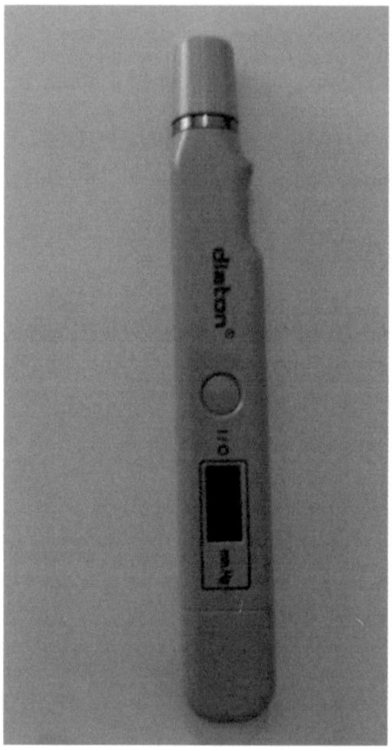

Figure 12. Self Tonometer

5.5. iCare tonometer

This tool is ideal for all patients treated with anti-glaucoma medications.

iCare tonometer is used in the diagnosis, follow-up and screening of intraocular pressure.

The iCare is an handheld tonometer, which is based on the impact-induction principle also known as rebound tonometry [31] The main advantages of this device include its quick and simple use, and that local anesthesia and slitlamp are not needed.

iCare tonometer has shown good reproducibility [31]and correlation with GAT and other tonometers in healthy and glaucomatous eyes. [31,32,33,34] Although iCare was designed not to be influenced by corneal properties, studies have shown that CCT and other corneal structural characteristics affect iCare IOP readings [32,33,34,35,36]

6. Sensory system lenses

This system consists of a soft contact lens attached to a micro-voltage detection unit connected to the external recording tool. It is still a prototype and several physiological parameters such as the tear film and eyelid movements need to be evaluated.

http://dx.doi.org/10.5772/58690

Another type of lens is the tonometric gonioscopic Smart Lens.

The values obtained are overestimated compared to those obtained with the Goldmann of approximately 4-5 mmHg.

6.1. The continuous measurement tonometry

Based on methods that allow evaluating the IOP through the application of a sensor to lens applied on the cornea, during the day, or to an intra-ocular lens (IOL). The latter system allows to obtain continuous values of IOP, without interference of the corneal thickness and curvature. This sensor, made of silicone, is applied on the IOL and has a plate shape divided into 4 parts where there are some cavities that generate a specific electrical voltage. The intraocular pressure fluctuations change the silicone structure and consequently the generate voltage. The chip present on the lens transforms the electric pulses into digital signals that are sent to a tool, called Photodisc, constituted by radio waves and a coil. The receiver is inserted in special glasses and is connected to a portable display. The values of IOP are sent to the photodisc and then displayed on the external display expressed in mmHg [37]

Conclusion Tonometry is the fastest, simple, and popular way to assess the IOP, which is the main risk factor for the glaucoma disease. The GAT is considered, the gold-standard for the assessment of IOP. Over the centuries it has been tried to develop accurate tonometers, searching for the true IOP value, and not altered from the biomechanical characteristics of the human eye. The way to the pursuit of the best tonometer is still long, but certainly the evolution of technology in ophthalmology will permit to develop more and more sophisticated and accurate tools to defeat the "thief of sight": glaucoma.

Author details

Felicia Ferreri[1], Rosa Minniti[1], Alessandra Polimeni[1], Lucia Zavettieri[1], Giuseppina Ferreri[1], Paolo Ferreri[2] and Pasquale Aragona[1]

1 Institute of Ophthalmology, University of Messina, Italy

2 Institute of Ophthalmology, University of Bari, Italy

References

[1] Dua HS, Faraj LA, Said DG, Gray T, Lowe J. Human corneal anatomy redefined: a novel pre-Descemet's layer (Dua's layer). Ophthalmology. 2013 Sep;120(9):1778-85.

[2] Shah S, Laiquzzaman M, Bhojwani R, Mantry S, Cunliffe I: Assessment of the biomechanical properties of the cornea with the ocular response analyzer in normal and keratoconic eyes. Invest Ophthalmol Vis Sci 2007, 48(7):3026-3031.

[3] Touboul D, Roberts C, Kerautret J, Garra C, Maurice-Tison S, Saubusse E, Colin J: Correlations between corneal hysteresis, intraocular pressure, and corneal central pachymetry. Journal of cataract and refractive surgery 2008, 34(4):616-622.

[4] .Moses RA, Grodzki WJ. Theory and calibration of the Schiötz tonometer. VII. Experimental results of tonometric measurements: scale reading versus indentation volume. Invest Ophthalmol. 1971 Sep;10(9):716-23.

[5] Friedenwald Js.: Jun;52:543-7

[6] Pemberton JW.: Schiötz-applanation disparity following retinal detachment surgery.Arch Ophthalmol. 1969 Apr;81(4):534-7.

[7] Friedenwald Js.: Some problems in the calibration of tonometers. Am J Ophthalmol. 1948 Aug;31(8):935-44.

[8] Goldmann H, Schmidt T. Applanation tonometry. Ophthalmologica. 1957 Oct;134(4): 221-42.

[9] Holladay JT, Allison ME, Prager TC.Goldmann applanation tonometry in patients with regular corneal astigmatism. Am J Ophthalmol. 1983 Jul;96(1):90-3.

[10] Johnson MW, Han DP, Hoffman KE. The effect of scleral buckling on ocular rigidity. Ophthalmology. 1990 Feb;97(2):190-5.

[11] Ehlers N, Bramsen T, Sperling S.: Applanation tonometry and central corneal thickness. Acta Ophthalmol. 1975 Mar;53(1):34-43.

[12] Doughty MJ, Jonuscheit S.: Effect of central corneal thickness on Goldmann applanation tonometry measures-a different result with different pachymeters. Graefes Arch Clin Exp Ophthalmol. 2007 Nov;245(11):1603-10.

[13] Kohlhaas M, Boehm AG, Spoerl E, Pürsten A, Grein HJ, Pillunat LE :Effect of central corneal thickness, corneal curvature, and axial length on applanation tonometry. Arch Ophthalmol. 2006 Apr;124(4):471-6.

[14] Whitacre MM, Stein R.:Sources of error with use of Goldmann-type tonometers. Surv Ophthalmol. 1993 Jul-Aug;38(1):1-30

[15] Dunn JS, Brubaker RF: Perkins applanation tonometer. Clinical and laboratory evaluation. Arch Ophthalmol. 1973 Feb;89(2):149-51

[16] Arora R, Bellamy H, Austin M. Applanation tonometry: a comparison of the Perkins handheld and Goldmann slit lamp-mounted methods. Clin Ophthalmol. 2014 Mar 26;8:605-10.

http://dx.doi.org/10.5772/58690

[17] Kaufman HE, Wind CA, Waltman SR: Validity of Mackay-Marg electronic applanation tonometer in patients with scarred irregular corneas. Am J Ophthalmol. 1970 Jun;69(6):1003-7.

[18] Moses Ra, Marg E, Oechsli R. Evaluation of the basic validity and clinical usefulness of the Mackay-Marg tonometer.Invest Ophthalmol. 1962 Feb;1:78-85.

[19] Hessemer V, Rössler R, Jacobi KW: Tono-Pen, a new tonometer. Int Ophthalmol. 1989 Jan;13(1-2):51-

[20] Deuter CM, Schlote T, Hahn GA, Bende T, Derse M.: Measurement of intraocular pressure using the Tono-Pen in comparison with Goldmann applanation tonometry-a clinical study in 100 eyes. Klin Monbl Augenheilkd. 2002 Mar;219(3):138-42.

[21] West CE, Capella JA, Kaufman HE.Measurement of intraocular pressure with a pneumatic applanation tonometer. Am J Ophthalmol. 1972 Sep;74(3):505-9.

[22] Pianka O Geyer O : Comparison of the pneumatonometry with applanation tonometry. Inv Ophthalmology Vis Sci 1998; 39: 4309

[23] Doughty MJ, Zaman ML Human corneal thickness and its impact on intraocular pressure measures: a review and meta-analysis approach. Surv Ophthalmol. 2000 Mar-Apr;44(5):367-408.

[24] Gunvant P, Baskaran M, Vijaya L, Joseph IS, Watkins RJ, Nallapothula M, Broadway DC, O'Leary DJ.Effect of corneal parameters on measurements using the pulsatile ocular blood flow tonograph and Goldmann applanation tonometer.Br J Ophthalmol. 2004 Apr;88(4):518-22.

[25] Shields MB. The non-contact tonometer. Its value and limitations. Surv Ophthalmol. 1980 Jan-Feb;24(4):211-9.

[26] Ku JY, Danesh-Meyer HV, Craig JP, Gamble GD, McGhee CN. Comparison of intraocular pressure measured by Pascal dynamic contour tonometry and Goldmann applanation tonometry.Eye (Lond). 2006 Feb;20(2):191-8.

[27] Fernandes P1, Díaz-Rey JA, Queirós A, Gonzalez-Meijome JM, Jorge J. Comparison of the ICare rebound tonometer with the Goldmann tonometer in a normal population. Ophthalmic Physiol Opt. 2005 Sep;25(5):436-40

[28] Groenhoff S, Draeger J, Deutsch C, Wiezorrek R, Hock B.: Self-tonometry: technical aspects of calibration and clinical application. Int Ophthalmol. 1992 Sep;16(4-5): 299-303.

[29] Avarez TL Gollance SA The Proview Phosphene tonometer fails to measure ocular pressure accurately in clinical practice,Ophthalmology 2004 Jun;111(6):1077-85

[30] Witte V, Glass Ä, Beck R, Guthoff R.Evaluation of the self-tonometer Icare ONE in comparison to Goldmann applanation tonometry.Ophthalmologe. 2012 Oct;109(10): 1008-13.

[31] Kontiola AI. A new induction-based impact method for measuring intraocular pressure. Acta Ophthalmol Scand. 2000;78:142–145.

[32] Martinez-de-la-Casa JM, Garcia-Feijoo J, Castillo A, Garcia-Sanchez J. Reproducibility and clinical evaluation of rebound tonometry. Invest Ophthalmol Vis Sci. 2005;46:4578–4580.

[33] Nakamura M, Darhad U, Tatsumi Y, Fujioka M, Kusuhara A, Maeda H, et al. Agreement of rebound tonometer in measuring intraocular pressure with three types of applanation tonometers. Am J Ophthalmol. 2006;142:332–334.

[34] Martinez-de-la-Casa JM, Garcia-Feijoo J, Vico E, Fernandez-Vidal A, Benitez del Castillo JM, Wasfi M, et al. Effect of corneal thickness on dynamic contour, rebound, and Goldmann tonometry. Ophthalmology. 2006;113:2156–2162.

[35] Brusini P, Salvetat ML, Zeppieri M, Tosoni C, Parisi L. Comparison of ICare tonometer with Goldmann applanation tonometer in glaucoma patients. J Glaucoma. 2006;15:213–217.

[36] Chui W, Lam A, Chen D, Chiu R. The influence of corneal properties on rebound tonometry. Ophthalmology. 2008;115:80–84.

[37] Mottet B, Aptel F, Romanet JP, Hubanova R, Pépin JL, Chiquet C. 24-hour intraocular pressure rhythm in young healthy subjects evaluated with continuous monitoring using a contact lens sensor. Jama Ophthalmol 2013 Dec;131(12):1507-16

Chapter 5

Clinical Ocular Electrophysiology

Fatih C. Gundogan and Umit Yolcu

Additional information is available at the end of the chapter

http://dx.doi.org/10.5772/57609

1. Introduction

Ocular electrodiagnostic tests are invaluable tools in most clinical circumstances in routine ophthalmology practice. Sometimes, these tests are the only methods exploring the functional deficits of the patient in otherwise normal structure. In contrast, ocular electrophysiological tests may explore normal function in cases with functional vision loss. In this chapter, we will focus on the clinical use of ocular electrophysiological tests after a short explanation about recording parameters. A basic clinical use of ocular electrophysiological tests will be discussed rather than detailed and theoretical explanations.

2. Full-field electroretinogram

Full-field electroretinogram (ERG) represents a mass-response of the retina to a full-field flash of light. The resultant single waveform is the total response of the retina. The details of full-field ERG recording techniques may be obtained from ISCEV (International Society for Clinical Electrophysiology of Vision) standards [1]. The functions of rod, cones and inner retinal layers may be recorded separately by changing stimulus parameters and the adaptive state of the eye to the light.

In a typical full-field ERG (Figure 1), five recordings are performed. At first, the patient is dark adapted for at least 20 minutes. A dim white or blue flash light [2.0 log unit below the standard flash intensity (Standard flash: 3.0 cds/m^2)] is used to stimulate the retina. This response is shown as 'DA 0.01 response' in the latest ISCEV guideline for full-field ERG recording. At that flash intensity, only rod photoreceptors are stimulated and the resultant waveform belongs to rod functions. In that response, only a positive b wave originated from rod ON-bipolar cells is recorded. This means that DA 0.01 response is an indirect indicator for rod photoreceptor function. Secondly, DA 3.0 response is recorded. A standard flash light is used to stimulate both rod and cone photoreceptors and combined response of rod and cone photoreceptors is recorded. The first negative peak, a-wave is caused by the hyperpolarization of photoreceptors. However, in DA 3.0 response, a-wave has a bifid configuration which makes the evaluation of photoreceptor function problematic. For this reason, ISCEV recommended the use of bright flash ERG recordings (DA 10.0 ERG or DA 30.0 ERG) for photoreceptor function evaluation. In these brighter light levels, a–wave has a clear single peak. Oscillatory potentials, which reflects amacrine cell function is recorded using standard flash light intensity under dark-or light-adapted (LA; at least 10-min of light adaptation using a background luminance of 30cd/m^2) conditions. LA 3.0 response is generated within cone system. LA 3.0 30 Hz flicker response is the most sensitive indicator of cone system however, it arises in the inner retina and cannot be used to localize the level of abnormality within the cone system [2].

Each retina consists of approximately 4-5 million of cone and 100-120 million of rod photoreceptors. The rods contain light-sensitive pigment rhodopsin with a spectral absorption peak at 496 nm. Each cone contains one of three types of color sensitive pigments. L, M and S-cones (L: long wavelength cones, M: middle wavelength cones, S: small wavelength cones) have peak absorption spectra at 558nm, 531nm and 419nm, respectively. L,M and S cones is also named as red cones, green cones and blue cones with respect to colors of peak-sensitized light [3].

It is apparent from the stimulation technique that small areas of retinal dysfunction cannot be explored by full-field ERG, such as cases with Stargardt macular dystrophy or age-related macular degeneration, macular edema, etc. The cone photoreceptors are the most heavily packed in the macula, however 85-90 percent of cone photoreceptors reside in extra-macular retina. For this reason, full-field ERG is not a good way to investigate functional status or follow-up of retinal diseases known to be restricted to the macular area. Full-field ERG should be used for generalized retinal dysfunction.

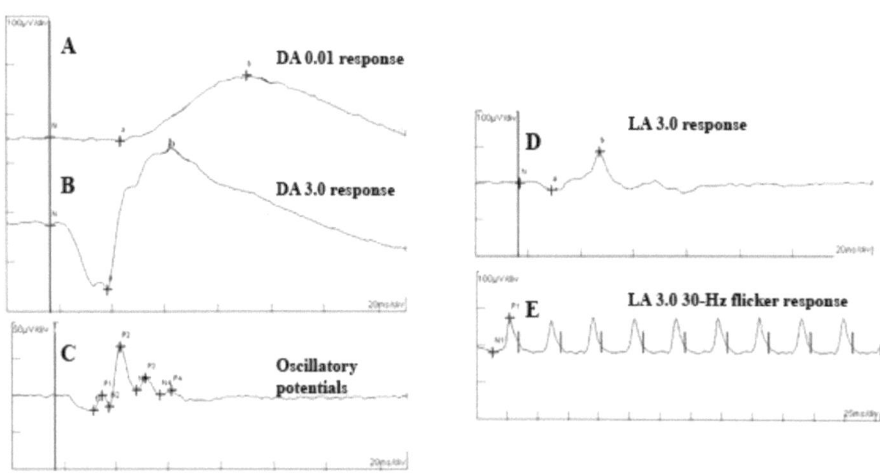

Figure 1. A representative full-field ERG response from a healthy subject.

Retinitis Pigmentosa: Retinitis pigmentosa refers to a large group of genetically heterogeneous disorders characterized by rod dysfunction in the early stages of the disease and progressive rod-cone dysfunction. In typical retinitis pigmentosa, full-field ERG is almost non-recordable in most clinical situations. Rod functions are generally deteriorated earlier and more severely than cone functions. Figure 2 shows a full-field ERG recording belonging to a 21-year-old male patient with retinitis pigmentosa.

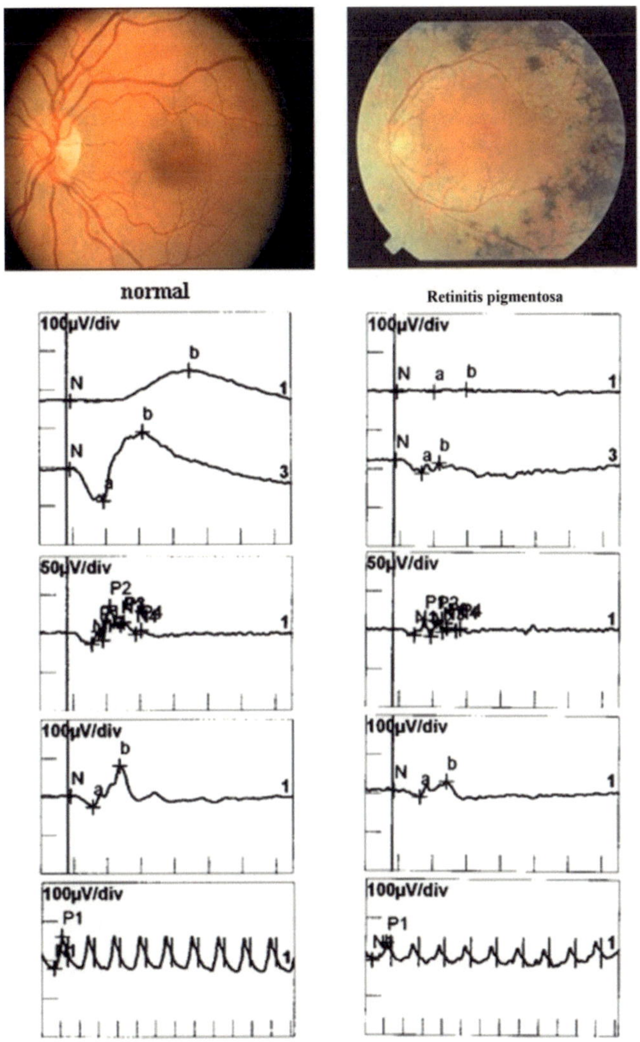

Figure 2. Full-field ERG responses belonging to a healthy subject and a 21-year old male with retinitis pigmentosa. DA 0.01 response is non-recordable. DA 3.0 response has a very low b wave amplitude. LA 3.0 and LA 3.0 30 Hz responses are reduced.

The original report of the ERG in primary retinitis pigmentosa revealed nondetectable or very small responses but these patients usually had advanced disease with attenuation of retinal vessels and extensive pigmentary changes in the retina. However, later studies showed that in the early stages of the disease, the ERG amplitudes are generally subnormal when the patient is asymptomatic. In that stage, however, delays in the implicit times helps in the establishing of widespread progressive forms of retinitis pigmentosa [4].

Retinitis pigmentosa has mainly three types of genetic transmission, autosomal dominant, autosomal recessive and X-linked recessive forms. Almost 50% of patients are sporadic retinitis pigmentosa patients which means that the most common form is this form of the disease. The worst prognosis is seen in X-linked recessive inheritance. These patients generally have non-recordable rod and cone ERG until the end of first decade. However, autosomal dominant type has the best prognosis, and patients with autosomal dominant inheritance may have good rod and cone functions until the fourth and fifth decades [4].

In cases with non-recordable full-field ERG, the follow-up of the macular function may be performed with multifocal ERG, focal ERG or pattern ERG. This will be discussed in the next parts of this chapter.

Cone dystrophies: Cone dystrophy refers to a large group of genetically heterogeneous disorders characterized by progressive diffuse cone dysfunction. Patients have progressive visual acuity loss, decreased color vision and, aversion to bright light. In cone dystrophies, rod function is normal in the early stages of the disease, however may deteriorate in the late stages. Combined rod-cone bright flash ERG shows a mild to moderately reduced a wave and b wave with variable prolongation and oscillatory potentials are also reduced. Single cone responses and 30 Hz cone responses are reduced and prolonged (Figure 3) [5].

Congenital Stationary Night Blindness (CSNB): In contrast to retinitis pigmentosa which is characterized by progressive night vision blindness and photoreceptor loss, CSNB refers to a group of congenital hereditary retinal diseases with non-progressive night blindness and no structural photoreceptor damage. The patient even may not recognize night blindness if the symptoms are mild. Schubert-Bornschein type of CSNB is the most frequent type and is characterized by negative full-field ERG. Negative ERG is told to occur when a b-wave amplitude lower than a-wave amplitude in combined rod-cone response. That is, the peak of the b-wave is under the isoelectric line of the full-field ERG and b/a ratio is under 1 (Figure 4). CSNB represents only one of the stationary night blinding disorders. Others are fundus albipunctatus, Oguchi disease and fleck retina of Kandori. However, CSNB may be said to be the only one with normal fundus, except myopic fundus changes in some subgroups.

Negative ERG is seen in stationary night blidness but is not limited to this condition. A normal a wave and reduced b wave means that there is problem in the transmission of electrical biopotential from the photoreceptors to the inner retinal layers. The retina has a dual circulation. Photoreceptors are nourished by choroidal circulation while inner retinal layers are nourished by retinal circulation. The biopotential cannot be transferred to inner retinal layers if a problem exist in the retinal circulation. For this reason, central retinal artery obstruction, central retinal vein obstruction may cause negative ERG. Similarly, juvenile retinoschisis is one of the causes of negative ERG.

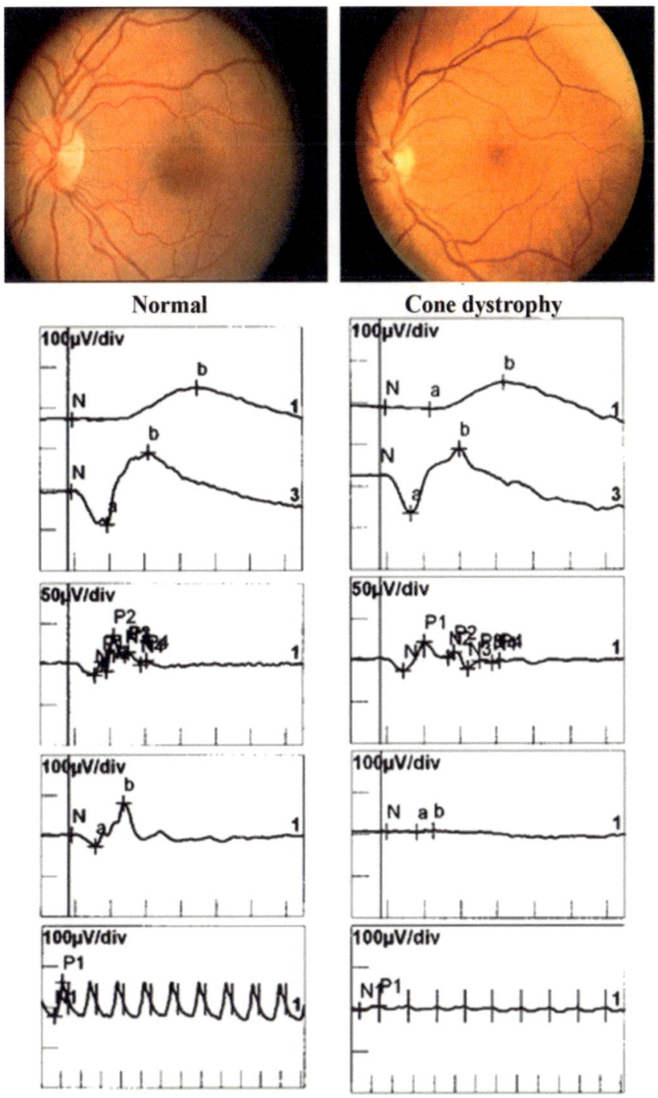

Figure 3. Full-field ERG responses belonging to a healthy subject and a 23-year old male with cone-dystrophy. DA 0.01 and DA 3.0 responses are normal. LA 3.0 response is almost non-recordable. LA 3.0 30 Hz responses are very much reduced.

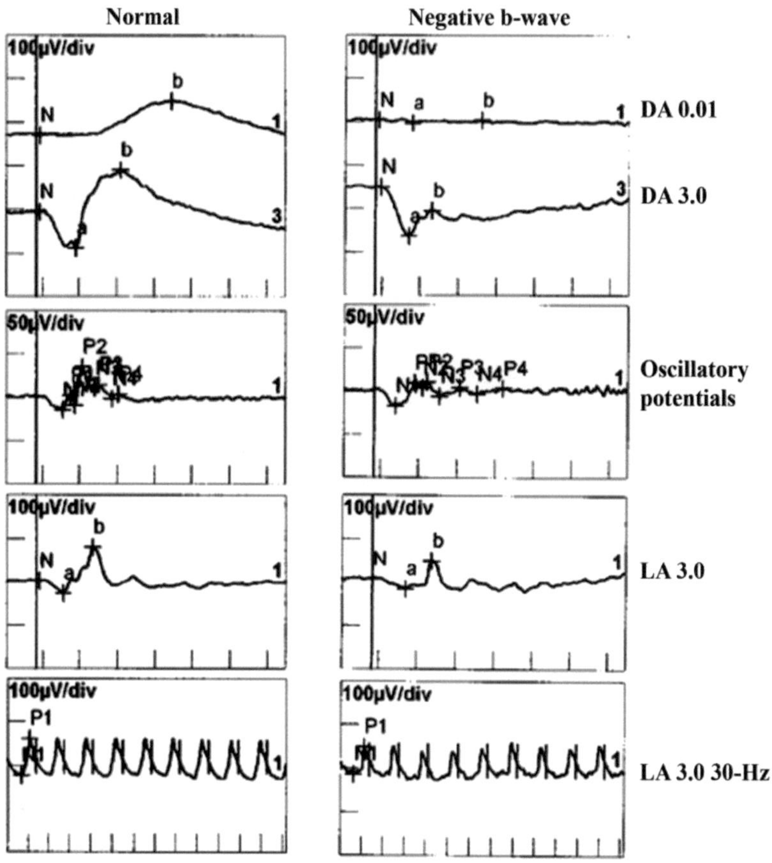

Figure 4. Full-field ERG responses belonging to a healthy subject and a 20-year old male with congenital stationary night blindness. DA 0.01 is non-recordable, DA 3.0 response has a negative configuration that is b-wave amplitude is lower than a-wave amplitude. LA 3.0 response and LA 3.0 30 Hz responses are mildly reduced.

Cone dystrophy with supernormal rod ERG. Cone dystrophy with supernormal ERG was first described by Gouras et al. in 1983 [6]. This autosomal recessively inherited syndrome is characterized by reduced visual acuity, abnormal color vision, discrete macular changes, and specific alterations of ERG responses. Full-field ERG changes are: (1) reduced and delayed cone responses, (2) a reduction and marked delay of rod b-waves at low light intensities, (3) elevated rod b-wave amplitudes at higher light intensities [7]. In the early stages of the disease, the fundus appearance may be normal, however macular pigmentary changes and macular atophy may occur in the later stages [8]. The dystrophy was shown to be caused by KCNV2 gene mutation [9-11]. This gene encodes a subunit of a voltage-gated potassium channel expressed in both rod and cone photoreceptors [9]. It is probable that the rapid increase in b-wave amplitude over a short range of stimulus may result from a 'gated' mechanism, occurring only after an abnormmally high threshold has been exceeded, enabling channel activation and ERG b-wave generation. Robson et al. reported that the ERG to the bright-flash showed a

http://dx.doi.org/10.5772/57609

broadened and delayed a-wave through with a rhomboid-like shape [8]. Figure 5 shows a cone dystrophy patient with supernormal rod ERG [12].

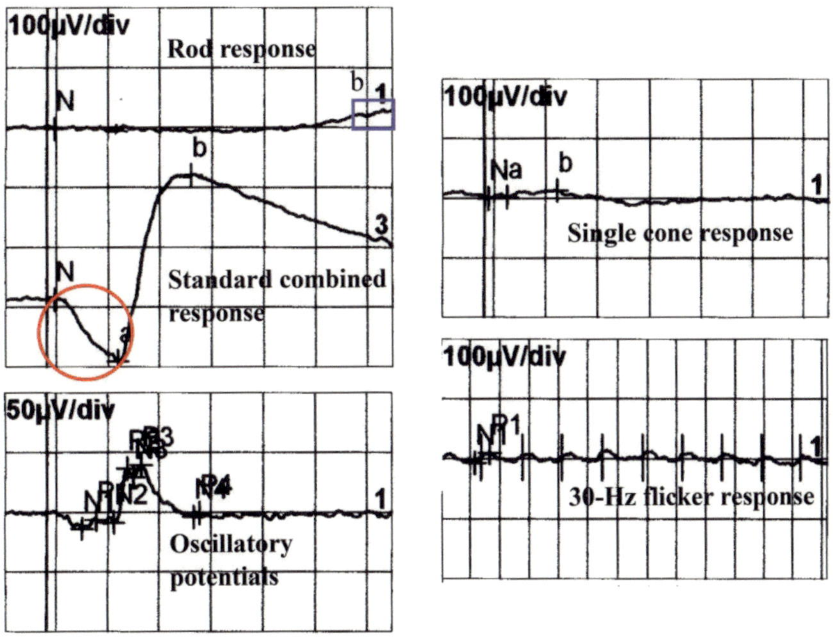

Figure 5. Full-field electroretinogram with very delayed rod response, a rhomboid a-wave and supernormal b-wave in bright-flash rod-cone response and very reduced cone responses in a patient with KCNV2 mutation (Used with permission of Journal of Retina-Vitreus, 2011).

Diabetic retinopathy. Full-field ERG changes are somewhat equivocal in diabetes mellitus. However, there are a number of studies reporting full-field ERG changes in diabetes mellitus. In one study, several ERG changes were reported in diabetics with or without retinopathy From the literature, it is apparent that full-field ERG changes were found in diabetic patients with and without diabetic retinopathy [13]. Holopigian et al. found several ERG parameters to be abnormal in early diabetic retinopathy [14]. Reductions in the oscillatory potentials were reported in diabetic retinopathy, [13, 15, 16] however there was no changes in one study [17]. Bresnick et al. found that oscillatory potential amplitudes predicted the progression of mild nonproliferative diabetic retinopathy to severe proliferative diabetic retinopathy [15, 18].

Toxic effects. Many drugs may have toxic effects on the retina, including choroquine/ hydroxychloroquine, chlorpromazine, thioridazine, indomethacine, quinine, methanol, gentamicin, cisplatin, vigabatrin, desferroxamine, sildenafil,..etc.

Chloroquine/hydroxychloroquine is used in the treatment of rheumatoid arthritis, systemic lupus erithematosis, and malarial fever. Both drugs have an affinity to melanin and tends to accumulate in the choroid, ciliary body, and retinal pigment epithelium. When the degenerative changes are limited to the macular area, normal or subnormal full-field ERG responses are obtained. In the late stages of the toxic effect, peripheral pigmentary changes become apparent. In this stage, minimal or non-recordable responses are obtained. Because full-field ERG responses are minimally affected in the early stages, this test is not recommended to detect early functional deficits. Instead, central 10/2 visual field testing and multifocal ERG is more appropriate for this purpose [19].

Photopic negative response. The photopic negative response is a negative-ongoing wave that occurs following the b-wave in response to a long flash. It is particularly easy to see in red flashes on blue backgrounds. Several studies indicated that the photopic negative response originates from the retinal ganglion cells. The photopic negative response is significantly reduced in patients with primary open-angle glaucoma,[20-24] anterior ischemic optic neuropathy, and other optic neuropathies,[25, 26] consistent with an origin in ganglion cells or their axons [27].

3. Multifocal electroretinogram

Multifocal ERG, first developed by Sutter and Tran in 1991 [28], provides a topographic map of the retinal function. As discussed above, full-field ERG is a mass response of the retina and small areas of retinal dysfunction cannot be explored with full-field ERG. At that point, multifocal ERG has its own advantages. By using a single electrode, multifocal ERG technique allows the recording of the functions of 61, 103 or even more retinal areas in less than 7-8 minutes. The recordings belong to central 30 to 50 degrees of the retina. For this reason, it is an excellent tool in detecting macular function. Multifocal ERG is a reproducible technique although very small responses are produced in each hexagonal area [29].

Multifocal ERG responses may be presented as single waveforms for each hexagonal area, ring analysis beginning from the most central to the periphery of the stimulated area and 3-D presentation (Figure 6).

The multifocal ERG stimulus is displayed on a video monitor. The stimulus consists of a pattern of hexagonal areas which are scaled to produce equal ERG responses from the retina (Figure 7). During stimulation, the display appears to flicker because each hexagon goes through a pseudo-random sequence (the m-sequence) of black and white presentations. Each hexagon has a probability of 0.5 of being white or black on each frame change [30]. Complex mathematical analyses between each retinal response and pseudo-random m sequence provide local retinal responses belonging to each hexagonal area.

http://dx.doi.org/10.5772/57609

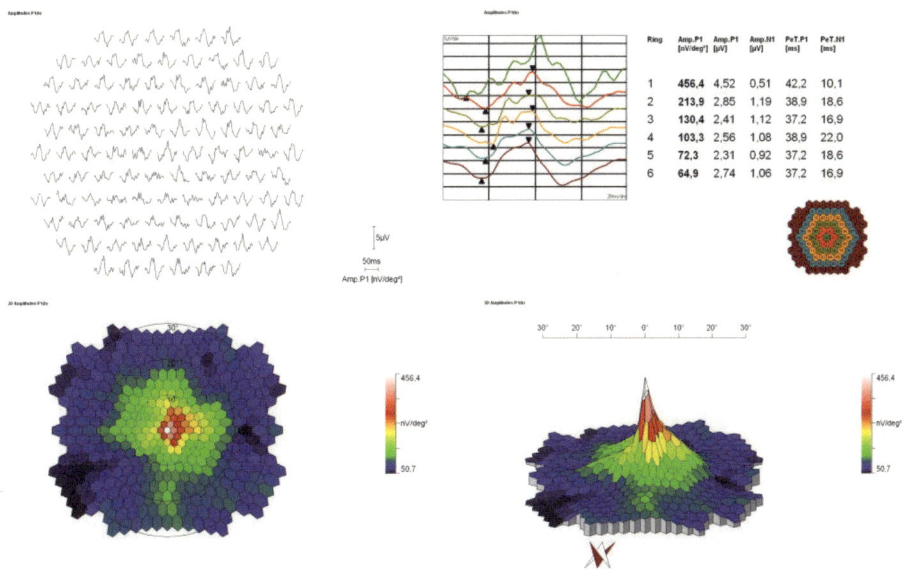

Figure 6. A normal multifocal ERG response output. Upper left: Plots diagram showing single responses from each retinal area. Upper right: Ring analyses. The upper rings show central retinal functions, the lower rings show peripheral functions. Lower right: 2-D amplitudes with color-coded diagram. Lower left: 3-D amplitudes.

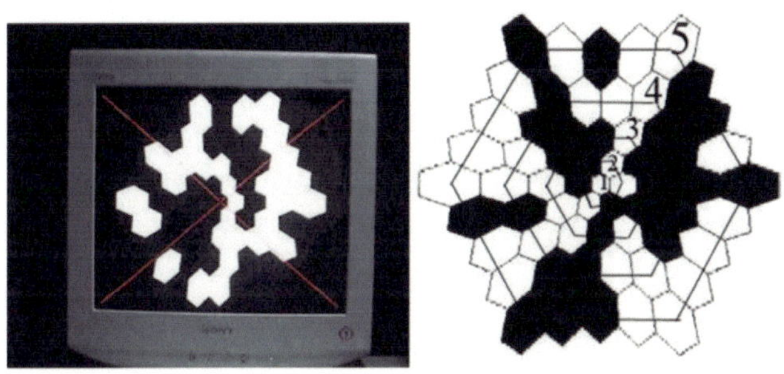

Figure 7. Multifocal ERG stimulus

Macular disease. One of the best uses of multifocal ERG is in Stargardt disease. The central responses are reduced and delayed and the better responses are obtained in the peripheral rings.

Central areolar choroidal dystrophy, first described by Nettleship in 1884, is a macular dystrophy characterized by the development of fine, mottled, depigmented retinal pigment epithelium in the macula. After several decades the pathognomonic zone of circumscript atrophy, affecting retina, retinal pigment epithelium and choriocapillaris, develops in the macular region of the eye [31, 32]. Although, most cases are sporadic, autosomal dominant and recessive inheritance patterns have been reported [33]. In a recent study, we have showed that mfERG responses were reduced corresponding to the areas of ophthalmoscopically visible lesion and there were significant correlations between foveal retinal sensitivity in the Humprey visual field and mfERG P1/N1 amplitudes (Figure 8) [34].

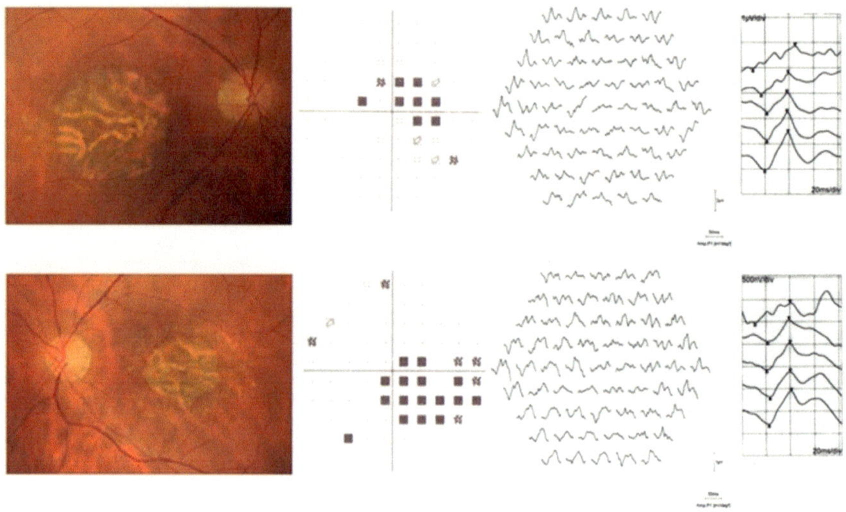

Figure 8. Color fundus photographs, pattern deviation of Humphrey visual fields and multifocal ERG results of four patients with central areolar choroidal dystrophy. Central responses are markedly reduced and delayed in multifocal ERG. (Used with permission of Wichtig Editore. From. 'Multifocal electroretinogram and central visual field testing in central areolar choroidal dystrophy'', Gundogan et al, European Journal of Ophthalmology, Volume 20, Number 5, 2010).

Multifocal ERG was used to evaluate macular function and the response of macular edema to different types of treatment in different types of macular edema. In one of them we showed that multifocal ERG is not a good way to monitor the macular function in *chronic* macular edema [35].

Diabetic retinopathy. One of the important features of early diabetic retinopathy is its focal nature. Full-field ERG is a mass response of all retinal areas. For this reason, full-field ERG recordings cannot detect smaller areas of focal retinopathy in early diabetic retinopathy. Because multifocal ERG records the function of very small retinal areas, it may be used to detect very early local retinal dysfunctions in diabetic retinopathy. Holm et al. showed that hard exudates prolongs the implicit times of the multifocal ERG independent from the macular thickness [36]. In accordance with this finding, Dhamdhere et al. found that local neuroretinal function is not associated with full retinal thickness measured locally in patients with diabetes and no retinopathy, even in abnormal locations. The authors concluded that full retinal thickness measured locally by OCT is not a surrogate for multifocal ERGs in early diabetic retinopathy [37].

Follow-up of retinitis pigmentosa. Multifocal electroretinography is a powerful tool in the follow-up of residual central cone functions in retinitis pigmentosa. In these cases, full-field ERG is generally not reproducible and cone functions are non-recordable. In one study, [38]

http://dx.doi.org/10.5772/57609

yearly progression according to the multifocal ERG values was found to be approximately 6% to 10% in the outer three rings. Ring 5 amplitudes of the multifocal electroretinogram correlated well with the scotopic full-field mixed rod-cone ERG response amplitude.

Glaucoma. Glaucoma primarily affects the inner retina, specifically the retinal ganglion cells, most likely with unremarkable signs or symptoms in the early stages. The damage to retinal ganglion cells results in visual field loss. However, approximately 30-35% of ganglion cells should be lost for an evidence of visual field loss. In recent years, retinal nerve fiber layer analysis by optical coherence tomography has become the most common technique for glaucoma detection [39]. Several studies have used multifocal ERG in detecting signs of glaucoma in terms of amplitude [40] and implicit times [41]. The amplitude of the multifocal ERG is also reduced in patients with ocular hypertension [42].

One of the most important studies on the use of multifocal ERG for glaucoma detection was performed by Sutter and Bearse [43]. The authors used a mathematical algorithm to extract a component with a latency, which increased in proportion to the estimated length of the ganglion cell axons from the site of stimulation to the optic nerve head. The authors found that glaucomatous damage may reduce the magnitude of this component (optic nerve head component) [39, 43].

4. Focal electroretinogram

Focal ERG is used to record local ERG response. In contrast to multifocal ERG stimulus, a direct focal light is used over the retinal area being tested, mostly the macular or foveal region. The response to such a stimulus is about a few microvolts, for this reason, signal-to-noise ratio is low in focal ERG. To overcome this issue, hundreds of stimulus should be used to have a reliable average response. Second problem in focal ERG is the scattered light. The original ring-shaped light is scattered in the eye and may easily stimulate the area outside the intended retinal area. For this reason, the stimulating light is encircled by an annulus ring of steady background light that is typically brighter than the test stimulus. However, this is not an unproblematic solution, because it use of a brighter background light prevents the recording of rod functions [44]. Focal ERG is generally not used in routine clinical practice in most electrophysiological units because of these difficulties and the emergence of multifocal ERG in 1992.

5. Pattern electroretinogram

Pattern ERG is a retinal response to a checkerboard pattern stimulus with alternating black and white squares. In low temporal frequencies (<6 reversals per second), a positive component, P50 (positive peak around 50th milliseconds), and a negative component, N95 (negative component around 95th milliseconds), are observed. Sometimes, a negative component around 35 milliseconds may be recorded (N35).This response to low-frequency stimulus is called 'transient PERG. (Figure 9)

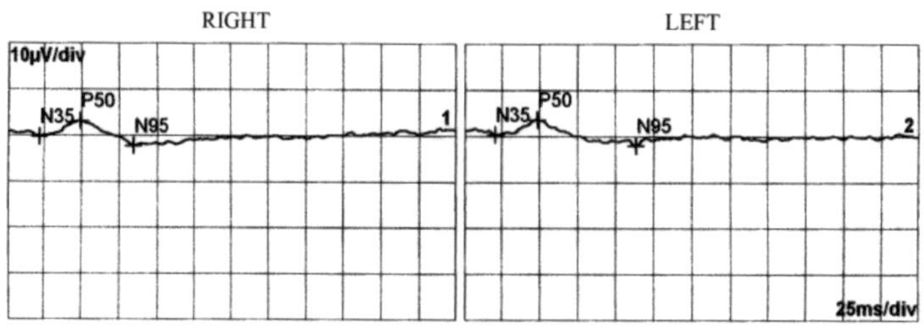

Figure 9. A typical pattern ERG recording.

In high temporal frequencies (>7 reversals per second), P50 and N95 peaks are merged into a sinusoidal waveform, dominated by the N95 component. This response is called 'steady-state pattern ERG'. In steady-state pattern ERG, it is impossible to distinguish the original P50 and N95 peaks [45].

Initially it was thought that PERG is almost totally originated from ganglion cell functions. However, later studies showed that P50 peak has an earlier component originated from cells distal to the ganglion cells and reflecting mostly the macular function [46-49]. In two reports [50, 51], it has been detected that some pattern ERG response still may be recorded after post-traumatic and surgical optic nerve section despite no light perception. In one of them, P50 amplitude reduction with P50 latency shortening was observed. These findings too imply that pattern ERG is not completely originated from ganglion cells. In addition, shortening of the P50 latency caused the theory that a later part of the P50 response is related with ganglion cell function and P50 latency shortens if ganglion cell function extinguishes.

It is apparent from the Figure 9 that P50 amplitude reduction is accompanied by a secondary N95 reduction, as N95 amplitude is measured from P50 peak to N95 trough. However, this is not the same for N95 amplitude reduction. N95 amplitude reduction may be selective. For this reason, the ratio of N95 amplitude to P50 amplitude has an importance in detecting whether the visual loss is related to macular disease or ganglion cell disease. If N95/P50 ratio is normal, then it may be thought that the visual loss may be attributed to macular disease. If the ratio is lower than normal (which is called as 'selective N95 reduction'), visual loss may be attributed to ganglion cell disease. N95/P50 ratio is about 1.5 in the author's electrophysiology laboratory.

5.1. Chronic effect of optic nerve disease to pattern ERG.

The first reports about N95 in optic nerve demyelination were presented by Holder. Holder reported that pattern ERG abnormalities could be limited to N95 component. The author also reported that there was a 40% pattern ERG abnormality among 200 patients with optic nerve demyelination, however 85% of the abnormalities were detected in N95 [52, 53].

http://dx.doi.org/10.5772/57609

Figure 10 and figure 11 show P50 and N95 results of 382 patients with optic nerve demyelination. As shown in Figure 10, most of the patients have normal P50 amplitudes despite prolonged P100 latency in pattern VEP. However Figure 11 shows that N95/P50 ratio decreases as P100 latency increases [52].

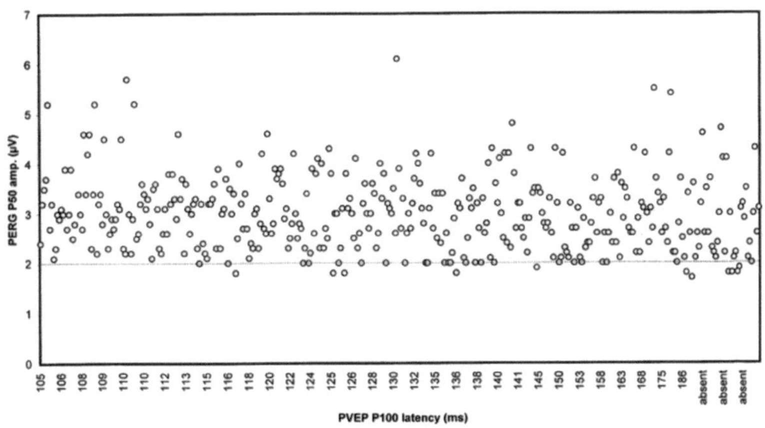

Figure 10. Pattern ERG P50 amplitudes in patients with optic nerve demyelination. (Used with permission of Pergamon. From. 'Pattern Electroretinography (PERG) and an Integrated Approach to Visual Pathway Diagnosis ", Holder GE, Progress in Retinal and Eye Research, Volume 20, Number 4, 2001).

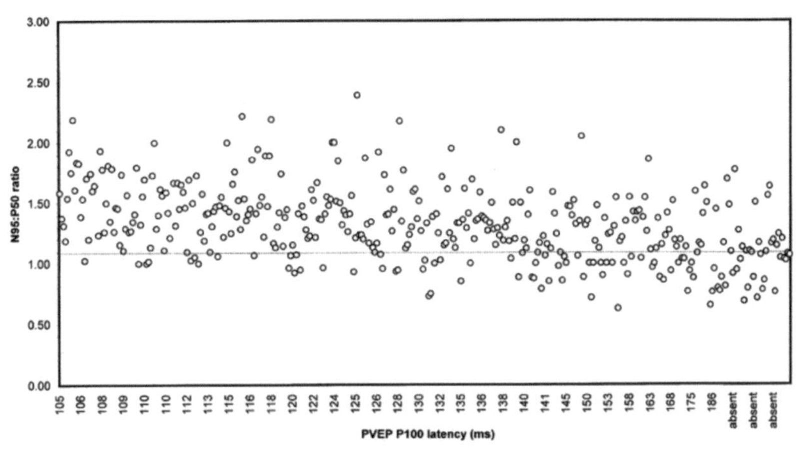

Figure 11. Pattern ERG N95/P50 ratio in patients with optic nerve demyelination. (Used with permission of Pergamon. From. 'Pattern Electroretinography (PERG) and an Integrated Approach to Visual Pathway Diagnosis ", Holder GE, Progress in Retinal and Eye Research, Volume 20, Number 4, 2001).

Acute effects of optic nerve disease on pattern ERG. Pattern ERG changes in the acute phase of the optic nerve inflammation is not simply as mentioned above. In the acute phase of the inflammation, P100 amplitude in pattern VEP is reduced with less latency changes while P50 in pattern ERG is also reduced. A few weeks later, as the inflammation subsides P50 amplitude in pattern ERG and P100 amplitude in pattern VEP recover, however, ganglion cell dysfunction or demyelination begin to appear. N95 is reduced (selectively as mentioned above) while P100 is delayed. N95/P50 ratio is lowered in the chronic phase of the inflammation. MRI findings in the acute and chronic phase of the inflammation was shown to be consistent with this theory [52, 54].

Glaucoma and pattern ERG. Hood et al. [55] studied pattern ERG in glaucoma patients with confirmed visual field deficits. The authors included 21 eyes of 15 patients with glaucoma. Pattern ERG was within normal limits for 4 of the worse eyes of 15 glaucoma patients. Overall, 6 of the 21 eyes that met the criteria for glaucomatous damage had normal pattern ERGs on both N95 amplitude and N95/P50 ratio. Second, the N95 amplitude was nonlinearly related to visual field sensitivity. Small field losses were associated with disproportionately large losses in pattern ERG amplitude. Third, the PERG from both eyes of a patient were very similar, even when the visual fields suggested very different levels of damage.

Ventura et al.[56] investigated the steady-state pattern ERG responses with PERGLA paradigm in 200 glaucoma suspects with increased optic disc cupping and normal visual field and in 42 patients with early manifest glaucoma. The PERG was abnormal in amplitude, phase, or inter-ocular asymmetry in amplitude and phase in 52% of glaucoma suspect patients and 69% of EMG patients. The pattern ERG amplitude was correlated weakly with both mean deviation and vertical C/D (p=0.05). The correlation between pattern ERG amplitude and MD and C/D was stronger for inter-ocular differences rather than absolute measures. Inter-ocular pattern ERG amplitude asymmetry was positively correlated with the severity of the disease. Compared to white glaucoma suspects, a lower pattern ERG amplitude was found in black glaucoma suspects and early manifest glaucoma patients, but not in black glaucoma controls.

6. Electro-oculogram

Unlike full-field ERG, electro-oculogram (EOG) is not a stimulated response. EOG records the continuous resting potential across the retinal pigment epithelium which is named as 'trans-epithelial potential'. This potential is only about a few millivolts. Transepithelial potential is mainly generated by retinal pigment epithelium. However, as well as the integrity of the retinal pigment epithelium, photoreceptor and interphotoreceptor matrix integrity and function should be intact. For this reason, EOG is decreased in photoreceptor diseases, retinal detachment and other generalized outer retinal damages in addition to primary retinal pigment diseases such as Best disease.

The resting potential across the retinal pigment epithelium is not a steady potential. In the dark-adaptation, transepithelial potential is decreased to a minimum value (dark trough) after about 12 minutes. In the light-adaptation, the transepithelial potential increases to a peak value (light-peak) after about 7-12 minutes [57]. The ratio of light-peak to dark-trough is called Arden ratio or 'EOG ratio'. This value should be 1.8 or greater in normal subjects and considered abnormal under 1.6. In the author's institution, Arden ratio is 2.35±0.44 (mean±SD) [58]. Figure 12 shows EOG recordings of a patient with Best disease. There is almost no light peak with light stimulation in EOG. Arden ratios are 1.18 in the right eye and 1.17 in the left eye.

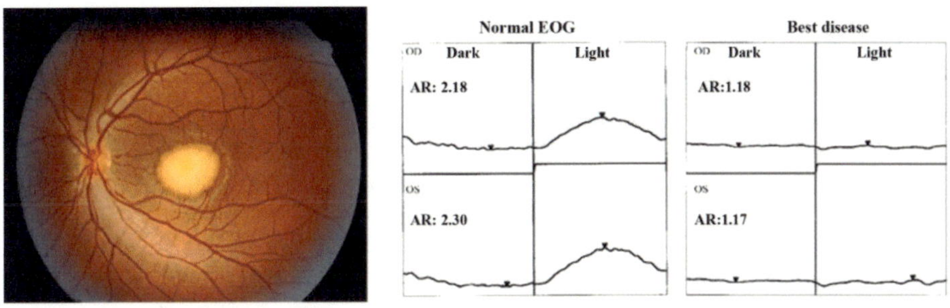

Figure 12. Fundus photo of a patient with Best disease and EOG recordings. Arden ratio is 1.18 in OD and 1.17 in OS. This implies very small change in transepithelial potential with light stimulation.

7. Visual evoked potential

Visual evoked potential (VEP) represents the cortical response to a checkerboard-pattern stimulus (pattern VEP) or a flash stimulus (flash VEP). Pattern VEP components that are commonly measured are N75, P100 and N135 peaks (Figure 13).

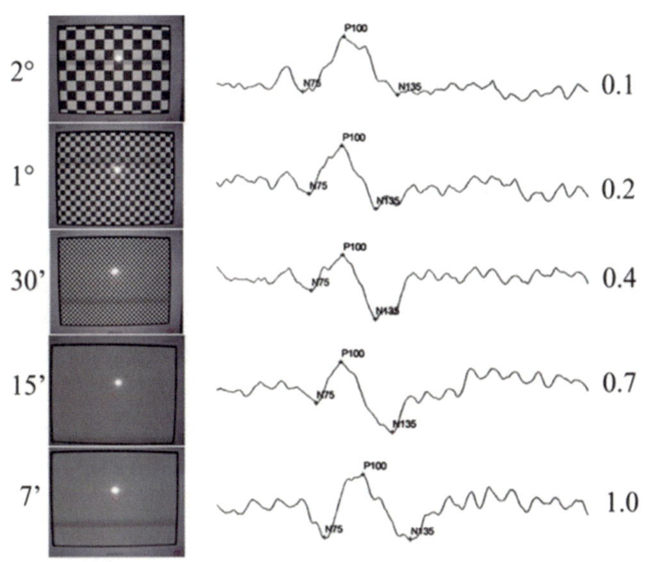

Figure 13. Representative pattern VEP waveforms to five consecutive check sizes.

The amplitudes of the peaks are measured from the peak of the one component to the trough of the preceding component. P and N refer to positive and negative voltages recorded at the occipital electrode with respect to the voltage at the reference electrode.

Flash VEP components are defined as N1, P1, N2, P2, etc (Figure 14).

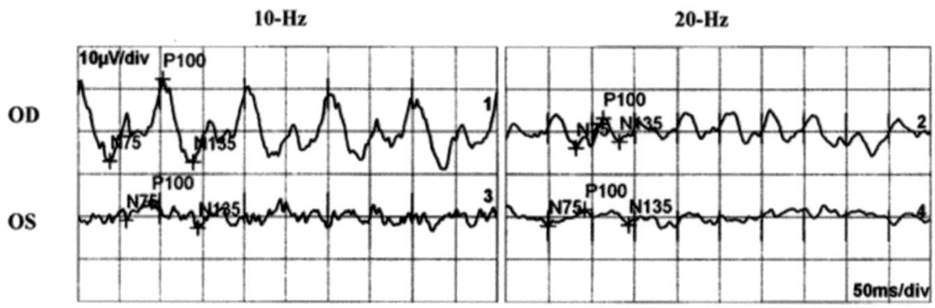

Figure 14. Flash VEP responses in a patient with intravitreal hemorrhage in the left eye. Left-eye flash VEP responses are very much reduced.

VEP response primarily reflects the central retinal function although the stimulated retinal area in pattern VEP and flash VEP is about 50 degrees and full retinal areas, respectively. There are three main reasons for this contribution of the central retina [59]. (1).The central visual field is represented at the outer surface of the visual cortex while peripheral retina is represented at the deep surfaces of the calcarine sulcus. Active electrode in VEP recordings is placed approximately 2 cm above the protuberentia occipitalis externa which is the nearest point to the surface of the visual cortex. (2) Cortical magnification phenomenon. In the central retina each photoreceptor transmits its signal almost to one ganglion cell, while many photoreceptors converges on a single ganglion cell in the peripheral retina. Thus, more than 50% of the cells in the visual cortex represent approximately central 10 degrees of the retina. (3) In PVEP testing, small checkerboard stimuli may be used. These small sized stimuli may only be resolved by the central retina which has the highest concentration of photoreceptors.

Because of the reflection of the central retinal function, pattern VEP is used to estimate visual acuity in many clinical situations besides optic nerve function [60]. An impaired VEP is anatomically non-specific. However, a through ocular examination including the retina, optic nerve and brain frequently explores the localization of the problem [61]. Pattern VEP is more valuable than flash VEP in the clinical evaluations of the visual pathway. However, flash VEP is valuable in the situations of fixation problem, mature cataract, intravitreal hemorrhage, ocular trauma or any other circumstance that prevents patient cooperation. In these situations, flash VEP gives important knowledge about visual status.

Pattern VEP recording requires fixation to a point in the screen. Impaired VEP responses may be produced by deliberate poor fixation, defocusing to the fixation point, or conscious suppression.[61-64] This is an important issue in the evaluation of patients with functional visual loss. Voluntary flash VEP suppression is more difficult, because it does not require fixation.

Optic nerve disease. VEP is commonly used to detect visual pathway deficits in patients with no apparent objective signs of ocular dysfunction. In a study on MS patients with no clinical history of optic nerve involvement, we showed that 21 of 39 patients had delayed P100 latency [65]. Figure 15 shows PVEP recording of an MS patient included in that study. Snellen visual acuity was 1.0 in both eyes although P100 latency was clearly prolonged in the left eye.

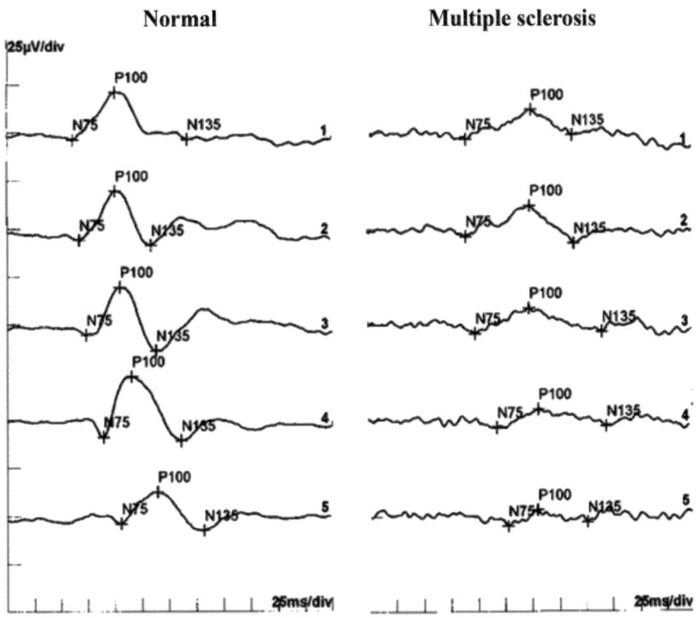

Figure 15. Pattern VEP traces belonging to a –normal and a multiple sclerosis patient. P100 latency to 2 degree check size is about 150 ms in the left eye while it is about 100 ms in the right eye.

Functional Visual Loss. The term 'functional visual loss' is used when the visual loss cannot be explained with organic lesions in the visual pathway. 'Vision' is a cortical function and the bio-potential change in the visual cortex after a visual stimulus is evaluated with visual evoked potentials. In a study, we showed that pattern VEP recordings to five check sizes (2 degree, 1 degree, 30 minute, 15 minute and 7 minute) may be used objectively to estimate visual acuities of the patients with suspected functional visual loss [66].

Figure 16 shows PVEP recordings to 5-consecutive check sizes of an African woman with no light perception in the left eye for 2 years. Biomicroscopic and fundoscopic examinations were unremarkable. No relative afferent pupillary defect was detected. Pattern VEP responses in both eyes were totally in the normal limits in terms of P100 amplitude and latency values. In this patient, we were able to show that the patient was capable of reading at least 0.3 in Snellen chart from 6 meters with the use of polaroid glasses.

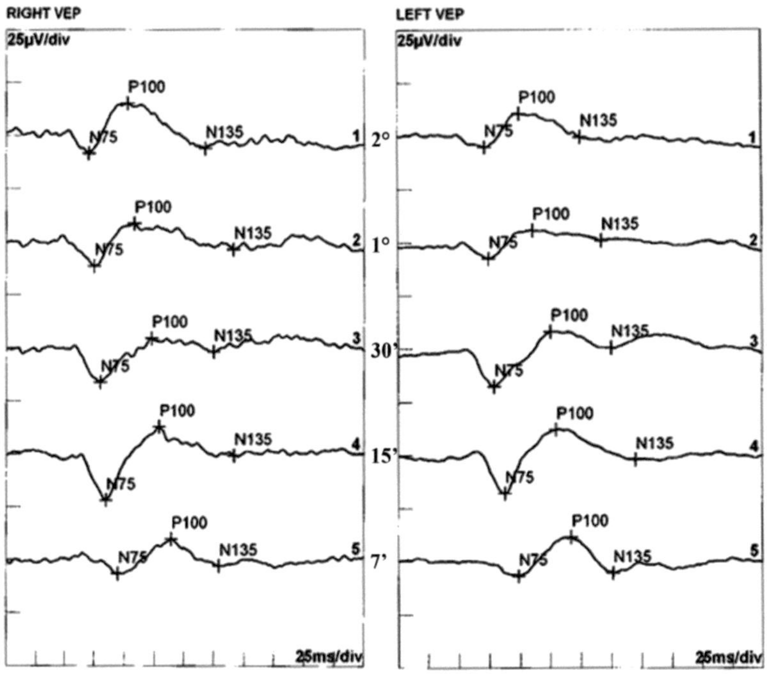

Figure 16. PVEP response to five consecutive check sizes in a malingerer who claimed no light perception in the left eye.

8. Conclusion

Full-field ERG is invaluable in generalized retinal diseases. Pattern ERG is complimentary test for full-field ERG, because it may localize the problem to macula or ganglion cells. Multifocal ERG is used to evaluate central retinal function. EOG is the recording of transepithelial potential. VEP is a cortical potential that is the end of visual pathway, for this reason it gives important knowledge about the 'vision' itself. The ophthalmologist can localize the visual problem with a thorough understanding of the origins of these tests.

Author details

Fatih C. Gundogan[1*] and Umit Yolcu[2]

*Address all correspondence to: fgundogan@yahoo.com

1 GATA Medical School, Ophthalmology, Ankara, Turkey

2 Siirt Military Hospital, Ophthalmology, Siirt, Turkey

References

[1] Marmor MF, Fulton AB, Holder GE, Miyake Y, Brigell M, Bach M, et al. ISCEV Standard for full-field clinical electroretinography (2008 update). Doc Ophthalmol 2009;118(1):69-77.

[2] Vincent A, Robson AG, Holder GE. Pathognomonic (diagnostic) ERGs. A review and update. Retina 2013;33(1):5-12.

[3] Lam BL. Full-field electroretinogram. In: Lam BL, editor. Lam, Byron L. Boca Raton: Taylor & Francis; 2005. p. 1-64.

[4] Berson EL. Retinitis pigmentosa and allied diseases: applications of electroretinographic testing. Int Ophthalmol 1981;4(1-2):7-22.

[5] Lam BL. Macular disorders. In: Lam BL, editor. Electrophysiology of vision : clinical testing and applications. Boca Raton: Taylor & Francis; 2005. p. 277-330.

[6] Gouras P, Eggers HM, MacKay CJ. Cone dystrophy, nyctalopia, and supernormal rod responses. A new retinal degeneration. Arch Ophthalmol 1983;101(5):718-24.

[7] Wissinger B, Dangel S, Jagle H, Hansen L, Baumann B, Rudolph G, et al. Cone dystrophy with supernormal rod response is strictly associated with mutations in KCNV2. Invest Ophthalmol Vis Sci 2008;49(2):751-7.

[8] Robson AG, Webster AR, Michaelides M, Downes SM, Cowing JA, Hunt DM, et al. "Cone dystrophy with supernormal rod electroretinogram": a comprehensive genotype/phenotype study including fundus autofluorescence and extensive electrophysiology. Retina 2010;30(1):51-62.

[9] Wu H, Cowing JA, Michaelides M, Wilkie SE, Jeffery G, Jenkins SA, et al. Mutations in the gene KCNV2 encoding a voltage-gated potassium channel subunit cause "cone dystrophy with supernormal rod electroretinogram" in humans. Am J Hum Genet 2006;79(3):574-9.

[10] Thiagalingam S, McGee TL, Weleber RG, Sandberg MA, Trzupek KM, Berson EL, et al. Novel mutations in the KCNV2 gene in patients with cone dystrophy and a supernormal rod electroretinogram. Ophthalmic Genet 2007;28(3):135-42.

[11] Ben Salah S, Kamei S, Senechal A, Lopez S, Bazalgette C, Bazalgette C, et al. Novel KCNV2 mutations in cone dystrophy with supernormal rod electroretinogram. Am J Ophthalmol 2008;145(6):1099-106.

[12] Gundogan FC, Tas, A., Sobaci, G. Cone Dytrophy with Rod Supernormal Electroretinogram: KCNV2 Mutation. Journal of Retina-Vitreus 2011;19(4):282-84.

[13] Juen S, Kieselbach GF. Electrophysiological changes in juvenile diabetics without retinopathy. Arch Ophthalmol 1990;108(3):372-5.

[14] Holopigian K, Seiple W, Lorenzo M, Carr R. A comparison of photopic and scotopic electroretinographic changes in early diabetic retinopathy. Invest Ophthalmol Vis Sci 1992;33(10):2773-80.

[15] Bresnick GH, Korth K, Groo A, Palta M. Electroretinographic oscillatory potentials predict progression of diabetic retinopathy. Preliminary report. Arch Ophthalmol 1984;102(9):1307-11.

[16] Bresnick GH, Palta M. Oscillatory potential amplitudes. Relation to severity of diabetic retinopathy. Arch Ophthalmol 1987;105(7):929-33.

[17] Wanger P, Persson HE. Early diagnosis of retinal changes in diabetes: a comparison between electroretinography and retinal biomicroscopy. Acta Ophthalmol (Copenh) 1985;63(6):716-20.

[18] Bresnick GH, Palta M. Predicting progression to severe proliferative diabetic retinopathy. Arch Ophthalmol 1987;105(6):810-4.

[19] Fischman GA. The electroretinogram. In: Fishman GA, Sokol S, Holder GE, Brigell M, editors. Electrophysiologic testing in disorders of the retina, optic nerve, and visual pathway. San Francisco, CA: American Academy of Ophthalmology; 2001. p. 1-156.

[20] Machida S, Tamada K, Oikawa T, Gotoh Y, Nishimura T, Kaneko M, et al. Comparison of photopic negative response of full-field and focal electroretinograms in detecting glaucomatous eyes. J Ophthalmol 2011;2011.

[21] Kiszkielis M, Lubinski W, Penkala K. The photopic negative response as a promising diagnostic tool in glaucoma. A review. Klin Oczna 2012;114(2):138-42.

[22] Gotoh Y. [Photopic negative response of eyes with normal-tension glaucoma]. Nihon Ganka Gakkai Zasshi 2002;106(8):481-7.

[23] Viswanathan S, Frishman LJ, Robson JG, Walters JW. The photopic negative response of the flash electroretinogram in primary open angle glaucoma. Invest Ophthalmol Vis Sci 2001;42(2):514-22.

[24] Colotto A, Falsini B, Salgarello T, Iarossi G, Galan ME, Scullica L. Photopic negative response of the human ERG: losses associated with glaucomatous damage. Invest Ophthalmol Vis Sci 2000;41(8):2205-11.

[25] Gotoh Y, Machida S, Tazawa Y. Selective loss of the photopic negative response in patients with optic nerve atrophy. Arch Ophthalmol 2004;122(3):341-6.

[26] Miyata K, Nakamura M, Kondo M, Lin J, Ueno S, Miyake Y, et al. Reduction of oscillatory potentials and photopic negative response in patients with autosomal dominant optic atrophy with OPA1 mutations. Invest Ophthalmol Vis Sci 2007;48(2):820-4.

[27] Frishman LJ. Origins of the electroretinogram. In: Heckenlively JR, Arden GB, editors. Principles and practice of clinical electrophysiology of vision. Cambridge, Mass.: MIT Press; 2006. p. 139-84.

[28] Sutter EE, Tran D. The field topography of ERG components in man--I. The photopic luminance response. Vision Res 1992;32(3):433-46.

[29] Gundogan FC, Sobaci G, Bayraktar MZ. Intra-sessional and inter-sessional variability of multifocal electroretinogram. Doc Ophthalmol 2008;117(3):175-83.

[30] Hood DC. Assessing retinal function with the multifocal technique. Prog Retin Eye Res 2000;19(5):607-46.

[31] Carr RE. Central Areolar Choroidal Dystrophy. Arch Ophthalmol 1965;73:32-5.

[32] Hoyng CB, Deutman AF. The development of central areolar choroidal dystrophy. Graefes Arch Clin Exp Ophthalmol 1996;234(2):87-93.

[33] Nagasaka K, Horiguchi M, Shimada Y, Yuzawa M. Multifocal electroretinograms in cases of central areolar choroidal dystrophy. Invest Ophthalmol Vis Sci 2003;44(4): 1673-9.

[34] Gundogan FC, Dinc UA, Erdem U, Ozge G, Sobaci G. Multifocal electroretinogram and central visual field testing in central areolar choroidal dystrophy. Eur J Ophthalmol 2010;20(5):919-24.

[35] Durukan AH, Memisoglu S, Gundogan FC. Is multifocal ERG a reliable index of macular function after triamcinolone acetonide injection in diffuse diabetic macular edema? Eur J Ophthalmol 2009;19(6):1017-27.

[36] Holm K, Ponjavic V, Lovestam-Adrian M. Using multifocal electroretinography hard exudates affect macular function in eyes with diabetic retinopathy. Graefes Arch Clin Exp Ophthalmol 2010;248(9):1241-7.

[37] Dhamdhere KP, Bearse MA, Jr., Harrison W, Barez S, Schneck ME, Adams AJ. Associations between local retinal thickness and function in early diabetes. Invest Ophthalmol Vis Sci 2012;53(10):6122-8.

[38] Nagy D, Schonfisch B, Zrenner E, Jagle H. Long-term follow-up of retinitis pigmentosa patients with multifocal electroretinography. Invest Ophthalmol Vis Sci 2008;49(10):4664-71.

[39] Chan HH, Ng YF, Chu PH. Applications of the multifocal electroretinogram in the detection of glaucoma. Clin Exp Optom 2011;94(3):247-58.

[40] Frishman LJ, Saszik S, Harwerth RS, Viswanathan S, Li Y, Smith EL, 3rd, et al. Effects of experimental glaucoma in macaques on the multifocal ERG. Multifocal ERG in laser-induced glaucoma. Doc Ophthalmol 2000;100(2-3):231-51.

[41] Hasegawa S, Takagi M, Usui T, Takada R, Abe H. Waveform changes of the first-order multifocal electroretinogram in patients with glaucoma. Invest Ophthalmol Vis Sci 2000;41(6):1597-603.

[42] Chan HH, Brown B. Pilot study of the multifocal electroretinogram in ocular hypertension. Br J Ophthalmol 2000;84(10):1147-53.

[43] Sutter EE, Bearse MA, Jr. The optic nerve head component of the human ERG. Vision Res 1999;39(3):419-36.

[44] Lam BL. Focal Electroretinogram. In: Lam BL, editor. Electrophysiology of vision : clinical testing and applications. Boca Raton: Taylor & Francis; 2005. p. 67-8.

[45] Holder GE. The Pattern Electroretinogram. In: Fishman GA, Birch DG, Holder GE, Brigell MG, editors. Electrophysiologic testing in disorders of the retina, optic nerve, and visual pathways. San Francisco, CA: American Academy of Ophthalmology; 2001. p. 197-237

[46] Berninger T, Schuurmans RP. Spatial tuning of the pattern ERG across temporal frequency. Doc Ophthalmol 1985;61(1):17-25.

[47] Schuurmans RP, Berninger T. Luminance and contrast responses recorded in man and cat. Doc Ophthalmol 1985;59(2):187-97.

[48] Trick GL, Wintermeyer DH. Spatial and temporal frequency tuning of pattern-reversal retinal potentials. Invest Ophthalmol Vis Sci 1982;23(6):774-9.

[49] Kirkham TH, Coupland SG. The pattern electroretinogram in optic nerve demyelination. Can J Neurol Sci 1983;10(4):256-60.

[50] Sherman J. Simultaneous pattern-reversal electroretinograms and visual evoked potentials in diseases of the macula and optic nerve. Ann N Y Acad Sci 1982;388:214-26.

[51] Harrison JM, O'Connor PS, Young RS, Kincaid M, Bentley R. The pattern ERG in man following surgical resection of the optic nerve. Invest Ophthalmol Vis Sci 1987;28(3):492-9.

[52] Holder GE. Pattern electroretinography (PERG) and an integrated approach to visual pathway diagnosis. Prog Retin Eye Res 2001;20(4):531-61.

[53] Holder GE. The incidence of abnormal pattern electroretinography in optic nerve demyelination. Electroencephalogr Clin Neurophysiol 1991;78(1):18-26.

[54] Youl BD, Turano G, Miller DH, Towell AD, MacManus DG, Moore SG, et al. The pathophysiology of acute optic neuritis. An association of gadolinium leakage with clinical and electrophysiological deficits. Brain 1991;114 (Pt 6):2437-50.

[55] Hood DC, Xu L, Thienprasiddhi P, Greenstein VC, Odel JG, Grippo TM, et al. The pattern electroretinogram in glaucoma patients with confirmed visual field deficits. Invest Ophthalmol Vis Sci 2005;46(7):2411-8.

[56] Ventura LM, Porciatti V, Ishida K, Feuer WJ, Parrish RK, 2nd. Pattern electroretinogram abnormality and glaucoma. Ophthalmology 2005;112(1):10-9.

[57] Lam BL. Electro-oculogram. In: Lam BL, editor. Electrophysiology of vision : clinical testing and applications. Boca Raton: Taylor & Francis; 2005. p. 105-22.

[58] Gundogan FC, Uysal Y, Erdem U, Sobaci G, Bayraktar MZ. Our normal values of electrooculogram. Gulhane Medical Journal 2006;48(2):79-82.

[59] Brigell M. The visual evoked potential. In: Fishman GA, Birch DG, Holder GE, Brigell M, editors. Electrophysiologic testing in disorders of the retina, optic nerve, and visual pathway. San Francisco, CA: American Academy of Ophthalmology; 1990. p. 237-81.

[60] Gundogan FC, Mutlu FM, Altinsoy HI, Tas A, Oz O, Sobaci G. Pattern visual evoked potentials in the assessment of objective visual acuity in amblyopic children. Int Ophthalmol 2010;30(4):377-83.

[61] Lam BL. Visual Evoked Potential. In: Lam BL, editor. Electrophysiology of vision : clinical testing and applications. Boca Raton: Taylor & Francis; 2005. p. 123-50.

[62] Ladenson PW, Stakes JW, Ridgway EC. Reversible alteration of the visual evoked potential in hypothyroidism. Am J Med 1984;77(6):1010-4.

[63] Tan CT, Murray NM, Sawyers D, Leonard TJ. Deliberate alteration of the visual evoked potential. J Neurol Neurosurg Psychiatry 1984;47(5):518-23.

[64] Sumskii LI, Guppa NS, Sklovskaia ML. [Alteration of the visual evoked potential following concussion]. Vopr Neirokhir 1976 (5):25-30.

[65] Gundogan FC, Demirkaya S, Sobaci G. Is optical coherence tomography really a new biomarker candidate in multiple sclerosis?--A structural and functional evaluation. Invest Ophthalmol Vis Sci 2007;48(12):5773-81.

[66] Gundogan FC, Sobaci G, Bayer A. Pattern visual evoked potentials in the assessment of visual acuity in malingering. Ophthalmology 2007;114(12):2332-7.

Chapter 6

Electronic Communication and Digital Images: Referral Pathways and Clinical Uses in Ophthalmology

Hannah Timlin and Roshini Sanders

Additional information is available at the end of the chapter

http://dx.doi.org/10.5772/58309

1. Introduction

Our eyes are the only place in the body where abnormalities such as blocked blood vessels and pale atrophied nerves can be directly visualised and subsequently diagnosed without further invasive tests. This is due to the transparent properties of the cornea, aqueous humour, lens and vitreous. This unique property of the eye lends itself well to being photographed. We now have the technology to image all the structures of the eye, all the way from the cornea, through the lens to the retina, choroid and optic nerve. This even includes anterior chamber cells and flair. We now live in a world where the average camera has superseded the resolution of the human eye, allowing the ability to visualise small retinal lesions such as exudates only when digital imaging and zooming is performed. Additionally, technology which uses optical coherence tomography and scanning lasers produce images, which show information and data on the layers of the retina and nerve fibre thickness which cannot be visualised by the ophthalmologists' examination. This chapter aims to describe how digital images and internet connections, including the roll out of 3G and 4G mobile networks, are utilised to aid ophthalmologists and benefit patients around the world.

Internet connections have grown exponentially over the last 20 years, connecting rural areas to cities, and developing countries to developed countries. The rapid adoption of smartphones has also helped to increase the number of doctors and patients who have easy access to the internet. This rapid adoption of smartphone internet access is particularly apparent in developing countries, who previously had little internet access due to a sparse fixed line telecommunication infrastructure. The cost of smartphone handsets and mobile data prices are dropping and thus becoming more affordable for many. Broadband, 3G and 4G connections allow these digital images to be sent anywhere around the world within seconds. Thus, eye conditions can be diagnosed in patients who are remote to the doctor, in both place and time.

Ophthalmology departments worldwide are under intensifying pressure to reduce referral waiting times and work at a faster pace to deliver new sight saving treatments. Studies increasingly demonstrate that treatment of potentially blinding conditions, such as wet age related macular degeneration (ARMD) and retinal vein occlusion are most efficacious in preventing sight loss when treatment is commenced promptly [1]. This strain on ophthalmology departments has been compounded by the exponential growth of wet ARMD in an aging population where life expectancy is increasing. This means that traditional systems for referring patients and reviewing them in clinics many weeks later need to be updated to adapt to these time pressures. Digital electronic communication, if embraced, can have a significant impact on ophthalmic service. Digital image referrals can be reviewed within seconds and can avoid an unnecessary wait for the clinic review before investigation or treatment can begin.

2. Benefits of electronic digital diagnosis

Electronic digital diagnoses in ophthalmology mean that the patient and the doctor do not have to meet face to face, nor at the same time. These two basic principles have widespread benefits for the patient, non-ophthalmic clinicians and ophthalmologists;

- The patient doesn't have to travel long distances to see the doctor, benefiting patients' time and reducing cost.
- The patient can be seen in a location and at a time which suits them best.
- The patient's images can be seen by the most appropriate subspecialty doctor, rather than the doctor in the hospital on the day that the patient visits, who may not be an expert in that subspecialty.
- It facilitates rapid discussion of difficult cases between multiple doctors around the world, rather than the patient travelling to different hospitals for multiple opinions.
- It facilitates the screening of referrals, leading to some patients not requiring hospital review.
- The patient can be triaged, ensuring that conditions requiring urgent review and treatment are given priority clinics.
- Doctors can monitor patients' progress through self-photographing and emailing to their consultant.

There are many examples of how Ophthalmology departments worldwide are starting to use digital images to aid with telemedicine, for diagnosis, triage and follow up communication with other ophthalmologists or non-ophthalmic clinicians. Additionally digital images are enhancing communication between patients and their ophthalmologist. Some of these are described below.

http://dx.doi.org/10.5772/58309

3. Anterior segment

3.1. Periocular skin abnormalities

There are many differential diagnoses to eyelid lumps, which may pose diagnostic difficulty for General Practitioners. These lesions are easily amenable to photography with either a standard camera at the GP practice or a slit lamp mounted camera at the optometry practice. The most important thing is to differentiate between benign and malignant lesions. Most benign lesions such as cysts, naevae, chalazia, molluscum contagiosum and xanthelasma need not be seen by an ophthalmologist, whereas malignant lesions require soon review and treatment in an appropriate oculoplastic oncology clinic. The most common eyelid tumour is a basal cell carcinoma, which can be diagnosed in many cases by an ophthalmologist from a photograph though signs such as a skin lump with rolled pearly edges, ulceration, crusting or loss of lashes. However, care must be taken with morphoeic basal cell carcinomas or sebaceous cell carcinomas as these have subtle signs and are often misdiagnosed as scarring or blepharitis from photographs or clinical examination. Patients with an obvious malignant lesion on a referral photograph can be directly booked into a one-stop minor procedure clinic. This misses out the assessment clinic step, thus reducing the time from referral to treatment.

It is important to estimate the size of a malignant lesion so that appropriate reconstruction can be planned in the correct location, such as theatre if the lesion is large rather than a clinical procedure room if the lesion is small. This can be difficult to do on digital images and we have found it extremely useful for referrers to place a ruler within the photograph.

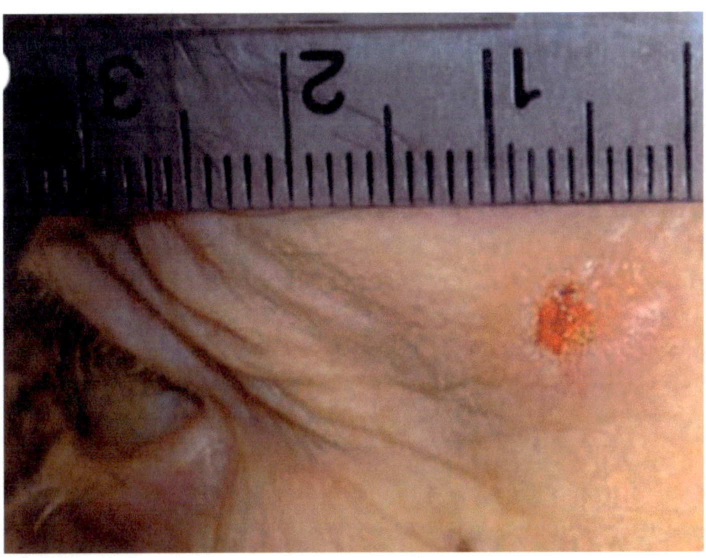

Figure 1. Photograph of a 10mm Periocular Basal Cell Carcinoma referred by an optometrist. This shows the classic signs of rolled pearly edges with central ulceration. This patient was booked directly into a minor procedure list for excision and rhomboid flap reconstruction.

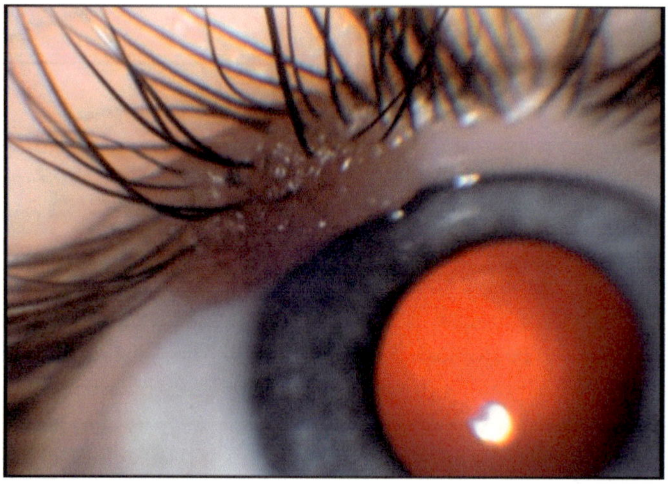

Figure 2. Photograph of an eyelid naevus, demonstrating normal growth of lashes though the benign lesion

3.1.1. Patient communication examples

Although there is limited published evidence of the use of electronic digital diagnosis in the periocular area of the skin by ophthalmologists, we can utilize the experience from dermatologists. In Brisbane, patient generated photographs of melanocytic skin lesions from camera phones showed 69% diagnostic concordance with face to face diagnosis, suggesting potential for remote diagnosis [2]. In Dundee, referrals of suspected malignant skin lesions from GPs which included digital images had reduced time to diagnosis by 81% and time to treatment by 30%, with diagnostic accuracy comparable to face to face diagnosis [3].

Digital images can also be useful for monitoring progress following skin surgery. In Heidelberg, plastic surgeons monitor post-operative skin flaps using smart phone images sent from the patient at home. Compared to traditional in-person clinic review, the response time to re-exploration was significantly shorter [4]. In Taiwan, this method enabled rapid and thus successful re-exploration [5].

It is relatively simple for patients to use their own phone to photograph themselves and email the image within a few seconds, without having to get off their sofa. This can be planned every day postoperatively, or as and when the patient has concerns. It is easy to foresee how this enables rapid detection of problems when compared with a planned one week follow up hospital appointment. It is not unimaginable that patients following ptosis surgery or periocular reconstruction could be monitored by their consultant through smartphone images, with a hospital visit only required if an abnormality is seen on the photographs such as erythema and discharge. Other potential examples of their use are; a patient emailing in a photograph showing over correction of a ptosis could be advised to perform lash traction over an email without needing to attend the hospital, or a patient emailing in a camera phone image of a graft showing contraction and ectropion can be advised to perform firm massage without having to attend the hospital.

http://dx.doi.org/10.5772/58309

3.2. Corneal, conjunctival and anterior chamber abnormalities

Many corneal and conjunctival images are amenable to digital imaging for example pterygium, pinguecula, conjunctival pigmentation, corneal scarring, corneal vascularisation, ulcers and hypopion. Larger lesions can be photographed with a standard camera, whereas smaller lesions, particularly of the cornea are best imaged using a slit lamp camera. Various illumination techniques commonly used by the ophthalmologist can be used for the slit lamp camera also. Direct diffuse illumination is most commonly used. However, more information can be gained by using the fine slit direct illumination or retroillumination using the red reflex from the fundus. Indirect and scleral scatter can be harder to photograph.

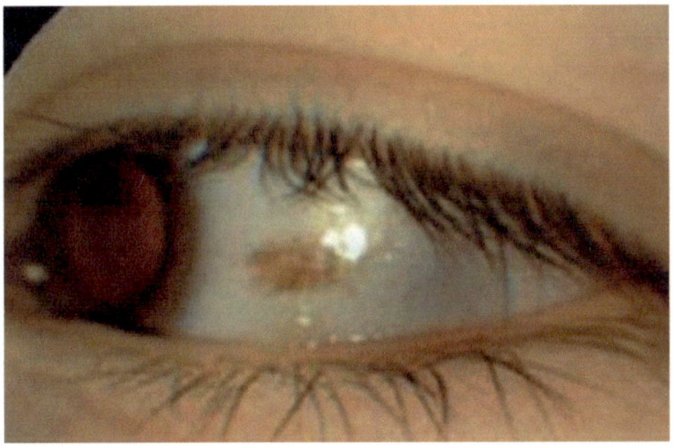

Figure 3. Photograph of a benign pigmented conjunctival naevus in a child

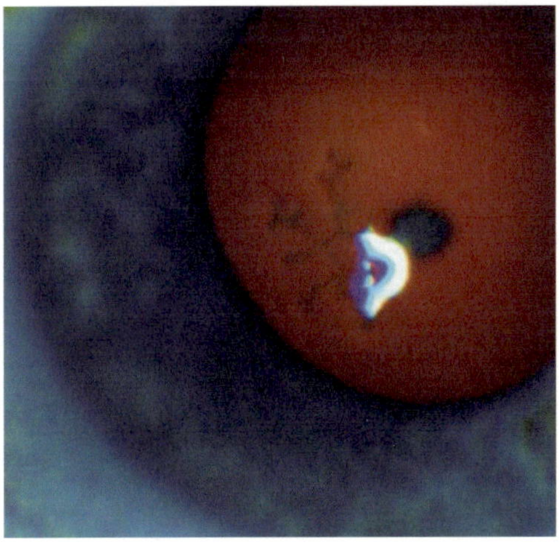

Figure 4. Slit lamp photograph of a dendritic ulcer seen with retroillumination, using the red reflex of the fundus to illuminate the corneal epithelial lesion.

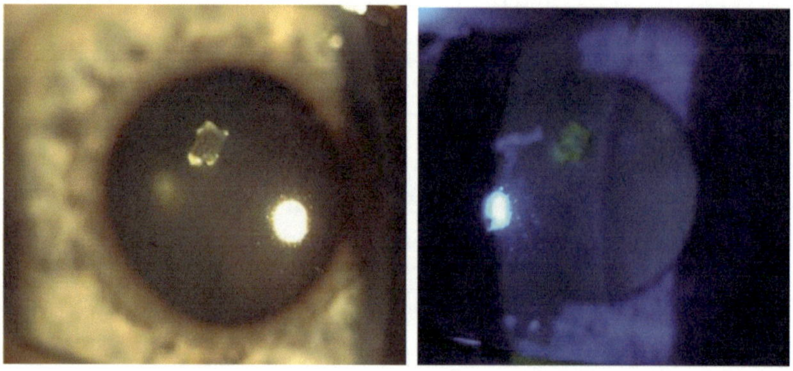

Figure 5. Slit lamp photographs using white light with no filter and cobalt blue filter showing a white foreign body on the cornea which stains with fluorescence.

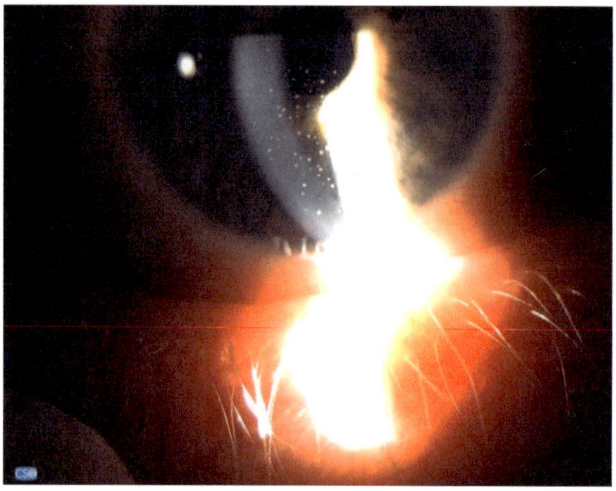

Figure 6. Slit lamp photograph using a broad beam of light showing keratic precipitates on the endothelium

3.2.1. Non-ophthalmic clinician communication example

In Perth, Western Australia, a portable hand held slit lamp camera has been created to be small, portable and simple to operate by health care workers across the large geographical area of Western Australia. They have demonstrated that this instrument had good correlation to slit lamp anterior segment image diagnoses [6].

3.2.2. Patient communication example

Perhaps ophthalmologists could learn from dermatologists in Austria, whose patients on biologics for psoriasis send in weekly camera phone images for monitoring [7]. This could potentially be used for conditions such as mucous membrane pemphigoid, where frequent

http://dx.doi.org/10.5772/58309

images over years can perhaps be made into a time-lapse video, which could potentially show clearer evidence of disease progression than clinical drawings. This technology is currently used in natural history programmes to demonstrate slowly changing environments such as sand dunes, within a few seconds of film, and could be easily adapted into the ophthalmic domain.

4. Posterior segment

4.1. Glaucoma

Glaucoma is a massive worldwide problem. The problem with open angle glaucoma is the lack of symptoms perceived by the patient. This means that patients will only self-present with end-stage glaucoma once central vision is being lost, when treatment is less effective. In poorer communities, most of the population is not examined regularly by an optometrist or ophthalmologist. In these places, the issue is the lack of diagnosis, which could be assisted with the use of health care assistants with camera phones, sending the images over the internet to a distant ophthalmologist for diagnosis.

In more affluent communities, optometrists are trained to rigorously screen for any sign or suspicion of glaucoma and refer to a hospital assessment e.g. raised intraocular pressure, field loss and abnormal optic disc appearance including thinned rim, change in cup disc ratio and disc haemorrhage. The main issues here are that of a high rate of false positives (the worried well) and the large volume of patients requiring long term hospital follow up. Many of these glaucoma suspects require hospital review over a few years only to then be discharged without requiring any treatment. Additionally, many ocular hypertensives are detected and require long term follow up without ever developing any field loss. These two examples constitute a large volume of patients seen in hospital eye services, and who would benefit from a digital electronic virtual clinic. All the data required by the consultant for the patients' management can be viewed digitally with computerised field of vision data sheets, intraocular pressure documentation and optic disc images with or without further ancillary glaucoma tests including red free photographs of the nerve fibre layer, optic disc Ocular Coherence Tomography, Heidelberg Retina Tomography and Scanning Laser Polarimetry. Thus large numbers of patients can be monitored by the consultant ophthalmologist virtually.

There is an obvious difference between slit lamp disc examination of the optic disc, which is binocular and thus 3D, and a standard fundus image which is 2D. The optic disc rim shape and cup disc ratio in 2D images are often interpreted using the colour change from the peach coloured optic rim to the whiter coloured optic cup and the distortion of blood vessels, rather than depth perception. This can lead to inaccurate interpretation of the optic disc. However, this can be accommodated for to some extent using serial photographs to identify subtle anatomical change over time and with stereo images where two photographs of the optic disc are taken from slightly different angles and viewed on a screen either side by side and viewed with specially designed goggles or displayed alternately with a fast flicker, where no goggles are required.

4.1.1. Allied ophthalmic professionals communication examples

Data from Virtual Glaucoma Clinics in Portsmouth have been published. These virtual clinics involve the glaucoma consultant electronically reviewing digital disc images, Humphrey visual field tests and Goldman intraocular pressure results to assess new glaucoma referrals without meeting the patients. 94% of disc photographs were gradable and only 32% of patients required to be accepted into the hospital eye clinic, thus saving 1400 clinic appointments per year [8]. Swansea performed a virtual glaucoma clinic trial using scanning laser ophthalmoscopy. Although 22% of images were unable to be graded, the remaining had 94% sensitivity and 87% specificity when compared to clinical assessment, with no case of glaucoma being misdiagnosed [9]. These two examples demonstrate how digital images can enable a consultant to review more glaucoma referrals in a shorter period of time than if examining the patient themselves thus saving money.

In these two published virtual glaucoma clinics, the patients still attended the hospital but were seen directly by photographers, nurses and hospital optometrists. There is potential for the tests to be performed at the patients' local optometry practice to save on travel time and costs. However, this would be limited by the costs of purchasing investigative equipment such as computerised field of vision analysers and fundus cameras.

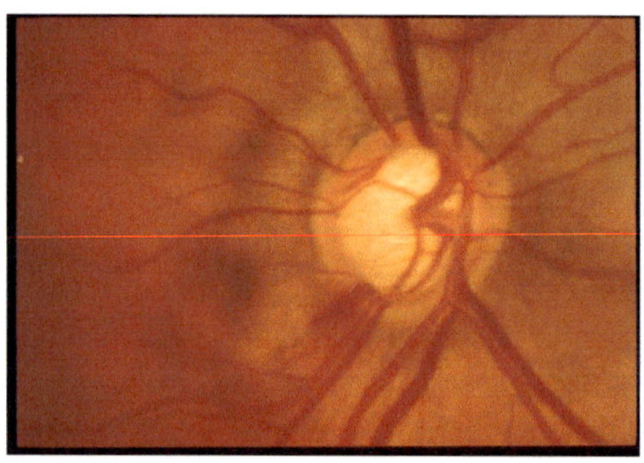

Figure 7. Right optic disc photograph taken by an optometrist at a local practise. This shows inferior temporal disc haemorrhage and rim thinning. This rim thinning is seen on this 2D image by the location of both the colour change and blood vessel distortion. This patient was given a glaucoma assessment clinic and diagnosed with glaucoma.

4.2. Disc anomalies

Normal optic discs have a huge range of appearances. Thus there is a large grey area where an unusual looking disc can either be at one end of the normal range or be showing pathology. Pattern recognition plays a large part in determining a diagnosis in these patients. Optometrists and General Practitioners see large volumes of normal optic discs and thus find it difficult to distinguish between disease and normal range. The main condition which causes concern in this area is bilateral swollen discs with diagnosis of possible raised intracranial pressure. This can trigger referral for a CT scan and lumbar puncture, both of which have side effects. Actual diagnoses are often myopic discs, where the large peripapillary atrophy is misinterpreted as disc oedema and swelling when performing a uniocular examination through a direct ophthalmoscope by a non-ophthalmologist, or optic disc drusen which can give a lumpy raised appearance and scalloped margins with anomalous vascular branching. Digital imaging and an ophthalmologist's opinion can negate the need for these unnecessary tests in many within a few seconds of seeing the image.

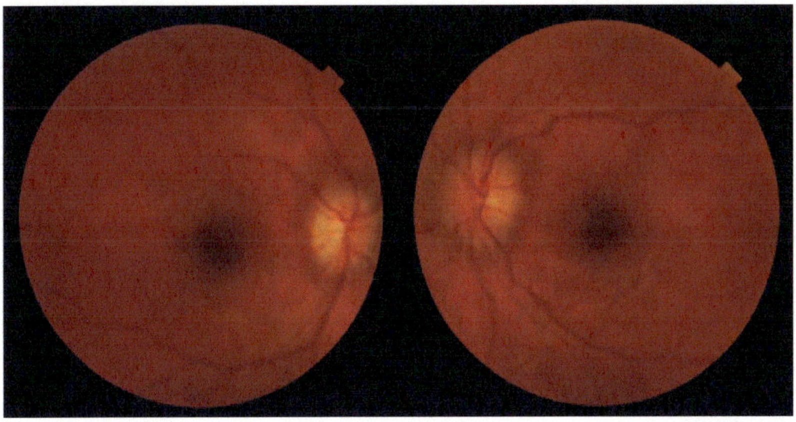

Figure 8. Fundus photographs of a child, taken at their local optometry practice showing bilateral disc swelling. This is characterised on digital 2D image as blurred disc margin due to oedema, curving of blood vessels over the swollen nerve with an angle as the vessel flattens onto the retina, reduced or no colour change from optic disc rim to cup due to swelling. The digital electronic referral of these images was seen within minutes by a consultant ophthalmologist who was able to arrange a CT scan and paediatric admission to the patient's local hospital all of which was performed within 2 hours, without the need for long travel and time delay to the regional Emergency Eye Clinic. The patient was diagnosed with a brain tumour and raised intracranial pressure.

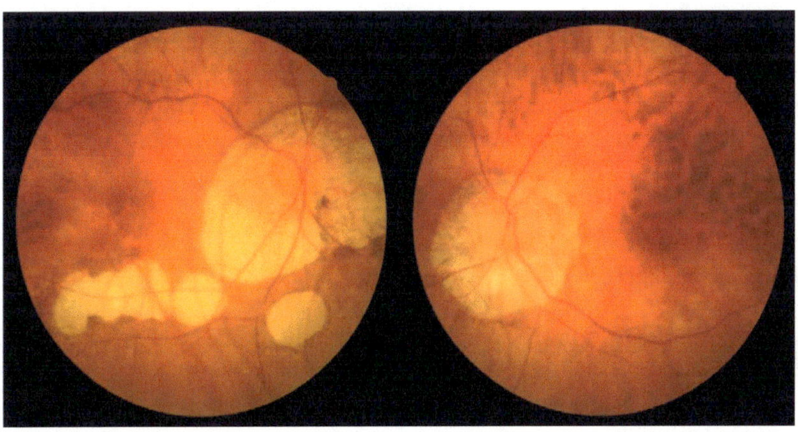

Figure 9. Fundus photographs of a patient with myopic discs. This patient was misdiagnosed as swollen discs due to the 'large' pale discs with no visible cup. An ophthalmologist can see in the photo that this is significant peripapillary atrophy and reassure the referrer. The digital image electronic referral means that a diagnosis is made quickly and the patient does not need to travel to the eye department or undergo CT scans or lumbar punctures.

4.3. Retinopathy of prematurity

Retinopathy of prematurity guidelines recommend fundus screening to be performed 1 to 2 weekly in babies of <32 weeks gestation or <=1.5kg at birth [10]. Physical examination with an indirect ophthalmoscope and indentation is a difficult skill to master and is thus done by very experienced ophthalmologists. Additionally, the process of examination can be distressing for the baby and often affects their vital signs. The guidelines recommend grading retinopathy according to the area of retina where normal vascular development has occurred as well as the extent of abnormal vessels that have grown, along with their sequelae. These grades dictate whether treatment of the peripheral retina with laser is recommended, which is done by an expert usually in a tertiary referral centre [10].

4.3.1. Non-ophthalmic clinician communication examples

However, these premature babies have multiple other comorbidities making transfer over long distances to tertiary hospitals precarious for their health and life. Studies have shown that only 6% of these babies actually develop sight threatening disease [10] and require treatment by a specialist ophthalmologist. Thus, this condition is ideally suited to digital image screening where babies in peripheral hospitals have their fundus photographs taken by trained nurses. These are then emailed to the specialist ophthalmologist in the distant tertiary centre for grading. This method of viewing the fundus is also potentially less distressing for the baby. For some time, the wide field 120 degrees camera Retcam has been used for this purpose, producing clear images and reliable grading [11-16]. The use of this digital screening system means that most babies can stay in their hospital surroundings without the instability of a transfer. The only babies requiring transfer are those 6% requiring laser treatment, without which vision loss and blindness can develop. More recently, the noncontact ultra-widefield Optos dual wavelength scanning laser ophthalmoscope Optomap is being used for this purpose in Oxford [17].

Recent advances in neonatology have led to an increase in the number of premature babies at risk of sight loss. However, the frequency of sight threatening retinopathy is low, meaning that experts in the field are small in number and often covering a large geographic area. In poorer, remote populations, these fundus cameras could allow robust and effective retinopathy of prematurity screening, where there had previously been none.

4.4. Diabetic retinopathy

4.4.1. Non-clinical personnel communication examples (medical photographers)

A national screening programme for diabetic retinopathy has been set up in the UK [18] with the use of mobile non-mydriatic fundus cameras operated by technicians. This programme enables all diabetic patients to have a fundus examination close to their home. These fundus images are graded electronically, with patients only needing to travel to the hospital ophthalmology clinic if there are signs of sight threatening retinopathy or maculopathy. In some regions, Optical Coherence Tomography images are also taken to screen for macula oedema, thus further reducing the number of patients requiring hospital appointments. The attendance rate is likely to be higher if the patients have to give up less time and money for travelling,

http://dx.doi.org/10.5772/58309

thus screening occurs in multiple locations with mobile cameras. Teleretinal screening data for diabetic retinopathy has also been published from the USA [19,20], Bahrain [21], Canada [22,23] and France [24].

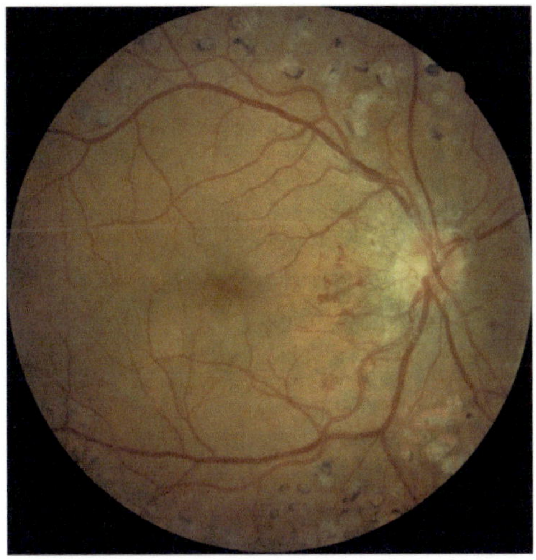

Figure 10. Diabetic Retinopathy screening photograph taken with a non-mydriatic fundus camera showing proliferative diabetic retinopathy with new vessels visible and previous pigmented pan retinal photocoagulation scars.

4.5. Wet age related macular degeneration

Age Related Macular Degeneration is a common condition causing visual loss. Unfortunately, only the less common wet subtype is treatable. Unnecessary referral and review of patients with the dry subtype are common and results in a large number of unnecessary hospital appointments. The wet type results from abnormal growth of vessels from the choroidal circulation into the retina and is identified clinically by intraretinal fluid and / or haemorrhage. Intraretinal fluid is best seen as retinal thickening when examining binocularly on the slit lamp, which cannot be perceived on a fundus photograph. However, photographic signs of fluid identifiable are a grey appearance, loss of focus of fine detail of the retina and distortion of blood vessels. Additionally Optical Coherence Tomography machines are becoming more widely available. These are now used routinely in the macular degeneration clinics as they can show even very small pockets of fluid within the retina which are not perceivable on slit lamp examination of the fundus. Use of these fundus and OCT images with referrals, has the scope to avoid the unnecessary hospital visit of a patient with dry age related macular degeneration.

4.5.1. Allied ophthalmic professionals communication examples

Evaluating colour retinal images of patients referred with suspected wet age related macular degeneration has been reported to have high sensitivity and specificity and facilitate more timely treatment [25]. In York, there is a Mobile Community Eye Care Clinic with OCT machines. This is relocated overnight on a 4 weekly location cycle around the region, with fundus and OCT images viewed at the central hospital [26]. In Salford, an optometry practise with an OCT machine refers in patient details with the OCT image via nhsmail, meaning that patients can attend directly for a treatment clinic [26]. Thus the patient's number of visits to the hospital is reduced.

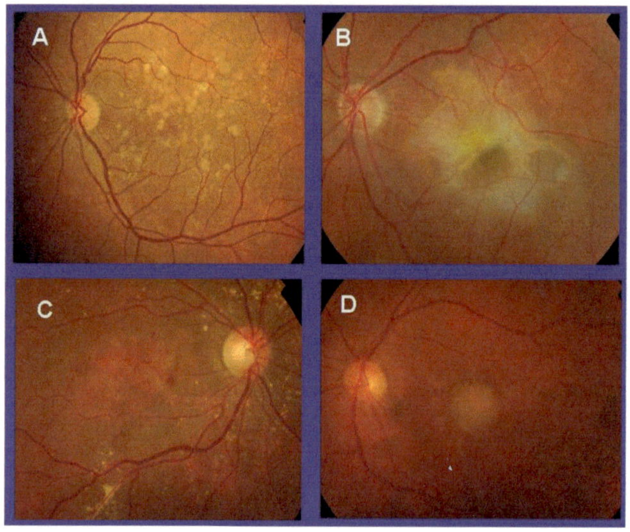

Figure 11. Four fundus photographs of patients referred by optometrists with macular degeneration, illustrating the benefit of fundus photographs when triaging hospital referrals. Figure 11A shows dry age related macular degeneration, which does not require hospital review. Figure 11B shows scaring from advanced wet age related macular degeneration with vision worse than 6/96, who can be directed to the low vision services. Figure 11C shows wet age related macular degeneration, which can be triaged to an urgent wet ARMD treatment clinic. Figure 11D shows a pigment epithelial detachment, which needs triage into an assessment clinic within 2 weeks. This last image illustrates the limitations of using images. In this case, the patient requires an Optical Coherence Tomography image, which their local optometrist did not have and thus required to be done at a hospital visit, in order to detect any intraretinal fluid that would require treatment.

Treatment of wet age related macular degeneration requires multiple intravitreal injections of anti vascular endothelial growth factor often over many years. Best visual outcomes occur when treatment is given within the first two weeks of disease onset. However, the number of wet age related macular degeneration patients are already greater than capacity, and with an aging population this is set to worsen. One solution to this crisis is a virtual clinic, which can be used to follow up patients who have been treated. Electronic Patient Databases have been shown to facilitate virtual wet age related macular degeneration diagnosis and monitoring by consultants, who can view a patient's vision, fundus image and OCT without face to face contact. This increases the number of patients monitored by a consultant within the same session [26].

4.6. Retinal vein occlusion

Central and branch retinal vein occlusions are common causes of reduced vision. The vast majority of cases do not require treatment. However, patients need to be monitored for the

http://dx.doi.org/10.5772/58309

growth of new vessels, which requires laser treatment. More recently, treatment with intravitreal steroid or anti vascular endothelial growth factor have shown benefit in patients with macular oedema. Additionally, manufacturers report better visual outcomes if treatment is commenced promptly. Therefore patients with a vein occlusion would benefit from a digital electronic referral from the optometrist in a similar way to those with wet age related macular degeneration, where the referral is made via a fundus image email along with an Optical Coherence Tomography image when available to demonstrate the macular oedema. This would enable rapid triage for a soon appointment directly into a treatment clinic when macular oedema is seen.

4.7. Retinal lesions

Abnormal pigmentary changes are commonly detected by optometrists at routine review in asymptomatic patients. Common lesions detected are choroidal naevae, chorioretinal scars, congenital hypertrophy of retinal pigmented epithelium, laser scars and myelinated nerve fibres. None of these lesions are visually significant and thus are best managed in the community with digital imaging. The digital image acts firstly as a referral to an ophthalmologist who will often be happy to diagnose the condition on the image alone. Secondly, the image acts as a record for long term monitoring. If a choroidal naevus shows even a small growth from one image to the next, then referral for investigation for melanoma is required. Subtle changes in lesion appearance are much easier to detect when comparing image to image, rather than fundus examination to a drawing. Thus digital imaging enables rapid diagnosis and accurate monitoring for malignant signs.

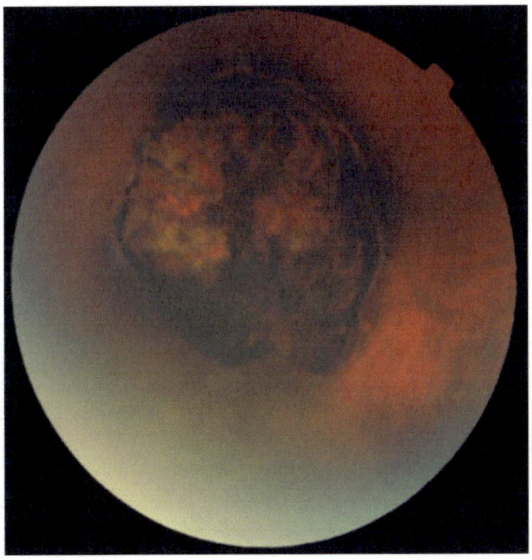

Figure 12. Fundus image showing pigmented chorioretinal scar. This is most likely a longstanding scar as the lesion has sharp pigmentary boundaries and no acute signs of haemorrhage or exudation. Therefore, the patient does not require hospital review.

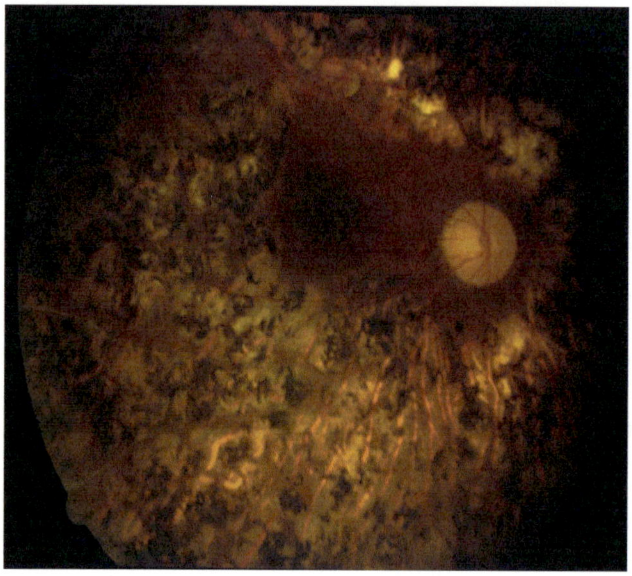

Figure 13. Fundus image showing heavy pan retinal photocoagulation, not requiring hospital review

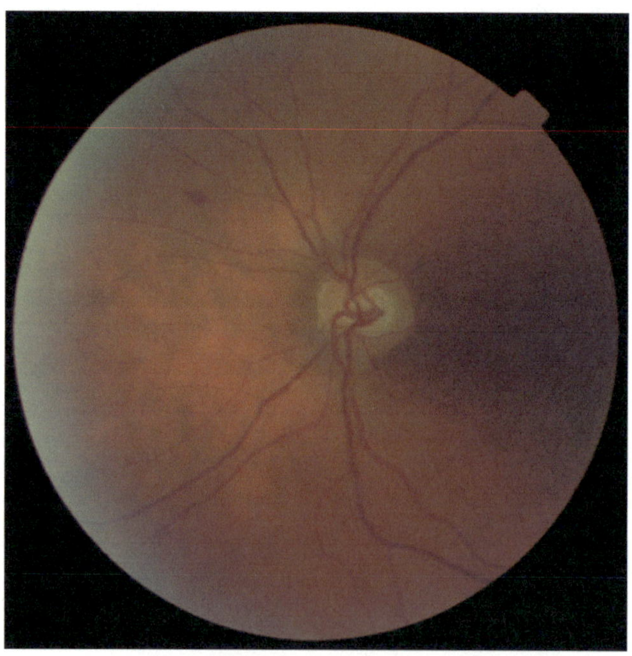

Figure 14. Fundus image showing an isolated small blot haemorrhage

http://dx.doi.org/10.5772/58309

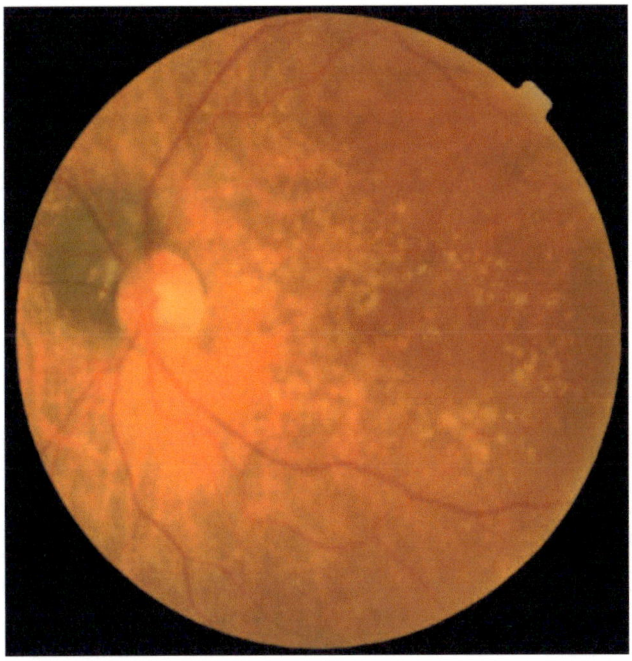

Figure 15. Fundus image showing a choroidal naevus at the disc and drusen. Careful monitoring is required and changes in the lesion are best detected by comparing fundus image to fundus image side by side.

4.8. Optos

One of the limitations of standard fundus imaging is the small field of view of 45 degrees, making it difficult to capture the mid peripheral and peripheral retina. Optos have developed the optomap ultra-widefield scanning laser ophthalmoscope which produces a pseudo-colour image [27].This is a significant addition to the current ophthalmic imaging tools. It has a 200 degree field of view enabling peripheral lesion imaging whilst simultaneously imaging the disc and macula, which enables the location of the lesion in relation to them. This is especially useful for picking up retinal detachments by non-ophthalmologists or documenting peripheral choroidal naevae or melanomas for long term follow up. The two main benefits to this system are that dilation is not required, and that it requires very little training to perform enabling a non-ophthalmologist to view large areas of the retina and share electronically via email.

4.8.1. Non clinical personnel example (medical photographers)

Studies in an emergency eye clinic have shown the Optos limitations at picking up only 33% of peripheral retinal tears and holes [28], although interestingly, this was the same accuracy as their casualty doctor's examination. However, it accurately photographed retinal detachments, which are commonly missed on conventional fundus imaging.

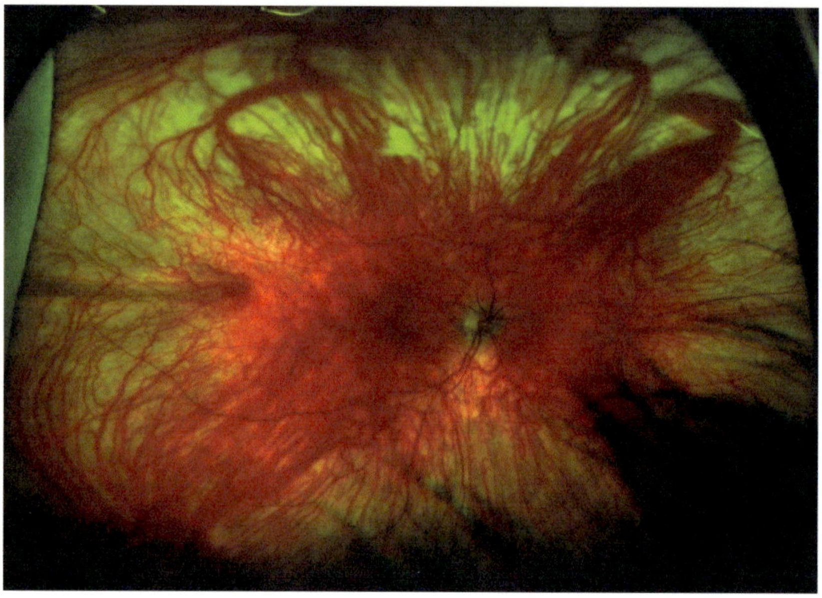

Figure 16. Optomap fundus image of a patient with ocular albinism showing more peripheral changes than can be visualised with standard fundus cameras.

5. Video conferencing

Live video conferencing facilitates live consultation between either doctor and patient or doctor and the doctor/optometrist/nurse currently examining a patient. It requires a faster internet connection than that needed for sending images via email, which is becoming increasingly available in more rural areas. Skype and FaceTime are commonly used software which are user friendly and regularly used non-professionally by the internet generation to communicate to friends and family. Thus it is an acceptable and non-frightening means of communication for both patients and doctors.

5.1. Non-ophthalmic clinicians example

Telemedicine video conferencing has been utilised in Western Australia, in a remote hospital where an ophthalmologist from Perth only visits twice a year. The average video conference length was 30 minutes and reduced emergency air evacuations to Perth from seven per year to none. This lead to a huge cost saving, better utilisation of air transfer staff and potentially increased patient satisfaction at remaining in their own home [29].

This is clearly a valuable resource in locations where there is no local ophthalmologist. Perhaps there will be increased access in Accident and Emergency Departments worldwide, which would most likely be utilised at night when ophthalmologists are on duty from home.

Video Technology is useful for conditions such as nystagmus and pupil abnormalities, which are difficult to capture with photographs.

6. Referrals to the hospital eye service

Trying to encompass all ophthalmic telemedical digital imaging techniques is the Central Ophthalmic electronic Referral Unit (COeRU) in Fife, Scotland. Here, patients have benefited from a Government financed set up of broadband connection from all community optometrists to the hospital. All referrals to the hospital Ophthalmology Department are done electronically by the local optometrist with electronic images from any machinery attached. It has demonstrated a global benefit to the hospital department of; a reduction in waiting times from 14 to 4 weeks, a reduction in the number of patients seen in the emergency clinic, and a reduction in 'Did Not Attend' patients [30]. This has had enormous benefit from patients who are now seen rapidly, especially patients with wet ARMD who are rapidly seen and treated.

The pilot study was set up in 2005 on 350 consecutive patients who were electronically referred with attached digital images by their community optometrists to the hospital using NHS mail [31]. The results were encouraging and showed that sight threatening disease could be identified early and that 37% of referral images allowed an electronic diagnosis which did not require a hospital appointment. Following the success of the pilot, the scheme was rolled out to the entire region in 2007 and a central ophthalmic electronic referral unit (COeRU) was created. In 2011, the five year data was studied, which analysed over 40,000 patient episodes [30]. The new electronic pathway meant that waiting times were reduced, which was mainly because the old tortuous paper referral pathway was bypassed by emailing the referral directly to the ophthalmology department and simultaneously copying in the GP. Significant changes to service delivery were achieved with all sight threatening disease seen within days rather than weeks, 15% of new patient referrals retained in the community and between 20 – 25% reduction in both the casualty attendance and DNA (did not attend) rate.

The Fife service data following implementation of COeRU was compelling and fed into three business case submissions to the Scottish government between 2009 – 2010 for electronic connection between community optometrists and hospital ophthalmic departments across the whole of Scotland.

In 2010 the Scottish government health department (SGHD) committed 6.6 million pounds for electronic connections between the community and the hospitals and in 2011 the Eyecare Integration Project was formed. The group has representation from Eyecare Scotland (all Scottish lead clinicians), Optometry Scotland, general practice (GP) and the Royal National Institute for the Blind. There is also representation from subdivisions of the SGHD that support the project to include the Practitioner Services Division (PSD), eHealth, SCI Gateway, ISD (information and statistics division) and National Information Systems Groups (NISG). The goals of this project are to provide a nationally supported electronic link between every community optometry practice and hospital ophthalmic department, which will enable electronic referrals with attached digital images. Concurrently the PSD are working on electronic software that will connect with the optometry practices' IT management systems to enable electronic payment verification [32].

The effect of this Scotland wide implementation of digital image referral is much awaited by other regions of the UK and worldwide.

7. Limitations of diagnoses with digital imaging

One of the main limitations of digital images is that they are 2D rather than the 3D image seen when using the slit lamp or indirect ophthalmoscope binocularly. This can make it difficult to identify oedema or raised suspicious choroidal naevae. However, the Optical Coherence Tomography images can help to overcome this concern, by providing a cross sectional view of the retina. Another difficulty in using digital images is the difficulty in imaging the peripheral retina, which is the common location of retinal tears. The Optomap ultrawide field images have improved peripheral retinal visualisation on images and have been shown to pick up lesions posterior to the equator with high specificity. However, they do not pick up all lesions anterior to the equator [33].

8. Conclusion

With the widespread access to camera phones in both developed and developing countries, imaging of eyes by patients and health carers becomes more accessible. Additionally, accessories have been designed to fit onto phone cameras to act as non mydriatic fundus cameras [34]. The new Portable Eye Examination Kit (PEEK) [35] is a smartphone App that enables health carers to perform detailed eye examinations including vision, fields, lens and fundus imaging in extremely rural homes with only a £300 iPhone and clip on camera hardware with little training. The diagnoses and management plans are then made remotely in the UK from the electronic data and images. Patients can then be located for treatment via the GPS coordinates of their home, which is automatically attached to smartphone photographs at the time of image capture.

The future of ophthalmology will undoubtedly involve more virtual clinics and perhaps more digital imaging from patients themselves. Perhaps there will be a time where all diabetics have a fundus camera phone accessory to photograph their own fundi and email their images to the hospital graders themselves.

In summary, electronic communication with digital images and teleconferencing has huge potential for eye care service delivery. It has the ability to overcome geographical barriers and pick up sight threatening disease at the earliest opportunity. With the exponential growth in global electronic communication there is no doubt that this will be incorporated into several health service delivery models. We have outlined the existing models within ophthalmology and have also outlined the future growth areas.

http://dx.doi.org/10.5772/58309

Author details

Hannah Timlin and Roshini Sanders

*Address all correspondence to: hannahtimlin@nhs.net.uk

Cataract Unit, Queen Margaret Hospital, Dunfermline, NHS Fife, UK

References

[1] Matthe E, Sandner D. Early treatment of exudative age-related macular degeneration with ranibizumab: the key to success. Ophthalmologe. 2011;108(3):237-43.

[2] Boyce Z, Gilmore S, Xu C, Soyer HP. The remote assessment of melanocytic skin lesions: a viable alternative to face-face consultation. Dermatology 2011;223(3):244-50.

[3] Tadros A, Murdoch R, Stevenson JH. Digital image referral for suspected skin malignancy – A pilot study of 300 patients. Journal of Plastic, Reconstructive & Aesthetic Surgery 2009;62:1048-1053.

[4] Engel H, Huang JJ, Tsao CK, Lin CY, Chou PY, Brey EM, Henry SL, Cheng MH. Remote real-time monitoring of free flaps via smartphone photography and 3G wireless Internet: a prospective study evidencing diagnostic accuracy. Microsurgery 2011;31(8):589-95.

[5] Varkey P, Tan NC, Girotto R, Tang WR, Liu YT, Chen HC. A picture speaks a thousand words: the use of digital photography and the internet as a cost-effective tool in monitoring free flaps. Annals of Plastic Surgery 2008;60(1):45-8.

[6] Kumar S, Yogesan K, Constable IJ. Telemedical diagnosis of anterior segment eye disease: validation of digital slit-lamp still images. Eye 2009;23(3):652-60.

[7] Koller S, Hofmann-Wellenhof R, Hayn D, Weger W, Kastner P, Schreier G, Salmhofer W. Acta Dermato-Venereologica 2011;91(6):680-5.

[8] Trikha S, Macgregor C, Jeffery, Kirwan J. The Portsmouth-based glaucoma refinement scheme: a role for virtual clinics in the future. Eye 2012;26(10):1288-94.

[9] Rathod D, Win T, Pickering S, Austin M. Incorporation of a virtual assessment into a care pathway for initial glaucoma management: feasibility study. Clinical & Experimental Ophthalmology 2008;36(6):543-6.

[10] Guidelines for the screening and treatment of retinopathy of prematurity. May 2008. Royal college of ophthalmologists and Royal college of Paediatrics and Child Health.

[11] Lorenz B, Spasovska K, Elflein H, Schneider N. Wide-field digital imaging based telemedicine for screening for acute retinopathy of prematurity. Six-year results of a

multicentre field study. Graefes Archive for Clinical & Experimental Ophthalmology 2009;247(9):1251-62.

[12] Weaver DT, Murdock TJ. Telemedicine detection of type 1 ROP in a distant neonatal intensive care unit. Journal of Aapos: American Association for Pediatric Ophthalmology & Strabismus 2012;16(3):229-33.

[13] Salcone EM, Johnston S, Vanderveen D. Review of the use of digital imaging in retinopathy of prematurity screening. Seminars in Ophthalmology 2010;25(5-6):214-7.

[14] Dai S, Chow K, Vincent A. Efficacy of wide-field digital retinal imaging for retinopathy of prematurity screening. Clinical & Experimental Ophthalmology 2011;39(1): 23-9.

[15] Ells AL, Holmes JM, Astle WF, Williams G, Leske DA, Fielden M, Uphill B, Jennett P, Hebert M. Telemedicine approach to screening for severe retinopathy of prematurity: a pilot study. Ophthalmology 2003;110(11):2113-7.

[16] Schwartz SD, Harrison SA, Ferrone PJ, Trese MT. Telemedical evaluation and management of retinopathy of prematurity using a fiberoptic digital fundus camera. Ophthalmology 2000;107(1):25-8.

[17] Patel CK, Fung THM, Muqit MMK, Mordant DJ, Brett J, Smith L, Adams E. Non-contact ultra-widefield imaging of retinopathy of prematurity using the Optos dual wavelength scanning laser ophthalmoscope. Eye 2013;27:589-596.

[18] www.diabeticeye.screening.nhs.uk/national

[19] Ogunyemi O, Terrien E, Eccles A, Patty L, George S, Fish A, Teklehaimanot S, Ilapakurthi R, Aimiuwu O, Baker R. Teleretinal screening for diabetic retinopathy in six Los Angeles urban safety-net clinics: Initial findings. AMIA Annual Symposium Proceedings / AMIA Symposium 2011:1027-35.

[20] Li Z, Wu C, Olayiwola JN, Hilaire DS, Huang JJ. Conneticut Medicine 2012;76(2): 85-90.

[21] Al alawi E, Ahmed AA. Screening for diabetic retinopathy: the first telemedicine approach in a primary care setting in Bahrain. Middle East African Journal of Ophthalmology 2012;19(3):295-8.

[22] Boucher MC, Nguyen QT, Angioi K. Mass Community Screening for diabetic retinopathy using a nonmydriatic camera with telemedicine. Canadian Journal of Ophthalmology 2005;40(6):734-42.

[23] Choremis J, Chow DR. Use of telemedicine in screening for diabetic retinopathy. Canadian Journal of Ophthalmology 2003;38(7):575-9.

[24] Massin P, Aubert JP, Erginay A, Bourovitch JC, Benmehidi A, Audran G, Bernit B, Jamet M, Collet C, Laloi-Michelin M, Guillausseau PJ, Gaudric A, Marre M. Screen-

ing for diabetic retinopathy: the first telemedical approach in a primary care setting in France. Diabetes & Metabolism 2004;30(5):451-7.

[25] Maberley DAL, Isbister C, MacKenzie P, Aralar A. An evaluation of photographic screening for neovascular age-related macular degeneration. Eye 2005;19:611-616.

[26] Amoaku W, Blakeney S, Freeman M, Gale R, Johnston R, Kelly SP, McLauglan, Sahu D, Varma D, Action on AMD Group. Action on AMD. Optimising patient management: act now to ensure current and continual delivery of best possible patient care. Eye 201; 26(S1)S2-S21.

[27] www.optos.com

[28] Khandhadia S, Madhusudhana KC, Kostakou A, Forrester JV, Newsom RSB. Use of optomap for retinal screening within an eye casualty setting. British Journal of Ophthalmology 2009;93(1):52-55.

[29] Kumar S, Yogesan K, Hudson B, Tay-Kearney ML, Constable IJ. Emergency eye care in rural Australia: role of internet. Eye 2006;20(12):1342-4.

[30] Borooah S, Grant B, Blaikie A, Styles C, Sutherland S, Forrest G, Curry P, Legg J, Walker A, Sanders R. Using electronic referral with digital imaging between primary and secondary ophthalmic services: a long term prospective analysis of regional service redesign. Eye 2013;27:392-397.

[31] Cameron JR, Ahmed S, Curry P, Forrest G, Sanders R. Impact of direct electronic referral with ocular imaging to a hospital eye service. Eye 2009;23:1134-1140

[32] Timlin H, Styles C, McPherson S, Sanders R. Eyecare Integration Project (Scotland); Electronic connections between primary and secondary sectors. Eye News 2013;20(1); 6-10.

[33] Mackenzie PJ, Russell M, Ma PE, Isbister CM, Maberley DA. Sensitivity and specificity of the optos optomap for detecting peripheral retinal lesions. Retina 2007;27(8): 1119-24.

[34] Lamirel C, Bruce BB, Wright DW, Newman, NJ, Biousse V. Nonmydriatic digital ocular fundus photography on the iPhone 3G: the FOTO-ED study. Archives of Ophthalmology 2012;130(7):939-40.

[35] www.peekvision.org

Section 2

Updates in Anterior Segment Diseases

Chapter 7

Dry eye — An Insight into Meibomian Gland Dysfunction

Vikas Tah, Kamran Saha, James Myerscough, Muhammad Ahad, Jason Ho, Pranev Sharma, Farihah Tariq and Stephen Tuft

Additional information is available at the end of the chapter

http://dx.doi.org/10.5772/58566

1. Introduction

The term 'Dry Eyes' was first coined in 1950 by the Ophthalmologist Andrew De Roeth (1893–1981): a dacryologist who introduced the term dry eye. For decades it was thought dry eyes was limited to a reduction in the aqueous phase of the tear film. It was as recent as 1995 that dry eyes was eventually recognised as a multifaceted ocular pathology which was due to decreased tear production and increased tear evaporation [1]. In this chapter we will focus on the latter, specifically looking at meibomian gland dysfunction.

An estimate of the prevalence of dry eyes is difficult given that many sufferers may be asymptomatic or dismissive of subjective questionnaires of their symptoms if mild. Various studies estimate the prevalence as between 7.4% to 33.7% [2-3]. The epidemiology of dry eye depends on the mode of diagnosis, population surveyed and study cited.

Large American epidemiological studies estimate symptomatic dry eyes to affect 7% of women and 4% of men over the age of 50 years in the United States [4]. Similar data is seen in Australian studies [3]. The far eastern studies report the largest proportion of dry eye sufferers with Taiwan having the highest at 33.7% [5] followed by Japan and Indonesia [6].

2. Meibomian gland dysfunction

The meibomian glands, named after the German physician Meibom in 1966, are specialised sebaceous glands within the eyelids. They number 20-5 on the lower lids and up to 50 on the upper lid. Meibomian glands are responsible for secretion of a lipid rich mixture call meibum onto the tear surface through small openings found on the lid margin. A single gland consists of a central duct linked to multiple acini via ductules. Meibum is loaded into acini and released into the central duct where it moves to the openings on the lid margin and ocular surface. The glands undergo constant renewal and are delicate owing to their holocrine nature.

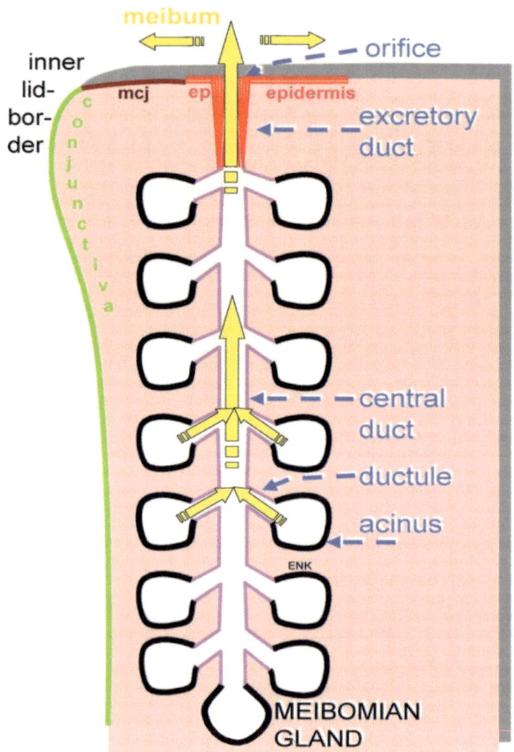

Scheme 1. Diagram courtesy of International Workshop on Meibomian Gland Dysfunction

It is widely thought that reduced meibum quality and quantity in addition to hyperkeratinisation of the ductal epithelium are the main reasons for meibomian gland dysfunction (MGD). Hyperkeratinised ducts and thicker meibum secretions lead to obstruction of the ducts. A progressive increase in pressure from continuous meibum secretion causes widening of the duct, acinar atrophy with cornification of duct epithelia. Ultimately there is reduced meibum secretion and gland drop out causing an unstable tear film. [7]

The tear film lubricates the ocular surface, which is vital to its maintaining its function and well being. It also forms a vital role in light refraction in the air-tear-cornea interface. Tear film is structured into 3 primary layers: The inner layer comprises mucin and a layer of glycocalyx that is synthesised by the conjunctiva and epithelial cells. The lacrimal gland primarily secretes the middle aqueous layer. The outermost lipid layer is secreted by the meibomian gland. This superficial layer stabilises the tear film by preventing its evaporation. Meibomian gland dysfunction is the most common cause of evaporative dry eye. Left untreated dry eye initially causes irritating ocular surface symptoms and signs that can threaten visual impairment, cause corneal perforation and blindness.[8]

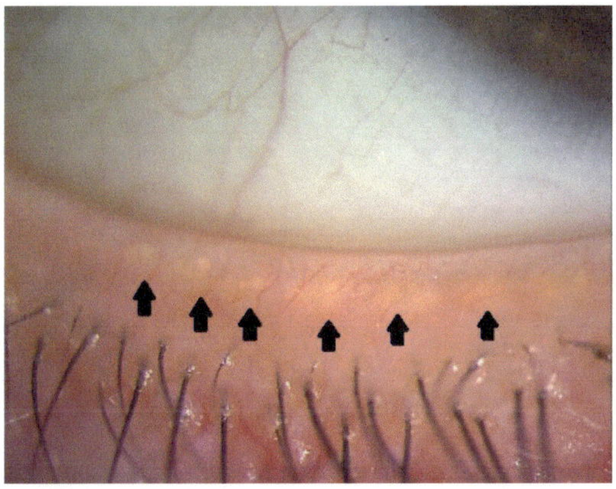

(courtesy of Stoke Mandeville Hospital)

Figure 1. Lower lid meibomian glands

Broadly meibomian gland dysfunction can be defined as *a chronic, diffuse abnormality of the meibomian glands commonly characterized by terminal duct obstruction and/or qualitative/quantitative changes in the glandular secretion. It may result in alteration of the tear film, symptoms of eye irritation, clinically apparent inflammation, and ocular surface disease[9-10].*

3. Aetiology

Meibomian gland dysfunction can affect many different groups.

Age is a major risk factor for the development of MGD. It is more common in the elderly. Studies in humans seem to mirror the effects in animals [9]. Decreased acinar proliferation, atrophy and altered localisation of the lipogenesis factor PPARγ (regulates meibomian differentiation and secretion) are seen in mice. Elderly patients have been noted to have a higher rate of meibomian glad dropout [10-11] with half as many functioning glands between 20 to 80 years of age. Human cadaveric studies show gland orifice metaplasia and narrowing [12-13] with hyperkeratinisation and lipogranulomatous inflammatory changes. Additionally meibum composition changes with age yielding a reduced volume and increased viscosity [10-14].

Androgens are known to be integrally involved in differentiation of sebaceous glands all over the body and have been shown to promote genes essential for meibomian function [13-14] Furthermore, complete androgen insensitivity syndrome has been shown to have altered meibomian glands and composition of lipid secretions that resulted in clinically apparent signs and symptoms of MGD [15-16].

Confusingly, chronic blepharitis has been suggested as a cause for MGD. Whilst MGD itself is a cause of chonic blepharitis, there is considerable overlap with other causes of chronic blepharitis that may accentuate MGD. One study showed 74% (42 of 57) chronic blepharitis sufferers had evidence of meibomian gland loss on meibography whereas 20% (4) of matched normal patients had any dropout. More detailed understanding is needed regarding the overlap of MGD with chronic blepharitis [18-19].

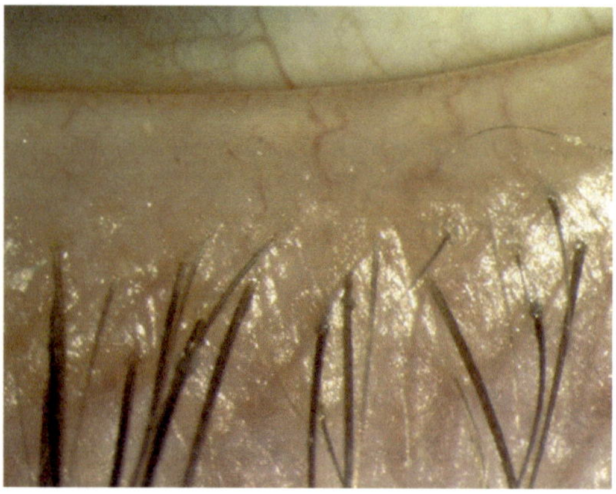

Figure 2. Lower lid meibomian glands and dropout in an elderly patient (courtesy of S Tuft)

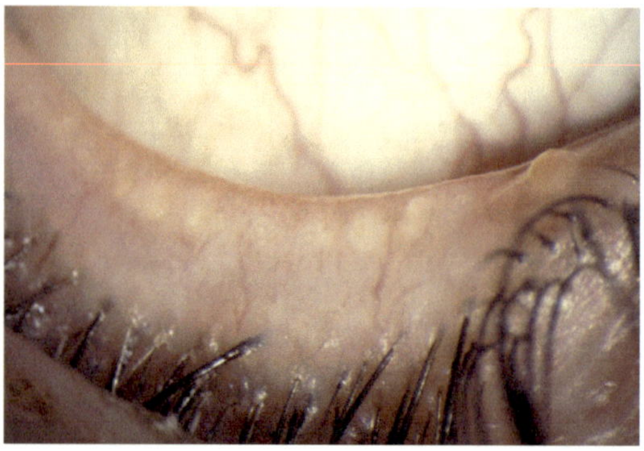

Figure 3. Meibum secretions of elderly patient showing increased plugging and viscosity (courtesy of S Tuft)

Demodex mites are the most common ectoparasites found in human skin. Of this species *D.brevis* is thought to be the most pertinent in MGD [20]. Current thinking is that the mite burrows deep into sebaceous and meibomian glands to feed on sebum and meibum respectively, as this forms as its main food source. Its chitinous exoskeleton causes a granulomatous reaction which ultimately leads to a mechanical blockage of the gland. *D.brevis* has been found in the centre of granulomatous meibomian glands surrounded by histocytes, epithelioid cells, fibroblasts and plasma cells which may thus offer a potential explanation for refractory and recurrent chalazia in some patients. [21]

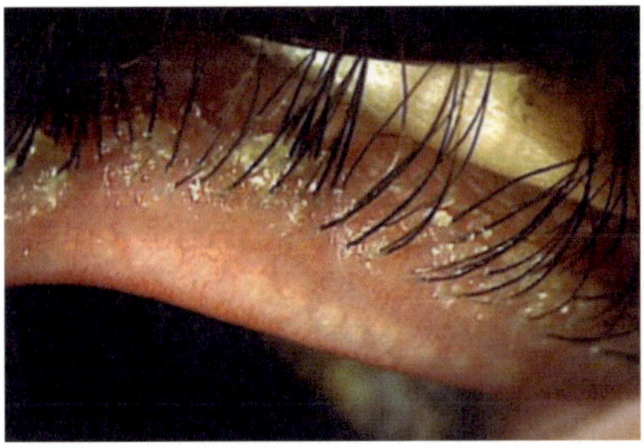

Figure 4. Desmodex infested lashes with meibomian gland dysfunction

Contact lens wear can increase the risk of MGD. Studies utilising meibography have shown that contact lenses alter meibomian gland morphology with greater rates of dropout than non-contact lens wearers. The duration and type of contact lens was weakly associated with this. By inserting and removing contact lenses, desquamated epithelial cells have been shown to obstruct the duct orifice leading to stagnation and atrophy [22-23]. While some studies show a statistically significant increase in MGD in contact lens wearers [22-24] others did not show significant differences [25-26]. It is important however to bear in mind these studies defined meibomain gland dysfunction differently. Damage to stem cells at the limbus is likely to be different based on duration on contact lens wear and may help account for the differences.

Environment may play a role in MGD. It is likely that factors such as temperature, humidity and visual undertaking have an accentuating impact rather than develop MGD. For example, concentrated computer use may be associated with reduced blink rate, exacerbating symptoms of MGD. One study of 70 patients found 74% of video display terminal users had MGD [27]. Decreased conjunctival temperature has been suggested to cause obstructive MGD through increased meibum viscosity [28-29].

Various medical conditions have been associated with MGD. Polycystic ovary syndrome (PCOS), where there is often insulin resistance and hyperinsulinaemia can result in increased androgen synthesis. Androgen receptors have been found in meibomian glands with a possible effect on function [30-33]. Twenty two (22)% of PCOS patients had MGD compared to 13% of normals in one study [34].

Dyslipidaemia appears to be associated with MGD. Patients with moderate to severe MGD have a higher incidence of dyslipidemia with respect to elevated total cholesterol than the general population [35-36]. Higher meibomian cholesterol ester levels are associated with MGD in humans [37].

Sjorgen's syndrome has been shown to have a higher incidence of MGD. One study found a higher incidence of MGD in MGD related dry eye to other causes of dry eye. The actual association, whether causative or a consequence of dry eye is not established and further study is needed [38-39]

Multiple medications have been implicated as possible risk factors for MGD. Studies looking at the acne treatment isotretinoin, 13-cis retinoic acid, have found that this resulted in altered meibum secretion, atrophy of the gland, reduced tear break up time and dry eye symptoms [40-41]. Other studies have looked at medication under the umbrella category of dry eye, not specially MGD. There may however be some overlap with MGD. Included in this category are antihistamines. One study has shown that treatment of allergic conjunctivitis with once daily loratidine resulted in signs of ocular dryness [42-43].

Post-menopausal hormone therapy has been associated with MGD [44-47] although the pathophysiology is not fully understood. Whilst established that sex hormone levels change from pre-to post-menopause, it is presumed that PMH results in changes to meibum gland secretions that can lead to MGD. Higher estrogen levels post-menopausally have been implicated in reduced tear function [45]. The largest of the studies, looking at 3500 patients from the Blue Mountain Study has shown a statistically significant 60% higher prevalence of dry eye in PMH users. A longer duration of use has been associated with longer symptoms [44].

Anitidepressant use has been associated with a higher risk of evaporative dry eye symptoms. Often many such medications simply have visual blurring only as a side effect without any mention of dry eye disease [48-51].

Omega 3 oils have been shown to have a beneficial effect on MGD whilst omega 6 oils have an opposite effect. Both are essential for growth and development. The omega 3 oils are found naturally in Mediterranean diets, flaxseed and cod liver oil [52]. Omega 6 oils are found typically in Northern European diets containing high red meat and less of the above [52]. The most detailed study to date showed a reduction in meibum thickness, dry eye signs and tear break up time in those with a high omega 3 to omega 6 ratio [53], agreeing with previous findings [52, 54. 55]. These oils compete for an enzyme involved in the inflammatory pathwaytherefore it is the ratio of omega 3 and 6 that is crucial. The ideal omega 6:3 ratio is 4:1 but typical Northern European and American diets are in the realm of 14:1 A higher omega 6 to 3 ratio results in overproduction of pro-inflammatory PGE2 from omega 6 and underproduction of anti-inflammatory PGE1 and PGE3 via omega 3 that induces MGD [53].

4. Presentation

Meibomian gland dysfunction is the leading cause of evaporative dry eye. As such patients will present with dry eye symptoms.

Most patients with MGD are likely to be asymptomatic. The vast majority will not experience any symptoms unless it is moderate in nature or exacerbated by other causes of evaporative dry eye. Burning, irritation, redness, watering or intermittent visual blur are frequently

http://dx.doi.org/10.5772/58566

described. It is important to ask what time of day this occurs to try to distinguish from other causes of dry eye. Blepharitis is typically worse in the morning with redness, crusting, puffiness, itchy lids or a 'gritty sensation' within the eyes.

5. Clinical assessment

There are different ways to assess meibomian gland dysfunction. Whilst a slit lamp is certainly beneficial and the commonest form of assessment, one can simply use a direct ophthalmoscope for those in primary care settings. Though it does not give as detailed a view the principles are the same as for slit lamp examination. The key is to observe the meibomian glands and ocular surface. With the ophthalmoscope one needs to place on high magnification to view the state of the meibomian glands which are located posterior to the greyline Often orifices can be seen to be plugged, or pouting. Surrounding tissue can be erythematous with telangiectatic vessels. Misdirected eyelashes can also be a sign of eyelid inflammatory changes. A good clinical examination will also include eversion of the eyelids which will often show white, hard deposits called concretions on the tarsal conjunctiva, follicles or granulomatous changes from previous chalazia. The ocular surface should also be assessed. Important to evaporative dry eyes is assessment of the tear film break up (TFBUT). This is done by instilling fluorescein sodium 2% (although 0.25% is an acceptable alternative) and asking the patient to blink a few times. The patient should then be asked to keep their eyes open and careful note of the time taken for vacuoles to appear in the tear film. A normal time frame is 10-15 seconds. The ocular surface should also be noted for punctate epithelial erosions which can be wide-spread or mainly inferior. In severe cases mucous filaments have been noted on the cornea. Abrasions can also be seen in those with associated in-turned eyelashes. The conjunctiva can be injected to varying degrees. As MGD is almost always bilateral, a unilateral presentation must alert the clinician of the possibility of basal cell carcinoma or meibomian cell carcinoma.

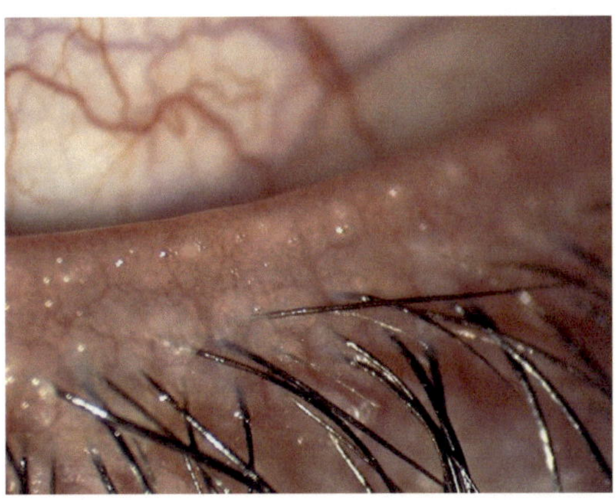

Figure 5. Thickened meibomian secretions i

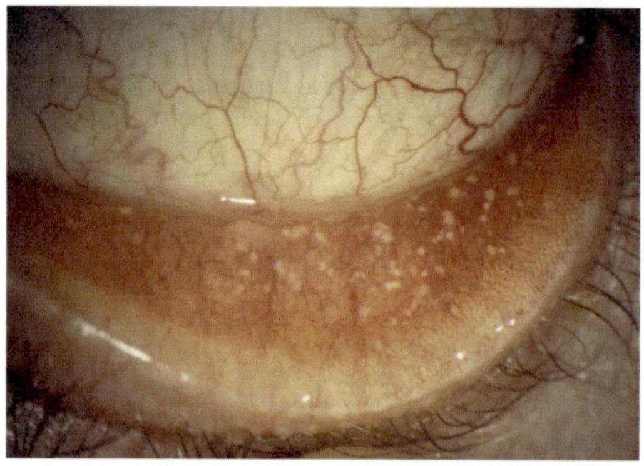

Figure 6. Concretions on the lower lid (courtesy of S Tuft)

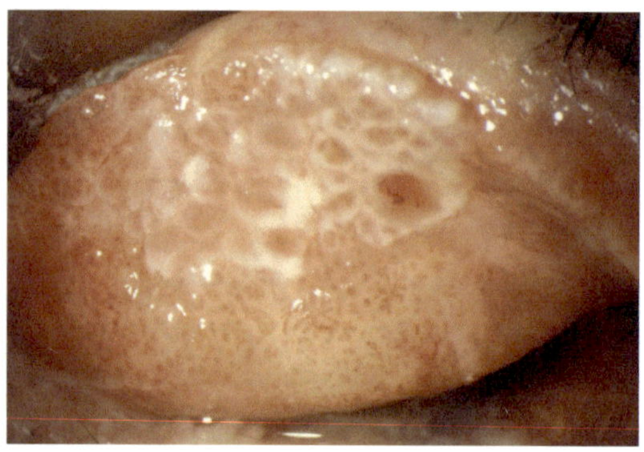

Figure 7. Follicles and sebaceous material (courtesy of S Tuft)

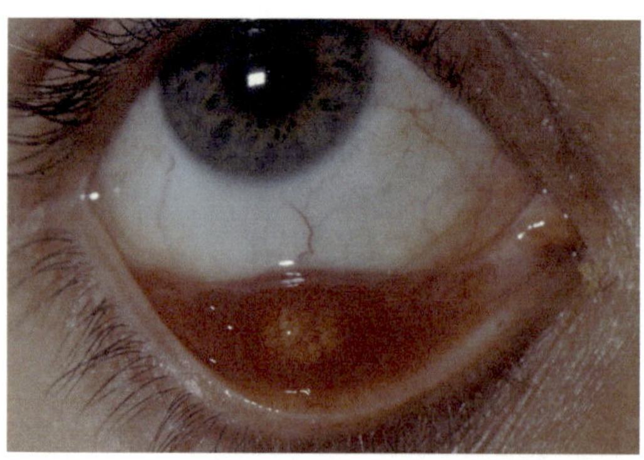

Figure 8. Chalazion on lower lid (courtesy of S Tuft)

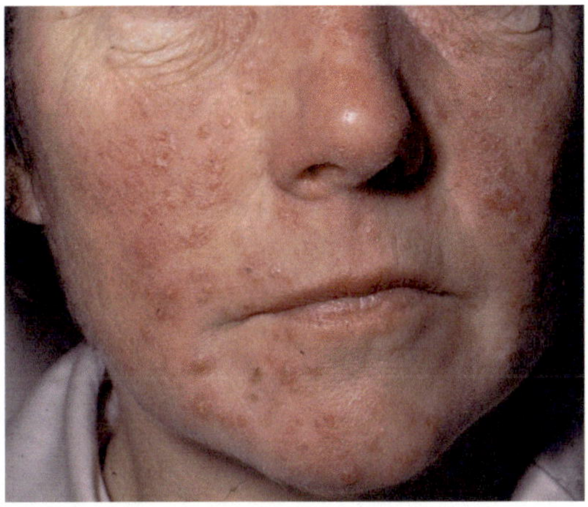

Figure 9. Rosacea above is associated with meibomian gland dysfunction (courtesy of S Tuft)

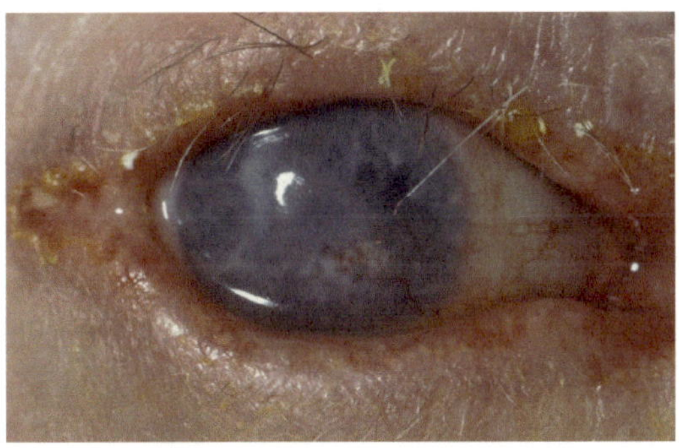

Figure 10. Trichiatic lashes resulting in corneal damage (courtesy of S Tuft)

There is no universal classification system of MGD. Different approaches have been used. The International Workshop Meibomian Gland subcommittee have recommended categorisation into 4 subtypes, although this is not universally applied.

1. MGD alone Asymptomatic Symptomatic (noncicatricial, cicatricial)

2. MGD with associated with ocular surface damage

3. MGD-related evaporative dry eye

4. MGD associated with other ocular disorders.

Alternatively, clinical measurement has been described. This is based on lid signs and meibum quality. Meibum can be graded on the Oxford score scale 0-3 (0=clear, 1=cloudy, 2=cloudy/particulate and 3=toothpaste like) [107].

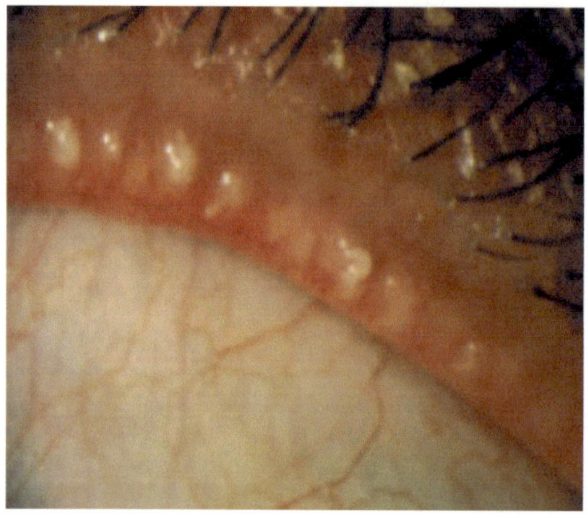

Figure 11. cloudy and particulate meibum: Oxford scale 2

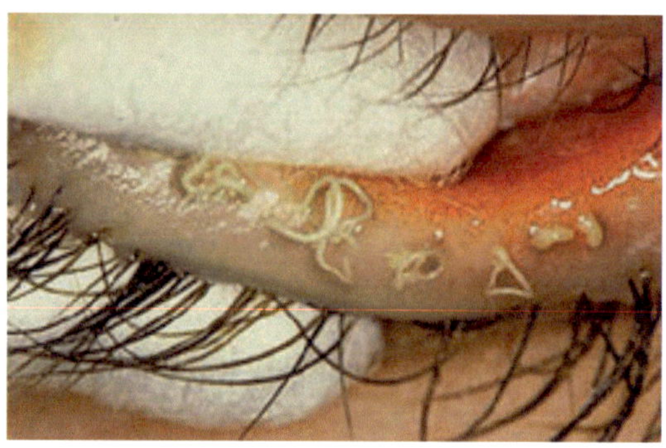

Figure 12. Toothpaste like meibum: Oxford score 3

5.1. Differential

A common misnomer is that MGD and posterior blepharitis are interchangeable terms [56-58]. Some previous literature has used the terms as such. MGD though, is one cause of posterior blepharitis (inflammation of the lid margins) and must be distinguished from other causes based on the anatomical structures of the posterior lid. Other causes include conjunctivitis (allergic or infective) and dermatological (acne rosacea or sebhorreic dermatitis).

Anterior blepharitis is another differential. This refers to inflammation anterior to the gray line, particularly around the lashes. The gray line anatomically subdivides the anterior and posterior lamellae of the lid. Anterior blepharitis can result in scurf on lashes, collarettes at the lash base and vascular changes of the eyelids.

5.2. Treatment principles

Typically treatment is predominantly based on the general term 'lid hygeine', ocular lubricants and antibiotics. There are more recent advances in the field and these are described further below.

Lid hygeine as a method varies across different centres [59]. Currently there is no standardised method. Commonly patients are told to either to place a warm compress over the lids at least twice daily or massage the lids for 10 minutes during each session. Compresses alone have been shown to cause transient visual blurring [60-61]. Active massage is encouraged. MGD secretions have been shown to have higher melting (35 C) points relative to normal (32C) [62-63]. The warmness melts the pathological meibum within the glands and active massage helps to unblock the glands. The authors feel that cotton wool whilst more gentle on the eye is often not firm enough to dislodge meibum that a flannel or towel is able to do. Lid hygeine is made more efficient by encouraging active massage just under the lashes themselves so the patient can directly affect the glands themselves. This needs to be demonstrated to patients directly. By pressing the lateral canthus firmly, traction can be provided and using a flannel the pulp of the finger swept gently over the inner aspect of the upper and lower lids. This needs to be balanced against any possible damage to the ocular and careful explanation and assessment of patient technique needs to be balanced against this [64-65]. The use of mild baby shampoo over the lids has also been advocated as part of lid hygeine. Ultimately patients need to be educated that lid hygiene is the basis upon which MGD will be controlled and that compliance is crucial in not only reducing symptoms but preventing recurrence.

Physical expression of the meibomian glands has been described [66-67]. Methods vary from gentle lid palpation to forceful squeezing of the lids. Use of a finger on the outer lid and a rigid object on the inner aspect like a metal paddle have been reported [68]. Often considerable force is needed to express pathological meibum and transient visual blurring owing to corneal distortion has been reported [60-61]. We believe that the risks involved and potential discomfort from this outweigh any benefit and do not recommend this.

Ocular lubricants are helpful to provide symptomatic relief. They help to alleviate symptoms experienced secondary to evaporative dry eye and do not treat the MGD itself. It is important for patients to realise that they are not a cure but give temporary respite. Ocular lubricants are helpful in bolstering the tear film volume, spreading of tears [69] and providing a layer over the cornea that reduced the possibility of corneal erosion from friction of the lid moving over the cornea by blinking [70-71]. The ocular lubricants may also help wash away pro-inflammatory molecules and dilute the concentration of inflammatory cytokines in tears. This has not been tested and remains a speculative theory presently.

Much research has been based around the contents of ocular lubricants. Preservatives can cause discomfort and toxicity to the corneal epithelium. Frequently used preservatives like benzylalkonium chloride and polyquaternium have been shown to decrease goblet cell density and thus affect tear film stability [72-77]. There is no evidence nor consensus on frequency of usage. It should be based on an individual level. Preservative free drops are recommended in severe dry eye where high frequency drops are required. More recently so called vanishing preservatives such as sodium perborate or sodium chlorite have been incorporated into artificial tears. There is a lack of data to date to suggest whether these have the intended less preservative toxicity than the traditional preservatives mentioned.

Lipid supplemented tears have been shown of benefit in MGD [79-84]. Patients have reported reduced symptoms with an increased tear break up time and thicker lipid layer of the tear film. Castor oil drops have been shown to reduce tear break up time in a randomised control trial [84]. Temporary visual blurring has been reported in older studies that used ointments but more recent formulations have not been shown to have this problem [84]

Leading from this is the viscosity of the ocular lubricant. The greater the viscosities the more benefit in bulking tear film thickness and volume in dry eyes [85-87] as well as increased transit time on the eye. This needs to be counterbalanced against visual blurring and inconvenience.

Antibiotics are often used in MGD. The exact pathogenesis of bacteria remains not entirely understood. However the presence of bacterial flora on the lid surface, notably staphylococcus epidermidis, staph aureus, propion acnes amongst others is known. It may be the case that the keratinisation of the meibum and abnormal lipids provide prime conditions for normal bacterial flora to produce enzymes such as lipases and exotoxins resulting in proinflammatory changes. Thus an antibiotic would need to be effective against common flora.

Macrolides are commonly used. Studies have shown that they exert many anti-inflammatory effects. Neutrophil activity is affected by downregulating adhesion protein expression [88]. Phagocytosis and chemotaxis are affected through this. A reduction in proinflammatory cytokines has been demonstrated [89-90].

Tetracyclines have multiple helpful anti-inflammatory properties, including influencing neutrophil chemotaxis and proliferation of lymphocytes [91-92]. Matrix metalloproteinases and inflammatory cytokines like IL1 are suppressed as are anti-angiogenesis properties [93-94]. Collagenase 2 (matrix metalloproteinase P8) is directly suppressed by doxycycline specifically. They have been established for treatment of acne rosacea. Lipase production of the typical bacterial flora such as S epidermidis is suppressed. The lipases are responsible for production of pro-inflammatory free fatty acids that can detstabilise the tear film and directly alter meibum composition. The tetracyclines as a group have varying lipophillicity that alters individual drug pharmacokinetics. The international workshop on meibomian gland dysfunction recommend the use of doxycycline and minocycline [96]. These have been shown to be clinically effective at lower doses relative to tetracycline, which is poorly lipophilic and has been found at lower relative concentrations in tears after 5 days [97-100]. Typically doxycycline or monocycline are given at 100mg dosage for 2 months.

Dietary modification have been popular treatments amongst patients. Omega 3 rich foods as can be found in flax seed or cod-liver oil have been shown to have improved meibum scores, tear break up time and surface signs [100-102]. Omega 6 rich foods such as red meat have a counter effect and should be discouraged [101].

Surgical management is reserved for complications from MGD. Typically this would occur where the MGD is severe. Chalazia can be treated with incision and curettage where they are inflamed and affecting vision. Eyelid cicatrisation may cause trichiatic lashes that can commonly undergo epilation or electrolysis. Lid laxity, ectropion or entropion may be treated surgically.

Recently, devices have been created to be worn by patients to help with lid hygiene. These include blepharitis goggles, which aim to provide heat and moisture via steam to unclog blocked meibomian glands [103-104].LipiFlow® Thermal Pulsation System is similar but provides heat therapy and physical pressure to express the meibomian glands [105]. These variables can be adjusted accordingly, and seems to offer more favourable outcomes over 12 months than typical lid hygiene and lubricating drops [105]. The evidence base for such devices is currently limited further studies on outcomes and potential side effects are needed.

5.3. Primary care setting

It is understandably difficult to make an unambiguous diagnosis of meibomian gland dysfunction without a slit lamp in primary care or on the ward.

However through careful history of symptoms and possible risk factors mentioned earlier, along with a direct ophthalmoscope on high magnification, an informed judgment can be made. Use of the direct ophthalmoscope does require practice to look at anterior surface structures in detail. Most hand held ophthalmoscopes have a cobalt blue mode, meaning that with available fluroscein drops an evaluation of the tear break up time and state of the corneal surface can be undertaken.

Where MGD is suspected, we would recommend starting lid hygiene, taking care to assess whether the patient is capable of performing this safely without damage to anterior structures. If there is suspicion of anterior surface structure damage from unsafe hygiene measures or possible other causes we recommend referral without starting lid hygiene. Prescribing suitable preservative free lubricating eye drops is recommended before ophthalmic referral.

6. Conclusion

Meibomian gland dysfunction is the most common ocular sign encountered in patients and cause of evaporative dry eye. Whilst awareness of the condition improves and research continues to be undertaken, a universal consensus on the definition, pathophysiology, signs and management is still being awaited. This is needed to allow for earlier detection and optimal structured treatment for MGD. Further questions do need to be answered regarding meibomian gland dysfunction too. Owing to a lack in consensus over definition and clinical tests performed in studies there is difficulty comparing results in different studies. The International Workshop for Meibomian Gland Dysfunction have suggested future research aim to prioritise a specific validated questionnaire for symptoms, a standard grading system of signs and validated outcomes for MGD [106]. It is hoped this will provide greater clarity in diagnosing, understanding the extent and severity of disease. Ultimately this would allow the most suitable treatment to be started improving the level of patient care in meibomian gland dysfunction.

Author details

Vikas Tah[1,2*], Kamran Saha[2], James Myerscough[3], Muhammad Ahad[1], Jason Ho[2], Pranev Sharma[4], Farihah Tariq[5] and Stephen Tuft[2]

1 Stoke Mandeville Hospital, UK

2 Moorfields Eye Hosptial London, UK

3 Colchester University Hospital NHS Foundation Trust, UK

4 Chelsea and Westminister Hospital, UK

5 Raigmore Hospital Inverness, UK

References

[1] CLAO J. 1995 Oct;21(4):221-32. Report of the National Eye Institute/Industry workshop on Clinical Trials in Dry Eyes. Lemp MA.

[2] Ophthalmology. 2003 Jun;110(6):1096-101. Prevalence of dry eye among an elderly Chinese population in Taiwan: the Shihpai Eye Study. Lin PY, Tsai SY, Cheng CY, Liu JH, Chou P, Hsu WM.

[3] Ophthalmology. 1998 Jun;105(6):1114-9. The epidemiology of dry eye in Melbourne, Australia. McCarty CA, Bansal AK, Livingston PM, Stanislavsky YL, Taylor HR.

[4] Am J Ophthalmol. 2003 Aug;136(2):318-26. Prevalence of dry eye syndrome among US women. Schaumberg DA, Sullivan DA, Buring JE, Dana MR.

[5] Results of a population-based questionnaire on the symptoms and lifestyles associated with dry eye. Shimmura S, Shimazaki J, Tsubota K. Br J Ophthalmol. 2002 Dec; 86(12):1347-51.

[6] Prevalence and risk factors associated with dry eye symptoms: a population based study in Indonesia. Lee AJ, Lee J, Saw SM, Gazzard G, Koh D, Widjaja D, Tan DT.

[7] The international workshop on meibomian gland dysfunction: report of the subcommittee on anatomy, physiology, and pathophysiology of the meibomian gland. Knop E, Knop N, Millar T, Obata H, Sullivan DA. Invest Ophthalmol Vis Sci. 2011 Mar 30;52(4):1938-78. doi: 10.1167/iovs.10-6997c. Print 2011 Mar. Review. No abstract available.

[8] Research in dry eye: report of the Research Subcommittee of the International Dry Eye WorkShop(2007). [No authors listed] Ocul Surf. 2007 Apr;5(2):179-93. Review. PMID:17508121

[9] Aging and dry eye disease. Ding J, Sullivan DA. Exp Gerontol. 2012 Jul;47(7):483-90. doi: 10.1016/j.exger.2012.03.020. Epub 2012 Apr 28. Review. PMID:22569356

[10] Norn, M., 1987. Expressibility of meibomian secretion. Relation to age, lipid precorneal film, scales, foam, hair and pigmentation. Acta Ophthalmol. 65, 137–142.

[11] Arita, R., Itoh, K., Inoue, K., Amano, S., 2008. Noncontact infrared meibography to document age-related changes of the meibomian glands in a normal population. Ophthalmology 115, 911–915

[12] Hykin, P.G., Bron, A.J., 1992. Age-related morphological changes in lid margin and meibomian gland anatomy. Cornea 11, 334–342

[13] Sullivan, B.D., Evans, J.E., Dana, M.R., Sullivan, D.A., 2006. Influence of aging on the polar and neutral lipid profiles in human meibomian gland secretions. Arch. Ophthalmol. 124, 1286–1292.

[14] Schirra, F., Richards, S.M., Liu, M., Suzuki, T., Yamagami, H., Sullivan, D.A., 2006. Androgen regulation of lipogenic pathways in the mouse meibomian gland. Exp. Eye Res.

[15] Krenzer, K.L., Dana, M.R., Ullman, M.D., Cermak, J.M., Tolls, D.B., Evans, J.E., Sullivan, D.A., 2000. Effect of androgen deficiency on the human meibomian gland and ocular surface. J. Clin. Endocrinol. Metab. 85, 4874–4882

[16] Sullivan, B.D., Evans, J.E., Cermak, J.M., Krenzer, K.L., Dana, M.R., Sullivan, D.A., 2002a. Complete androgen insensitivity syndrome: effect on human meibomian gland secretions. Arch. Ophthalmol. 120, 1689–1699.

[17] Sullivan, B.D., Evans, J.E., Dana, M.R., Sullivan, D.A., 2002b. Impact of androgen deficiency on the lipid profiles

[18] Mathers WD, Shields WJ, Sachdev MS, Petroll WM, Jester JV. Meibomian gland dysfunction in chronic blepharitis. Cornea. 1991;10:277–285

[19] The international workshop on meibomian gland dysfunction: report of the subcommittee on the epidemiology of, and associated risk factors for, MGD. Schaumberg DA, Nichols JJ, Papas EB, Tong L, Uchino M, Nichols KK. Invest Ophthalmol Vis Sci. 2011 Mar 30;52(4):1994-2005. doi: 10.1167/iovs.10-6997e. Print 2011 Mar. Review. No abstract available.

[20] Corneal manifestations of ocular demodex infestation. Clinical treatment of ocular demodecosis by lid scrub with tea tree oil. Gao YY, Di Pascuale MA, Elizondo A, Tseng SC Cornea. 2007 Feb; 26(2):136-43.

[21] Am J Ophthalmol. 1985 Sep 15;100(3):482-3.Desmodectic mites and chalazion. English FP, Cohn D, Groeneveld ER.

[22] Korb DR, Henriquez AS. Meibomian gland dysfunction and contact lens intolerance. J Am Optom Assoc. 1980;51:243–251

[23] Henriquez AS, Korb DR. Meibomian glands and contact lens wear. Br J Ophthalmol. 1981;65:108–111

[24] Ong BL, Larke JR. Meibomian gland dysfunction: some clinical, biochemical and physical observations. Ophthalmic Physiol Opt. 1990;10:144–148

[25] Prevalence of Meibomian gland dysfunction. Hom MM, Martinson JR, Knapp LL, Paugh JR Optom Vis Sci. 1990 Sep; 67(9):710-2.

[26] Relation between contact lens wear and Meibomian gland dysfunction. Ong BL Optom Vis Sci. 1996 Mar; 73(3):208-10.

[27] Meibomian gland dysfunction and ocular discomfort in video display terminal workers.

[28] Fenga C, Aragona P, Cacciola A, Spinella R, Di Nola C, Ferreri F, Rania L Eye (Lond). 2008 Jan; 22(1):91-5.

[29] Nagymiha′lyi A, Dikstein S, Tiffany JM. The influence of eyelid temperature on the delivery of meibomian oil. *Exp Eye Res*. 2004;78(3):367-370

[30] Baudouin C. The pathology of dry eye. *Surv Ophthalmol*. 2001;45:211–220.

[31] McCulley JP, Shine WE. The lipid layer of tears: Dependent on meibomian gland function. *Exp Eye Res*. 2004;78:361–365.

[32] Sutphin JE, Chodosh J, Dana MR, et al. Normal physiology of the ocular surface. In: Liesegang TJ, Skuta GL, Cantor LB, eds. *Basic and Clinical Science Course External Disease and Cornea*. San Francisco: American Academy of Ophthalmology; 2005: 47–52.

[33] Sullivan DA, Sullivan BD, Ullman MD, et al. Androgen influence on the meibomian gland. *Invest Ophthalmol Vis Sci*. 2000;41:3732–3742.

[34] Curr Eye Res. 2008 Feb;33(2):133-8. Meibomian gland alterations in polycystic ovary syndrome. Yavas GF, Ozturk F, Kusbeci T, Ermis SS, Yilmazer M, Cevrioglu S, Aktepe F, Kose S.

[35] Association of dyslipidemia in moderate to severe meibomian gland dysfunction. Dao AH, Spindle JD, Harp BA, Jacob A, Chuang AZ, Yee RW. Am J Ophthalmol. 2010 Sep;150(3):371-375.e1. doi: 10.1016/j.ajo.2010.04.016

[36] Ophthal Plast Reconstr Surg. 2013 Mar-Apr;29(2):101-3. doi: 10.1097/IOP.0b013e31827a007d. Associations between the grade of meibomian gland dysfunction and dyslipidemia. Bukhari AA.

[37] Shine WE, McCulley JP. The role of cholesterol in chronic blepharitis. *Invest Ophthalmol Vis Sci* 1991;32: 2272–2280.

[38] Meibomian gland dysfunction in patients with Sjögren syndrome. Shimazaki J, Goto E, Ono M, Shimmura S, Tsubota K Ophthalmology. 1998 Aug; 105(8):1485-8.

[39] Tear evaporation rates in Sjögren syndrome and non-Sjögren dry eye patients. Goto E, Matsumoto Y, Kamoi M, Endo K, Ishida R, Dogru M, Kaido M, Kojima T, Tsubota K Am J Ophthalmol. 2007 Jul; 144(1):81-85

[40] Ocular side effects associated with 13-cis-retinoic acid therapy for acne vulgaris: clinical features, alterations of tearfilm and conjunctival flora. Egger SF, Huber-Spitzy V, Böhler K, Raff M, Scholda C, Barisani T, Vecsei VP. Acta Ophthalmol Scand. 1995 Aug; 73(4):355-7.

[41] Ocular side effects of isotretinoin therapy.[J Am Optom Assoc. 1988] Caffery BE, Josephson JE J Am Optom Assoc. 1988 Mar; 59(3):221-4.

[42] Prevalence of and risk factors for dry eye syndrome.[Arch Ophthalmol. 2000] Moss SE, Klein R, Klein BE Arch Ophthalmol. 2000 Sep; 118(9):1264-8.

[43] An open-label, investigator-masked, crossover study of the ocular drying effects of two antihistamines, topical epinastine and systemic loratadine, in adult volunteers with seasonal allergic conjunctivitis.Ousler GW 3rd, Workman DA, Torkildsen GL. Clin Ther. 2007 Apr; 29(4):611-6.

[44] Dry eye in post-menopausal women using hormone replacement therapy.[Maturitas. 2007] Erdem U, Ozdegirmenci O, Sobaci E, Sobaci G, Göktolga U, Dagli S Maturitas. 2007 Mar 20; 56(3):257-62.

[45] W.D. Mathers, D. Strovall, J.A. Lane, M.B. Zimmerman Menopause and tear function: the influence of prolactin and sex hormones on human tear production Cornea, 17 (4) (1998), pp. 353–358

[46] B.E. Klein, R. Klein, L.L. Ritter Is there evidence of estrogen effect on age-related lens opacities? The Beaver Dam Eye Study Arch Ophthalmol, 112 (1994), pp. 85–91

[47] Chia EM, Mitchell P, Rochtchina E, Lee AJ, Maroun R, Wang JJ. Prevalence and associations of dry eye syndrome in an older population: The Blue Mountains Eye Study. Clin Exp Ophthalmol. 2003;31:229–232

[48] Schaumberg DA, Dana R, Buring JE, Sullivan DA. Prevalence of dry eye disease among US men: estimates from the Physicians' Health Studies. Arch Ophthalmol. 2009;127:763–768

[49] Long-term incidence of dry eye in an older population. Moss SE, Klein R, Klein BE Optom Vis Sci. 2008 Aug; 85(8):668-74.

[50] Wilkes S Bupropion. Drugs Today (Barc) 2006;42 (10) 671-681 PubMed

[51] Hudson JIPerahia DGGilaberte IWang FWatkin JGDetke MJ Duloxetine in the treatment of major depressive disorder: an open-label study. *BMC Psychiatry* 2007;743 PubMed

[52] Omega-3 Dietary Supplementation in Dry Eye and Blepharitis Trans Am Ophthalmol Soc / Vol 106 / 2008 338

[53] Calder PC. N-3 Polyunsaturated fatty acids and inflammation: from molecular biology to the clinic. Lipids 2003;38:343-352

[54] Simopoulos AP. The Mediterranean diets: what is so special about the diet of Greece? The scientific evidence. J Nutr 2001;131:3065-3073S.

[55] Am J Clin Nutr. 2005 Oct;82(4):887-93. Relation between dietary n-3 and n-6 fatty acids and clinically diagnosed dry eye syndrome in women. Miljanović B, Trivedi KA, Dana MR, Gilbard JP, Buring JE, Schaumberg DA.

[56] Meibomian keratoconjunctivitis. McCulley JP, Sciallis GF Am J Ophthalmol. 1977 Dec; 84(6):788-93.

[57] McCulley JP, Dougherty JM, Deneau DG. Classification of chronic blepharitis. Ophthalmology. 1982;89:1173–1180

[58] Luchs J. Efficacy of topical azithromycin ophthalmic solution 1% in the treatment of posterior blepharitis. Adv Ther. 2008;25:858–870

[59] The international workshop on meibomian gland dysfunction: report of the subcommittee on management and treatment of meibomian gland dysfunction. Geerling G, Tauber J, Baudouin C, Goto E, Matsumoto Y, O'Brien T, Rolando M, Tsubota K, Nichols KK. Invest Ophthalmol Vis Sci. 2011 Mar 30;52(4):2050-64. doi: 10.1167/iovs. 10-6997g. Review

[60] Warm compress induced visual degradation and Fischer-Schweitzer polygonal reflex. Solomon JD, Case CL, Greiner JV, Blackie CA, Herman JP, Korb DR Optom Vis Sci. 2007 Jul; 84(7):580-7.

[61] Goto E, Monden Y, Takano Y, et al. Treatment of non-inflamed obstructive meibomian gland dysfunction by an infrared warm compression device. Br J Ophthalmol. 2002;86:1403–1407

[62] Assessment of meibomian gland function in dry eye using meibometry. Yokoi N, Mossa F, Tiffany JM, Bron AJ. Arch Ophthalmol. 1999 Jun; 117(6):723-9

[63] Review Meibomian secretions in chronic blepharitis. McCulley JP, Shine WE Adv Exp Med Biol. 1998; 438():319-26.

[64] Smith GT, Dart J. External eye disease. In: Jackson TL, editor. ed. Moorfields Manual of Ophthalmology. Philadelphia: Mosby Elsevier; Chap 4:2008

[65] Ehler J, Shah ChP. Wills Eye Manual. Philadelphia: Lippincott Williams & Wilkins; 2008

[66] Krenzer, K.L., Dana, M.R., Ullman, M.D., Cermak, J.M., Tolls, D.B., Evans, J.E., Sullivan, D.A., 2000. Effect of androgen deficiency on the human meibomian gland and ocular surface. J. Clin. Endocrinol. Metab. 85, 4874–4882

[67] Sullivan, B.D., Evans, J.E., Cermak, J.M., Krenzer, K.L., Dana, M.R., Sullivan, D.A., 2002a. Complete androgen insensitivity syndrome: effect on human meibomian gland secretions. Arch. Ophthalmol. 120, 1689–1699.

[68] Mastrota K. The meibomian Mastrota paddle. Rosenberg, TX: Cynacon/Ocusoft, Inc., 2006. Available at http://www.ocusoft.com/for-eye-care-professionals/surgical/misc-surgical-instruments/mastrota-meibomian-paddle.html Accessed: July 16, 2010

[69] Rheology of tear film lipid layer spread in normal and aqueous tear-deficient dry eyes. Yokoi N, Yamada H, Mizukusa Y, Bron AJ, Tiffany JM, Kato T, Kinoshita S Invest Ophthalmol Vis Sci. 2008 Dec; 49(12):5319-24

[70] Lid-wiper epitheliopathy and dry-eye symptoms in contact lens wearers. Korb DR, Greiner JV, Herman JP, Hebert E, Finnemore VM, Exford JM, Glonek T, Olson MC CLAO J. 2002 Oct; 28(4):211-6.

[71] Prevalence of lid wiper epitheliopathy in subjects with dry eye signs and symptoms. Korb DR, Herman JP, Blackie CA, Scaffidi RC, Greiner JV, Exford JM, Finnemore VM Cornea. 2010 Apr; 29(4):377-83

[72] Labbe A, Pauly A, Liang H, et al. Comparison of toxicological profiles of benzalkonium chloride and polyquaternium-1: an experimental study. J Ocul Pharmacol Ther. 2006;22:267–278

[73] Fraunfelder FW. Corneal toxicity from topical ocular and systemic medications. Cornea. 2006;25:1133–1138. [PubMed]

[74] Debbasch C, Brignole F, Pisella PJ, Warnet JM, Rat P, Baudouin C. Quaternary ammoniums and other preservatives' contribution in oxidative stress and apoptosis on Chang conjunctival cells. Invest Ophthalmol Vis Sci. 2001;42:642–652. [PubMed]

[75] Furrer P, Mayer JM, Plazonnet B, Gurny R. Ocular tolerance of preservatives on the murine cornea. Eur J Pharm Biopharm. 1999;47:105–112. [PubMed]

[76] Palmer RM, Kaufman HE. Tear film, pharmacology of eye drops, and toxicity. Curr Opin Ophthalmol. 1995;6:11–16. [PubMed]

[77] Lapalus P, Ettaiche M, Fredj-Reygrobellet D, Jambou D, Elena PP. Cytotoxicity studies in ophthalmology. Lens Eye Toxic Res. 1990;7:231–242. [PubMed]

[78] Burstein NL. Corneal cytotoxicity of topically applied drugs, vehicles and preservatives. Surv Ophthalmol. 1980;25:15–30

[79] Low-concentration homogenized castor oil eye drops for noninflamed obstructive meibomian gland dysfunction. Goto E, Shimazaki J, Monden Y, Takano Y, Yagi Y, Shimmura S, Tsubota K Ophthalmology. 2002 Nov; 109(11):2030-5.

[80] Topical omega-3 and omega-6 fatty acids for treatment of dry eye. Rashid S, Jin Y, Ecoiffier T, Barabino S, Schaumberg DA, Dana MR Arch Ophthalmol. 2008 Feb; 126(2):219-25.

[81] Rieger G. Lipid-containing eye drops: a step closer to natural tears. Ophthalmologica. 1990;201:206–212. [PubMed]

[82] Tiffany JM. Lipid-containing eye drops. Ophthalmologica. 1991;203:47–49. [PubMed]

[83] Korb DR, Scaffidi RC, Greiner JV, et al. The effect of two novel lubricant eye drops on tear film lipid layer thickness in subjects with dry eye symptoms. Optom Vis Sci. 2005;82:594–601. [PubMed]

[84] Craig JP, Purslow C, Murphy PJ, Wolffsohn JS. Effect of a liposomal spray on the pre-ocular tear film. Cont Lens Anterior Eye. 2010;33:83–87

[85] Dynamic distribution of artificial tears on the ocular surface. Wang J, Simmons P, Aquavella J, Vehige J, Palakuru J, Chung S, Feng C Arch Ophthalmol. 2008 May; 126(5):619-25.

[86] Simmons PA, Vehige JG. Clinical performance of a mid-viscosity artificial tear for dry eye treatment. Cornea. 2007;26:294–302

[87] Khanal S, Tomlinson A, Pearce EI, Simmons PA. Effect of an oil-in-water emulsion on the tear physiology of patients with mild to moderate dry eye. Cornea. 2007;26:175–181.

[88] Sanz MJ, Nabah YN, Cerda-Nicolas M, et al. Erythromycin exerts in vivo anti-inflammatory activity downregulating cell adhesion molecule expression. *Br J Pharmacol.* 2005;144:190–201.

[89] Bosnar M, Bosnjak B, Cuzic S, et al. Azithromycin and clarithromycin inhibit lipopolysaccharide-induced murine pulmonary neutrophilia mainly through effects on macrophage-derived granulocyte-macrophage colony-stimulating factor and interleukin-1beta. *J Pharmacol Exp Ther.* 2009;331:104–113.

[90] Yamaryo T, Oishi K, Yoshimine H, Tsuchihashi Y, Matsushima K, Nagatake T. Fourteen-member macrolides promote the phosphatidylserine receptor-dependent phagocytosis of apoptotic neutrophils by alveolar macrophages. *Antimicrob Agents Chemother.* 2003;47:48 –53.

[91] Sanchez J, Somolinos AL, Almodovar PI, Webster G, Bradshaw M, Powala C. A randomized, double-blind, placebo-controlled trial of the combined effect of doxycycline hyclate 20-mg tablets and metronidazole 0.75% topical lotion in the treatment of rosacea. *J Am Acad Dermatol.* 2005;53:791–797.

[92] Sneddon IB. A clinical trial of tetracycline in rosacea. *Br J Dermatol.* 1966;7

[93] Li DQ, Lokeshwar BL, Solomon A, Monroy D, Ji Z, Pflugfelder SC. Regulation of MMP-9 production by human corneal epithelial cells. *Exp Eye Res.* 2001;73:449–459.8:649–652.

[94] Sobrin L, Liu Z, Monroy DC, et al. Regulation of MMP-9 activity in human tear fluid and corneal epithelial culture supernatant. *Invest Ophthalmol Vis Sci.* 2000;41:1703–1709.

[95] Beardsley RM, De Paiva CS, Power DF, Pflugfelder SC. Desiccating stress decreases apical corneal epithelial cell size–modulation by the metalloproteinase inhibitor doxycycline. *Cornea.* 2008;27: 935–940.

[96] The international workshop on meibomian gland dysfunction: report of the subcommittee on management and treatment of meibomian gland dysfunction. Geerling G, Tauber J, Baudouin C, Goto E, Matsumoto Y, O'Brien T, Rolando M, Tsubota K, Nichols KK. Invest Ophthalmol Vis Sci. 2011 Mar 30;52(4):2050-64.

[97] Ta CN, Shine WE, McCulley JP, Pandya A, Trattler W, Norbury JW. Effects of minocycline on the ocular flora of patients with acne rosacea or seborrheic blepharitis. *Cornea.* 2003;22:545–548.

[98] Aronowicz JD, Shine WE, Oral D, Vargas JM, McCulley JP. Short term oral minocycline treatment of meibomianitis. *Br J Ophthalmol.* 2006;90:856–860.

[99] Hoeprich PD, Warshauer DM. Entry of four tetracyclines into saliva and tears. *Antimicrob Agents Chemother.* 1974;5:330–

[100] Pinna A, Piccinini P, Carta F. Effect of oral linoleic and gammalinolenic acid on meibomian gland dysfunction. *Cornea.* 2007; 26:260–264

[101] Miljanovic B, Trivedi KA, Dana MR, Gilbard JP, Buring JE, Schaumberg DA. Relation between dietary n-3 and n-6 fatty acids and clinically diagnosed dry eye syndrome in women. *Am J Clin Nutr.* 2005;82:887–893.

[102] Macsai MS. The role of omega-3 dietary supplementation in blepharitis and meibomian gland dysfunction (an AOS thesis). *Trans Am Ophthalmol Soc.* 2008;106:336–356.

[103] http://www.spectrum-thea.co.uk/apps/content/html/ViewContent.aspx?fid=31

[104] http://www.butterflies-eyecare.co.uk/Blephasteam-Blephasteam.html

[105] *Current Eye Research, 37(4), 272–278, 2012*A Single LipiFlow® Thermal Pulsation System Treatment Improves Meibomian Gland Function and Reduces Dry Eye Symptoms for 9 Months Jack V. Greiner DO, PhD1,2

[106] Invest Ophthalmol Vis Sci. 2011 Mar 30;52(4):1922-9. doi: 10.1167/iovs.10-6997a. The international workshop on meibomian gland dysfunction: executive summary. Nichols KK, Foulks GN, Bron AJ, Glasgow BJ, Dogru M, Tsubota K, Lemp MA, Sullivan DA.

[107] Meibomian gland disease. Classification and grading of lid changes. Bron AJ, Benjamin L, Snibson GR. Eye (Lond). 1991;5 (Pt 4):395-411. Review.

Chapter 8

Ocular Aberrations and Image Quality, Contact Lens and MYOPIA Progression

Jie Shen

Additional information is available at the end of the chapter

http://dx.doi.org/10.5772/58456

1. Introduction

The eye as an optical instrument is imperfect with defocus, astigmatism and higher-order aberrations being common. The image formed on the retina is affected by these optical deficiencies. Refractive errors (myopia, hyperopia and astigmatism) are the most common ocular aberrations, and they are called lower-order aberrations. There are numerous higher-order aberrations, of which spherical aberration and coma are most of clinical interest. Refractive errors have been studied for many years and clinicians devote themselves to correct these focusing errors.

Compared to the efforts to understand and optimize the central vision, peripheral vision is not well understood. However, peripheral vision is important for motion and pattern detection and fundus imaging. Also, interest in studying the off-axis optical performance and image quality of humane eye has increased dramatically in recent years because the previous studies suggest a possibility that off-axis aberrations in human eye is important for the development of central refractive error.

Given the hypothesis that off-axis aberrations and image quality may affect central refractive error development, it is important to understand how ordinary ophthalmic lenses, which are used to correct foveal vision, influence the peripheral optics of human eye.

In this chapter, we will describe and discuss the following six major topics: 1) control of ocular growth, 2) axial ocular aberrations, 3) off-axis aberrations, 4) contact lens and myopia progression, 5) peripheral refractions and contact lens correction, and 6) peripheral image quality and contact lens correction.

2. Control of ocular growth

Animal studies have demonstrated that the eyes growth is controlled by local retina mechanism. [1-3] Local retinal mechanism refers to a condition that local retina could minimize the image degradation on the corresponding retinal location by changing the axial eye growth rate. [4] The homeostatic control signals of the eyes growth try to keep the image sharply focused on the retina ("grow to clarity" model). [5] If the eye is in myopic status, the image of a distant object falls in front of the retina and if the eye is hyperopic, the image falls behind the retina. These two situations are simulated in Fig. 1A, inserting a positive lens put the image in front of the retina (myopic focus) and negative lens focus the image behind the retina (hyperopic focus). By increasing the thickness of choroids or slowing the rate of eye's elongation, the eye can grow to counteract the effect of the lens, regaining a sharp focus (for small amount of myopic defocus). For hyperopic defocus, the choroids will become thinning and the rate of eye's elongation will increase in order to focus the image on retina again (Fig. 1B). [6-8] These were proved by previous animal studies. [9-13] For example, animals, like birds, consistently experience near objects in their inferior visual field have longer superior ocular length. [14, 15]

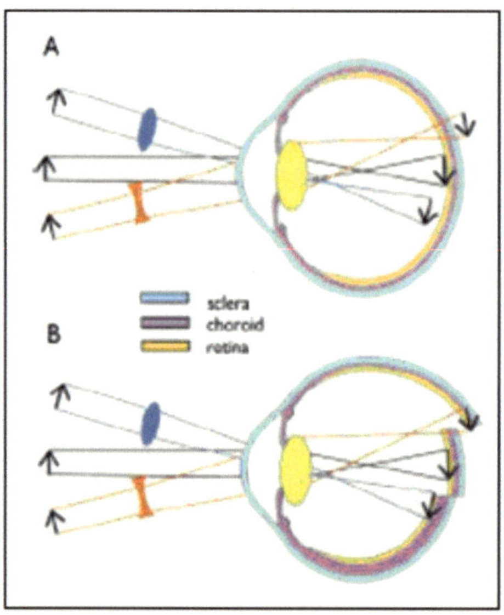

Figure 1. Ocular Compensation for lens-Induced Defocus

a. A positive lens (blue, convex) causes the image to form in front of the retina (myopic defocus), whereas a negative lens (red, concave) pushes the image plane behind the retina (hyperopic defocus). With no lens (black rays), the image of a distant objects is focused on the retina.

b. The eye compensates for positive lenses by slowing its rate of elongation and by thickening the choroid, pushing the retina forward toward the image plane. It compensates of negative lenses by increasing the rate of elongation and thinning the choroid, pulling the retina back toward the image plane. The emmetropic eye is intermediate in length and in choroid thickness. (Figure and legend from [1])

As a development of local retina mechanism model in animal study, data from human beings also suggested that peripheral refractive error can influence the ocular growth. [16-19] For example, young pilots that had relatively hyperopic refractive status in both horizontal and vertical meridian, which potentially contributes to the eye's elongation, were more likely to develop adult-onset myopia than those who showed myopic refractive status at least in one meridian. [16] More recently, Smith and colleagues [20] have tested the hypothesis that the peripheral visual experiences contribute for the ocular growth and central refractive development in primates. Their study provided strong evidence that the peripheral retinal mechanism can influence the refractive development at the fovea and this, most likely, also happens in human beings.

3. Axial ocular aberration

Aberrations are classified as monochromatic and chromatic aberrations. Chromatic aberrations occur when light source has multi-wavelength components. Monochromatic aberrations occur when only one wavelength light source is refracted. The aberration discussed in this chapter is monochromatic aberration.

3.1. Representation of aberration

It is useful to understand wavefront and wavefront aberration before we discuss the measurement and representation of aberration. A wavefront is a surface which is orthogonal to light rays. The wavefront aberration is the distance, in optical path length (product of the refractive index and path length), from the reference plane to wavefront plane at the exit pupil (Figure 2).

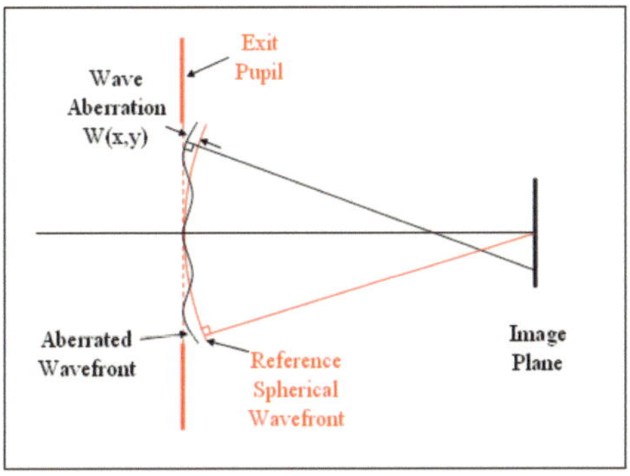

Figure 2. The concept of wavefront aberration: wavefront aberration is the departure of the measured wavefront from the ideal spherical wavefront at the exit pupil.

There are different ways to represent wavefront aberrations such as Taylor series and Zernike polynomials. The Taylor series are rarely used these days since each individual term are not orthonormal. [21] People usually use Zernike series which were recommended by Optical Society of America to describe the eye's wavefront error (Figure 3 & Table 1). [22]

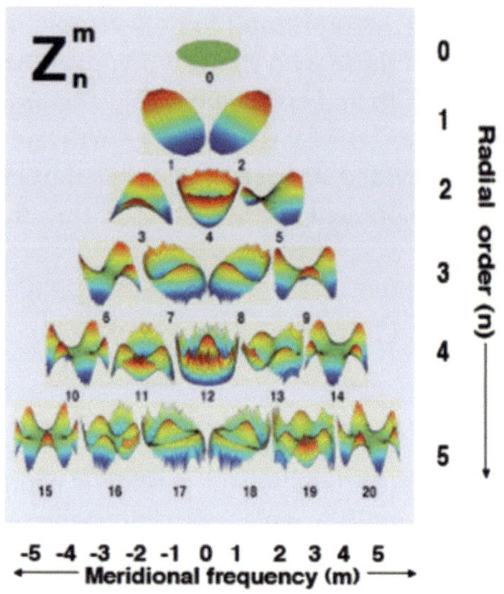

Figure 3. Zernike polynomials: Each row is a radial order. Each column is a meridional frequency. Each function is defined over the circular domain of the pupil and is mathematically orthogonal to all other functions in the table.

The normalized Zernike polynomial has two major advantages when applied to quantify the optical aberrations. First, the magnitude of the Zernike coefficient represents the wavefront error in that mode and usually given in the unit micrometers (μm). Second, in the Zernike series, each mode is orthogonal to the other mode, so the coefficients are independent of each other. This will allow us to manipulate each mode individually. RMS (root mean square) error is widely used to indicate the human eyes' wavefront error in each mode or combined modes. RMS is defined as

$$RMS = \sqrt{\sum_{n>1,m} (C_n^m)^2} \tag{1}$$

First and second order aberrations are regarded as lower-order aberrations. 1st-order Zernike terms are tilts which do not cause image blur therefore are usually ignored. Traditional refractive errors refer to 2nd-order Zernike terms. The relationship between 2nd-order Zernike coefficients and sphero-cylindrical components M, J_0, J_{45} (M: the spherical equivalent, J_0: with-the-rule (WTR) and against-the-rule (ATR) astigmatism, J_{45}: oblique astigmatism with axes at 45 deg and 135 deg) is given by the following equations. [23]

mode j	order n	frequency m	$Z_n^m(\rho,\theta)$
0	0	0	1
1	1	-1	$2\rho\sin(\theta)$
2	1	1	$2\rho\cos(\theta)$
3	2	-2	$\sqrt{6}\rho^2\sin(2\theta)$
4	2	0	$\sqrt{3}(2\rho^2-1)$
5	2	2	$\sqrt{6}\rho^2\cos(2\theta)$
6	3	-3	$\sqrt{8}\rho^3\sin(3\theta)$
7	3	-1	$\sqrt{8}(3\rho^3-2\rho)\sin(\theta)$
8	3	1	$\sqrt{8}(3\rho^3-2\rho)\cos(\theta)$
9	3	3	$\sqrt{8}\rho^3\cos(3\theta)$
10	4	-4	$\sqrt{10}\rho^4\sin(4\theta)$
11	4	-2	$\sqrt{10}(4\rho^4-3\rho^2)\sin(2\theta)$
12	4	0	$\sqrt{5}(6\rho^4-6\rho^2+1)$
13	4	2	$\sqrt{10}(4\rho^4-3\rho^2)\cos(2\theta)$
14	4	4	$\sqrt{10}\rho^4\cos(4\theta)$
⋮	⋮	⋮	⋮

Table 1. List of Zernike Polynomials

$$
\begin{aligned}
M &= \frac{-4\sqrt{3}}{r^2}C_2^0 \\
J_0 &= \frac{-2\sqrt{6}}{r^2}C_2^2 \\
J_{45} &= \frac{-2\sqrt{6}}{r^2}C_2^{-2}
\end{aligned}
\tag{2}
$$

Where C_{20}, C_{22}, C_{2-2} are Zernike coefficients for defocus, WTR/ATR astigmatism and oblique astigmatism terms, and r is pupil radius. We can also use the following equation to convert rectangular Fourier form (M, J_0, J_{45}) to conventional clinical negative-cylinder form. [24]

$$
\begin{aligned}
S &= M + \sqrt{J_0^2 + J_{45}^2} \\
C &= -2\sqrt{J_0^2 + J_{45}^2} \\
\alpha &= \frac{1}{2}\tan^{-1}(J_{45}/J_0)
\end{aligned}
\tag{3}
$$

Start from 3rd order Zernike terms, aberrations are referred as higher-order aberrations. Coma ($C_{3\pm1}$) and spherical aberration (C_{40}) are the most important higher-order aberrations since they present in higher amounts than the other higher-order aberrations in the population. [25, 26]

3.2. Measurement of aberrations

As a development of autorefractors, aberration measuring instruments bear the same principle (Scheiner disc principle) which illustrated in Figure 4. [27, 28] Aberrations can be measured by "into-the-eye" or "out-of-the-eye" aberrometry technique. [28, 29] "Into-the-eye" aberrometry means an image is formed on the retina and re-imaged out of the eye for analysis, like laser ray tracing and Tscherning aberrometer. "Out-of-the-eye" aberrometry refers to an instrument which project a narrow beam into the eye and trace the rays from the retina out of the eye, like Hartmann-Shack wavefront sensor. [28] Aberrometer measure aberrations either sequentially or simultaneously. Sequential aberrometry, like laser ray tracing, measures aberration in one location of the pupil once a time but simultaneous aberrometer (Hartman-Shack wavefront aberrometer) can measure aberration at multiple locations of the pupil at the same time.

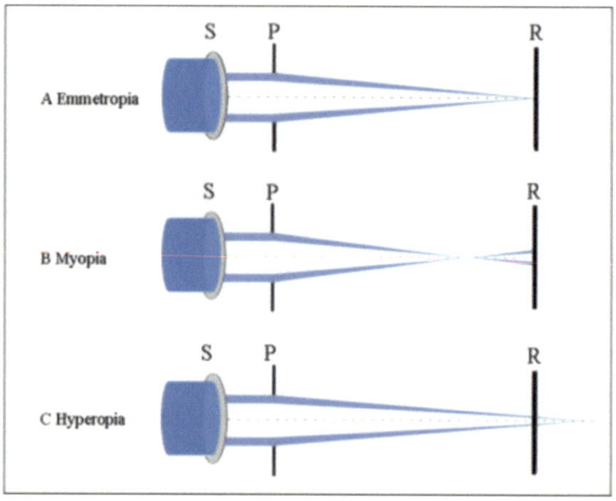

Figure 4. Scheiner disc principle: Light comes from a distant object reduce to two small bundles of light by two pinholes on Scheiner disc. These two rays focus to be a single image on the retina if the eye is emmetropia (Figure 4 a). Double images will be sensed if the eye is myopia or hyperopia (Figure 4 b&c). By adjusting the position of the object until on image is seen, the far point and refractive error of the patient's eye can be determined. S: Scheiner disc; P: Pupil; R: Retina

Most commercial aberrometers use Hartmann-Shack wavefront sensor. Hartmann-Shack technology can be tracked back to early 20th century when Hartmann test was used to measure aberration of optical system. [30, 31] Shack and Platt modified Hartmann technique to invent the Hartmann-Shack aberrometer. [32] This technique was originally developed by astronomers for improving the image quality of the stars and satellites and Liang et al. [33] adapted it to measure conventional refractive errors as well as higher-order aberrations of the eyes. The principle of operation of the Hartmann-Shack aberrometer is shown in Figure 5.

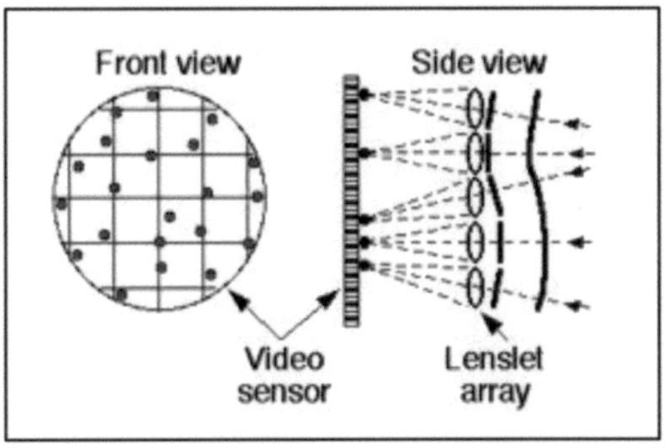

Figure 5. Principle of the Hartmann-Shack (HS) wavefront sensor. HS sensor subdivides the wavefront into hundred small beams which are focused on to a CCD video sensor by an array of small lenses. The displacement of each image relative to the grid of optical axes is determined by the local slope of the wavefront in x-and y-direction at the face of the corresponding lenslet. [Adapted from Thibos [34]]

The critical part of Hartmann-Shack wavefront sensor is a micro-lenslet array. A CCD video sensor is placed in one focal length of those small lenses behind the lenslet array. The reflected wavefront of light emerging from the eye will be partitioned to hundred smaller wavefront and will be focused on the CCD sensor. If the measured eye is a perfect optical system, the wavefront emerging from the eye will be a plane and will be focused perfectly on the intersections of the grids. In the real situation, the aberrated wavefront coming back from the eye will be focused by each lenslet on CCD sensor with displacement corresponding to lenslet axis. The local slopes of the wavefront can be deduced from this displacement.

Hartmann-Shack aberrometer have been widely used to measure aberrations in different area of clinical research [34-40] due to its fast measuring and less affected by scattering of light compared to most other aberrometers. [41] Hartmann-Shack wavefront aberrometer has been reported as a robust and reliable instrument to measure both lower and higher order aberrations. [34, 42, 43]

4. Off-axis aberration

While previous studies concentrated on foveal aberrations, investigations of off-axis (peripheral) vision increased dramatically in recent years because the quality of off-axis optics is important for retina imaging, motion and orientation detection, and development of refractive error. [20, 44-48]

4.1. Measurement of Off-axis aberration

Little is known about off-axis wavefront aberrations and image quality in the eccentric visual fields, for which most studies only reported the changes of defocus and astigmatism in the peripheral visual angle. [16, 46, 47, 49-51] Different techniques, such as retinoscopy, [46, 49, 51, 52] subjective refraction, [47, 50],photorefraction [53] and autorefraction, [54] were used to measure these lower-order aberrations in the peripheral visual field.

The published studies on peripheral refraction [16, 17, 28, 53, 55-58] suggested that hyperopes had relative less hyperopic error in the periphery, while myopes usually had relative less myopic error in periphery. These experimental data was consistent with the previous predictions made by Charman and Jennings [59] and Dunne et al. [60, 61] which used simple models with ray tracing technique on the schematic eye.

In 1998, Navarro et al. first measured higher-order aberrations in four naked eyes using laser ray-tracing method and described aberrations using Zernike polynomials. [62] They measured nasal visual field only and reported that despite large variation between subjects, the four subjects showed the same pattern of the change of the aberrations across the visual field. They found both 3rd-and 4_{th}-order aberrations increasing from center to periphery. Atchison and Scott were the first to use Shack-Hartmann wavefront aberrometer to measure off-axis higher-order aberrations in human eye. [63] They measured aberrations both in nasal and temporal visual field up to 40_0. Like Navarro's study, Atchison's data also showed large between-subject variability. They reported that 3rd-order aberration increased to both nasal and temporal visual field and with nasal-temporal asymmetry. Unlike Navarro's study, they didn't report the large change of 4_{th}-order aberration across the horizontal visual field. Both these two studies only recruited small number of subjects.

In the previous studies, [62-67] researchers didn't attempt to quantify the image quality in the peripheral visual field. Most researchers talked about the peripheral image quality, speculated that off-axis IQ would drop fast and become worse based on the measurements of peripheral refraction (defocus and astigmatism). They neglected the complex interaction between these lower-order and the higher-order aberrations in eyes. [68] In order to investigate the off-axis image quality, to study the interaction between lower-order aberrations and higher-order aberrations in the large visual angle and to study the potential contributions of the off-axis image quality to the whole eyes refractive development, the first step is to measure the monochromatic aberrations in the peripheral visual field accurately.

4.2. Peripheral vision and development of refractive error

The rationale that peripheral refraction can influence the development of refractive error is pointed out by Wallman [1] that if the peripheral retina is relatively hyperopic, this relatively hyperopic defocus will cause the elongation of the eyeball no matter what the foveal refractive status is. As mentioned above, the homeostatic signals from the hyperopic periphery will guide the eye to elongate. If the fovea retina is emmetropic or myopic, the homeostatic signals from the central retina will direct the eye to elongate less. These two signals, from central retina and from the peripheral retina, will try to keep balance. Although the neurons density is higher in the central than in the peripheral retina, considering the total area of the central retina is quite small, the homeostatic signals from peripheral retina directing the eye to elongate more will be stronger than the signals from central retina that directing the eye to elongate less if these signals have spatial summation. If the larger area of the retina become elongated surrounding the fovea area, the mechanical constrains in eye growth will also make the fovea axially elongated. [1] This mechanism has been hypothesized by several studies. [53, 58, 69]

The critical step to understand the above mechanism is that the peripheral retina has the capacity to detect the changes of image quality which are produced by the off-axis aberrations.

[47, 70, 71] Peripheral vision is limited by two factors: the optical image quality and the neurons density in the periphery. It is already known that in large visual angles, the oblique astigmatism increases dramatically. However, these refractive errors can be corrected by ordinary ophthalmic lenses. There are other higher-order aberrations such as coma and spherical aberrations in the off-axis visual field which can also deteriorate the image quality but are difficult to correct. [72] The neurons density (including cones and ganglion cells) is at maximum near the fovea and drops quickly in the periphery. [73] This neurons density constitutes an upper limit of the visual acuity at higher retinal field angles when the off-axis optics is corrected.

The resolution acuity becomes worse with the increasing of the retina eccentricity, but the detection acuity remains high at large eccentricities given the peripheral optics are well corrected. [71, 74] Detection acuity is significantly influenced by the optical defocus and is lower when the retina image is formed by the eye's natural optics, these suggest that the detection acuity is optically limited. [74, 75] But after correct the major off-axis aberrations (defocus and astigmatism), the detection acuity becomes quite good in the peripheral visual field. [70, 76]

Besides evidences supported by other human studies, [16, 17, 19, 77] Smith and colleagues [20] provided further evidence that visual experience in peripheral retina can influence the refractive development at the fovea. And as a development, other studies made a hypothesis that high level of aberrations will guide ocular elongation by degradation of the retinal image. [78-82] Growth of the eye tends to minimize the image blur on the most part of the retina (known as "grow to clarity" model). [5] Thus peripheral vision is closely related with development of central refractive error.

5. Contact lens and myopia progression

Contact lenses are widely used treatments for refractive errors. They had long been used as an optical correction since their introduction by Eugen Fick in 1888. [83] A large number of studies investigated the effect of different types of contact lenses (silicone acrylate contact lenses, hydrophilic contact lenses, hydrogel lenses) on the progression of myopia had been done. [84-90] Though most of the studies had small sample size or were not randomized, they did suggest that wearing soft contact lenses induced increasing in myopia progression. [84, 91, 92] Another large sample size, randomized study done by Horner et al. suggested that there were no significant different in the rate of myopia progression between the children who wore SCLs and spectacles. [93]

Hard contact lenses have longer history than the SCLs. PMMA (polymethyl methacrylate) hard contact lenses were widely prescribed in the clinic although they have side effects caused by low oxygen permeability. After 1970', Rigid-Gas-Permeable (RGP) lens becomes popular. These lenses have higher oxygen permeability than soft contact lens, clinically proved to be a suitable and safer alternative for correcting refractive error. [89] In a three years study, 100 children with myopia were fitted with RGP and compared with control group who wore spectacles, significant reduction of myopia progression was found. [94] Another study also reported a similar results. [95]

Although in 2003, a larger randomized clinical trial of rigid contact lenses conducted in Singapore Children didn't report significant difference of myopia progression between RGP wearers and spectacles wearers, [96] the more recent CLAMP (Contact Lens and Myopia Progression) study [18] has shown that RGP produced a significant slower rate of progression of myopia in children, although this was largely due to flattening of the cornea rather than slowing of axial elongation. [97]

No matter whether the SCLs or RGP lenses can slow the progression of myopia or not, all of the SCLs and RGP studies above tried to relate the lens' efficacy with the ocular physiological changes. No studies have examined the peripheral optical quality after these ophthalmic corrections although there were attempts to evaluate on-axis optical performance of these lenses. [39, 98] Since the peripheral vision is an important factor to contribute for the development of myopia, experimentally measure the monochromatic off-axis aberrations with these ophthalmic lenses on-eye is my proposed experiment and will discussed in detail in later chapters.

5.1. Contact lens and on-axis ocular aberration

The on-axis optical quality after wearing RGP lenses has been well studied both by theoretically calculation and experimental measurements. [99-101] It is widely accepted in clinic that RGP lenses provided the best optical performance for the central vision compared to SCLs and spectacles. RGP lens can smooth the irregularities of the corneal front surface with its rigidity and smooth lens surface. With the correction of moderate astigmatism by the tear lens between RGP and cornea, RGP lenses provide the best on-axis optical performance. Due to the conformity of SCLs, the corneal astigmatism and corneal irregularity will be preserved in some extent for the SCLs wearer (Fig. 6). Theoretically calculation of the on-axis aberrations of RGP lenses always ignores the interaction between the cornea and contact lenses, also without considering the contribution of inner components of the eye to the total optical aberrations. Only Hong et al. [100] and Dorronsoro et al. [98] have measured aberrations in subjects wearing RGP lenses, finding that RGP lenses provided lower aberrations than SCLs and spectacle lenses. They concluded that wearing RGP lenses can significantly reduce the ocular aberrations, not only defocus and astigmatism, but also higher-order aberrations.

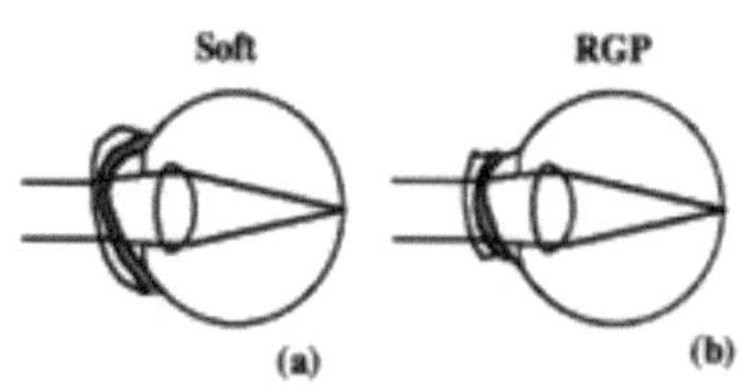

Figure 6. Schematic diagram of the eye with a) soft contact lens, b) rigid gas-permeable (RGP) contact lens. The shaded regions indicated the tear layer. Corneal distortions are exaggerated to illustrate the differences between different optical corrections. [Adapted from [39]]

http://dx.doi.org/10.5772/58456

5.2. Contact lens and off-axis aberrations

Since contact lens correct central refractive error by adding an appropriate compensating power across the entire eye, it will affect the peripheral vision as well while foveal refractive errors are corrected. And due to the potential role of peripheral vision in the development of central refractive error, it is possible that the ophthalmic corrective methods which only correct the central vision but ignoring peripheral image quality will be less successful for controlling myopia progression. Since the myopic eyes have a relative hyperopic periphery, correcting the central myopic will leave the periphery hyperopic (if the correcting lenses have the same power everywhere across the lens piece). The hyperopic periphery will continue to guide the elongation of the eye and the progression of myopia will not stop. Thus the contact lens correction which only corrects the central vision might actually have no effect or even increase the progression of myopia. However, we lack the knowledge of how contact lenses affect peripheral optics of the eye. Although knowledge of off-axis aberrations of CL in isolation is important to help understanding the effect of CLs on peripheral optics of the eye, [102] to obtain a definitive result of how the peripheral refractive error and image quality changes across the visual field with CLs correction requires that the CLs be worn by a human eye.

6. Peripheral refractions and contact lens correction

Multiple studies [53, 103-105] have shown that hyperopic and emmetropic eyes tend to have peripheral refractive errors that are myopic relative to the fovea. The image shell from a distant, extended object is therefore more curved than the retinal surface, resulting in an increasing amount of myopic blur at greater retinal eccentricities. In this chapter, we will refer to this condition as "myopic field curvature" or "relative peripheral myopia". By contrast, myopic eyes tend to have less myopia in the peripheral visual field than foveally. Most authors agree on this point for the horizontal field, but there is some controversy regarding the generality of the finding at the other meridian. [53, 54, 106] The image shell from a distant, extended object is less curved than the retinal surface in myopic eyes, resulting in a decreasing amount of myopic blur at greater retinal eccentricities. Thus, relative to foveal refractive error, the eye has an increasing amount of hyperopic blur at greater retinal eccentricities. In this chapter, we will refer to this condition as "hyperopic field curvature" or "relative peripheral hyperopia".

The rationale that peripheral refraction can influence the development of refractive error is that if the peripheral retina is relatively hyperopic, this relatively hyperopic defocus will cause the elongation of the eyeball no matter what the foveal refractive status is. As mentioned above, the homeostatic signals from the hyperopic periphery will guide the eye to elongate. If the fovea retina is emmetropic or myopic, the homeostatic signals from the central retina will direct the eye to elongate less. These two signals, from central retina and from the peripheral retina, will try to keep balance. Although the neurons density is higher in the central than in the peripheral retina, considering the total area of the central retina is quite small, the homeostatic signals from peripheral retina directing the eye to elongate more will be stronger than the signals from central retina that directing the eye to elongate less if these signals have spatial summation. If the larger area of the retina become elongated surrounding the fovea area, the mechanical constrains in eye growth will also make the fovea axially elongated. This also demonstrated by the local retina mechanism. [58, 69, 107].

More recently, Smith and colleagues [108] have tested the hypothesis that the peripheral visual experiences contribute for the ocular growth and central refractive development in primates. Their study provided strong evidence that the peripheral retinal mechanism can influence the refractive development at the fovea and this, most likely, also happens in human beings.

6.1. Curvature of field and peripheral astigmatism for the naked eye

Consistent with most previous studies, emmetropic eyes showed myopic shift into the periphery (Fig.7 a & b) whereas myopic subjects showed relatively hyperopic shift (Fig.8 a & b). Greater myopia and higher astigmatism in the nasal visual field than in the temporal visual field were found in most of the subjects in the study (Fig.7, 8, 9, 10 & Fig.11). This asymmetry of the changes of M, J_0 and J_{45} across horizontal visual field has been noted in previous, large-scale studies of peripheral refraction. However, the larger error bar indicated that there were considerable differences occur among the subjects. (Within-subject variance was small as indicated from the Fig.7a and Fig.8a, but this might be due to the lack of necessary realignments of the instrument between the measurements in each visual angle position.) A more apparent hyperopic shift beyond 20 degree eccentricity was found (Fig.7). (Previous, Atchison et al. reported a subtle changes in refraction across the central 10º of the retina, with changes in M varying by up to half a diopter and with smaller changes in astigmatism [109].)

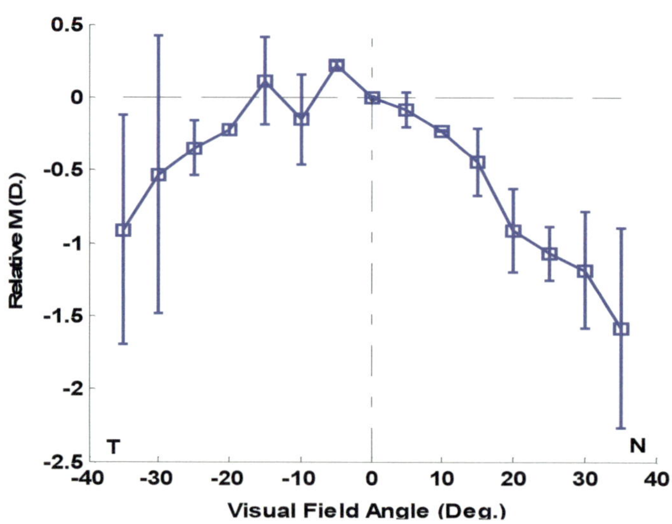

Figure 7. a) Spherical equivalent refractive error (M) relative to the fovea as a function of visual field angle for Sub.1 and Sub.2. Both of these two subjects are emmetropes. Symbols show the means and Error bar indicate the standard deviation of 5 repeated measurements. b) The mean value of Spherical equivalent (M) as a function of visual field angle for the two emmetropes. Error bar indicate the standard deviation of the two emmetropic subjects.

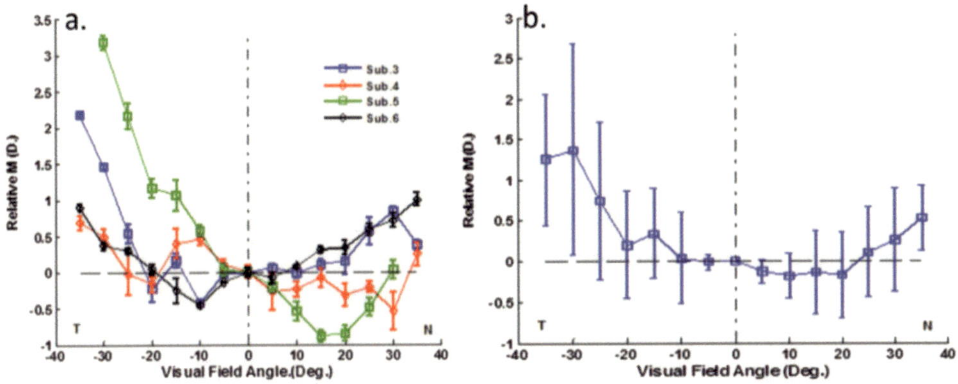

Figure 8. a) Relative M as a function of visual field angle for the naked eye of 4 myopic subjects separately. Error bar indicate the within-subject variance of 5 repeated measurements. b) Relative M as a function of retina eccentricity for myopes. Error bar indicate the standard deviation of the four myopic subjects.

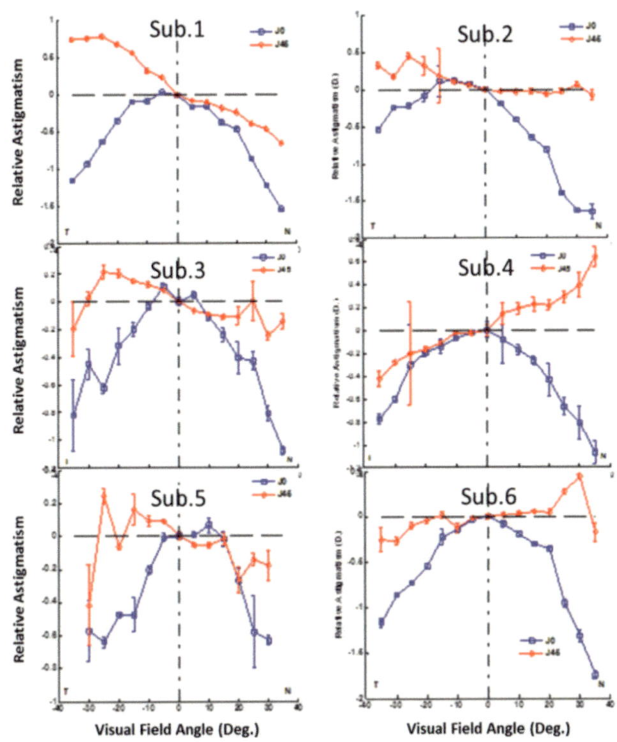

Figure 9. a) Relative J_0 and J_{45} as a function of visual field angle for the six naked eye. Symbols show the mean and error bar indicate the standard deviation of 5 repeated measurements. b) Mean value of the relative J_0 and J_{45} of the six subjects. Error bar indicate the standard deviation of these six subjects.

In another published study, the mean data show a monotonic increase in PRM with eccentricity that is approximately linear with a slope of 0.01 diopters/deg of eccentricity. Thus for an eccentricity of E degrees, PRM is approximately E percent of foveal refractive error in the naked eye. [110]

6.2. Effect of contact lenses on field curvature and peripheral astigmatism

In the group with 4 myopic subjects, the mean value of the change of mean spherical and astigmatism across the horizontal visual field without any correction and with full SCLs correction were shown in Fig. 10 and Fig. 11. With the SCLs corrections, which rendered the fovea conjugate to infinity, the M component still showed a relatively hyperopic shift to the peripheral visual field away from the center. In most of the measurement positions, spherical equivalent had larger hyperopic value after subjects wearing SCLs than their naked eye's data. This suggested that using Acuvue 2 SCLs in this experiment to fully correct the foveal refractive error might cause more hyperopic shift in the peripheral visual field. The nasal-temporal asymmetry after wearing the SCL was not apparent anymore (Fig.10). This result suggested that either corneal shape was responsible for the asymmetry or it was an artifact of CL movement. In the new experiment, the measurements will be taken by rotate subject's head instead of eye rotation. This can eliminate the artifact of SCLs movement and will give us answer about this issue. J_0 was the major contributor for the increase of astigmatism in large visual angle. After full correction with SCLs, J_{45} did not change much across the horizontal visual field, but greater J_0 (more negative) was found in the experiment (especially across the temporal retina) (Fig.11). However, large between-subject differences were found. Only 4 subjects who had very different center refractive error participated in the study. Hopefully, the variance will be reduced by recruiting more subjects who have similar central refractive status in the future study.

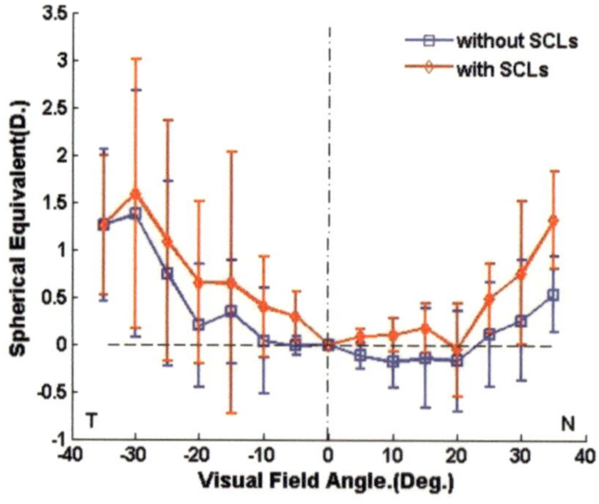

Figure 10. The effect of SCLs on relative M as a function of visual field angle with and without SCLs correction. Error bar indicate the standard deviation.

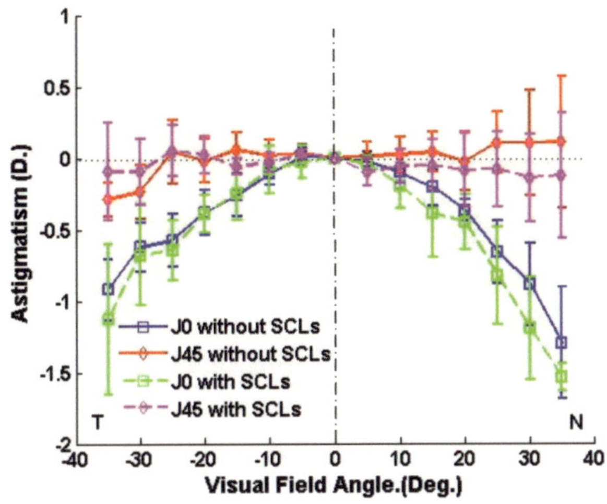

Figure 11. The effect of SCLs on relative J_0 and J_{45} across the horizontal visual field with and without SCLs. Red lines are $J_{45,}$ blue lines are $J_{0.}$ Dash lines indicate the astigmatisms after subjects wear the SCLs. Error bar shows the standard deviation.

Compared to the naked eye, curvature of field was reduced, and in some cases reversed in sign, by contact lenses.

6.3. Contact lens effect on total sphero-cylindrical blur

The results described above show that defocus (M) and astigmatism (J_0) both vary across the visual field. If image quality is a driving force for myopia progression as suggested previously, [78-82] then it is important to determine the combined effects of M and J_0. The effect of contact lenses may be complex because, as shown above, relative hyperopic defocus is reduced by contact lenses, but peripheral astigmatism increases. Therefore, to determine the effect of contact lenses on peripheral image quality, we need to quantify and compare the total sphero-cylindrical image blur on the peripheral retina before and after wearing contact lenses.

In one of our published studies, [110] the average image blur caused by sphere and cylinder in naked eye increased to 2 D at 35° periphery relative to the eye's optical axis. SCLs did not have a consistent effect on sphero-cylindrical blur but RGP lenses consistently reduced the blur across the visual field ($p < 0.01$, non-parametric sign test) by approximately 0.25 diopter.

7. Peripheral image quality and contact lens correction

7.1. Variation of higher-order aberrations with visual field eccentricity

The data was also analyzed in Zernike coefficient terms in order to study the change of high-order aberrations as a function of the visual field angle. Coefficients from 2nd-to 6th-order were used to describe the wavefront aberrations. The change of mean (all 6 subjects) relative 2nd-

order aberration as a function of visual field angle was shown in Fig.12. The 2nd-order aberration increased with the visual field angle. Across the horizontal visual field, C_2^2 was the major contributor for the change of 2nd-order aberration (Fig.13 b). Since positive value of C_2^2 indicates Against-The-Rule (ATR) astigmatism and negative value of C_2^2 indicates With-The-Rule (WTR) astigmatism, mean value of C_2^2 in this experiment suggested that the astigmatism changed from WTR to ATR with the increasing of visual field angle from center to periphery (Fig.13 a). Considerable differences occurred among the 6 subjects. This might partly due to the different center refractive error of these six subjects had effects on the peripheral refraction shift.

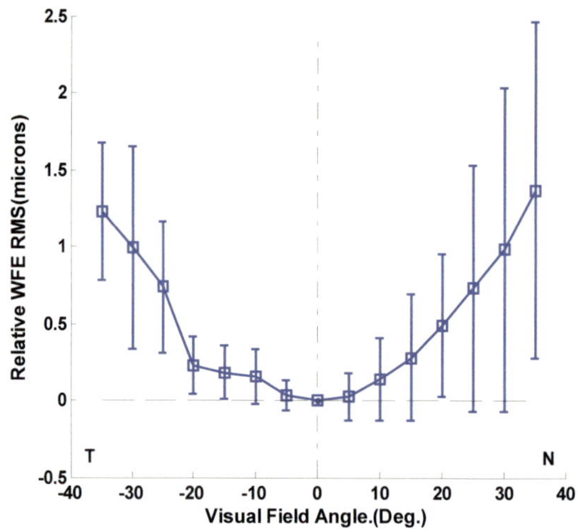

Figure 12. Relative RMS in 2nd-order aberration across the horizontal visual field of the naked eye. Error bar indicate the standard deviation among the six subjects.

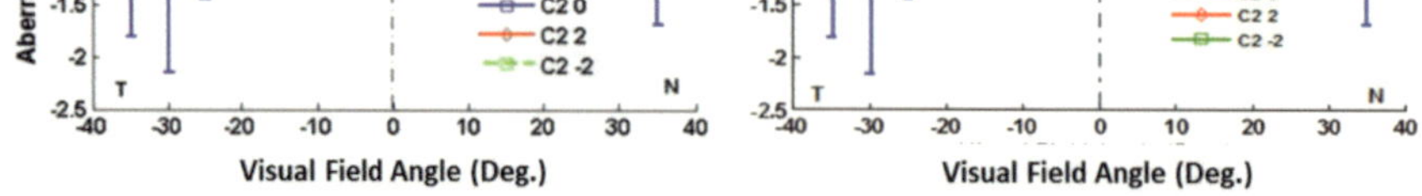

Figure 13. a) The change of Zernike coefficients in the 2nd-order aberration without any correction with the increasing of visual field angle. The data is the mean value of six subjects. Error bar indicate the standard deviation. b) Relative Zernike coefficients in 2nd-order aberration as a function of visual field angle. Error bar indicate the standard deviation.

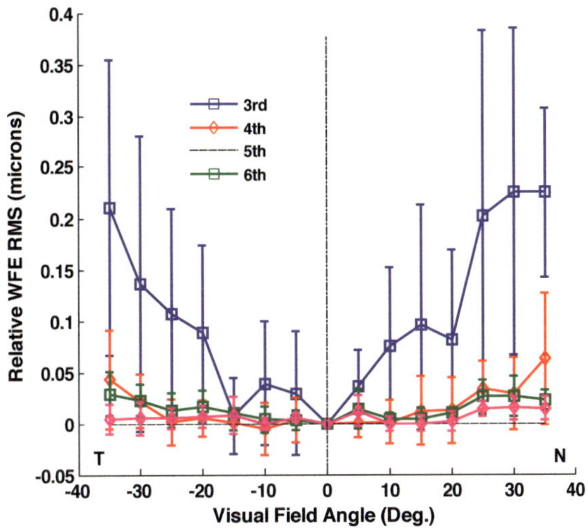

Figure 14. Relative RMS value of high order aberrations' change across the horizontal visual field without any correction for the all six subjects. Error bar indicate the standard deviation.

The high order aberrations (3rd-to-6th-, in this experiment) basically showed the same pattern with Atchison & Navarro's data [62, 111]. The 3rd-, 4th-and 5th-order aberrations showed an increasing magnitude with the visual field angle. Changes of 6th-order aberration were quite small across the horizontal visual field. The nasal-temporal asymmetry of 3rd-order aberration was not as apparent as Atchison's data. In the nasal visual field, there was a factor of 2.8 increasing in 3rd-order aberration. Which reported by Atchison was 5 and by Navarro was 2.5. For temporal visual field, there was a factor of 2.6 for 3rd-order aberration, which reported by Atchison was 3. For 4th-and 5th-order aberrations, a small increase of magnitude with the increasing visual field angle was also noticed. Big individual variance was found in our data as well as in Atchison and Navarro's data (Fig. 14). The sample size was small both in this experiment and previous studies.

Horizontal coma (C_3^1) was a major contributor to the increase of 3rd-order aberration in the peripheral visual field and it showed a linear dependence on the visual field position. This contrasted with changes of vertical coma (C_3^{-1}) and trefoils (C_3^3 and C_3^{-3}), which were quite flat across the visual field. This linear relationship between horizontal coma and retina eccentricity was predicted by Seidel theory [112], and both Atchison's data and my data showed this relationship in the human eye (Fig.15). Although there were large individual variances, both spherical aberrations (C_4^0) and secondary astigmatism (C_4^2) showed a quadratic dependence on visual field position. This relationship between C_4^0, C_4^2 and visual field position was also predicted by Seidel Theory. The spherical aberration (C_4^0) showed a positive value in the fovea (most people have positive spherical aberration in the un-accommodated state for foveal vision [28]). However, the magnitude of spherical aberration reduced into the horizontal periphery and finally became negative (Fig. 16).

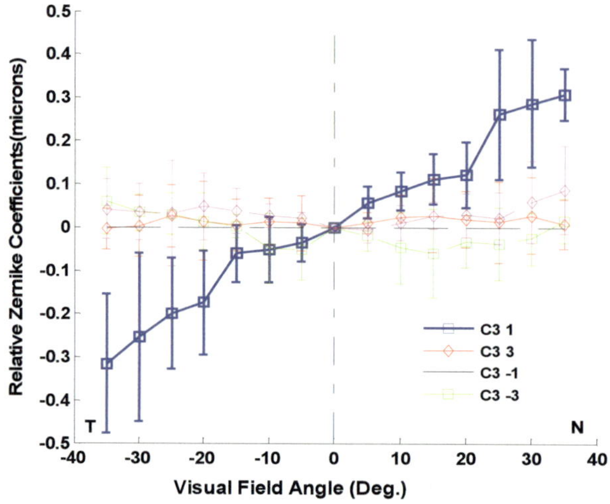

Figure 15. Relative Zernike coefficients in 3rd-order aberration across the horizontal visual field without any correction. Data is mean value of 6 subjects. The blue line is the horizontal coma (C_3^1). Error bar indicate the standard deviation.

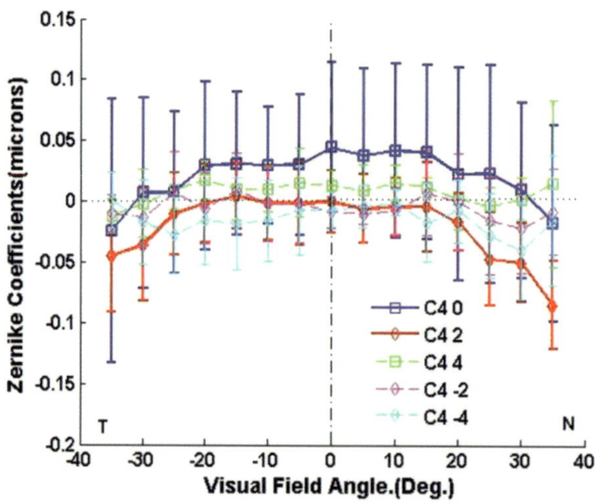

Figure 16. a) The change of Zernike coefficients in 4th-order aberration across the horizontal visual field without any correction. Blue line and red line are spherical aberration (C_4^0) and secondary astigmatism (C_4^2), respectively. Data is mean value of 6 subjects. Error bar indicate the standard deviation. (From the figure, we can notice the C_4^0 is positive value in the fovea and finally become negative in the far periphery) b) Relative Zernike coefficients in the 4th-order aberration. Error bars was omitted in order only to show the change pattern of C_4^0 and C_4^2 more clearly.

After wearing SCLs, the changes of 2nd-to 6th-order aberrations kept the similar pattern from center to periphery as those uncorrected eyes. Large individual variances still existed, and the 2nd-to 5th-order aberration increased with the visual field angle. The nasal-temporal asymmetry was not apparent as well. In the 3rd-order aberration, after wearing soft contact lens, the horizontal coma still somehow showed a linear dependence with the horizontal visual angle. The spherical aberration and secondary astigmatism continued to show quadratic dependences on the visual field positions after soft contact lenses wearing. (Fig. 17 a, b, c & d)

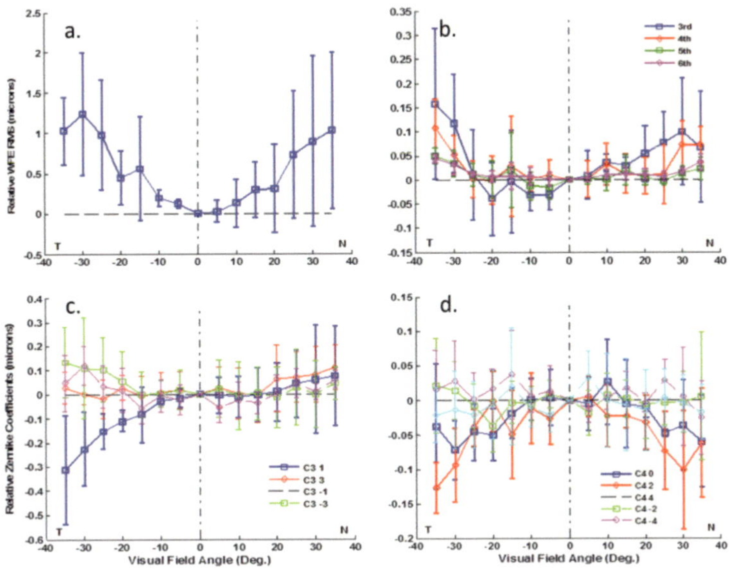

Figure 17. The relative value of 2nd-to 6th-order aberrations and Zernike coefficients across the horizontal visual field with SCLs fully corrected the subjects' foveal vision. Error bar indicate the standard deviation of the 4 SCL wearer subjects. a). Mean relative value of 2nd-order aberration. b). Mean relative value of 3rd-to 4th-order aberrations. c). Relative Zernike coefficients in the 3rd-order aberration. d). Relative Zernike coefficients in the 4th-order aberration.

7.2. Effect of contact lens correction on ocular higher-order aberrations

After wearing SCLs to fully correct the foveal refractive error, 2nd-order aberration increased in the most positions in temporal visual field but decreased in most positions in nasal visual field (Fig. 18 a & b). This was consistent with the data shown in Fig.7 & 8.

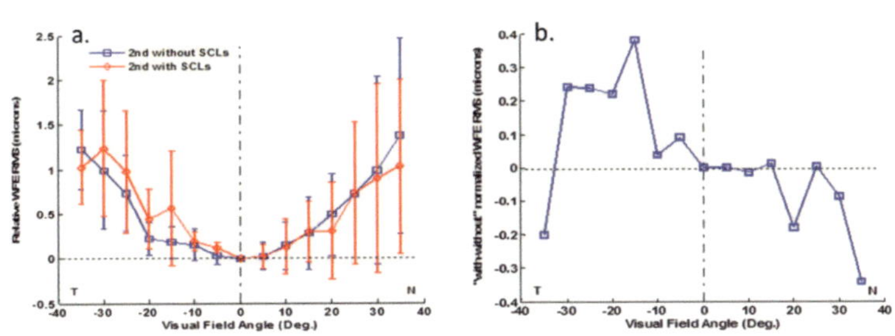

Figure 18. a) The change of 2nd-order aberrations across the horizontal visual field with and without SCL correction. Error bar indicate the standard deviation. b) By subtracting the naked eye's data, the curves in the figure indicate the effect of SCLs on relative wavefront RMS of the subjects. Negative value means the RMS becomes smaller after wearing SCL.

When comparing 3rd-to 6th-order aberrations before and after wearing soft contact lenses, we found that the magnitude increasing rate of 3rd-order aberration decreased after SCLs correction compared to that in the naked eyes, especially beyond 20 degree nasal visual field (Fig. 19 a & b). A 1.4 fold increase in 3rd-order aberration of the nasal visual field after wearing soft contact lenses compared to the 2.5 fold before wearing the soft contact lenses was found. Since the irregular corneal anterior surface contributed significantly to the asymmetric aberrations, the eye with soft contact lenses more or less smoothed the anterior corneal surface, thus the reduction of 3rd-order aberration after contact lens fitting was anticipated. Another more possible reason might be the movement of SCLs in the eye. When the eye turned around to the far periphery to fixate on the target, SCLs would move in the opposite direction, thus the measurements taken by aberrometer in these visual angles would not be the exact reading taken if the SCLs could move with the eyes perfectly but this might be a great advantage of SCLs in real life. RGP lens can probably reduce 3rd-order aberration more since RGP lenses have larger movement than SCLs (if the measurements are still taken in the same way with the eye rotation to fixate on target in different visual angle). After wearing SCLs, the 4th-order aberration increased to the far horizontal periphery beyond center 50 degrees. This, again, might be caused by the movement of the contact lenses. The 5th-and 6th-order aberrations also slightly increased after wearing soft contact lenses in the temporal visual field (Fig. 19 a & b).

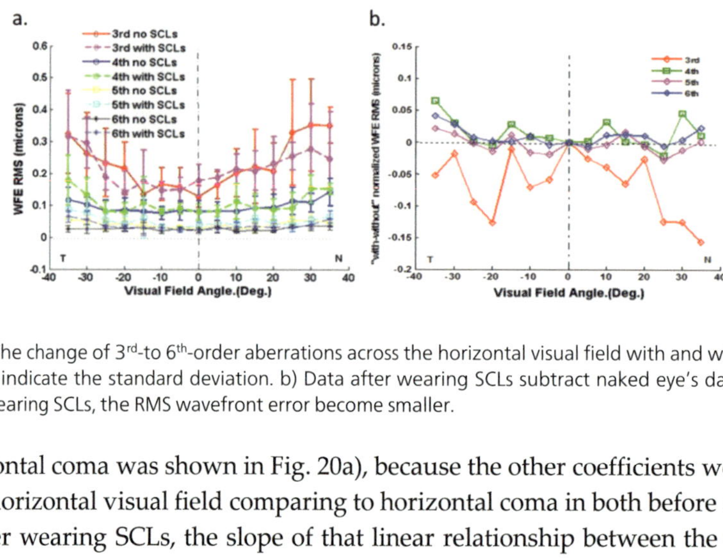

Figure 19. a) The change of 3rd-to 6th-order aberrations across the horizontal visual field with and without SCLs correction. Error bar indicate the standard deviation. b) Data after wearing SCLs subtract naked eye's data. Negative value means after wearing SCLs, the RMS wavefront error become smaller.

Only horizontal coma was shown in Fig. 20a), because the other coefficients were quite small across the horizontal visual field comparing to horizontal coma in both before and after SCLs fitting. After wearing SCLs, the slope of that linear relationship between the C_3^1 and visual field angle became flatter (Fig.20 a). This contributed to the overall decrease of 3rd-order aberration after wearing SCLs. For the 4th-order aberration, since the spherical aberration (C_4^0) and secondary astigmatism (C_4^2) were the two major components which contributed to the 4th-order aberration change across the horizontal visual field, data were plotted of these two coefficients only with and without SCLs correction (Fig.20 b & c). The spherical aberration (C_4^0) did not show significant differences across all the retina eccentricity before and after contact lenses fitting. However, secondary astigmatism (C_4^2) showed larger magnitudes to the horizontal periphery compared to the uncorrected eye (Fig.20 b & c). This might help to explain

http://dx.doi.org/10.5772/58456

the increase in the magnitude of 4th-order aberration in the far periphery. Both the primary astigmatism and secondary astigmatism became larger in the large off-axis visual angle after wearing SCLs, but there was no adequate explanation currently to explain this.

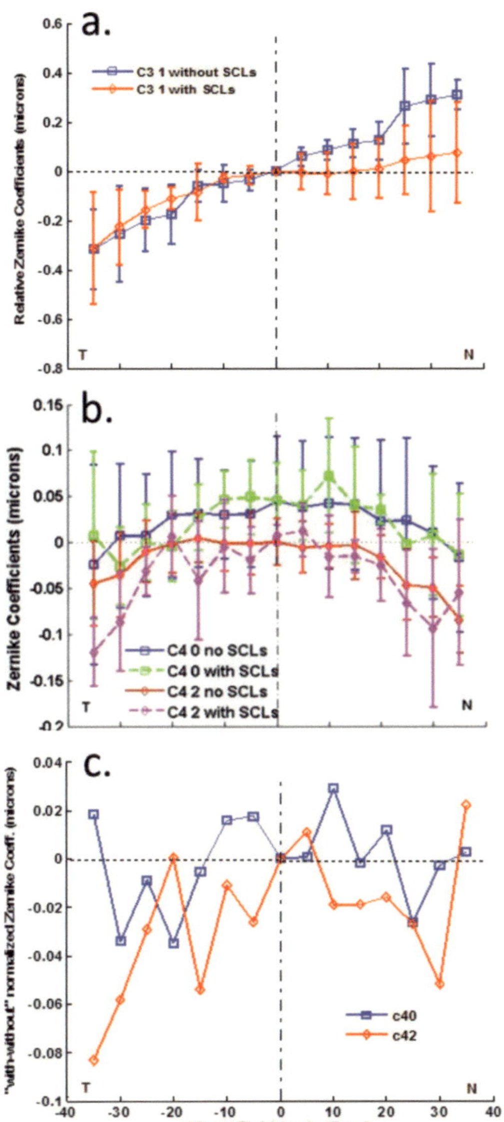

Figure 20. The change of Zernike coefficients as a function of visual field angle. The data are the mean value got from 4 myopic subjects with and without SCL correction. Error bar indicate the standard deviation. a). Change of the relative horizontal coma (C_3^1) across the horizontal visual field before and after SCLs correction. b). Change of spherical aberration (C_4^0) and secondary astigmatism (C_4^2) across the horizontal visual field before (solid lines) and after (dash lines) SCLs correction. c). Data after wearing SCLs subtract naked eye's data. Negative value means Zernike coefficients of C_4^2 became larger after wearing SCLs comparing to naked eyes.

7.3. Peripheral image quality with and without contact lens correction

Image quality was assessed with the VSOTF metric [113, 114] for the complete wavefront aberration (including 2nd order aberrations) measured over the full entrance pupil of each eye in another published study Without contact lens correction, VSOTF gradually decreases from center to periphery. With contact lens correction, image quality improves greatly both in the center and in the periphery. This improvement is due mainly to a reduction in 2nd order aberrations. RGP lens correction shows a trend of better image quality than SCLs across the whole visual field. Image quality drops quickly from center to the periphery after contact lens correction.

8. Conclusion

Both SCL and RGP lenses reduce the degree of hyperopic field curvature present in myopic eyes, but only RGPs reduce the relative amount of image blur on the peripheral retina. Although our study was motivated by the myopia question, the results pertain also to the perceptual quality of peripheral vision. The visual benefit of improved image contrast for peripheral vision obtained by RGP lenses should outweigh the visual benefit of SCLs. The tradeoff between reduced field curvature but increased peripheral astigmatism with RGP correction limits the net improvement of image blur on the peripheral retina that might, in turn, limit RGP lens effectiveness for improving vision or controlling myopia progression. Our results suggest that axial growth mechanisms that depend on retinal image quality will be affected more by RGP than by SCL lenses. These results provide some guidance for future designs of contact lenses to control myopia progression.

Contact lens increases higher-order aberrations in the peripheral visual field except 3rd-order Zernike terms. RGP lenses improve peripheral image quality for objects located at the foveal far point. Increased HOA after contact lens correction reduces image quality by an amount that depends on the eye's initial IQ. If the eye has good IQ initially, changes in HOA have a relatively large effect on IQ. But if the eye has poor IQ initially, HOA will have relatively small effect on IQ. These results suggest contact lens designer and manufacturers should aim to improve the capabilities of contact lens for correcting HOA while simultaneously providing best sphero-cylinder correction for the eye across the visual field.

Author details

Jie Shen*

Address all correspondence to: jshen@westernu.edu

College of Optometry, Western University of Health Sciences, USA

http://dx.doi.org/10.5772/58456

References

[1] Wallman, J.J.W., *Homeostasis of Eye Growth and the Question of Myopia.* Neuron, 2004. 43: p. 447-468.

[2] Hodos, W. and W.J. Kuenzel, *Retinal-image degradation produces ocular enlargement in chicks.* Invest Ophthalmol Vis Sci, 1984. 25: p. 652-659.

[3] Diether, S. and F. Schaeffel, *Local changes in eye growth induced by imposed local refractive error despite active accommodation.* Vision Res, 1997. 37 (6): p. 659-68.

[4] Bartmann, M. and F. Schaeffel, *A simple mechanism for emmetropization without cues from accommodation or colour.* Vision Res, 1994. 34 (7): p. 873-6.

[5] Wildsoet, C.F., *Active emmetropization--evidence for its existence and ramifications for clinical practice.* Ophthalmic Physiol Opt, 1997. 17 (4): p. 279-90.

[6] Gentle, A. and N. McBrien, *Modulation of scleral DNA synthesis in development and recovery from induced axial myopia in the tree shrew.* Exp. Eye Res., 1999. 68: p. 155-163.

[7] Wallman, J., et al., *Moving the retina: choroidal moduation of refractive state.* Vision Res, 1995. 35: p. 37-50.

[8] Wildsoet, C. and J. Wallman, *Choroid and scleral mechanisms of compensation for spectacle lenses in chicks.* Vision Res, 1995. 35: p. 1175-1194.

[9] Graham, B. and S.J. Judge, *The effects of spectacle wear in infancy on eye growth and refractive error in the marmoset (Callithrix jacchus).* Vision Res, 1999. 39 (2): p. 189-206.

[10] Hung, L.F., M.L. Crawford, and E.L. Smith, *Spectacle lenses alter eye growth and the refractive status of young monkeys.* Nat Med, 1995. 1 (8): p. 761-5.

[11] Irving, E.L., M.G. Callender, and J.G. Sivak, *Inducing myopia, hyperopia, and astigmatism in chicks.* Optom Vis Sci, 1991. 68 (5): p. 364-8.

[12] Schaeffel, F. and H.C. Howland, *Properties of the feedback loops controlling eye growth and refractive state in the chicken.* Vision Res, 1991. 31 (4): p. 717-34.

[13] Siegwart, J.T., Jr. and T.T. Norton, *Regulation of the mechanical properties of tree shrew sclera by the visual environment.* Vision Res, 1999. 39 (2): p. 387-407.

[14] Hodos, W. and J.T. Erichsen, *Lower-field myopia in birds: an adaptation that keeps the ground in focus.* Vision Res, 1990. 30 (5): p. 653-7.

[15] Fitzke, F.W., et al., *Refractive sectors in the visual field of the pigeon eye.* J Physiol., 1985. 369: p. 33-34.

[16] Hoogerheide, J., F. Rempt, and W.P. Hoogenboom, *Acquired myopia in young pilots.* Ophthalmologica, 1971. 163 (4): p. 209-15.

[17] Mutti, D.O., et al., *Peripheral refraction and ocular shape in children.* Invest Ophthalmol Vis Sci, 2000. 41 (5): p. 1022-30.

[18] Walline, J., et al., *A randomized trial of the effects of rigid contact lenses on myopia progression.* Arch Ophthalmol., 2004. 122: p. 1760-1766.

[19] Schmid, G.F., *Retinal steepness vs. myopic shift in children (Abstract).* Optom Vis Sci, 2004. 12 (suppl) (23).

[20] Smith, E.L., 3rd, et al., *Peripheral vision can influence eye growth and refractive development in infant monkeys.* Invest Ophthalmol Vis Sci, 2005. 46 (11): p. 3965-72.

[21] Atchison, D.A., *Recent advances in representation of monochromatic aberrations of human eyes.* Clin Exp Optom, 2004. 87 (3): p. 138-48.

[22] Thibos, L.N., et al., *Standards for reporting the optical aberrations of eyes.* J Refract Surg, 2002. 18 (5): p. S652-60.

[23] Thibos, L.N., et al., *Accuracy and precision of objective refraction from wavefront aberrations.* J. Vis.,, 2004. 4: p. 329-351.

[24] Thibos, L.N., W. Wheeler, and D. Horner, *Power vectors: an application of Fourier analysis to the description and statistical analysis of refractive error.* Optom Vis Sci, 1997. 74 (6): p. 367-75.

[25] Thibos, L.N., A. Bradley, and X. Hong, *A statistical model of the aberration structure of normal, well-corrected eyes.* Ophthalmic Physiol Opt, 2002. 22 (5): p. 427-33.

[26] Wang, L. and D.D. Koch, *Ocular higher-order aberrations in individuals screened for refractive surgery.* J Cataract Refract Surg, 2003. 29 (10): p. 1896-903.

[27] Thibos, L.N., R.A. Applegate, and S. Marcos, *Aberrometry: the past, present, and future of optometry.* Optom Vis Sci, 2003. 80 (1): p. 1-2.

[28] Atchison, D.A., *Recent advances in measurements of monochromatic aberrations of human eye.* Clin. Exp. Optom., 2005. 88: p. 5-27.

[29] MacRae, S., R. Krueger, and R. Applegate, *Customized Corneal Ablation: The Quest for Super Vision II.* Thorofare: Slack Incorporated, 2001.

[30] Hartmann, J., *Bemerkungen uber den Bau und die Justirung von Spektrographen.* Z Instrumentenkd, 1900. 20 (47).

[31] Hartmann, J., *Objektuvuntersuchungen.* Z Instrumentenkd, 1904. 24 (1).

[32] Shack, R. and B. Platt, *Production and use of a lenticular Hartmann screen.* J Opt Soc Am A., 1971. 61 (656).

[33] Liang, J., et al., *Objective measurement of wave aberrations of the human eye with the use of a Hartmann-Shack wave-front sensor.* J Opt Soc Am A., 1994. 11: p. 1949-57.

[34] Thibos, L.N. and X. Hong, *Clinical applications of the Shack-Hartmann aberrometer.* Optom Vis Sci, 1999. 76 (12): p. 817-25.

[35] Cheng, X., et al., *Relationship between refractive error and monochromatic aberrations of the eye.* Optom Vis Sci, 2003. 80 (1): p. 43-9.

[36] Klein, S.A., *Optimal corneal ablation for eyes with arbitrary Hartmann-Shack aberrations.* J Opt Soc Am A Opt Image Sci Vis, 1998. 15 (9): p. 2580-8.

[37] Miller, J.M., et al., *Higher order aberrations in normal, dilated, intraocular lens, and laser in situ keratomileusis corneas.* J Refract Surg, 2002. 18 (5): p. S579-83.

[38] Guirao, A., et al., *Calculated impact of higher-order monochromatic aberrations on retinal image quality in a population of human eyes.* J Opt Soc Am A Opt Image Sci Vis, 2002. 19 (3): p. 620-8.

[39] Munson, K., X. Hong, and L.N. Thibos, *Use of a Shack-Hartmann aberrometer to assess the optical outcome of corneal transplantation in a keratoconic eye.* Optom Vis Sci, 2001. 78 (12): p. 866-71.

[40] Hong, X. and L.N. Thibos, *Longitudinal evaluation of optical aberrations following laser in situ keratomileusis surgery.* J Refract Surg, 2000. 16 (5): p. S647-50.

[41] Dai, G., *Wavefront optics for vision correction.* Bellingham: SPIE, 2008.

[42] Cheng, X., et al., *Validation of a clinical Shack-Hartmann aberrometer.* Optom Vis Sci., 2003b. 80: p. 587-595.

[43] Cheng, X., et al., *Test-retest reliability of clinical Shack-Hartmann measurements.* Invest Ophthalmol Vis Sci, 2004. 45 (1): p. 351-60.

[44] Atchison, D.A., *Effect of defocus on visual field measurement.* Ophthalmic Physiol Opt, 1987. 7 (3): p. 259-65.

[45] Fankhauser, F. and J.M. Enoch, *The effects of blur upon perimetric thresholds. A method for determining a quantitative estimate of retinal contour.* Arch Ophthalmol, 1962. 68: p. 240-51.

[46] Johnson, C. and H. Leibowitz, *Practice, refractive error, and feedback as factors influencing peripheral motion thresholds.* Percept Psychophys, 1974. 15 (2): p. 276-280.

[47] Wang, Y.Z., et al., *Subjective refraction of the peripheral field using contrast detection acuity.* Journal of the American Optometric Association., 1996. 67: p. 584-589.

[48] Smith, E.L., 3rd, et al., *Effects of foveal ablation on emmetropization and form-deprivation myopia.* Invest Ophthalmol Vis Sci, 2007. 48 (9): p. 3914-22.

[49] Ferree, C., G. Rand, and C. Hardy, *Refraction for the peripheral field of vision.* Arch Ophthalmol., 1931. 5: p. 717-731.

[50] Millodot, M. and A. Lamont, *Refraction of the periphery of the eye.* J. Opt. Soc. Am., 1974. 64: p. 110-111.

[51] Anderson, R.S. and L.N. Thibos, *Relationship between acuity for gratings and for tumbling-E letters in peripheral vision.* J Opt Soc Am A Opt Image Sci Vis, 1999. 16 (10): p. 2321-33.

[52] Rempt, F., Hoogerheide, J., & Hoogenboom, W.P.H., *Peripheral retinoscopy and the skiagram.* Ophthalmologica., 1971. 162: p. 1-10.

[53] Seidemann, A., et al., *Peripheral refractive errors in myopic, emmetropic, and hyperopic young subjects.* J Opt Soc Am A Opt Image Sci Vis, 2002. 19 (12): p. 2363-73.

[54] Atchison, D.A., *Higher order aberrations across the horizontal visual field.* J Biomed Opt, 2006. 11 (3): p. 34026.

[55] Logan, N.S., Gilmartin, B., Wildsoet, C.F., & Dunne, M.C., *Posterior retinal contour in adult human anisomyopia.* Invest Ophthalmol Vis Sci, 2004. 45: p. 2152-2162.

[56] Love, J., Gilmartin, B., & Dunne, M.C.M., *Relative peripheral refractive error in adult and emmetropia.* Invest Ophthalmol Vis Sci, 2000. 41: p. s302.

[57] Millodot, M., *Effect of ametropia on peripheral refraction.* American Journal of Optometry and Physiological Optics., 1981. 58: p. 691-695.

[58] Schmid, G.F., *Variability of retinal steepness at the posterior pole in children 7-15 years of age.* Current Eye Research., 2003. 27: p. 61-68.

[59] Charman, W.N. and J.A. Jennings, *Ametropia and peripheral refraction.* Am J Optom Physiol Opt, 1982. 59 (11): p. 922-3.

[60] Dunne, M.C. and D.A. Barnes, *Schematic modelling of peripheral astigmatism in real eyes.* Ophthalmic Physiol Opt, 1987. 7 (3): p. 235-9.

[61] Dunne, M.C., D.A. Barnes, and R.A. Clement, *A model for retinal shape changes in ametropia.* Ophthalmic Physiol Opt, 1987. 7 (2): p. 159-60.

[62] Navarro, R., E. Moreno, and C. Dorronsoro, *Monochromatic aberrations and point-spread functions of the human eye across the visual field.* J. Opt. Soc. Am. A, 1998. 15: p. 2522-9.

[63] Atchison, D.A. and D.H. Scott, *Monochromatic aberrations of human eyes in the horizontal visual field.* J Opt Soc Am A Opt Image Sci Vis, 2002. 19 (11): p. 2180-4.

[64] Atchison, D.A., N. Pritchard, and K.L. Schmid, *Peripheral refraction along the horizontal and vertical visual fields in myopia.* Vision Res, 2006. 46 (8-9): p. 1450-8.

[65] Guirao, A. and P. Artal, *Off-axis monochromatic aberrations estimated from double pass measurements in the human eye.* Vision Res,, 1999. 39: p. 207-217.

[66] Lundstrom, L., P. Unsbo, and J. Gustafsson, *Off-axis wave front measurements for optical correction in eccentric viewing.* J Biomed Opt, 2005. 10: p. 034002.

[67] Sheehan, M.T., et al., *Population study of the variation in monochromatic aberrations of the normal human eye over the central visual field.* Opt Express, 2007. 15 (12): p. 7367-80.

[68] Applegate, R.A., et al., *Interaction between aberrations to improve or reduce visual performance.* J Cataract Refractive Surg., 2003. 29: p. 1487-1495.

[69] Stone, R.A. and D.I. Flitcroft, *Ocular shape and myopia.* Ann Acad Med Singapore, 2004. 33: p. 7-15.

[70] Thibos, L.N., *Calculation of the influence of lateral chromatic aberration on image quality across the visual field.* Journal of the Optical Society of America, A,, 1987. 4: p. 1673-1680.

[71] Wang, Y.Z., L.N. Thibos, and A. Bradley, *Effects of refractive error on detection acuity and resolution acuity in peripheral vision.* Invest Ophthalmol Vis Sci., 1997. 38: p. 2134-2143.

[72] Williams, D.R., et al., *Off-axis optical quality and retinal sampling in the human eye.* Vision Res, 1996. 36: p. 1103-1114.

[73] Curcio, C.A., et al., *Human photoreceptor topography.* J Comp Neurol, 1990. 292 (4): p. 497-523.

[74] Artal, P., A.M. Derrington, and E. Colombo, *Refraction, aliasing, and the absence of motion reversals in peripheral vision.* Vision Res., 1995. 35: p. 939-947.

[75] Thibos, L.N., D.L. Still, and A. Bradley, *Characterization of spatial aliasing and contrast sensitivity in peripheral visual.* Vision Res., 1996. 36: p. 249-258.

[76] Still, D.L., L.N. Thibos, and A. Bradley, *Peripheral image quality is almost as good as central image quality.* Invest Ophthalmol Vis Sci., 1989. 30 (suppl):52.

[77] Mutti, D.O., et al., *Refractive error, axial length, and relative peripheral refractive error before and after the onset of myopia.* Invest Ophthalmol Vis Sci, 2007. 48 (6): p. 2510-9.

[78] Charman, W.N., *Aberrations and myopia.* Ophthalmic Physiol Opt, 2005. 25 (4): p. 285-301.

[79] Marcos, S., S. Barbero, and L. Llorente, *The sources of optical aberrations in myopic eyes.* Invest. Ophthalmol. Vis. Sci. (suppl.), 2002. 43: p. Abstract 1510.

[80] Thorn, F., et al. *The vision of myopic children: how wavefront aberrations alter the image of school book text..* in *Myopia 2000, Proceedings of the VIII international conference in Myopia.* 2000. Boston.

[81] Wildsoet, C., *Structural correlates of myopia. In: Myopia and nearwork,* M.R.a.B. Gilmartin, Editor. 1998, Butterworth-Heinemann, Oxford. p. 31-56.

[82] Kee, C.S., et al., *Effects of optically imposed astigmatism on emmetropization in infant monkeys.* Invest Ophthalmol Vis Sci, 2004. 45 (6): p. 1647-59.

[83] Haugwitz, T. and F. Blodi, *Hirschberg's history of ophthalmology.* Optical instruments Postage stamps. West Germany, 1986. 11: p. 77.

[84] Dumbleton, K., et al., *Changes in myopic refractive error with nine months' extended wear of hydrogel lenses with high and low oxygen permeability.* Optom Vis Sci., 1999. 76: p. 845-9.

[85] Grosvenor, T., D. Perrigin, and J. Perrigin, *Rigid gas-permeable contact lenses for myoipia control: effects of discontination of lens wear.*. Optom Vis Sci., 1991. 68: p. 385-9.

[86] Kemmetmuller, H., *Contact lenses versus spectacles in myopia.* Contact lens Med Bull, 1972. 5: p. 14-17.

[87] Miller, B., *Can progressive myopia be prevented by contact lenses.* Contacto, 1962. 6: p. 196-9.

[88] Nolan, J., *Myopia control with contact lenses.* Contacto, 1967. 11: p. 24-7.

[89] Perrigin, J., D. Perrigin, and e.a. Quintero S, *Silicone-acrylate contact lenses for myopia control: 3-year results.* Optom Vis Sci., 1990. 67: p. 764-9.

[90] Stone, J., *Myopia control after contact lens wear.*. Br J Physiol Opt., 1974. 29: p. 93-108.

[91] Harris, M., M. Sarver, and K. Polse, *Corneal curvature and refractive error changes associated with wearing hydrogel contact lenses.* Am J Optom Physiol Optics., 1975. 52: p. 313-9.

[92] Binder, P., *Myopic extended wear with the Hydrocurve 2 soft contact lens.* Ophthalmology., 1983. 90: p. 623-6.

[93] Horner, D., P. Soni, and T. Salmon, *Myopia progression in adolenscent wearers of soft contact lenses and spectacles.* Optom Vis Sci., 1999. 76: p. 474-9.

[94] Grosvenor, T., D. Perrigin, and J. Perrigin, *Do rigid gas permeable contact lenses control the progress of myopia?* Spectrum, 1991: p. 29-35.

[95] Khoo, C., J. Chong, and U. Rajan, *A 3-year study on the effect of RGP contact lenses on myopic children.* Singapore Med J., 1999. 40: p. 230-7.

[96] Katz, J., O. Schein, and B. Levy, *Arandomized trial of rigid gas permeable contact lenses to reduce progression of children's myopia.* Am J Ophthalmol., 2003. 136: p. 82-90.

[97] Walline, J.J., et al., *A randomized trial of the effects of rigid contact lenses on myopia progression.* Arch Ophthalmol, 2004. 122 (12): p. 1760-6.

[98] Dorronsoro, C., S. Barbero, and L. Llorente, *On-eye measurement of optical perfomance of rigid gas permeable contact lenses based on ocular and corneal aberrometry.* Optom Vis Sci., 2003. 80 (2): p. 115-125.

[99] Atchison, D.A., *Aberrations associated with rigid contact lenses.* J Opt Soc Am A., 1995. 12: p. 2267-73.

[100] Hong, X., N. Himebaugh, and L.N. Thibos, *On-eye evaluation of optical performance of rigid and soft contact lenses.* Optom Vis Sci., 2001. 78: p. 872-80.

[101] Lu, F., et al., *Monochromatic wavefront aberrations in the human eye with contact lenses.* Optom Vis Sci., 2003. 80: p. 135-141.

[102] Atchison, D.A., *Aberrations associated with rigid contact lenses.* J Opt Soc Am A Opt Image Sci Vis, 1995. 12 (10): p. 2267-73.

[103] Logan, N.S., et al., *Posterior retinal contour in adult human anisomyopia.* Invest Ophthalmol Vis Sci, 2004. 45 (7): p. 2152-62.

[104] Millodot, M., *Effect of ametropia on peripheral refraction.* Am J Optom Physiol Opt, 1981. 58 (9): p. 691-5.

[105] Schmid, G.F., *Axial and peripheral eye length measured with optical low coherence reflectometry.* J Biomed Opt, 2003. 8 (4): p. 655-62.

[106] Schmid, G.F., *Variability of retinal steepness at the posterior pole in children 7-15 years of age.* Curr Eye Res, 2003. 27 (1): p. 61-8.

[107] Seidemann, A., Schaeffel, F., Guirao, A., Lopez-Gil, N., & Artal, P., *Peripheral refractive errors in myopic, emmetropic, and hyperopic young subjects.* Journal of the Optical Society of America A. Optics and Image Science, 2002. 19: p. 2363-2373.

[108] Smith, E.L., et al., *Peripheral vision can influence eye growth and refractive developement in infant monkeys.* invest Ophthalmol Vis Sci., 2005. 46 (11): p. 3965-72.

[109] Atchison, D.A., et al., *Refraction and aberration across the horizontal central 10 degree of the visual field.* Optom Vis Sci., 2006. 83 (4): p. 213-221.

[110] Shen, J., et al., *Peripheral refraction with and without contact lens correction.* Optom Vis Sci., 2009.

[111] Atchison, D.A. and D.H. Scott, *Monochromatic aberrations of human eyes in the horizontal visual field..* J Opt Soc Am A Opt Image Sci Vis,, 2002. 19 (2180-2184).

[112] Smith, G. and D.A. Atchison, *The eye and visual optical instruments.* Cambridge University Press, New York, 1997: p. 601-606.

[113] Cheng, X., A. Bradley, and L.N. Thibos, *Predicting subjective judgment of best focu*s with objective image quality metrics. J Vis, 2004. 4 (4): p. 310-21.

[114] Cheng, X., L.N. Thibos, and A. Bradley, Estimating visual quality from wavefront aberration measurements. J Refract Surg, 2003. 19 (5): p. S579-84.

Chapter 9

Keratitis — A Clinical Approach

Patricio A. Pacheco

Additional information is available at the end of the chapter

http://dx.doi.org/10.5772/58411

1. Introduction

Any inflammatory reaction of the cornea of the eye is known as keratitis. The concept originates from the Greek word "κέϱας-(kerat)" that means "horn" and "itis" which represents the classical suffix in medicine for inflammation. Since early civilization, the cornea was considered to be "strong as a horn". Its highly complex, almost indestructible, collagen conformation gives it strong physical properties that made the ancients to name it like that.

Keratitis is a frequent clinical condition. A correct initial diagnosis and treatment are critical in limiting the amount of residual damage and scarring left to the cornea, as the preservation of its transparent property is critical in the recovery and maintenance of useful vision in any affected patient.

In the present chapter a description of the clinical findings in different forms of keratits, intend to illustrate ophthalmic practitioners with the different potential diagnosis associated to this condition and through this, to orientate them in the useful investigations that will lead to the correct diagnosis.

2. Anatomy and physiology

The cornea has five layers: a superficial one called "epithelial", an intermediate one or "stromal", an internal named "endothelial" and two limiting membranes: Bowman's and Descemet's (Fig.1). Each of these layers is conformed by different structures and types of cells that give them unique properties and different responses when affected by disease, this difference between the layers produces an inflammatory response that is typical to each layer, with clinical findings that can orientate to the primarily affected site.

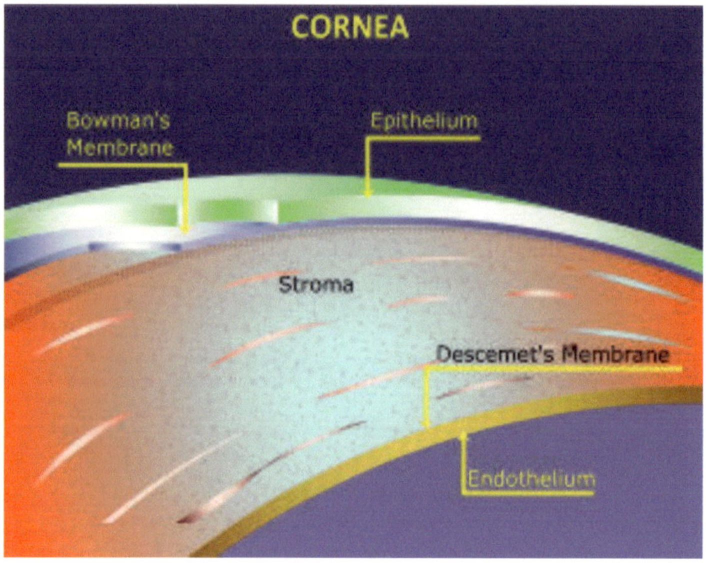

Figure 1. Corneal layers

The epithelial layer is formed by a stratified, squamous and non-keratinized epithelium that comprises a single layer of basal columnar cells attached by hemi-desmosomes to the underlying basement membrane followed by two to three rows of epithelial wing cells and two external layers of squamous surface cells which surface area is increased by microplicae and microvilli that facilitates the attachment of the mucin layer of the tear film. After a lifespan of approximately twenty-four hours the superficial cells are often shed into the tear film. The epithelial stem cells are located in the limbal region (this is the area between the cornea and the sclera), within the palisades of Vogt mainly located in the superior and inferior limbus. The indemnity of the corneal stem cells is essential for the maintenance of a healthy corneal epithelium and they also act as a barrier, preventing conjunctival epithelium from growing on to the clear cornea.

The stromal layer makes up to 90% of the corneal thickness, it is composed of regularly orientated collagen type I and V fibrils layers whose space is maintained by proteoglycan ground substance (chondroitin and keratan sulphate) with interspread modified fibroblast cells (keratocytes). The superficial portion of the stroma is called the Bowman membrane that constitutes an acellular portion of the stroma. It is, in part, the congruent and precise distribution of the collagen fibers of the stromal layer that permits the structure of the cornea to be transparent, letting the spectrum of visible light to pass through into the inner structures of the eye to finally allowing us to see.

The endothelial layer consists of a single layer of hexagonal cells that sits on a fine basal membrane made of a latticework of collagen fibers named the Descemet membrane. This layer and its indemnity is also crucial in keeping the transparency of the cornea by reducing the amount of water in the corneal stroma through an active membrane channels mechanism that

http://dx.doi.org/10.5772/58411

allows the movement of water from the stroma into the anterior chamber of the eye. The endothelial cells cannot regenerate as they are arrested in the G1 phase of the cell cycle; the normal adult cell density is about 2500 cells/mm^2, this amount of cells decreases at a rate of 0.6% per year. When the cell density falls to about 500 cells/mm^2, corneal edema develops and then corneal transparency is reduced.

In 2013, the Dua's layer was described for the first time. In a paper published by Dua et al., experimental and electron microscopy studies revealed the existence of a thin layer (15 microns) of corneal collagen between the corneal stroma and the Descemet membrane. This layer has physical properties that are different to the stromal layer and the Descemet membrane, having the highest resistance to pressure among the corneal layers. Its discovery has implications in corneal surgical procedures.

Macrophages and dendritic antigen presenting cells are present mainly in the epithelium and the anterior stroma. Small numbers of macrophages are also present in the posterior stroma.

The sensory innervation of the cornea derives from the trigeminal nerve (V_1) and it is mainly distributed in the sub-epithelial region and anterior stroma as sub-epithelial plexus, it is therefore at this level that we can find most nerves in the corneal structure.

3. Keratitis: Clinical history

A detailed clinical history is crucial in the diagnosis keratitis. Demographic aspects like age, sex, ethnicity and occupation are always needed and can orientate to certain specific associated pathologies or risk factors. The use of contact lenses is important to note in detail including the type of lenses, length of use, cleaning systems used and daily routines (i.e. tap water washing, swimming, etc). History of any recent injury to the eye or systemic disease that might relate to corneal compromise is also needed. History of recent infections, cold sores or flu can be helpful in orientating a diagnosis. The use of topical eye drops or any other medication needs to be recorded as the use of topical steroids, anesthetics, etc can be significant as a risk factor for infections and anatomical/ functional changes of the corneal surface.

4. Keratitis: Anatomical classification

Keratitis can be classified on the portion of the cornea affected. It is important to note that perhaps most of the cases have more than one layer involved and in some cases all three are compromised, however this classification can help the diagnosis of more pure forms of keratitis.

Epithelial: when the most superficial layer of the cornea is affected, a characteristic epithelial defect or epithelial cellular infiltrate can be seen, fluorescein staining can help in the diagnosis, there are multiple sizes and possible shapes for both the defect and/or the infiltration. Some of the epithelial defects are pathognomonic as it is the dendriform seen in herpes simplex virus keratitis, it is therefore important to note the size, shape and depth of the defect in any epithelial form, as it will certainly help not only in the diagnosis but also in the assessment of the progression or recovery of the affected patient. In the case of the infiltrate, it is important to note the size, color and quality of the borders that can be of help in diagnosis and follow up. Any satellite lesions need also to be assessed as well as the upper and lower tarsal plates in search for any foreign bodies or other associated lesions like calcareous concretions, meibomian gland cysts, papillae or follicles. The epithelial form of keratitis is extremely painful and at times enlarged or infiltrated corneal nerves can be seen. Usually the anterior stroma is also affected with an inflammatory cellular infiltrate surrounding the epithelial lesions, it has in general poorly defined borders. Corneal pannus can be seen as a result of previous episodes of epithelial keratitis in some cases. Examples include herpetic epithelial keratitis, adenoviral keratoconjunctivitis, microbial corneal ulcers and contact lens related keratitis.

Stromal: this is the keratitis that has primarily a compromise of the corneal stroma. An associated epithelial defect may be or not detected at initial presentation. The main finding in this type of keratitis is an infiltration of the collagen layers in the stroma by inflammatory cells, this can be seen at any depth, it can be unifocal or multifocal, with many different shapes and sizes, but usually has a very well defined and regular edge. There is in general some degree of anterior chamber cell reaction and at times keratic precipitates can be seen. Thickening of the cornea is another way to appreciate the cellular infiltration seen in these cases. Examples are herpetic stromal keratitis, sclero-keratitis and fungal/atypical microorganisms' related keratitis.

Endothelial: the main structure affected in these cases is the endothelial layer. Characteristic features include keratic precipitates, descemet folds and almost invariably a significant anterior chamber cells reaction. Secondary diffuse corneal thickening at later stages can be seen as a result of impaired endothelial function. Examples include corneal graft rejection, herpetic endothelial keratitis, any form of kerato-uveitis, and post-traumatic/post-surgical endothelial damage.

5. Keratitis: Causes

The cornea is sometimes the target of one direct pathophysiological condition, others, the compromise is secondary to an external indirect event in the complex functional anatomical triad between the lids, the cornea and the tear film.

There are multiple different causes of keratitis; these can be grouped in three major groups including infectious, autoimmune/inflammatory, neoplastic and traumatic causes.

http://dx.doi.org/10.5772/58411

5.1. Infectious keratitis

As an important component of the anatomical anterior wall of the eye, the cornea is a structure highly exposed and vulnerable to external pathogens. The use of contact lenses constitutes an accumulative risk for developing infectious keratitis, as it is also any history of chronic corneal disease or the use of topical steroids. Any corneal epithelial disruption as seen sometimes in dry eye syndrome, severe blepharitis and injuries are able to cause disruptions of the epithelial barrier as seen in corneal abrasions, post-surgical procedures or corneal foreign bodies that can predispose to corneal infections. Sometimes it is the result of highly pathogenic microorganisms with high affinity to the epithelial cells the ones that can cause a direct involvement as it is frequently seen with the herpes virus family.

5.1.1. Viral

By far the most frequent cause of viral keratitis is the one caused by herpes viruses type 1 and 2, also varicella-zoster virus can sometimes be responsible in the context of herpes zoster ophthalmicus. The typical form of viral keratitis is epithelial, with a characteristic dendritiform epithelial defect and secondary infiltrate very easy to diagnose with fluorescein staining (Fig 2). The epithelial defect seen in herpes zoster infection is classically described as geographic rather than dendritiform. In less than 10% of the cases the compromise can be primarily stromal or endothelial that typically is associated with elevated intraocular pressure (Fig 3). A PCR for virology in a swab of the epithelial lesion usually confirms diagnosis. Recent history of herpes zoster or recurrent cold sores can also orientate the clinician. If PCR is not available, another way of confirming diagnosis is by performing antibodies serology (IgG / IgM) for HSV and VZV at the time of presentation, an elevated IgM would confirm the diagnosis of recent infection and an elevated IgG a recurrence. This form of keratitis leaves behind sometimes significant corneal scarring with pannus, this clinical finding, in the context of an atypical recurrent hypertensive stromal or endothelial keratouveitis, can help sometimes achieve the correct clinical diagnosis.

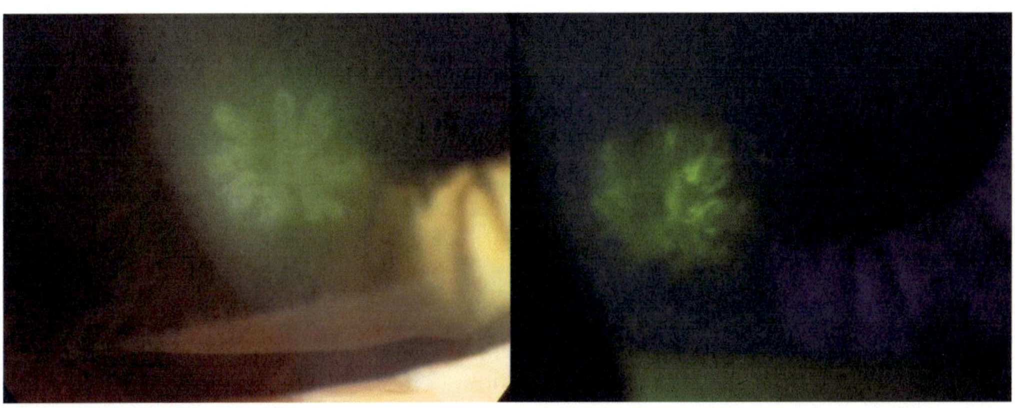

Figure 2. Herpes simplex virus epithelial keratitis as typical dendrite.

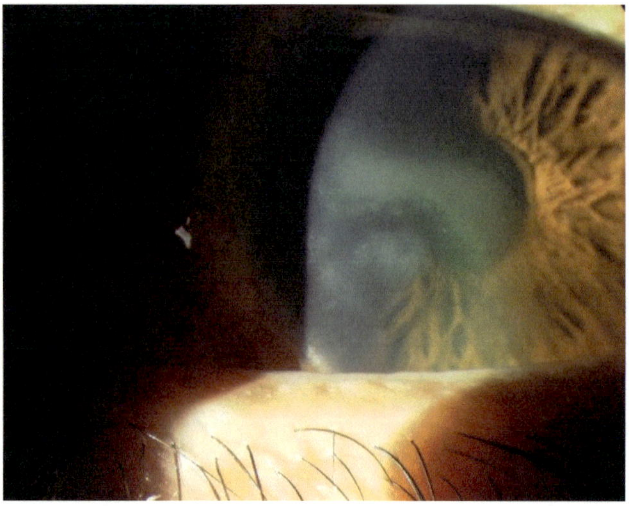

Figure 3. Herpes simplex virus stromal keratitis.

5.1.2. Bacterial

For bacteria to act as a pathogen in the cornea, it is necessary a disruption in the epithelial barrier like the ones seen in injuries (corneal foreign bodies and corneal abrasions) or a significant risk factor like contact lens wear or use of topical steroids. Almost any bacterium is able to cause keratitis, the most frequently involved are the ones that are the gram positive microorganisms found in the eyelids margin and skin (staphylococcus sp, streptococcus sp), sometimes gram negative bacteria like pseudomonas sp can be isolated. The typical keratitis caused by bacteria is epithelial and the presentation is acute; it usually has a well-defined epithelial defect surrounded by a stromal grayish infiltrate, which has a depth and extension proportional to the time of onset to presentation. Often a level of hypopyon and anterior chamber reaction are seen. The speed and extension of the compromise also depends on the pathogenicity of the bacteria involved, often being worse in the case of gram-negative microorganisms (Fig 4). Slow growth bacteria like streptococcus viridans can give the aspect of crystalline keratitis, as the invasion of the corneal stroma is very slow following the branching of the collagen layers. The diagnosis is usually confirmed by a corneal scrape of the lesion that can be sent for microbiological studies; in any ophthalmic setting it is crucial to perform a gram stain, blood agar, brain heart infusion (BHI) and cooked meat broth (CMB) cultures to be able to isolate the pathogen and determine the sensitivities to antibiotic therapy. The gram stain can give immediate initial information of the type of microorganism excluding other causes of keratitis. In contact lens wearers is important also to send for culture the contact lenses container and the last pair of lenses used.

http://dx.doi.org/10.5772/58411

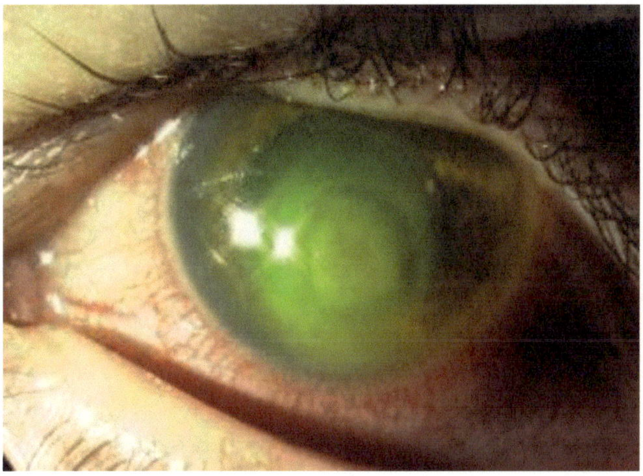

Figure 4. A patient with pseudomonas sp keratitis.

5.1.3. Fungal

It is a rare cause of keratitis in temperate climates but common cause of keratitis in tropical countries. It is difficult to treat. Usually occurs following trauma to the cornea especially the one caused by vegetable matter. Also contact lens wearing is emerging as a significant risk factor. The course is indolent sub-acute, it takes weeks for the patient to seek help as it does not cause significant discomfort in the early stages as fungi are slow in replicate. The clinical presentation is that of a stromal form of keratitis, an epithelial defect can or not be present, but usually is small compared to the amount of stromal infiltrate associated. The stromal infiltrate is always irregular in the borders and poorly defined, it has a 'fluffy' aspect and very white (Fig 5). In very advanced cases the infiltration of the stroma can be full thickness with associated anterior chamber whitish solid hypopyon. The diagnosis is often confirmed by a corneal scrape or a corneal biopsy sent for microbiological studies; the gram stain can be very useful in identifying hyphae, filaments or microorganisms very quickly, for the culture it is important to repeat the cultures described for bacteria (in case of mixed infection) and also a Sabouraud's media that is more specific for fungal growth.

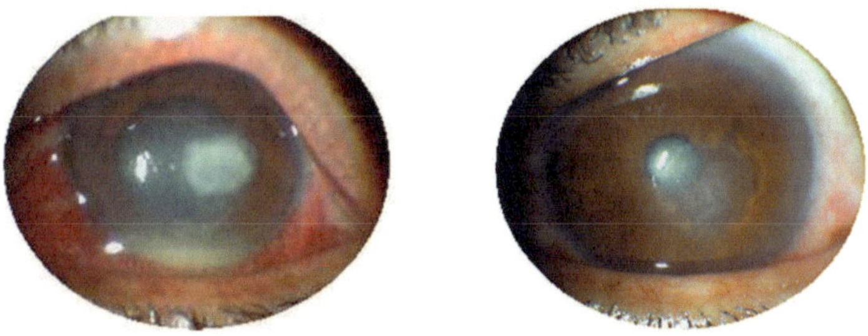

Figure 5. Fungal keratitis pre / post treatment.

5.1.4. Acanthamoeba

It is a rare cause of keratitis caused by one of the most common protozoa found in soil and water. In 90% of the cases a history of contact lens wear is found. Clinically this form of keratitis is combined with an epithelial and stromal component. The epithelial component is characteristically a large epithelial defect with abundant sub-epithelial infiltrate and enlargement of the corneal nerves that have been described as invaded by the pathogen at some stages of the disease, causing intense pain; this is perhaps the most painful form of keratitis, and this is regarded as a significant clinical finding at the time of diagnosing contact lens related keratitis. The stromal infiltrate is grey-whitish with irregular, multiple or single lesions, sometimes satellite areas can be seen (Fig 6 a & b). The diagnosis is confirmed by scrape or corneal epithelial biopsy sent for microbiological studies, it is important to repeat the gram and all the previously described medias (blood, BHI, CMB, Sabouraud's) and add the E. coli enriched non-nutrient agar media where this pathogen can be detected easily.

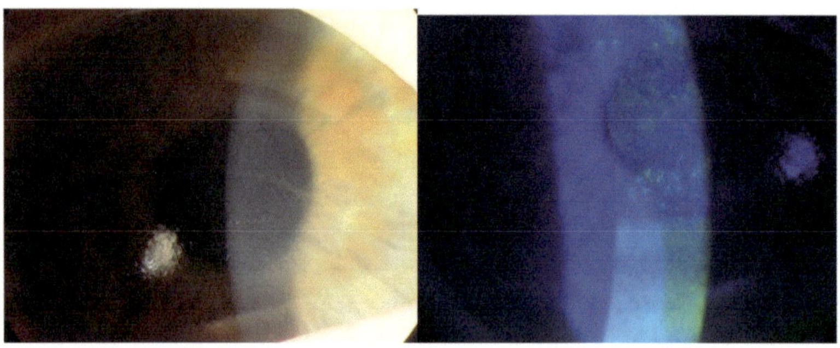

a)

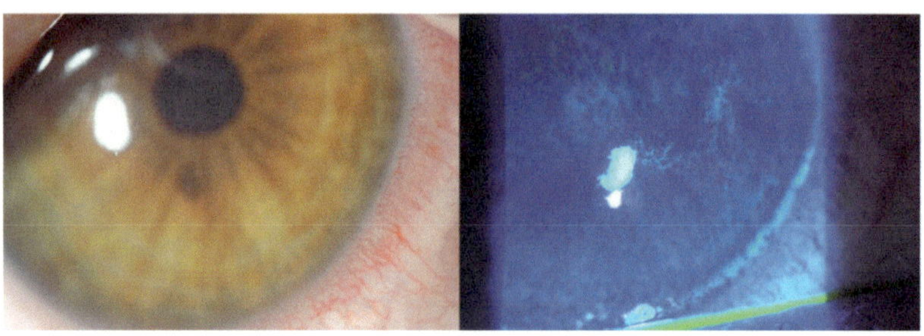

b)

Figure 6. a) Epithelial infiltrate with perineuritis in a patient with acanthamoeba keratitis. b) Diffuse stromal infiltrate in early acanthamoeba keratitis.

5.1.5. Atypical

This term is used to describe an infectious keratitis caused by atypical microorganisms like mycobacterium. The pattern of keratitis can be very confusing as it occurs usually in the context

http://dx.doi.org/10.5772/58411

of postoperative, traumatic or previous corneal pathology situations. The course is always chronic, unresponsive to multiple previous treatments and the clinical picture varies between an epithelial and stromal form of keratitis with atypical features (Fig 7). Perhaps the most important aspect is the invariable presence of a significant risk factor like previous surgery, as this pathogen needs a significant break in the epithelial barrier to be able to invade and cause the condition due to its relative large size. The isolation of mycobacterium to confirm diagnosis depends on a high level of suspicion and the scrape or corneal biopsy culture that needs all the previously described media plus a Zhiel-Neelsen gram stain for identification of acid-fast bacteria and Lowenstein-Jensen agar for culture growth.

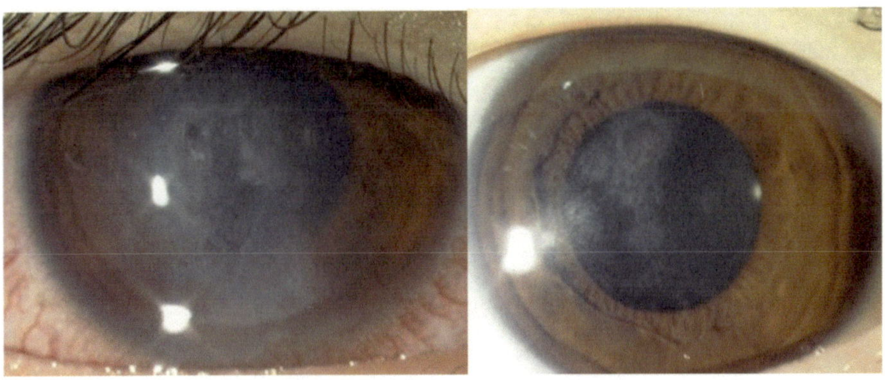

Figure 7. Atypical keratitis caused by mycobacterium abscessus after LASIK pre / post treatment.

5.2. Inflammatory — Autoimmune keratitis (Non suppurative keratitis)

Any condition that can induce an inflammatory response of the cornea can be classified in this group of causes of keratitis. There are autoimmune and no autoimmune related diseases.

5.2.1. Autoimmune

Like in any other autoimmune condition where the main target is the collagen in the body, the so-called autoimmune collagen or connective tissue diseases can be responsible for various forms of inflammatory keratitis, due to the high content of collagen seen in the corneal and scleral tissue. In some patients the cornea is the initial manifestation of the autoimmune process sometimes well in advance before the systemic condition manifests. The collagen diseases related to peripheral corneo-scleral ulceration or sclero-keratitis, include systemic lupus erythematosus, rheumatoid arthritis, Wegener's granullomatosis and polyarteritis nodosa. The form of keratitis seen in theses cases is epithelial with a significant stromal component mainly in the form of subtle infiltrate with severe stromal melting and associated episcleral or scleral vasculitis (Fig 8). In other circumstances the cornea is the only affected structure as it is seen in Mooren's or peripheral ulcerative keratitis, the characteristic clinical finding is corneal stromal melting associated to inflammation (Fig 9 a & b).

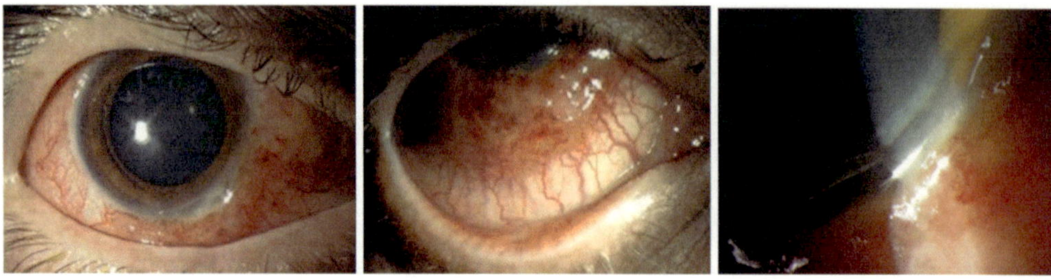

Figure 8. Sclerokeratitis in a patient with Wegener's granullomatosis.

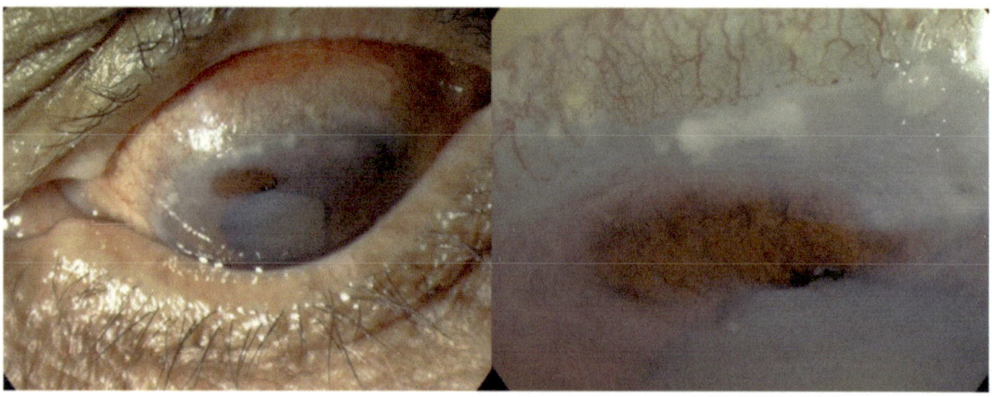

a)

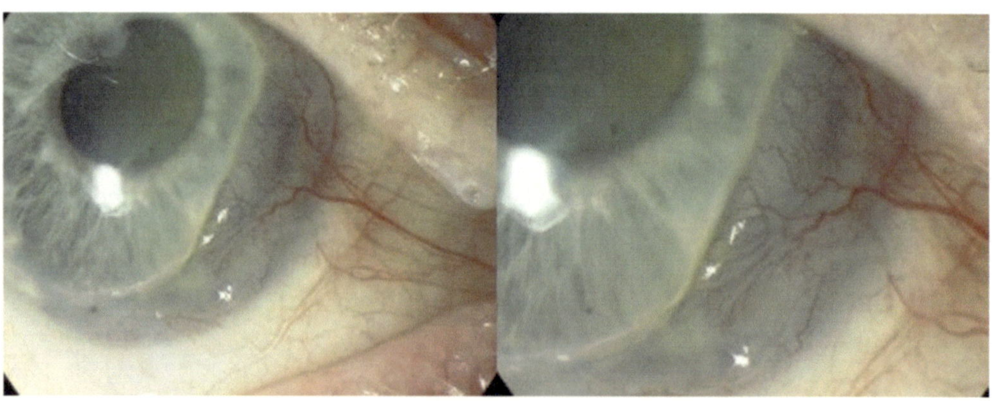

b)

Figure 9. a) Peripheral ulcerative keratitis with associated scleritis and corneal stromal corneal infiltrate. b) Typical case of Mooren's keratitis.

http://dx.doi.org/10.5772/58411

5.2.2. Non autoimmune

In this group, we find conditions that can compromise the delicate functional triad between the cornea, the tear film and the lids. If any of these is affected it will indirectly affect the anatomy and function of the other, potentially causing an inflammatory keratitis. Lids conditions like blepharitis, rosacea, lagophthalmos, entropion, ectropion, tarsal calcareous concretions or tear film dysfunctions like the ones seen in Sjogren's or severe dry eye syndrome can directly or indirectly cause keratitis in the form of marginal keratitis (Fig 10), phlyctenular keratoconjunctivitis and sometimes diffuse punctate keratitis as seen in Thygeson's keratitis. Usually the clinical pattern in this form of keratitis is epithelial with isolated or multiple epithelial defects and sub-epithelial superficial mild infiltrates (Fig 11), filaments can also sometimes be seen. When chronically affected a peripheral corneal pannus can often be seen (Fig 12).

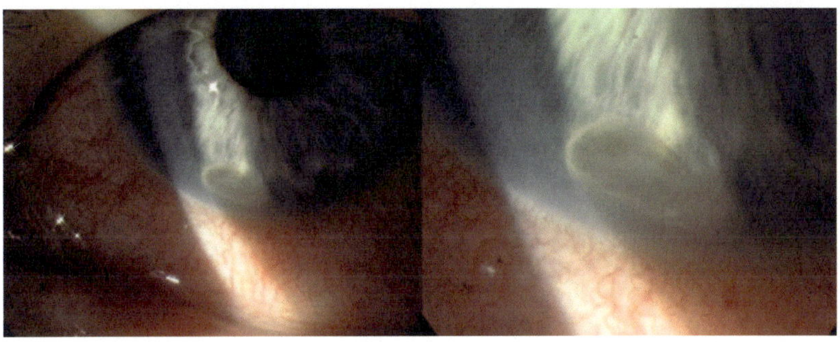

Figure 10. Typical marginal keratitis associated to rosacea.

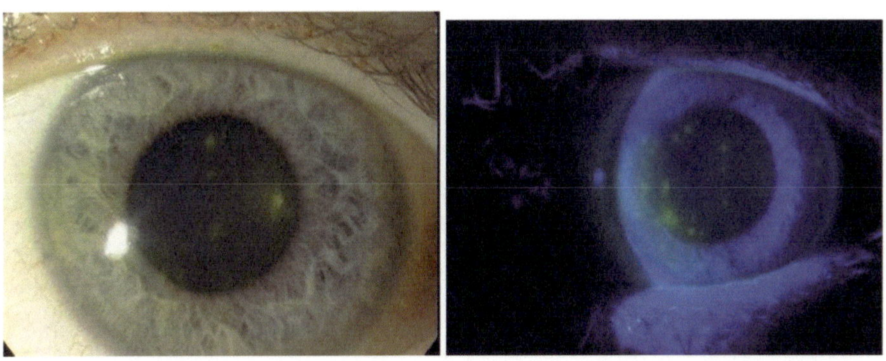

Figure 11. Superficial epithelial defects in dry eye syndrome.

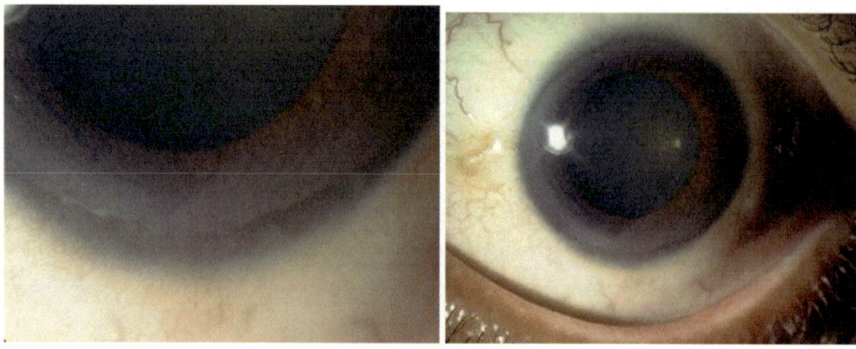

Figure 12. Peripheral pannus in chronic dry eye syndrome.

5.3. Neoplasia associated inflammatory corneal involvement

Any neoplastic process in the limbal region and surrounding conjunctiva can indirectly extend to the cornea and cause an inflammatory reaction, this is generally not considered in the differential diagnosis of keratitis and is perhaps the most rare and less suspected cause of corneal and limbal inflammation, however it is important to consider it in order to achieve an early diagnosis, as this type of conditions untreated can extend quickly with some mortality rate.

5.3.1. Conjunctival intraepithelial neoplasia and squamous carcinoma

Neoplasia of the conjunctival epithelial cells is more commonly seen in the elderly. There are different grades of penetration in the underlying tissue and the amount of cellular atypical cells defines also the degree of malignancy ranging from grade 1 to a carcinoma in situ. The more invasive the type of neoplasia, the more likely this will extend to the adjacent corneal tissue and regional lymphonodes; the corneal involvement always remains superficial (Fig 13, 14).

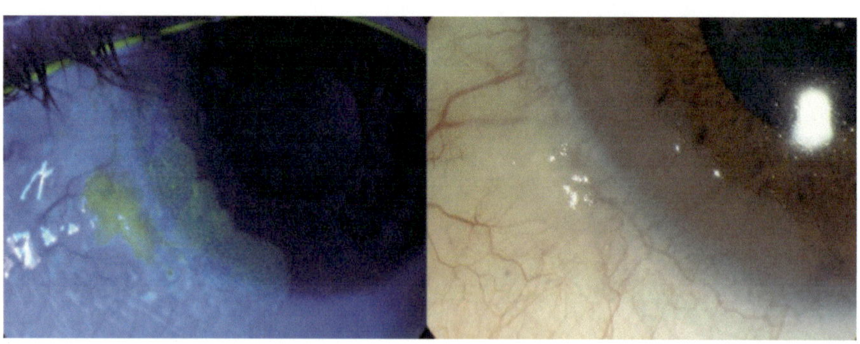

Figure 13. Conjunctival intraepithelial neoplasia (CIN) grade 3 with and without fluorescein staining.

http://dx.doi.org/10.5772/58411

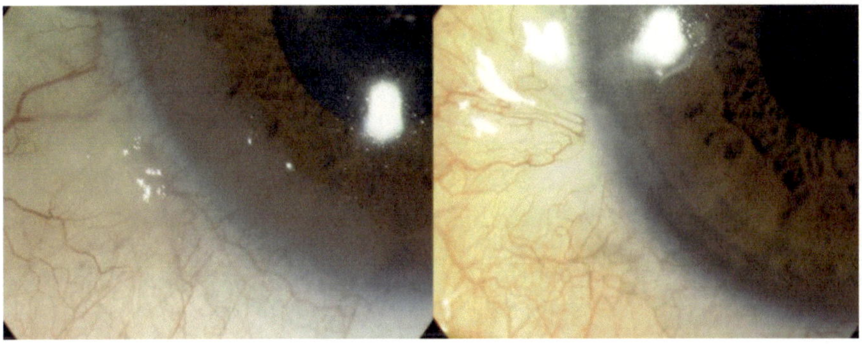

Figure 14. Conjunctival intraepithelial neoplasia (CIN) grade 3 treated with topical mytomicin C.

5.3.2. Conjunctival / limbal melanomas

They are rare but lethal. They can be very polymorphic with multiple types of different clinical presentation, pigmented (melanotic) or not pigmented (amelanotic), they are of rapid growth and can invade distant organs especially lungs and liver. The most likely origin is at the conjunctival epithelial cells when some pigmentation is associated. Isolated or multiple sentinel vessels are a pathognomonic feature (Fig. 15).

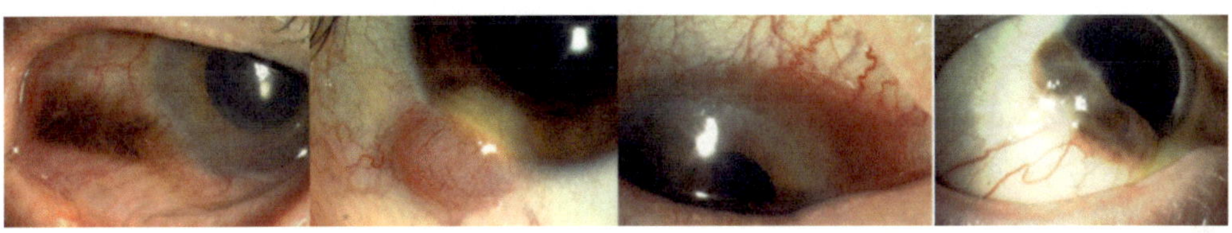

Figure 15. Four different conjunctival melanomas with corneal involvement, notice the polymorphism in clinical presentation.

5.4. Traumatic keratitis

In this group we can consider trauma by direct blunt injury with secondary corneal abrasion and corneal edema, or a surgical injury that damages the endothelial layer causing secondary corneal edema and endothelial failure with concurrent bullous keratopathy. The type of keratitis seen in these situations is mainly endothelial and stromal with multiple descemet folds, stromal collagen fibers disorganization, keratic precipitates and often associated anterior chamber reaction. At later stages if the endothelial layer does not recover from the insult, a severe corneal edema may lead to epithelial bullous formation and consequent epithelial keratitis. A clear history of trauma might not be obvious and the clinicians are encouraged to obtain it from the clinical history remembering that sometimes the traumatic event can precede the clinical manifestation for many years (i.e. previous cataract surgery, etc)

6. Keratitis: Treatment

The treatment of keratitis will depend on the direct cause; it is for this reason that an appropriate diagnosis is crucial at the moment of deciding the initial treatment.

6.1. Infectious causes

In viral herpetic keratitis cases, the drug of choice is acyclovir in topical or oral form depending on the extension of the keratitis within the corneal layers. A typical dose is ointment acyclovir 3% five times daily for one week or 400 mg orally five times a day for the same period. In severe cases both forms can be used to maximize effect. In children and the elderly the oral formulation is recommended due to difficulties in the application of the ointment. In resistant cases the alternative treatment will be topical trifluorthymidine 1% (F3T) or vidarabine 3% (Vira-A^{tm}). If high intraocular pressure (IOP) is detected this also need to be treated with lowering IOP agents. Other antiviral agents like topical ganciclovir 0.15% (Zirgan^{tm}) have started to be used more widely in recent years.

In bacterial suspected infections the initial treatment of choice is topical ciprofloxacin 0.3%, Ofloxacin 0.3% or levofloxacin 0.3% hourly, when significant anterior chamber reaction is found a cycloplegic/dilating drop to minimize pain and reduce the formation of posterior synechias is recommended and depending on the bacterial sensitivities results the treatment should be adjusted accordingly.

In acanthamoeba the treatment requires a combination of poly-hexyl-methyl-biguanide 0.02% (PHMB) and propamide isethionate 0.1% (Brolene^{tm}), alternatively preparations of chlorhexidine 0.02% can be used as well.

In atypical keratitis one can start treatment based on the suspicious on the most likely clinically apparent etyiological cause and adequate it based on the findings from the sampling.

6.2. Inflammatory / autoimmune

For autoimmune keratitis usually systemic therapy is needed, the important approach in the treatment is to identify corneal limbal ischemia and/or corneal melting as these are reasons not to use topical steroids due to the high risk of perforation. Severe cases will need high dose of oral steroids and immunosuppressant agents. No autoimmune cases, presenting with inflammatory features due to blepharitis and/or dry eyes with marginal infiltrates do benefit from topical steroids, however is also very important to treat the initial cause of corneal inflammation as this is usually secondary, i.e. removal of concretions and ectopic eyelashes, repair lagophthalmos or other lids malpositions, treat dry eyes with topical lubricants, etc.

6.3. Neoplasia associated

Surgical removal and biopsy is important as it is based on the histological diagnosis that further interventions like cryotherapy or radiotherapy might be indicated and planned. The excision

http://dx.doi.org/10.5772/58411

of any suspicious lesion ideally has to have a margin of two centimeters of healthy tissue to prevent recurrences. In CIN cases concomitant cryotherapy is useful as well as topical mytomicin C or 5 – fluorouracil at different concentrations. In melanomas a systemic workup including chest CT scan and liver function tests at regular intervals to detect metastasis is important, concomitant local radiotherapy has been advocated as well at the time of removal of the lesion.

6.4. Traumatic

In cases of corneal abrasion the treatment of choice is to use topical antibiotic ointments to prevent infections and to pad the eye for 24 hours to allow epithelisation of the cornea, the use of preservative free cycloplegic drops initially to relief pain is recommended before padding. In blunt injuries the use of topical anti-inflammatory or steroid drops is useful depending on the severity of the inflammation. In cases of bullose keratopathy, endothelial corneal transplantation is highly successful, the use of highly osmotic drops like NACL 5% or bandage contact lenses can sometimes clear the corneal stroma and relief pain while waiting for a corneal donor.

7. Conclusion

A clear and simple approach to the differential diagnosis of keratitis has been presented. The methodological clinical diagnostic remains the cornerstone of medicine at anytime, the clinical history, examination of the patient and auxiliary diagnostic methods to confirm a suspected diagnosis are all crucial in achieving a clinical improvement of the clinical condition known as keratitis.

The simple classification based on clinical findings will help ophthalmologists, general practitioners to assess patients with this condition and start an adequate initial investigation and treatment

Keratitis remains one of the most frequent diagnoses in ophthalmology and a comprehensive review like the one here presented is useful for any levels of clinical practice.

Author details

Patricio A. Pacheco[1,2]

1 Moorfields Eye Hospital, London, UK

2 West Hertfordshire Hospitals, NHS trust, UK

References

[1] Chow, C.Y.; Foster, C.S. (1996). Mooren's ulcer. *International Ophthalmology clinics*, Vol. 36, (Winter 1996), pp. 1-13

[2] Donzis, P.B.; Mondino, B.J. (1987). Management of non infectious corneal ulcers. *Survey Ophthalmology*, Vol. 32, (January 1987), pp. 94-110

[3] Dua, H.S.; Faraj, L.A.; Said, D.G.; Gray, T.; Lowe, J. *Ophthalmology*, Vol. 120 (9), (September 2013), pp. 1778-1785

[4] Holland, E.J.; Schwartz, G.S. (1999). Classification of herpes simplex virus keratitis, *Cornea*, Vol. 18, (March 1999), pp. 144-154

[5] Kanski, J.; Pavesio C. & Tuft S. (2006). Ocular Inflammatory Disease, Mosby-Elsevier, ISBN 0-323-03737, 1st edition, Philadelphia, USA

[6] Ladas, J.G.; Mondino, B.J. (2000). Systemic disorders associated with peripheral corneal ulcération. *Current opinion Ophthalmology*, Vol. 11, (December 2000), pp. 468-471

[7] Radford, C.F.; Minassian, D.C. & Dart, J.K. (2002). Acanthamoeba keratitis in England and Wales: incidence, outcomes and risk factors. *British Journal Ophthalmology*, Vol. 86, (May 2002), pp. 536-542

[8] Rohatgi, J.; Dhaliwal, U. (2000). Phlyctenular eye disease. *Japanese Journal Ophthalmology*, Vol. 44, (March-April 2000), pp. 146-150

[9] Suchecki, J.K. ; Donshik, P. & Ehlers W.H. (2003). Contact lens complications. *Ophthalmology Clinics North America*, Vol. 16, (March 2003), pp. 471-484

[10] Solomon, A.; Karp, C.L. & Miller, D. (2001). Mycobacterium interface keratitis after laser in situ keratomileusis. *Ophthalmology*, Vol. 108, (December 2001), pp. 2201-2208

[11] Stern, M.; Gao, J & Siemasko, K. F. (2004). The rôle of the lacrimal functional unit in the pathophysiology of dry eye. *Experimental Eye Research*, Vol. 78, (March 2004), pp. 409-416

Section 3

Updates in Posterior Segment Diseases

Chapter 10

Structure and Function Relationship in Glaucoma-Historical Perspective to a Practical Approach

Elliot M. Kirstein

Additional information is available at the end of the chapter

http://dx.doi.org/10.5772/57601

1. Introduction

Physicians, by nature, seem to strive for more precise means to diagnose, quantify and manage chronic disease. It seems intuitive that doing so will help us diagnose earlier, have an increased understanding for the relative severity of disease in individual patients and, ultimately, through more timely diagnosis, mitigate morbidities associated with that disease. In the example of diabetes, we can now look at glycosylated hemoglobin levels (HbA1c) and derive a reasonable understanding of risk level and relative treatment success for individual patients. While the HbA1c value is not flawless as a metric, it has become an extremely robust and accepted tool in diabetes management. Our efforts to coalesce ocular physical measurements with functional values seem to point to our desire to define glaucoma in one simple value. While the effort itself has already shed great benefits to our understanding of this complex disease, it ultimately seems unlikely that we will ever be able to adequately define glaucoma in terms of a singular value.

During the past century, the metrics used to diagnose and manage glaucoma have varied and evolved. In the 1950's, using Schiotz tonometry, Leydecker showed that approximately 2.5% of the population had intraocular pressures greater than 21mm Hg. It was also determined that a similar number of people in that study had glaucoma. From that point forward, 21mm Hg became the empirical metric for determining who was at risk. More than fifty years has passed since the publication of Leydecker's study and a cornucopia of compelling scientific literature has been presented which has shed light on the diversity and complexity of glaucoma and clearly diminishes its relevance as a stand-alone diagnostic feature. Ironically, the vast body of evidence which clearly discourages reliance of the old 21 mm red flag in glaucoma diagnosis seems not to have been sufficient to clear it from the minds and hearts of too many eye doctors in this century. It would appear that we have an inner need to strive for and adhere to simple answers to even the most complex problems.

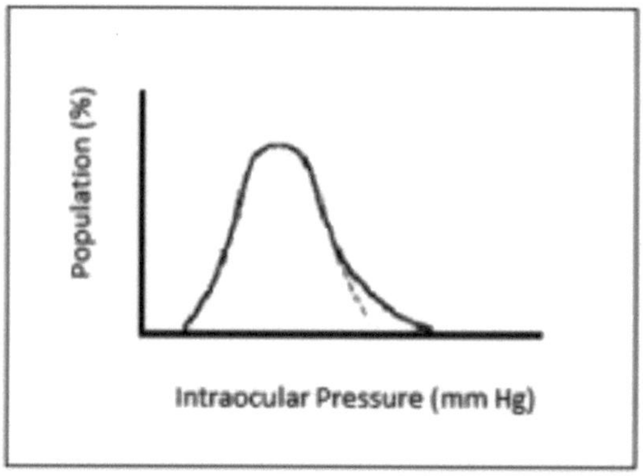

Figure 1. CURRENT SIGNIFICANCE OF 21 mmHg: The distribution of IOP in the general population as studied by Leydecker (normal IOP was statistically defined two standard deviations above and below mean, as 11-21 mmHg) is not Gaussian, but is slightly skewed towards higher IOP's [1]

Beyond the early observation that glaucomatous vision loss is generally accompanied with high intraocular pressure, scientists began to observe the physical changes within the eye that seemed to occur in concert with that loss. In 1885, Priestley Smith elegantly defined glaucoma, stating that "The excavation of the disc in glaucoma is not a purely mechanical result of exalted pressure; it is, in part at least, an atrophic condition which, though primarily due to pressure, includes vascular changes and impaired nutrition of the substance of the optic disc... which may possibly progress even though all excessive pressure be removed". Given this understanding, eye doctors started to look for tools to study the eye and its function in greater detail.

Today, eye doctors are challenged with a new puzzle. In current clinical practive we can obtain physical and psychometric data that was previously unimaginable. We are still attempting to determine which of the vast data has the greatest utility and specificity in regard to the diagnosis, quantification and management of glaucoma.

2. Observation and measurement of structure

2.1. Ophthalmoscopy

Understandably, long before doctors could document the eye's interior contents with imaging techniques, observation and evaluation of the nerve was performed by ophthalmoscopy. Observations were recorded with drawings. Though others produced earlier versions of the ophthalmoscope, in 1851, Hermann von Helmholtz reported its usefulness and, therein, revolutionized ophthalmology.

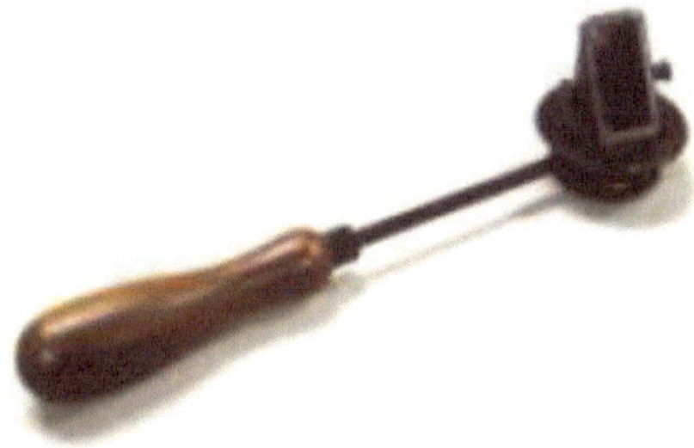

Figure 2. Early Welsh Allyn ophthalmoscope

In 1915, Francis A. Welch and William Noah Allyn invented the world's first hand-held direct illuminating ophthalmoscope, precursor to the device now used by clinicians around the world. This refinement and updating of von Helmholtz's invention enabled ophthalmoscopy to become one of the most ubiquitous medical screening techniques in the world today. The company started as a result of this invention is Welch Allyn. [2]

The need for stereopsis arose soon after the discovery of the ophthalmoscope. Given the limitations of a two dimensional view, the glaucomatous cup was, at first, mistaken for a swelling. At that time, Brewster's popular stereoscope was introduced, and its theory and method were then applied to ophthalmoscopy by Giraud-Teulon. His was the first binocular instrument, subsequently much improved by Zachariah Laurence. Binocular indirect ophthalmoscopy was abandoned toward the end of the 19th century in favor of direct monocular ophthalmoscopy, until it was revived in the 1950s by Schepens. More recently, hand held biomicroscopic lenses, which were popularized in the late 1980's by Volk Optical, Inc., are now a clinical standard for indirect three dimensional observations and evaluation of the nerve. [3]

3. Disc documentation

3.1. Drawings

Having the ability to view the nerve in vivo, proper scientific method deemed it necessary to document of these observations. For the better part of the twentieth century, manual drawing of the disc remained the clinical standard.

While disc drawing and careful direct observation of the nerve still have significant benefits, our scientific curiosity and our frank understanding of the likelihood of human variability and error with manual drawings, has driven us to develop methods of observation and recording which yield information down to the cellular level and render documentation which is relatively free of the obvious variability in individual observer skill and methodology.

Before the mid 1970's, eye doctors, in training, could not yet see photographs of the live human retina. Ophthalmic texts traditionally included drawings of normal and pathological eyes, which were rendered by professional medical artists.

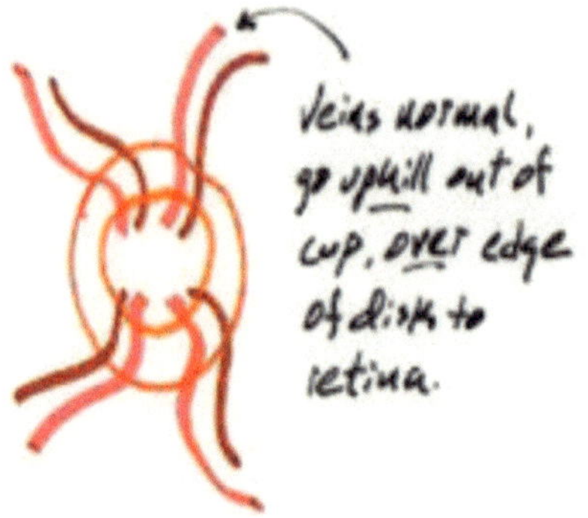

Figure 3. Typical clinician's disc drawing

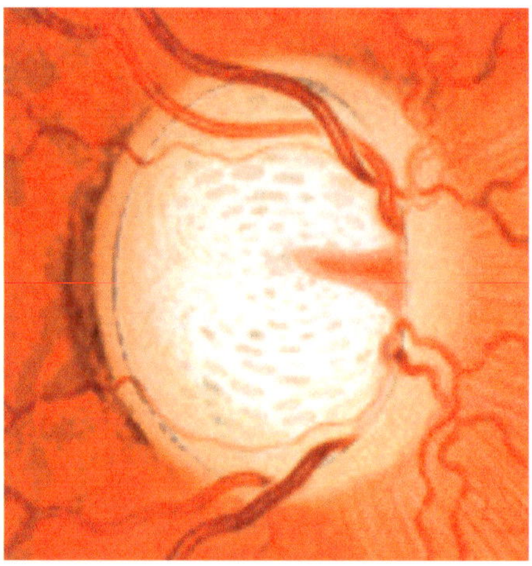

Figure 4. Medical artist's disc drawing of glaucomatous optic nerve

3.2. Photography

With fundus photography becoming commonplace by the early 1980's, stereo disc photography became possible and earned its place as the clinical gold standard in optic nerve documentation for the remainder of the twentieth century.

Recently, digital two and three dimensional photography have quickly outpaced conventional film photography of the nerve because of its obvious advantages in efficiency, economy and portability.

http://dx.doi.org/10.5772/57601

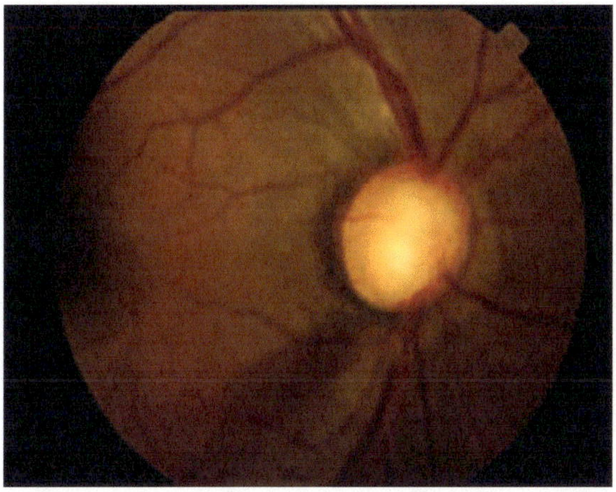

Figure 5. Optic nerve photograph

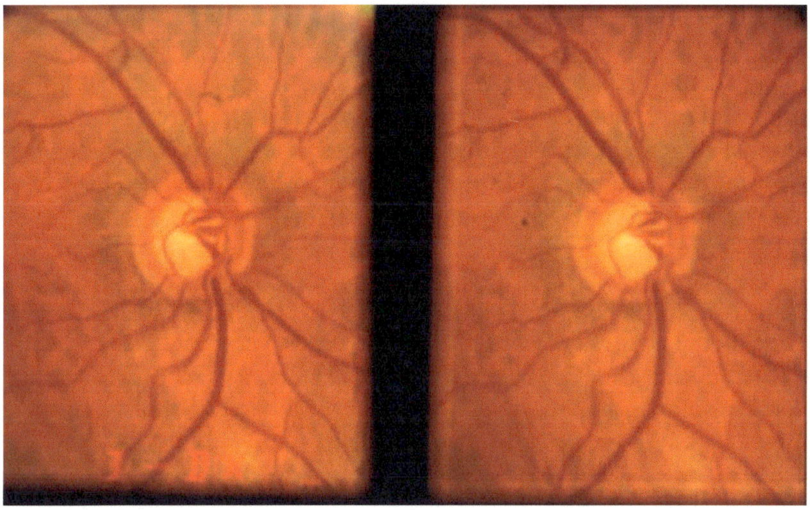

Figure 6. Simultaneous digital stereo disc photograph captured using the Nidek 3-DX system

3.3. Beyond photography

While photography had given us robust methodology for documentation of the appearance of the optic nerve head, it seemed natural to look for ways to numerically quantify various nerve attributes. An early attempt called the Glaucomascope, cast a series of infrared bars across the surface of the nerve. The variation in line contours signaled the instrument to make calculations regarding cup dimensions and, hopefully, track topographical change in concordance with glaucoma progression. The next generation of devices including the GDX (Carl Ziess) and the Heidelberg Retinal Tomograph (HRT) (Heidelberg Engineering), provided a more comprehensive perspective of nerve attributes and, with GDX, added new measurements of the nerve fiber layer surrounding the papilla. The HRT was the first to incorporate nerve progression analysis.

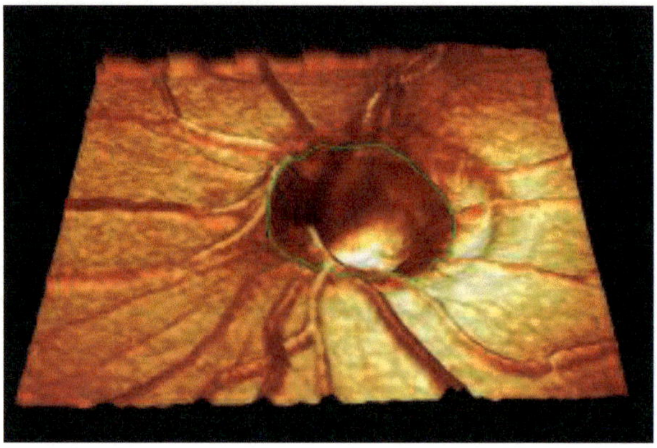

Figure 7. HRT 3-D image of the optic nerve and retinal nerve fiber layer (RNFL)

The Heidelberg Retina Tomograph (HRT) is a confocal scanning laser ophthalmoscope. A laser light scans the retina in 24 millisecond sequential scans, starting above the retinal surface, then capturing parallel images at increasing depths. The stacks of images can be combined to create a three-dimensional (3-D) topographic image of the retina. Images are aligned and compared using TruTrack™ software for both individual examinations and for detecting change between examinations.

When applying the technology to glaucoma, the HRT takes data from a 3-D stack of tomographic images of the optic nerve and retinal nerve fiber layer (RNFL), aligns the images and computes a 3-D topographic map of the surface of the retina. This 3-D topographic map is analyzed for signs of glaucomatous damage and the results are displayed on either a single eye examination report or on an OU examination report.

The GDx nerve fiber analyzers measures the retinal nerve fiber layer (RNFL) thickness with a scanning laser polarimeter based on the birefringent properties of the RNFL. Measurement is obtained from a band 1.75 disc diameters concentric to the disc.

The GDx projects a polarized beam of a light into the eye. As this light passes through the NFL tissue, it changes in speed. The detectors measure the change and convert it into thickness units that are graphically displayed. The GDx measures modulation around an ellipse just outside the optics disc and ratios of the thickest points either superiorly or inferiorly to the temporal or nasal regions.

The state of polarization of the light is change (retardation) as it passes through birefringent tissue (cornea and RNFL). Corneal birefringence is eliminated (in part) by a propriety 'corneal compensator'. The amount of retardation of light reflected from the fundus is converted to RNFL thickness.

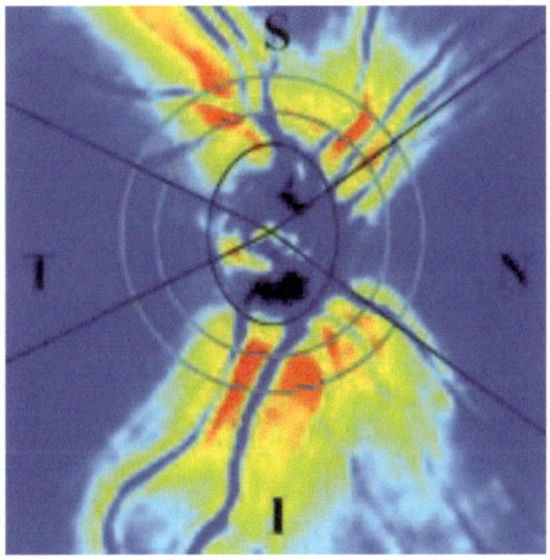

Figure 8. GDX ONH image

A Dutch study found that while there is a correlation between standard automated perimetry and GDx, variable corneal compensation (VCC) measurements in patients with glaucoma, suggesting that GDx VCC measurements relate well with functional loss in glaucoma. In healthy subjects, they found virtually no correlation between perimetry and GDx VCC measurements. This would cast doubt on its predictive value and suggests false positives. [4]

4. Ocular Coherence Tomography (OCT) – the new gold standard

Optical coherence tomography (OCT) has advanced considerably since it was first applied to the eye. It is an extension of a technique called low-coherence interferometry, which was initially applied to ophthalmology for in vivo measurements of eye axial length. OCT cross sections are used to evaluate the optic disc and retinal layers such as the retinal nerve fiber layer (RNFL). Scan patterns that enabled reproducible measurements were developed, and these eventually became incorporated into commercial systems. In 2000 Zangwill et al published a study comparing OCT nerve fiber thickness values against stereo photography and threshold visual field results showing that the OCT shows promise for providing quantitative measures of RNFL thickness for diagnosing and monitoring glaucoma. [5]

With these improvements in speed and sensitivity as seen in spectral domain OCT, it is now feasible to collect volumetric (three-dimensional; 3D) scans of tissue, whereas in the past, the amount of time required to do this would have been prohibitive. Broadband volumetric retinal imaging with SD-OCT have demonstrated speeds of up to 312,500. To date, most clinical systems operate at an acquisition rate of ~27,000 A-scans/s and an axial resolution of 5 to 6 μm.

The unprecedented speed and versatility of current forms of OCT have given us a new and vast data set, allowing us to seek out specific retinal measurements that are most highly specific for the diagnosis and observation of glaucomatous progression. Having the capacity to observe tissue at a cellular level, we now can more aptly compare between individuals and with specific individuals over time. The additional information at hand also allows us to emerge from cup/disc ratio, the age old and weather beaten descriptive of the nerve in the context of glaucoma. It is now possible to look far deeper into retinal and nerve attributes and across a wider diameter of retina, to look for structural changes that are most highly pathognomonic of glaucoma and its progression. [6]

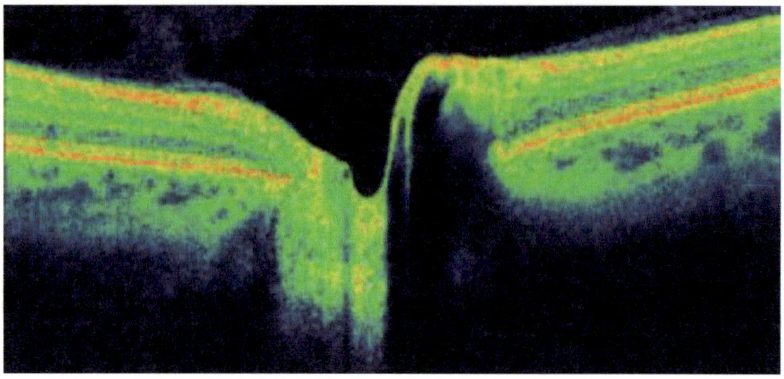

Figure 9. OCT crossectional view of the optic nerve

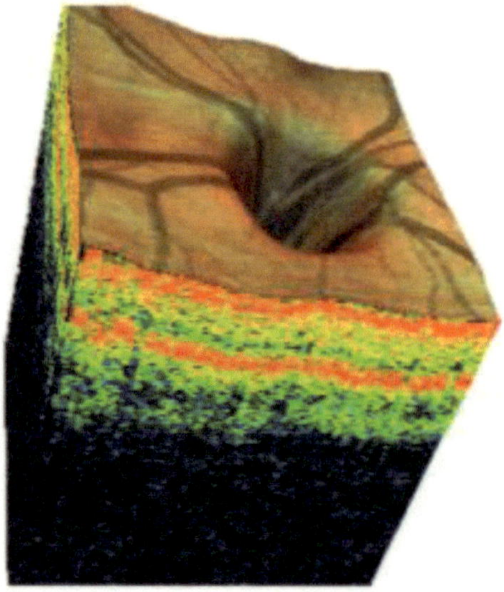

Figure 10. OCT three dimensional optic nerve scan

http://dx.doi.org/10.5772/57601

5. Measuring the nerve

5.1. Cup Disc Ratio (C/D)

In quantifying glaucoma risk and severity, the C/D ratio of the optic nerve has been the standard bearer during the past one hundred years. An eye with a low ratio was considered less apt to be glaucomatous and, if glaucoma was diagnosed, was known to be less advanced. High ratios implied high risk and or advanced disease. Some investigators noted that that the significance of a specific C/D value would vary widely depending on the diameter of the nerve itself. Investigators also began to note that nerve attributes such as rim thickness can be quite meaningful. For example, given two nerves with C/D=.50, one may have a well centered cup and no glaucomatous visual field loss, while another,.50 nerve, with loss if the inferior margin may show a severe superior nasal field defect. To further confuse the notion of C/D, more recent attention has been given to disc diameter and its implications on the significance of C/D in individual patients. Our current understanding is that nerve diameter plays a large role in the relative value of C/D. A C/D of.60 with a relatively small nerve is likely to have far greater implications with regard to glaucoma than the same C/D in a large nerve.

Given the additional perspective of the influence of cup position and nerve diameter, it should be easy to understand the now diminished value of C/D as a singular descriptive value of the state of disease. Reminiscent of the loss of relevance of the age old "21 mm Hg" standard, our current understanding of the scope of changes that occur within the nerve, surrounding the nerve and, more recently, those changes in the axonal bed and the peri papillary ganglion cell layer, further disenfranchises C/D and the meaningful descriptive of structural change in glaucoma.

5.2. Retinal nerve fiber layer

Technologies such as GDX and, more recently, OCT provide nerve fiber measurements outside of the boundaries of the disc and it has become evident that axonal changes in the area surrounding the nerve are important in understanding the nature and severity of glaucoma. [7, 8]

In a study performed by Bowd et al, clearly revealed that OCT revealed statistically significant quantitative differences in RNFL thickness between OHT and normal eyes within their study population. [9]

Additional studies such as those performed by Garas (2009), Sehi (2009) and Savini (2009) (table 1) have helped develop greater confidence in our ability to clinically determine RNFL thickness and to evaluate those findings in comparison to a reasonable field of normative data. [10-12]

Similar investigations in the following years helped give confidence that there was finally a method of determining RNFL thickness that was reliable enough so that meaningful comparisons could be made between normal and glaucomatous subjects. Beyond that general comparison, investigators could search for specific nerve and other retinal attributes which are more specific to the diagnosis and management of glaucoma. In 2010, Mansoori et al showed that SD-OCT identified differences in most parameters between eyes with glaucoma and normal eyes and also between eyes with glaucoma and OHT. It was important to note that they also observed that there was overlap of RNFL thickness between normal and OHT eyes, which somewhat limits the ability of this instrument to differentiate between normal and OHT subjects.[13]

	Garas			Sehi			Savini		
	Mean	Std. Dev.	95% Normal Range	Mean	Std.	95% Normal Range	Mean	Std. Dev.	95% Normal Range
Average RNFL	106.7	7.5	91.7 to 121.7	103.3	12.6	78.1 to 128.5	105.8	14.9	76.7 to 135.6
Superior	128.8	12.8	103.2 to 154.4	134.5	18.6	97.3 to 171.1	128.44	24.48	83.48 to 173.4
Inferior	136.6	12.7	111.2 to 162	129.7	16.9	95.9 to 163.5	137.15	21.99	93.17 to 181.13
S/I Ratio	0.943			1.037			0.936		

Table 1. Retinal nerve fiber layer thickness averages in normal patients. Garas et al 2009 (14 normals), Sehi et al (20 normals) and Savini et al (23 normals)

5.3. Ganglion cell layer

Most recently, the new abundant source of data rendered via spectral domain OCT measurements, allow us to document structural changes in the axonal bed as well as other retinal layers which were thought to, possibly, have close association with some types of glaucomatous progression. It seems intuitive that failing nerves might show changes at their endpoints before doing so in their mid-sections. Additionally, it seemed likely that axonal ganglia might show changes in concert with various types of axonal demise. Studies such as those conducted Desatnik et al and Ziemer et al in the 1990's helped point us to our new appreciation of the value of perimacular measurements. [14, 15]

Determining the extent of retinal ganglion cell loss may prove to be a superior method for identifying glaucomatous progression. The loss of these cells leads to functional deficits and structural changes in the retinal nerve fiber layer (RNFL). In their efforts to correlate structural and functional loss in glaucoma, Harwerth and associates showed that the number of retinal ganglion cells can be reliably estimated from either visual field sensitivity data or from OCT RNFL analysis. [16]

6. Functional measurement

6.1. Subjective testing

The first record of a visual field defect is found in Hippocrates description of a hemianopia from the late fifth century B.C. Ptolemy (150 B.C.) first attempted to quantify the visual field

http://dx.doi.org/10.5772/57601

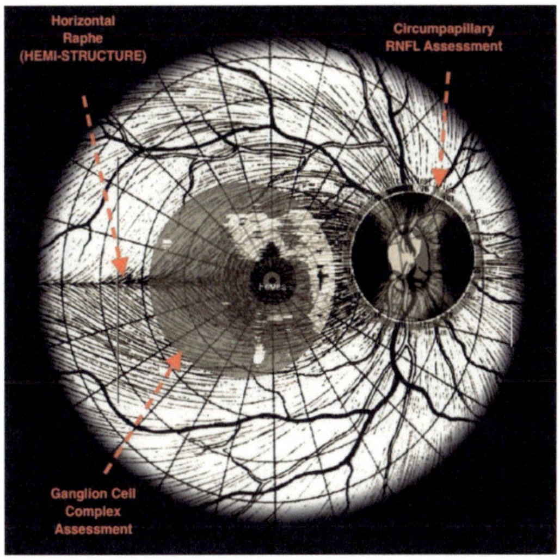

Figure 11. The RTVue scanning zones for assessment of the peripapillary retinal nerve fiber layer (RNFL) and the ganglion cell complex (GCC)

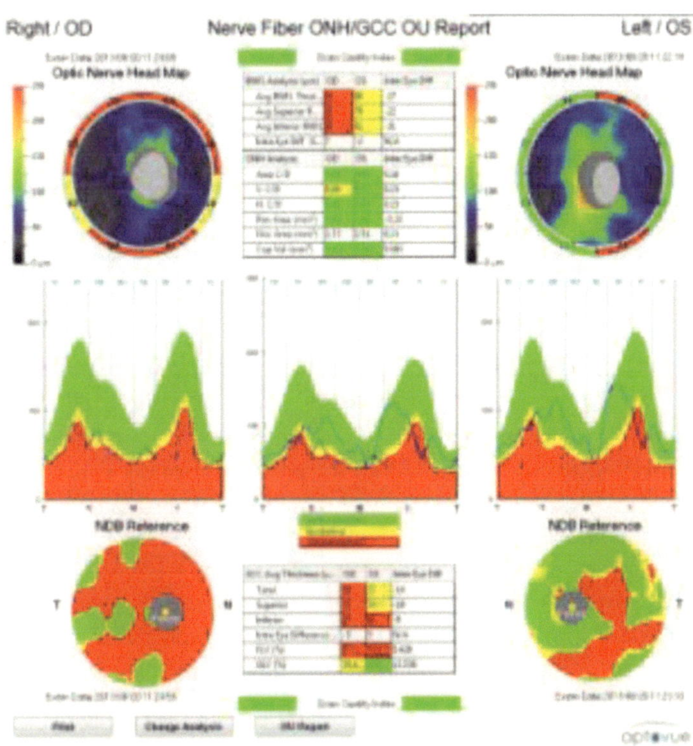

Figure 12. Optovue OCT report showing RNFL and GCC thickness. Colors green, yellow and red indicate normal, borderline and abnormal (low) findings.

and noted its circular form. According to Lloyd, Galen was the first physician "to record a recognition of Extramacular fields." He suggests the first illustration of the visual field was published in an article by Ulmus of Padua in 1602.

Early in the sixteenth century (about 1510) Leonardo da Vinci recognized that temporally the visual field reaches around more than 90 degrees from fixation. He said (Manuscript D. folio 8 verso), "the eye sees those objects behind it that are placed in lateral areas." He suggested that the cornea and the aqueous served to bend the light rays into the eye.

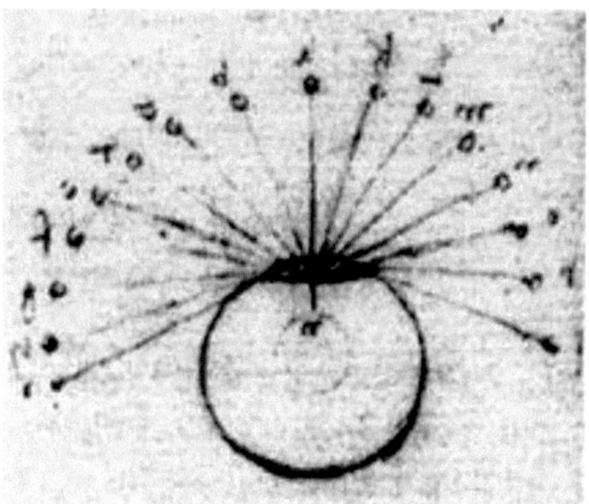

Figure 13. DaVinci's Illustration of rays approaching the cornea from different directions

Von Graefe (below) is credited with introducing perimetry into clinical medicine. In 1855, at the age of 28, he published "Examination of the Visual Functions in Amblyopic Affections." Von Graefe built on the work of Helmholtz. Helmholtz had recommended that, in order to keep one's bearing during the examination of the ocular fundus, a numbered grid be placed in front of the patient to direct the patient's eye into certain known directions of gaze. It was a piece of blackboard marked in this way that von Graefe used as a tangent screen. He worked at a distance of 18 inches and used as a test object a piece of white chalk, about 1 cm across, held in a wire. He made use of various symbols and dots as a fixation point so that the patient could recognize his deficits more easily. [17]

It was not until the late 1980's, when automated perimetry became widely available, that manual methods of visual field assessment were finally outpaced as the clinical standard. With the newfound ability to determine the relative depth of defect of a given point, clinicians had the ability to appreciate a three dimensional plot of one's visual status.

The introduction of computers and automation heralded a new era in perimetric testing. Static testing can be performed in an objective and standardized fashion with minimal perimetrist bias. A quantitative representation of the visual field can be obtained more rapidly than with manual testing. The computer allows stimuli to be presented in a pseudorandom, unpredictable fashion. Patients do not know where the next stimulus will appear, so fixation is improved, thereby increasing the reliability of the test. Random presentations also increase the speed with

http://dx.doi.org/10.5772/57601

which perimetry can be performed by bypassing the problem of local retinal adaptation, which requires a 2-second interval between stimuli if adjacent locations are tested.

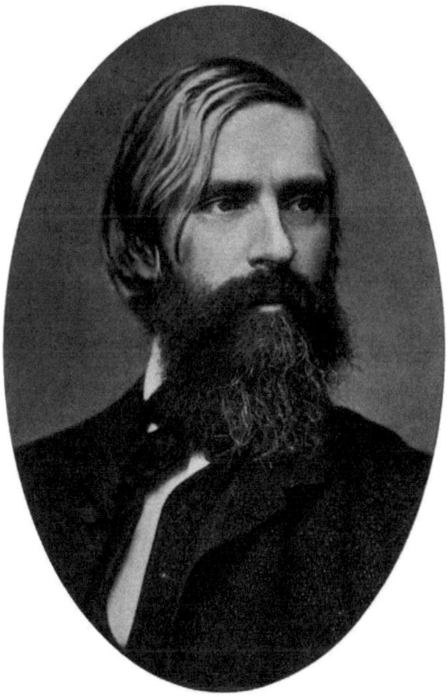

Figure 14. Albrecht von Graefe

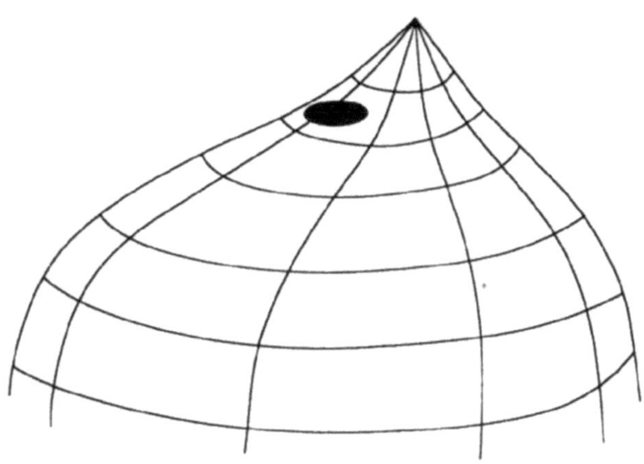

Figure 15. The normal island of vision. The hill is highest at fixation, where visual sensitivity is greatest. The height of the hill of vision declines toward the periphery as visual sensitivity diminishes.

Any clinically or statistically significant deviation from the normal shape of the hill of vision can be considered a visual field defect. In glaucoma, these defects are either diffuse depressions of the visual field or localized defects that conform to nerve fiber bundle patterns. [18]

6.2. Current choices in subjective functional testing

The addition of computerization to assessment of the eyes functional performance led the way to the development of several testing alternatives. Early white on white threshold testing strategies were followed with faster and more efficient programs such as Humphries Swedish Interactive Testing Algorithm (SITA) and the Haag-Streit Tendency Oriented Perimetry (TOP), Along with unenhanced test specificity, both strategies significantly reduce testing times by over 70%. The TOP strategy requires less than three minutes per eye per test.

A daunting point of frustration with the limits of threshold analysis came from the understanding that significant axonal loss had to have occurred before a repeatable threshold could be demonstrated. In 1982, Quigley reported that as much as 40% of optic nerve fibers may be lost before significant threshold visual field loss. [19]

Alternatives more recent methods in subjective field analysis, such as short wavelength (blue – yellow) and flicker strategies, were developed with the goal of reliably eliciting subject glaucomatous defects at an earlier point the progression of the disease. It is now shown that the flicker type tests such as Frequency Doubling Technology will have a role to play as a glaucoma screening tests, where as the the blue-yellow tests may not be as predictive as once throught. 20 Recently, there has been increased inteest in 10 degree white on white threshold fields because of its greater test point density and its apparent structure relationship to new OCT ganglion cell complex (GCC) imaging analyses. 14, 15

6.3. Objective testing

Objective methods such as Visual Evoked Potential (VEP), pattern electroretinography (pERG) (Diopsys, Inc.), and Relative Afferent Pupillary Defect (RAPDx) (Konan, USA) offer the potential of earlier and more specific functional testing but here continues to be a need to more reliably access functional loss at an earlier point in glaucomagenesis. While VEP and pERG measure the relative integrity of the electrical signal that passes through the nerve during the visual process,

RAPDx expands on the notion of diminished afferent pupillary reflex that may occur as nerve integrity is lost and glaucoma progresses.

With newer imaging methods such as OCT, we have made significant strides in earlier detection of structural loss, while our ability to detect functional loss earlier than what we achieve via white on white threshold field analysis remains a challenge. Given early evidence that VEP, pERG and RAPDx may offer some reliable evidence of early functional change, one can only hope that robust scientific evidence paired with more technical advancement of these types of tools may help us get a bit closer. [21-23]

http://dx.doi.org/10.5772/57601

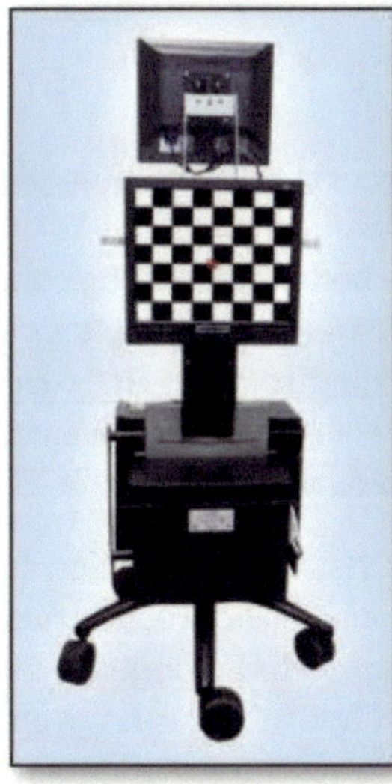

Figure 16. Visual Evoked Potential (VEP), pattern electroretinography (pERG) (Diopsys, Inc.)

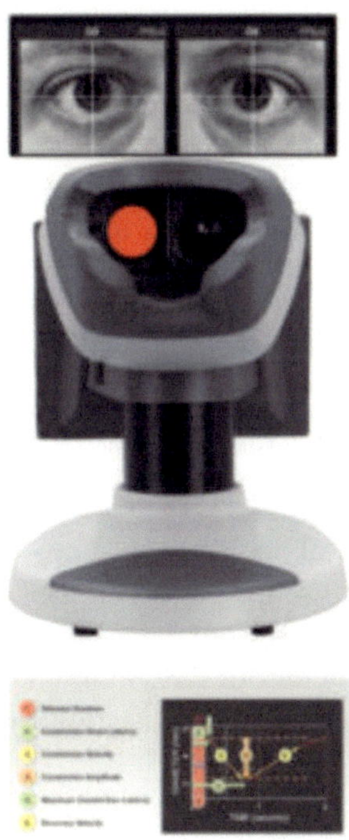

Figure 17. RAPDx (Konan, USA) measures Relative Afferent Pupillary Defect

7. Combining structural and functional data to optimize specificity in diagnosis

Along with our better understanding of the various limitations of either structural or functional analysis as a singular metric for glaucoma management, the obvious question has become can we, somehow, fortuitously coalesce both data sets? By combining the two, can we apprehend glaucoma earlier in its progression and develop better methods of dividing glaucoma into more meaningful subtypes? Will doing so allow us to treat more promptly, effectively and more specifically? Finally, is there a way to combine structural tests with functional tests to give us some type of unified glaucoma value?

Several investigators pioneered early structure function studies with the goal of establishing a better understanding of the relationships between various structural and functional values. In 1976, Stephen Drance described optic disc changes as they correlated to visual field defects in chronic open-angle glaucoma. Drance's studies were followed by Hoskins et al and Hitchings et al who also observed the nature of optic changes which occurred in concert with glaucomatous visual field changes (ref's). [24-26] These investigations were conducted with the goal of pairing specific anatomical changes commonly associated with glaucoma with associated functional (visual field) changes. Others tried to find a common more useful value in combining structural and functional data in different ways. [24-26]

Perhaps, the most renowned investigations which have established the foundations of our current understanding of the structure function relationship were performed by Quigley et al during the 1980's. Glaucomatous eyes were studied posthumously to determine how the number and distribution of human optic nerve axons compared with clinical measurements available the same eyes, including visual acuity, disc appearance, and visual field studies. Quigley reported that definite loss of axons occurs prior to reproducible visual field defects in some patients suspected of having glaucoma. In glaucoma, the superior and inferior poles of the nerve lose nerve fibers at a selectively greater rate, leading to an hourglass-shaped atrophy. He also reported that the pattern of atrophy in examples of toxic amblyopia, ischemic optic neuropathy and chronic papilledema differ from that of glaucoma, suggesting different mechanisms of damage in these conditions.

In later investigations, Harwerth et al described relationships between field loss and retinal ganglion cells. The data were analyzed by a model that predicted ganglion cell densities from standard clinical perimetry, which were then compared to histologic cell counts. Their work became part of the foundation for our current interest and understanding of functional loss in the context of retinal tissue changes beyond the losses previously described in retinal axons. [27-30]

In 2005, Gardiner et al produced a topographical map to demonstrate how sectors of the optic nerve head (ONH) are related to locations in the visual field, using empiric cross-sectional patient data. They observed one hundred nine subjects with healthy eyes and 166 subjects with diagnosed or suspected glaucoma (one test per patient) were evaluated using a Heidelberg Retina tomograph (HRT) and white-on-white standard automated perimetry (SAP). The

Tomograph ONH images were divided into 36 sectors; and the sector rim areas normalized to account for changes in the total rim area. These were then correlated with SAP thresholds. For each visual field location, a map was produced indicating the strength of correlation between the normalized sector rim areas and thresholds. Their efforts resulted in a map relating regions of the ONH to SAP test locations. This map may be useful in elucidating the structure-function relationship, particularly for cases of localized glaucomatous loss.

Their results also indicate that narrowing of the neuroretinal rim in some areas appeared to be more significant than in others, in terms of predicting functional loss; in particular in the polar areas of the ONH. This may account for some of the limitations of predictive power that has been shown of global HRT indices. [31]

In 2010, Harwerth et al attempted to build a model of these linking propositions using data from investigations of the relationships between losses of visual sensitivity and thinning of retinal nerve fiber layer over progressive stages of glaucoma severity. A foundation for the model was laid through the pointwise relationships between visual sensitivities (behavioral perimetry in monkeys with experimental glaucoma) and histological analyses of retinal ganglion cell densities in corresponding retinal locations. The subsequent blocks of the model were constructed from clinical studies of aging in normal human subjects and of clinical glaucoma in patients to provide a direct comparison of the results from standard clinical perimetry and optical coherence tomography. The final formulation is a nonlinear structure-function model that was evaluated by the accuracy and precision of translating visual sensitivities in a region of the visual field to produce a predicted thickness of the retinal nerve fiber layer in the peripapillary sector that corresponded to the region of reduced visual sensitivity. The model was tested on two independent patient populations, with results that confirmed the predictive relationship between the retinal nerve fiber layer thickness and visual sensitivities from clinical perimetry. Thus, the proposed model for linking structure and function in glaucoma has provided information that is important in understanding the results of standard clinical testing and the neuronal losses caused by glaucoma, which may have clinical application for inter-test comparisons of the stage of disease. The model was tested on two independent patient populations, with results that confirmed the predictive relationship between the retinal nerve fiber layer thickness and visual sensitivities from clinical perimetry. Thus, the proposed model for linking structure and function in glaucoma has provided information that is important in understanding the results of standard clinical testing and the neuronal losses caused by glaucoma, which may have clinical application for inter-test comparisons of the stage of disease. [16]

In 2012, Medeiros et al confirmed that an index combining structure and function performed better than isolated structural and functional measures for detection of perimetric and preperimetric glaucoma as well as for discriminating different stages of the disease. Observational study included 333 glaucomatous eyes (295 with perimetric glaucoma and 38 with preperimetric glaucoma) and 330 eyes of healthy subjects. All the eyes were tested with standard automated perimetry and spectral domain optical coherence tomography within 6 months. Estimates of the number of retinal ganglion cells (RGCs) were obtained from standard automated perimetry and spectral domain optical coherence tomography and a weighted averaging scheme was used to obtain a final estimate of the number of RGCs for each eye. The CSFI was calculated as the percent loss of RGCs obtained by subtracting estimated from expected RGC numbers. The performance of the CSFI for discriminating glaucoma from normal eyes and the different stages of disease was evaluated by receiver operating characteristic curves. [32, 33]

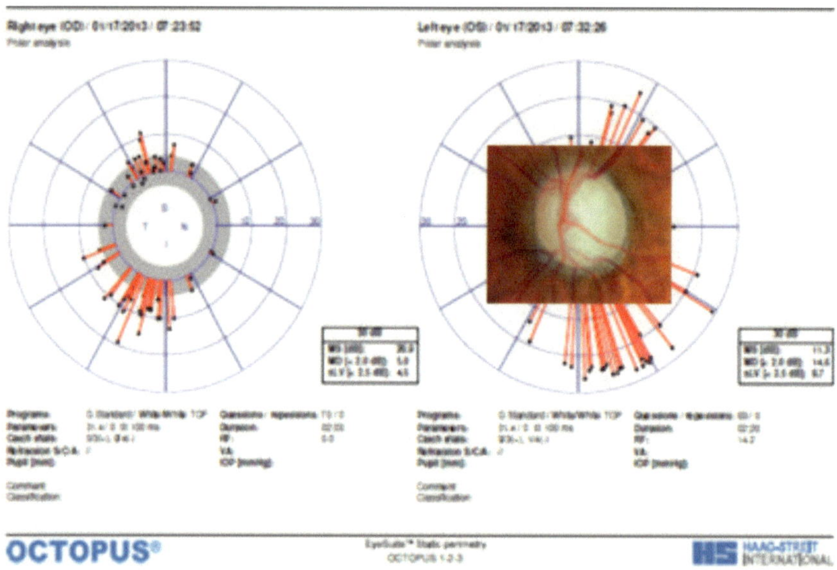

Figure 18. Polar analysis of a threshold visual field showing severity of the defect in concert with nerve anatomy. While traditional graphical reports of field analysis show projected (inverted) findings, the polar analysis is anatomically correct.

In 2013, Meira-Freitas et al demonstrated that baseline and longitudinal estimates of retinal ganglion cell counts based on combined structure and function tests may be helpful in predicting progression, and performed significantly better than conventional approaches for risk stratification of glaucoma suspects. The study included 288 glaucoma suspect eyes of 288 patients followed for an average of 3.8 ± 1.0 years. Estimates of RGC counts were obtained by combining data from SAP and OCT according to previously described method. Joint longitudinal survival models were used to evaluate the ability of baseline and rates of change in estimated RGC counts for predicting progression over time, adjusting for confounding variables. [34]

Also, in 2013, Le et al implemented fourier-domain optical coherence tomography (FD-OCT) system to map the macula and peripapillary regions of the retina in 56 eyes of 38 patients with perimetric glaucoma. The macular GCC and peripapillary NFL thicknesses were mapped and standard automated perimetry (SAP) was performed. Loss of GCC and NFL were correlated with the VF map on both a point-by-point and regional basis, showing that there are significant point-specific and regional correlations between GCC loss, NFL loss, and deficits on SAP. Their findings suggest that using these different data sources together may improve our understanding of glaucomatous damage and aid in the management of patients with glaucoma. [35]

In 2013, Hye-Young Shin et al Two hundred and thirteen eyes of 213 patients with glaucoma were observed to explore and compare the relationships between the visual field (VF) sensitivities assessed by standard automated perimetry (SAP) and the ganglion cell inner plexiform layer (GCIPL) and peripapillary retinal nerve fiber layer (pRNFL) thicknesses as measured by Cirrus high-definition optical coherence tomography (HD-OCT) in glaucomatous eyes.

The average and sectorial GCIPL thicknesses determined by Cirrus HD-OCT were significantly associated with global and regional VF sensitivity in patients with glaucoma. They concluded that the macular GCIPL thickness values may provide more valuable information than temporal profile thickness values for understanding the structure–function relationships of the macular region. [35]

In 2013, Marín-Franch et al reported their comparison structural and functional damage from glaucoma often using statistical methods such as linear regression, which was agreed to have limitations that can lead to inadequate clinical recommendations. These limitations were analyzed, using examples from the literature. Inferences from linear regression are model dependent. They concluded that tests of linear relations between structure and function in glaucoma may be improved by the use of Deming regression, although its application requires knowledge about test-retest variability of measures of glaucomatous damage. [37, 38]

8. Summary

It has been said that in Einstein's Grand Quest for a Unified Theory "He failed, of course, but he didn't exactly waste his time." Similarly, our search for a simplified common denominator to describe glaucoma in a simple way is likely to fail. Our methods of documenting the optic nerve and various ocular structures related to the genesis of glaucoma have evolved from direct observation paired with hand drawings to ocular corherance tomographic devices, which render elegant cross sectional views with as little as 5 microns of resolution. Quantification of the visual field has also evolved to sophisticated threshold subjective analyses and promising new objective strategies. In spite of this impressive technical evolution, we have yet to agree upon a practical combination of structural and functional data that can provide a single metric for risk of glaucoma and the level of its progression.

Perhaps, the solution to this conundrum can be derived from our acceptance that glaucoma does not appear to be one simple disease, but rather one that is the result of a litany of risk factors that commonly result in the untimely deterioration of the optic nerve. As investigators have and continue to examine the many structural and functional changes that may occur in the process of glaucoma, the field of clinical variables ironically seems to expand rather than contract. Physical changes may be observed at the neural retinal rim first, while in other patients changes in the peri macular ganglion cell layer may be the first signal of glaucomatous change. Some patients might show degradation in their peripheral visual fields while others seem to start with central changes. Recent investigators have even suggested that early changes, in glaucoma, may occur within the brain.

As with Einstein's Grand Quest, it can be argued that the efforts of researchers to find a "unified glaucoma value" have not been a waste of time. While there seems to be no simple solution to this puzzle in sight, we have been given a far better understanding of glaucoma's multivariate etiology which should enable more specific and prompt diagnosis and, ultimately, more specific and effective glaucoma therapies.

Author details

Elliot M. Kirstein*

Address all correspondence to: drkirstein@drkirstein.com

Harper's Point Eye Associates, Cincinnati, Ohio, USA

References

[1] The phasic variations in the ocular tension in primary glaucoma. Am J Ophthalmol. 1952 Jan;35(1):1–21.

[2] Ophthalmoscopes Part 1 http://www.college-optometrists.org/en/college/museyeum/online_exhibitions/optical_instruments/ophthalmoscopes/

[3] Mark HH, On the Evolution of Binocular Ophthalmoscopy. Ophthalmol. 2007;125(6): 830-833. doi:10.1001/archopht.125.6.830

[4] Reus NJ and Lemij HG. The Relationship between Standard Automated Perimetry and GDx VCC Measurements. Investigative Ophthalmology & Visual Science, March 2004, Vol. 45, No. 3

[5] Zangwill LM, Williams J, A comparison of optical coherence tomography and retinal nerve fiber layer photography for detection of nerve fiber layer damage in glaucoma. Ophthalmology Volume 113, Issue 9, Pages 1593-1602, September 2006

[6] Gabriele ML, Wollstein G, Ishikawa H, Kagemann L, Xu J, Folio L S and Schuman J S. Optical Coherence Tomography: History, Current Status, and Laboratory Work Investigative Ophthalmology & Visual Science, April 2011, Vol. 52, No. 5

[7] Bendschneider D, Tornow RP, Horn FK, Laemmer R, Roessler CW, Juenemann AG, Kruse FE, Mardin CY.Retinal nerve fiber layer thickness in normals measured by

spectral domain OCT.J Glaucoma. 2010 Sep;19(7):475-82. doi: 10.1097/IJG.0b013e3181c4b0c7

[8] Varma R, Skaf M, Barron E. Retinal nerve fiber layer thickness in normal human eyes. Ophthalmology. 1996 Dec;103(12):2114-9

[9] Bowd C, Weinreb RN; Williams JM, Zangwill LM. The Retinal Nerve Fiber Layer Thickness in Ocular Hypertensive, Normal, and Glaucomatous Eyes With Optical Coherence Tomography Arch Ophthalmol. 2000;118(1):22-26. doi:10.1001/archopht.118.1.22

[10] Garas A, Tóth M, Vargha P, Holló G. Comparison of repeatability of retinal nerve fiber layer thickness measurement made using the RTVue Fourier-domain optical coherence tomograph and the GDx scanning laser polarimeter with variable or enhanced corneal compensation. J Glaucoma. 2010 Aug;19(6):412-7. doi: 10.1097/IJG.0b013e3181bdb549

[11] Sehi M, Grewal DS, Sheets CW, Greenfield DS. Diagnostic ability of Fourier-domain vs time-domain optical coherence tomography for glaucoma detection. Am J Ophthalmol. 2009 Oct;148(4):597-605. doi: 10.1016/j.ajo.2009.05.030. Epub 2009 Jul 9.

[12] Savini G, Carbonelli M, Barboni P. Retinal nerve fiber layer thickness measurement by Fourier-domain optical coherence tomography: a comparison between cirrus-HD OCT and RTVue in healthy eyes. J Glaucoma. 2010 Aug;19(6):369-72. doi: 10.1097/IJG.0b013e3181bdb55d.

[13] Tarannum Mansoori, MS; Kalluri Viswanath, MS; Nagalla Balakrishna, PhD Quantification of Retinal Nerve Fiber Layer Thickness in Normal Eyes, Eyes With Ocular Hypertension, and Glaucomatous Eyes With SD-OCT Ophthalmic Surgery, Lasers & Imaging • Vol. 41, No. 6 (Suppl), 2010

[14] Desatnik H, Quigley HA, Glovinsky Y. Study of central retinal ganglion loss in experimental glaucoma in monkey eyes. J Glaucoma. 1996;5(1):46-53.

[15] Zeimer R, Asrani S, Zou S, et al. Quantitative detection of glaucomatous damage at the posterior pole by retinal thickness mapping: a pilot study. Ophthalmology. 1998;105(2):224-231.

[16] Harwerth RS, Wheat JL, Fredette MJ, Anderson DR. Linking structure and function in glaucoma. Prog Retin Eye Res. 2010 Jul;29(4):249-71. doi: 10.1016/j.preteyeres.2010.02.001. Epub 2010 Mar 11.

[17] Imaging and Perimetry Society History of the visual field before perimetry http://www.perimetry.org/PerimetryHistory/1-pre-perimetry.htm

[18] Piltz-Seymour J R, Heath Phillip O, Drance S M. Visual Fields in Glaucoma http://www.oculist.net/downaton502/prof/ebook/duanes/pages/v3/v3c049.html

[19] Quigley HA, Addicks EM, Green WR. Optic nerve damage in human glaucoma. III. Quantitative correlation of nerve fiber loss and visual field defect in glaucoma, ische-

mic neuropathy, papilledema, and toxic neuropathy. Arch Ophthalmol 1982 Jan; 100(1):135-46.

[20] Yoshiyama KK and Johnson CA. Which Method of Flicker Perimetry Is Most Effective for

[21] Detection of Glaucomatous Visual Field Loss? Investigative Ophthalmology & Visual Science, October 1997, Vol. 38, No. 11

[22] Pillai C, Ritch R, Derr P, Gonzalez A, Cox LK, Siegfried J, Liebmann JS and Tello C. Sensitivity and Specificity of Short-Duration Transient Visual Evolked Potentials in Discriminating Normal From Glaucomatous Eyes. Invest Ophthalmol Vis Sci. 2013 Apr 23;54(4):2847-52. doi: 10.1167/iovs.12-10097. f Short-Duration Transient Visual Evoked Potentials (SD-tVEP)

[23] Chang DS, Boland MV, Arora KS, Supakontanasan W, Chen BB, Friedman D. Wilmur Institute, Johns Hopkins August 2013 Symmetry of the Pupillary Light Reflex and its Relationship to Retinal Nerve Fiber Layer Thickness and Visual Field Defect Invest Ophthalmol Vis Sci. 2013 Aug 19;54(8):5596-601. doi: 10.1167/iovs.13-12142.

[24] Meira-Freitas D, Weinreb RN, Marvasti AH, Zangwill LM, and Madeiros FA. Estimation of retinal ganglion cell loss in glaucomatous eyes with a relative afferent pupillary defect. Ophthalmol. Vis. Sci. published 26 November 2013, 10.1167/iovs.13-12921

[25] Drance SM. Correlation between optic disc changes and visual field defects in chronic open-angle glaucoma. Trans Am Acad Ophthalmol Otolaryngol. 1976;81:224-226.

[26] Hoskins HD Jr, Gelber EC. Optic disk topography and visual field defects in patients with increased intraocular pressure. Am J Ophthalmol. 1975;80:284-290

[27] Hitchings RA, Spaeth GL. The optic disc in glaucoma II: Correlation of the appearance of the optic disc with the visual field. Br J Ophthalmol. 1977;61:107-113.

[28] Quigley HA, Addicks EM, Green WR. Optic nerve damage in human glaucoma. III. Quantitative correlation of nerve fiber loss and visual field defect in glaucoma, ischemic neuropathy, papilledema and toxic neuropathy. Arch Ophthalmol. 1982;100:135-146.

[29] Quigley HA, Dunkelberger GR, Green WR. Retinal ganglion cell atrophy correlated with automated perimetry in human eyes with glaucoma. Am J Ophthalmol. 1989;107:453-464.

[30] Harwerth RS, Carter-Dawson L, Smith EL 3rd, Crawford ML. Scaling the structure--function relationship for clinical perimetry. Acta Ophthalmol Scand. 2005;83:448-455.

[31] Harwerth RS, Quigley HA. Visual field defects and retinal ganglion cell losses in patients with glaucoma. Arch Ophthalmol. 2006;124:853-859.

[32] Gardiner SK, Johnson CA and Cioffi CA. Evaluation of the Structure-Function Relationship in Glaucoma. Copyright 2005 The Association for Research in Vision and Ophthalmology, Inc.

[33] Medeiros FA, Lisboa R, Weinreb RN, Girkin CA, Liebmann JM, Zangwill LM. A combined index of structure and function for staging glaucomatous damage. A combined index of structure and function for staging glaucomatous damage. Arch Ophthalmol. 2012 May;130(5):E1-10

[34] Medeiros FA, Zangwill LM, Anderson DR, Liebmann JM, Girkin CA, Harwerth RS, Fredette MJ, Weinreb RN. Estimating the rate of retinal ganglion cell loss in glaucoma. Am J Ophthalmol. 2012 Nov;154(5):814-824.e1. doi: 10.1016/j.ajo.2012.04.022. Epub 2012 Jul 27.

[35] Meira-Freitas D, Lisboa R, Tatham A, Zangwill LM, Weinreb RN, Girkin CA, Liebmann LM, and Medeiros FA. Predicting Progression in Glaucoma Suspects With Longitudinal Estimates of Retinal Ganglion Cell Counts Invest. Ophthalmol. Vis. Sci. 2013;54 4174-4183 7/2013 http://www.iovs.org/cgi/content/abstract/54/6/4174

[36] Phuc V. Le, Ou Tan, Vikas Chopra, Brian A. Francis, Omar Ragab, Rohit Varma, and David Huang. Regional Correlation Among Ganglion Cell Complex, Nerve Fiber Layer, and Visual Field Loss in GlaucomaInvest. Ophthalmol. Vis. Sci. 2013;54 4287-4295 http://www.iovs.org/cgi/content/abstract/54/6/4287

[37] Shin HY, Lopilly Park HY, Jung KI and Park CK. Comparative Study of Macular Ganglion Cell-Inner Plexiform Layer and Retinal Nerve Fiber Layer Measurement : Structure-Function Analysis IOVS IOVS-13-12667; published ahead of print October 15, 2013

[38] Marín-Franch I, Malik R, Crabb DP, and Swanson WH. Choice of Statistical Method Influences Apparent Association Between Structure and Function in Glaucoma Invest. Ophthalmol. Vis. Sci. 2013;54 4189-4196 7/2013 http://www.iovs.org/cgi/content/abstract/54/6/4189

[39] Mwanza JC, Warren JL, and BudenzInvest DL. Combining Spectral Domain Optical Coherence Tomography Structural Parameters for the Diagnosis of Glaucoma with Early Visual Field Loss Ophthalmol. Vis. Sci. published 26 November 2013, 10.1167/iovs.13-12749 http://www.iovs.org/cgi/content/abstract/iovs.13-12749v1

Chapter 11

Diabetic Retinopathy – An Update on Pathophysiology, Classification, Investigation and Treatment

Vikas Tah, Sonia Mall, James Myerscough,
Kamran Saha, Elizabeth Emsley, Andrew Swampillai,
Ganeshan Ramsamy, Daren Hanumunthadu and
Mandeep Bindra

Additional information is available at the end of the chapter

http://dx.doi.org/10.5772/58567

1. Introduction

The global prevalence of diabetes was estimated at 285 million in 2010.[1] The countries with the most significant number of sufferers in 2010 were India, China, United States, Russia and Brazil.[1] Countries with a low and middle income experience the worst burden of diabetes, compared with higher income countries.[1]

The total prevalence of diabetes in children and adults in the United States was 25.8 million in 2011, which is 8.3% of the entire population.[2] It is estimated that 18.8 million of this figure are diagnosed and 7 million remain undiagnosed.[2] 79 million individuals in the United States are expected to be at risk of diabetes.[2] The overall cost of diabetes in the United States in 2012 was $245 billion, with $176 being directly related to medical costs and $69 billion related to reduced productivity.[2] In the UK, 2.6 million individuals were diagnosed with diabetes in 2009,[3] and this is expected to exceed 4 million in 2024.[4] It is also expected that up to 500,000 other UK individuals remain undiagnosed.[5] An estimated one in 20 individuals in England have diabetes-both diagnosed and undiagnosed, and this is marginally reduced UK-wide.[1] For adults in the UK it is estimated that 10% of individuals with diabetes mellitus (DM) have Type 1 diabetes mellitus and 90% have type 2 diabetes mellitus.[1, 6]

Effective management of diabetes reduces complication risk.[7] However failure to control the condition can lead to microvascular and macrovascular complications. At the time of diagnosis, 50% of those with type 2 diabetes mellitus face complications.[8] Complications may begin five to six years prior to diagnosis, whilst the onset of diabetes itself may precede the clinical diagnosis by a decade.[9]

Diabetic retinopathy (DR) is the most frequent complication associated with diabetes mellitus, and is the number one cause of blindness in individuals of working age in developed nations.[10] Indeed individuals with diabetes are 10 to 20 times at greater risk of developing blindness than those without the diagnosis.[11] DR prevalence in the Wisconsin Epidemiological Study of Diabetic Retinopathy (WESDR) was identified as 50.1% and 54.2% in the diabetes control and complications trial (DCCT) in insulin-dependent diabetes mellitus (IDDM)[12, 13] DR prevalence in non-insulin dependent diabetes mellitus (NIDDM) was found to be 35-39% in the United Kingdom Prospective Diabetes Study.[14] During 2005-2008, 4.2 million (28.5%) of diabetics in the United States aged 40 years and above suffered from diabetic retinopathy, with 0.7 million (4.4% of these diabetics) experiencing advanced DR, thus risking severe loss of vision.[2] In the WESDR, 1.4% of patients with IDDM were able to achieve a best-corrected visual acuity of 20/80 to 20/160, with 3.6% having an acuity of 20/200 or worse in the better eye.[15] 3% of the older-onset group had vision ranging from 20/80 to 20/160, and 1.6% were 20/200 or worse in the best eye.[15]

1.1. Incidence of visual impairment

10 years following diabetes mellitus (DM) onset, blindness (a visual acuity of equal to or worse than 20/200 in the best eye) was 1.8% in the type 1 cohort, 4.0% in the insulin-treated type 2 group and 4.8% in the non-insulin-treated type 2 patients.[16] Further, in these groups the incidence of visual impairment at 10 years (loss of 15 letters on a 0-70 letter scale) was identified as 9.4, 37.2 and 23.9 respectively.[16]

There appear to be few paediatric cases of DR, though it has been identified in children as young as 5.5 years in an American study, and severe blindness has also been described in adolescents as the microvascular effects of diabetes, including DR, can develop during puberty years.[17]

1.2. Historical developments

The Diabetic Retinopathy Study in the 1970s and the Early Treatment Diabetic Retinopathy Study in the 1980s, identified the major effects of retinal photocoagulation on visual loss associated with proliferative diabetic retinopathy and macular oedema, as well as influencing guideline and screening programme development for early identification and management of diabetic retinopathy.[18, 19, 20] Following this, both the incidence and progression risk of diabetic retinopathy has reduced from an estimated 90% of patients with diabetes, to less than 50%.[20] In the WESDR, which focused on individuals with type 1 diabetes mellitus, the yearly incidence of proliferative diabetic retinopathy reduced by 77% from 1980 to 2007, with a 57% reduction in visual impairment during this same time period.[21] Evidence from a range of international studies, including those from Sweden, Denmark and the United States, indicate that individuals recently diagnosed with type 1 or type 2 diabetes mellitus have a significantly reduced risk of proliferative diabetic retinopathy, macular oedema and visual impairment, compared with those diagnosed in the past.[22, 23, 24, 25, 26] The considerable decrease in the prevalence and incidence of diabetic retinopathy and visual impairment over the previous few decades suggests improved glycaemic, blood pressure and lipid level management.[26]

1.3. A global epidemic

However the number of individuals with diabetes is expected to exponentially increase internationally to 429 million by 2030, attributed to the increased prevalence of obesity, an ageing population and enhanced identification of the disease.[27, 28] This represents a major public health concern. As an exemplar, in India 32 million individuals were diagnosed with diabetes in 2000 and an estimated 79 million will be affected by 2030, and if complication prevalence remains the same, around 0.7 million Indians will suffer from proliferative diabetic retinopathy and 1.8 million with have macular oedema with clinical manifestations.[29] This identifies a large population at risk of visual impairment attributed to their diabetes, and highlights the importance of effective epidemiological surveillance of developing countries as there may be reduced delivery of health care capacity compared with developed nations.[20]

2. Pathophysiology

The DCCT and United Kingdom Prospective Diabetes Study (UKPDS) both support the significant association between a long-term hyperglycaemic status and the establishment, as well as progression, of DR.[36, 37] However the mechanism which result in microvascular injury attributed to hyperglycaemia is uncertain.[36, 37] Several interlinking molecular pathways have been discussed as being possibly involved in the mechanism, and these include enhanced polyol pathway activity, diacylglycerol-(DAG-)PKC pathway activation, enhanced growth factor expression for example vascular endothelial growth factor (VEGF) and insulin-like growth factor-1 (IGF-1), haemodynamic alterations, faster advanced glycation endproducts (AGEs) production, oxidative stress, renin-angiotensin-aldosterone system (RAAS) activation, inflammation and leukostasis.[38] However the final metabolic pathway resulting in the establishment of DR is uncertain.[39]

2.1. Polyol pathway

The polyol pathway is involved in the metabolism of surplus glucose.[38]

Aldose reductase (AR), which exists in the retina, is involved in the reduction of glucose into sorbitol, employing nicotinamide adenine dinucleotide phosphate (NADPH) as a cofactor.[38] Sorbitol is then converted to fructose using sorbital dehydrogenase (SDH).[38] Sorbitol is impermeable to cellular membranes, and therefore there is an intracellular accumulation of it, which is followed by the gradual metabolism of sorbitol to fructose.[40] NADPH is also employed as a cofactor for glutathione reductase in the regeneration of intracellular glutathione, therefore limiting the antioxidant capability of the cells.[38]

Sorbitol accumulation may have multi-injurious effects on retinal cells, such as osmotic injury.[41] Further, the fructose formed in the polyol pathway can undergo a phosphorylation

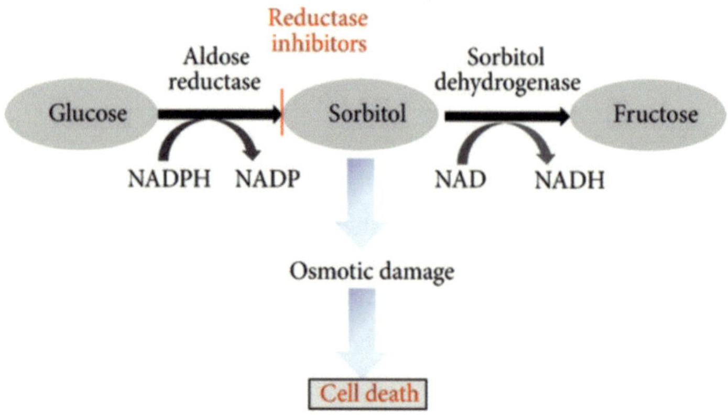

Figure 1. Polyol pathway

reaction, forming fructose-3-phosphate, with the potential for further degradation to 3-deoxyglucosone.[42] Both of these products are potent glycating mediators and can support the production of AGEs.[42] Moreover employment of NADPH in the polyol pathway, reduces NADPH availability for glutathione reductase, thereby preventing the production of reduced glutathione, resulting in reduced protection against oxidative stress.[43]

More recently, evidence suggests that AR is localised in retinal cells such as pericytes,[44] retinal endothelial cells,[45] ganglion cells,[45] Muller cells,[45] retinal pigment epithelial cells and neurons.[45, 46] Enhanced AR activity may be involved in retinal cell destruction.[43] Importantly, pericyte or endothelial cell exposure to enhanced concentrations of glucose or galactose reduces the survivability of these cells,[38] with reversal of this cell death on the administration of ARIs.[47] Generally, electrolye imbalance attributed to high aldose reductase levels results in cellular death, in particular retinal pericytes, which contribute to microaneurysm formation.[48]

The polyol pathway is also associated with other pathophysiological characteristics in DR, including a thickened retinal capillary basement membrane,[49] with ARI preventing this thickening in rat models.[50] ARIs are also effective in reducing leukocyte adhesion in endothelial cells,[51] which results in leukostasis and is discussed later, as well as preventing enhanced vascular permeability and blood retinal barrier breakdown which is a hallmark feature of DR.[46] Genetically, AR may also contribute to DR establishment.[52]

Thus far, ARIs employed in animal models at the onset of diabetes has been useful in preventing DR, though limited clinical benefit has been shown.[38]

2.2. Protein glycation

The establishment and accumulation of AGEs is a significant contributor to DR.[53] AGEs are molecules produced non-enzymatically when sugars are reduced with free amino groups of proteins, lipids and nucleic acids.[38] Normally, AGEs are produced at a constant and gradual rate, commencing at the embryonic stage and accumulating with time.[38] In the context of increased glucose availability in diabetes, their production is accelerated.[54]

AGEs are important in several diabetic complications.[38] For example, they have been identified in the retinal vessels of diabetics, and these AGE levels have been correlated with those found in the serum, as well as retinopathy severity.[55] AGE interaction with certain cell surface receptors such as RAGE, CD36 and the macrophage scavenger receptor have been described in DR development.[55]

Animal studies suggest significantly high AGE exposure is contributory to renal and vascular complications.[56, 57] In rats which developed diabetes, retinal capillaries had enhanced AGE accumulation, as well as a loss of pericytes.[53] Treatment with AGE formation inhibitors considerably reduced AGE accumulation, and stopped microaneurysm formation, acellular capillaries and pericyte loss.[53] In another study, rats with a diabetes duration of 29 weeks, there was an increase in acellular capillaries by more than three times compared to previously, and there was increased thickening of the basement membrane.[56] A thickened capillary basement membrane and enhanced deposition of extracellular matrix components is a contributor to the development of abnormal retinal haemodynamics.[58] Again, treatment with an AGE formation inhibitor prevented capillary dropout and reduced basement membrane protein formation.[56]

These studies, which are still in their infancy, identify AGE formation and activation of their respective receptors as important targets for pharmacotherapeutic strategies.[38]

2.3. Activation of Protein Kinase C (PKC)

PKC is a kinase involved in signal transduction activity in response to a stimulus which may be hormonal, neuronal or growth factor in origin.[38] The Beta1/2 isoform of PKC is associated with DR development.[59] Raised blood glucose increases glucose flux in the glycolysis pathway, thereby increasing diacylglycerol (DAG) production. DAG is a major PKC activator.[60] Clinical and experimental research has identified an increase in DAG and PKC activation in diabetes.[59]

PKC can also influence other physiological pathways therefore having the capability to alter endothelial permeability, retinal haemodynamics and expression of vascular endothelial growth factor (VEGF) in the retina and enhanced leukostasis.[59, 61, 62]

In particular, the expression of the PKC beta1/2 isoform is increased in diabetics, thereby contributing to DR pathogenesis by extracellular matrix (ECM) protein synthesis, remodeling of the ECM, increased angiogenic factor production, endothelial and leukocyte cell abnormalities, ultimately resulting in occluded capillaries and leukostasis, with alterations in retinal blood flow.[38] The PKC pathway also influences other activities such as inflammatory changes, neovascularisation and abberant haemodynamics.[38] This further progresses the pathogenic changes in DR. Experimentally, PKC-beta1/2 inhibitors significantly reduce DR progression.[63] In clinical trials, inhibitors do not prevent DR but considerably reduce the associated vision loss.[64]

2.4. Haemodynamic alterations

Hypertension, which has a high incidence in diabetes, is likely to contribute to DR progression.[38] This may involve the mechanical stretch and sheer stresses associated with hypertension, injuring endothelial cells. Enhanced retinal perfusion and increased blood viscosity can also lead to endothelial dysfunction.[65] Further, the endocrine mechanisms which have regulatory influences over blood pressure are also independently involved in DR pathogenesis.[66]

2.5. Renin-angiotensin-aldosterone system involvement

RAAS is fundamental in blood pressure and fluid regulation, with aberrant changes identified in this system in diabetics.[66] There is an increase in the expression of certain receptors and signaling molecules in the retina, in PDR, including renin, angiotensin converting enzymes (ACE) and angiotensin receptors.[66, 67] This is independent of systemic blood pressure.[38] In experimental studies, ACE inhibitor use prevents neovascularization and several clinical studies suggest that targeting of RAAS reduces the incidence of retinopathy in type 1 diabetes and prevents progression of DR.[68]-[70]

The exact mechanism of RAAS involvement in DR is uncertain, though in vitro evidence identifies association with PKC activation and VEGF signaling.[71]

2.6. Inflammatory changes and Leukostasis

The importance of inflammation, in particular subclinical inflammation in DR development is considerable, though complex.[38] The hyperglycaemic state, oxidative stress, AGE production and hypertension are all contributory to the inflammation. Moreover, the inflammation is self-propagating by means of cytokines, adhesion molecules, VEGF activity, increased RAGE expression, nitric oxide regulatory changes and NF-kB signaling.[38] This subclinical retinal inflammation increases intraocular blood pressure by the involvement of endothelial nitric oxide synthase (eNOS), formation of new but weak vessels and their enhanced VEGF permeability which results in retinal haemorrhages, as well as leukostasis attributed to multiple proinflammatory agents.[38] Leukostasis is crucial in DR pathogenesis, resulting in capillary occlusion, reactive oxygen species (ROS)-related cellular death and local retinal amplification of the inflammatory activities.[72]-[75]

There is a considerable increase in systemic proinflammatory cytokine expression, soluble and cell surface adhesion molecule activation and chemokine expression in the DR retina.[76] The increase in serum proinflammatory cytokines, adhesion agents and immune cell activation in diabetes correlates with DR progression.[77, 78] Endothelial abnormalities, as well as increased proinflammatory cytokines and adhesion molecules, contribute to leukostasis by increasing leukocyte and endothelial cell interaction.[79, 80] Localised inflammation including the activation of microglia, macrophages and immune cells is considered important in DR pathogenesis.[81] This is corroborated by the use of minocycline, an antibiotic and anti-inflammatory agent, which prevents microglial activation and thereby prevents DR.[81]

2.7. Oxidative stress

Oxidative stress occurs when the level of ROS or oxygen radicals increase to a degree where the antioxidant defences are unable to cope.[82] Oxidative stress established by hyperglycaemia is pivotal in microvascular complications.[83] Correlation between hyperglycaemia, alterations in redox homeostasis and oxidative stress is essential in DR pathogenesis.[84, 85] Increased ROS are likely to be involved in both the development and progression of DR.[86] It has been proposed that oxidative stress may be a "unifying mechanism" linking several injurious pathways induced by the hyperglycaemic state in DR.[87] ROS derived from mitochondria cause DNA breaks, which activate poly-(ADP-ribose)-polymerase (PARP).[87] PARP activation results in inhibition of glyceraldehyde phosphate dehydrogenase (GAPDH) activity, causing glycolytic metabolite accumulation.[87] These metabolites cause the activation of AGE, PKC-beta-2, polyol and hexosamine pathways.[87] NADPH oxidase-derived ROS may also be involved in the pathogenesis.[87]

2.8. Growth factor involvement

The importance of growth factors in DR is confirmed by the rare observation of serious DR in growth hormone deficient diabetic dwarfs,[88] and this is further corroborated by slowed DR progression in individuals with pituitary ablation in the 1970s.[89]

The growth factor most frequently considered in DR is VEGF, which promotes angiogenesis, causes blood-retinal barrier breakdown, endothelial cell growth stimulation and neovascularization, as well as increased vascular permeability in an ischaemic retina.[90]-[92] Ischaemia in the retina causes angiogenic factors, such as vascular endothelial growth factor (VEGF) to establish neovascularization, resulting in proliferative diabetic retinopathy (PDR). VEGFs are produced by retinal pigment epithelium, pericytes and retinal endothelial cells.[39] Animal and clinical evidence suggests VEGF, especially the 165 isoform, is important in the development and progression of DR.[93, 94]

Anti-VEGF agents have clinical efficacy in the treatment of DMO, but are not effective in all patients.[38] Further long-term use of anti-VEGF agents should be considered with caution in DR.[38]

2.9. Carbonic Anhydrase (CA)

Enhanced intraocular VEGF concentrations correlates with increased vascular permeability, contributing to haemorrhage, exudate formation, vascular leakage, and ultimately leading to NPDR, angiogenesis and vasculogenesis leading to PDR.[38]

CAs are ubiquitous metalloenzymes which cause conversion of carbon dioxide to bicarbonate and protons.[38] Diabetics have considerably higher CA concentrations than controls,[95] and CA inhibitors reduce DR progression and prevents visual loss in animal and clinical research.[96] The mechanisms involved may include reduced humour secretion, induction of vasodilatation and improved ocular blood flow, platelet aggregation inhibition and reduction in vascular permeability.[95]

2.10. Neurodegeneration in the retina

As well as the changes already described, structural and functional alterations can injure certain non-vascular cells.[38] It is believed that neurodegeneration of retinal neurons and glia may even precede microaneurysm development.[97]

3. Risk factors

Epidemiologic studies have shown several risk factors associated with the incidence of diabetic retinopathy and subsequent macular oedema (table 1). Several other risk factors have also been implicated in disease progression such as sleep apnoea [98], non-alcoholic fatty liver disease, genetic mutations[21, 99] and serum prolactin, homocysteine and adinopectin levels [33, 31, 34]. However the exact contribution of these factors to disease progression remains unknown. The precise association of smoking with diabetic retinopathy appears complex and is unclear.

Type of diabetes
Duration of diabetes
Poor glycaemic control
Hyperlipidaemia
Hypertension
Pregnancy

Table 1. Recognised risk factors associated with diabetic retinopathy

3.1. Type of diabetes

Type 1 diabetic patients are at substantially higher risk than type 2, which is independent of the duration of the disease process[100, 101]. Both severity and prevalence increase with age in the former group but not the later.

3.2. Duration of diabetes

A clear correlation exists between diabetic retinopathy and disease duration[1]. This risk factor has influenced the formation of guidelines for early examination of suspected patients to decrease disease progression. In two studies [100, 102] evidence was shown that after 15 years retinopathy would be present in virtually all type 1 diabetics and up to 75% of type 2 diabetics, with 2% becoming blind and up to 10% developing severe visual impairment. Puberty is now an accepted risk factor for retinopathy in type 1 diabetes, due to the acceleration of microvascular compromise as a result of physiological changes post puberty [103]. One study found that younger post-menarchal subjects were up to 3.2 times more likely to develop retinopathy, in comparison to pre-menarchal subjects[104]. Subjects older than 13 years at the time of diagnosis were more likely to suffer from retinopathy, than those younger. A four year follow-up also showed that the same post-menarchal had greater progression of their retinopathy than pre-menarchal (P=0.06). While the exact mechanism is not known, hormonal factors have been speculated to play a part.

3.3. Glycaemic control

The relationship between glycaemic control and onset/progression of diabetic retinopathy is well documented. Intensive metabolic control has shown a decreased in diabetic related complications [105]. Studies such as the Early Treatment of Diabetic Retinopathy Study (ETDRS) and Diabetes Control and Complication Trial (DCCT)[13] show that risk of progression is reduced with aggressive glycaemic control. Glycosylated haemoglobin levels have shown a relationship with the severity of proliferative diabetic retinopathy[106]. However, while glycosylated haemoglobin remains a formidable risk factor, it only accounted for 11% of all risks for retinopathy in DCCT [107].

3.4. Hyperlipidaemia

Association of hyperlipidaemia and diabetes is well documented [108]. A statistically significant association between elevated serum total cholesterol and low density lipoprotein cholesterol and the severity of retinal hard exudation in patients with diabetic retinopathy was confirmed by the ETDRS group and the Wisconsin Epidemiologic Study of Diabetic Retinopathy (WESDR) found [109]. As reported by Chew found patients with serum cholesterol level more than 240mg/dl were twice as likely to have more hard exudates as those patients with serum cholesterol level 200 mg/dl [110].

3.5. Hypertension

A major risk factor of cardiovascular disease in diabetics is hypertension. An age-adjusted 82% increase in risk of diabetes-related death is thought to come from this risk factor alone.[111] This is accorded with the theory that increased blood pressure is implicated in the onset of diabetic retinopathy [112, 113]. The UK Prospective Diabetic Study (UKPDS) showed that tight blood pressure control (144/82 vs 155/87) was associated with a 34% reduction in retinopathy with a 47% reduction in deterioration of visual acuity of three lines [14]. The use of angiotensin-converting-enzyme (ACE) inhibitors and their role in directly affecting the progression of retinopathy (as opposed to their therapeutic effects in hypertension) was the subject of much debate. ACE inhibitors were found to be associated with reduced levels of vascular endothelial growth factor in diabetic retinopathy patients[114]. However in the UKDPS group demonstrated an overall reduction of blood pressure was proven to be effective in slowing down the progression of retinopathy, rather than the type of antihypertensive drug used [115]. More recently, the '**DI**abetic **RE**tinopathy **C**andesartan **T**rial' (DIRECT) study recently posited that while candesartan did not have any beneficial effect on the progression of retinopathy in type 1 diabetic patients, it did yield improvement in type 2 patients with mild to moderate retinopathy [69, 68].

3.6. Pregnancy

Many studies have concluded that diabetic women in pregnancy have a substantial risk of worsening their retinopathy [116, 117] although resolution of ocular changes in post-partum period is reported [116, 118]. Studies by Phelps et al [119] and the Diabetes in Early Pregnancy Study (DIEP) group [120] concluded that retinopathy was most likely to progress in those who had the poorest control at baseline. DIEP also found that a disease duration of more than 15 years and severity of existing retinopathy were the most important factors in the development and progression of retinopathy in pregnancy. Type 1 diabetic women are most at risk and should be undergo an ophthalmic examination prior to pregnancy and counselled on good glycaemic control. The exact mechanism of progressive retinopathy in pregnant diabetic woman is the subject of much debate. Factors thought to be involved include duration of diabetes, co-existing hypertension, poor glycaemic control and its rapid normalisation during pregnancy [121].

4. Signs

Microaneurysms are out-pouchings of the capillary wall that form by either focal dilatation of the capillary wall in the absence of pericytes, or fusion of the two arms of a capillary loop. Clinically these are seen as tiny red dots. Retinal haemorrhages are divided into intraretinal, retinal nerve fibre layer and deeper dark round haemorrhages. Intraretinal haemorrhages are located in the middle layers of the retina and give rise to dot/blot configuration. Retinal nerve fibre layer haemorrhages are flame-shaped and arise from larger superficial pre-capillary arterioles. Deeper dark round haemorrhages represent retinal infarcts within the middle layers and are marker for progression to retinal neovascularisation. Cotton wool spots result from nerve fibre layer infarcts. Axon disruption causes accumulation of neuronal debris in the nerve fibre layer. Clinically these are seen as small fluffy lesions that can obscure underlying blood vessels. Exudates are composed of lipoprotein and lipid-filled macrophages located within the outerplexiform layer. They are seen as waxy yellow lesions with relatively distinct margins. They tend to progress as retinopathy worsens and can affect the macula resulting in macular oedema. Exudates reabsorb spontaneously when leakage ceases over a period of months. Venous changes include beading of blood vessels, tortuosity, and focal narrowing with dilatation called 'beading'. The extent of venous change correlates well with the proliferative change. IRMA, or intraretinal microvascular abnormalities are arteriolar venous shunts that run from retinal arterioles to venules. They bypass capillary beds and are seen in areas of capillary hypoperfusion. Arteriolar narrowing often can be marker for ischaemic dysfunction. Proliferative retinopathy is seen as new preretinal vessels that may arise at the optic disc or elsewhere in the retina or iris. There are fine fragile vessels that can develop fibrous tissue over time.

Diabetic macula oedema is one of or a combination of focal, diffuse or ischaemia. It is the main reason for visual impairment and represents foveal oedema, exudates or ischaemia. Focal maculopathy has retinal thickening and exudates. Fluoroscein angiogram shows late focal

http://dx.doi.org/10.5772/58567

hypofluorescence from leakage. Diffuse maculopathy can be associated with cystoids changes and diffuse retinal thickening. Fluoroscein angiogram shows late hypofluorescence with a flower petal pattern if cystoids macula oedema is present. Ischaemic maculopathy often has a relatively normal looking macula in the presence of reduced visual acuity. Fluoroscein angiogram shows non-perfusion and an enlarged foveal avascular zone.

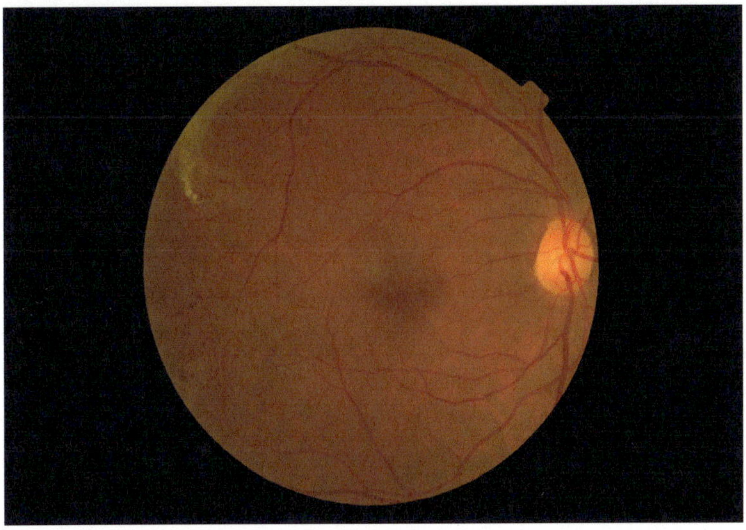

Figure 2. Microaneurysms at the macular and blot haemorrhages temporally

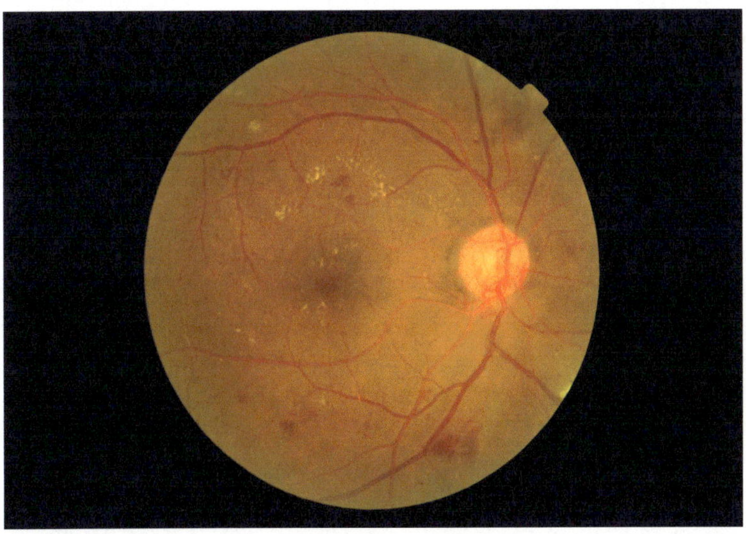

Figure 3. Exudates and microaneurysms at the macula, blot haemorrhages at the arcades, new vessels on the disc and cotton wool spots, IRMA and venous beading supoertemporally.

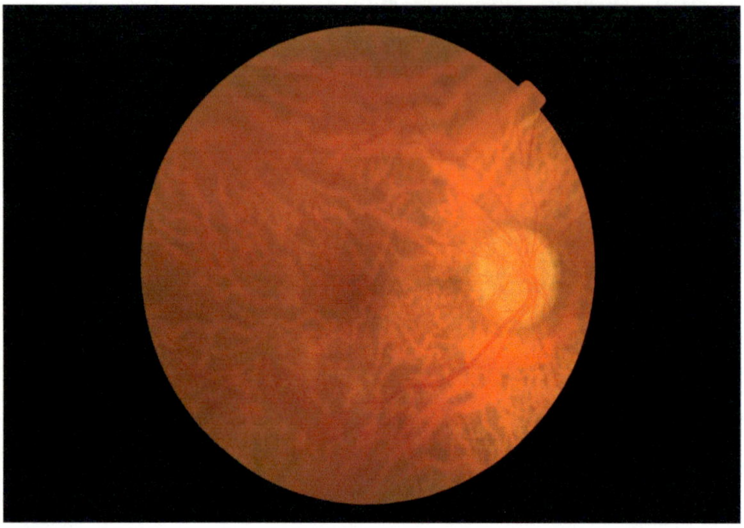

Figure 4. New vessels on disc and elsewhere inferotemporally

5. Classification

Diabetic retinopathy classification is based on who is classifying the disease. One approach has been for screening and one is based on grading severity in the context of ophthalmic signs. There are different screening systems in different parts of the developed world. In the UK, the English National Screening Criteria[122] is used to merit ophthalmological referral, seen in the table below. Two commonly used classification systems for classification in the context of ophthalmic signs are the Airlie House Classification [123] and the international (AAO) classification [124]. There are similarities and overlap in both. For the purpose of this chapter we will focus on the Airlie House classification.

The Airlie House classification was the original classification that has subsequently undergone modification in the Early Treatment of Diabetic Retinopathy Study (EDTRS)[125] aimed at grading retinopathy in the context of ophthalmic signs. EDTRS was first developed in 1997, but has undergone change and development for countries without significant screening and programmes and for the purpose of research. The sight threatening risk of diabetic retinopathy was incorporated into the later clinical grading system. Broadly this incorporates low risk non-proliferative retinopathy (3 substages), severe non-proliferative diabetic retinopathy, proliferative retinopathy and the presence of macula oedema.

Below is based on the Airlie House classification:

Mild Nonproliferative Diabetic Retinopathy (NPDR): At least one microaneurysm

Moderate NPDR: Severe retinal haemorrhages in at least one quadrant, cotton wool spots, venous beading or IRMA.

http://dx.doi.org/10.5772/58567

Severe NPDR: Severe retinal haemorrhages in four quadrants or venous beading in two quadrants; or extensive IRMA in one quadrant

Proliferative diabetic retinopathy: based on location and risk

Location: new vessels at disc (NVD) or elsewhere (NVE)

Risk: Low risk where neovascularisation of the optic disc is less than one-quarter to a third of the disc area with no vitreous haemorrhage.

High risk: mild NVD with vitreous haemorrhage.

Moderate to severe NVD (one quarter to a third disc areas)

New vessels elsewhere more than one half disc areas with vitreous haemorrhage.

ENSC Grade	Features
Retinopathy grade	
R0	No retinopathy
R1	Retinal microaneurysms, haemorrhages and or exudates not within the definition of maculopathy
R2	(Pre-proliferative) venous beading, venous loop or IRMA, dot or blot haemorrhages and cotton wool spots
R3	Proliferative: NVD, NVE or pre-retinal or vitreous haemorrhage, pre-retinal fibrosis and tractional retinal detachment
M0	No maculopathy
M1	Exudate within 1 disc diameter of fovea centre, or circinate exudates within the macula, or retinal thickening within 1 disc of fovea centre only if associated with vision of 6/12 or worse
P	Focal/grid laser to macula or peripheral scatter
U	Unobtainable

Table 2. The English National Screenin Committee Guidelines

Maculopathy

Focal: Well circumscribed areas of leakage with oedema and exudates, that may surround microaneurysms

Diffuse: Generalised leaking with oedema

Ischaemic: Reduced visual acuity with relatively normal clinical appearance but macula ischaemia on FFA.

Mixed: A combination of the above

Clinical significant macula oedema (CSMO)

- Retinal thickening at or within 500μm of the centre of the macula
- Hard exudates at or within 500μ of the centre of the macula if associated with adjacent retinal thickening
- Retinal thickening of > 1 disc area any part of which is within one disc diameter of the centre of the macula.

More recently the terms centre involving and non-centre involving macula oedema have been used.

6. Investigations

Diabetes Mellitus is a complex disease requiring a multidisciplinary approach. The systemic investigations requested for a patient identified with ocular manifestations of the disease may provide valuable information regarding other organ systems affected which are not yet clinically apparent. Some of the general investigations below may be requested by an ophthalmologist depending on the local health setting but require referral for result interpretation and subsequent management by diabetologist colleagues.

6.1. Systemic Investigations

6.1.1. HbA1C

The Diabetes Control and Complication Trial (DCCT) [126] and subsequent follow-up study, Epidemiology of Diabetes Interventions and Complications (EDIC), highlighted that the effect of good glycaemic control on progression of retinopathy is significant and persists for at least 10 years. Due to the 8-12 week turnover of erythrocytes the glycosylated haemoglobin molecule is a more useful marker of glucose control than a random blood glucose measurement.

6.1.2. Lipids

Recent studies [127] have identified the importance of cholesterol lowering medications to both treatment naïve and previously treated hypercholestrolaemic type 2 diabetics in reducing the risk of clinically significant macular edema (CSME), and diabetic retinopathy progression[127, 128]. Fasting lipids should therefore be requested in new patients.

6.1.3. Urea & electrolytes

Diabetic nephropathy is an important consequence of microvascular disease and all patients should be screened for any renal dysfunction.

6.1.4. Genetic markers

Various clinical studies have looked at retinopathy clusters in families with type 1 diabetes. Genetic studies have analysed risk genes for retinopathy [The Diabetes Control and Complications Trial Research Group, 1997][126]. No study has provided an evidence base for genetic testing in diabetic patients to predict the rate of retinopathy progression and therefore genetic testing is not currently recommended for routine practice.

6.1.5. Blood pressure

Patients should be referred to a physician for investigation of all modifiable risk factors including blood pressure and smoking cessation, both known to contribute to the rate of diabetic retinopathy progression. [Gaede *et al.* 2008][129].

7. Imaging

7.1. Fundus Photography

Fundus photography provides a useful photographic record of the posterior pole and is useful in the Diabetic Screening Programme, but relies on 2-dimensional surrogate markers of macular thickening since it cannot quantify actual thickening.

7.2. Optical Coherence Tomography (OCT)

Optical Coherence Tomography is a non-invasive imaging technique which is non-contact and facilitates high resolution cross-sectional imaging of the anterior segment, vitreous, retina and optic nerve head. Rather than the sound waves of B-scan ultrasonography, OCT uses light interferometry (near-infrared) to interpret the interference patterns of wave superposition.

OCT is useful is very sensitive in detecting change in macula thickness and therefore useful in the diagnosis of diabetic macula oedema. It is also able to identify the loss of ganglion cells in the retina, which precedes vascular changes. Because OCT gives a quantitative measure of retinal thickness it is critical in monitoring retinal thickness in response to treatment e.g. Macula laser or Anti-VEGF agents.

Different tissue reflectivities are depicted by different colours; red denotes high reflectivity, green-yellow intermediate reflectivity and blue-black low reflectivity. In addition to numerical measures of retinal thickness a topographical map is created which is colour coded according to thickness.

7.3. Fundus Fluorescein Angiography (FFA)

Fundus Fluorescein Angiography involves the injection of an orange water-soluble dye; sodium fluorescein into the systemic circulation. It remains predominantly intravascular and is fluorescent; i.e. it emits light of a longer wavelength when stimulated by light of a lower wavelength. After intravenous injection, fundus photography is performed in a rapid sequence. Blue filtered light is absorbed by the molecule as it enters the retinal circulation and in turn emits yellow-green light.

The FFA image maps the retinal vasculature and the structural and functional integrity of the vessels.

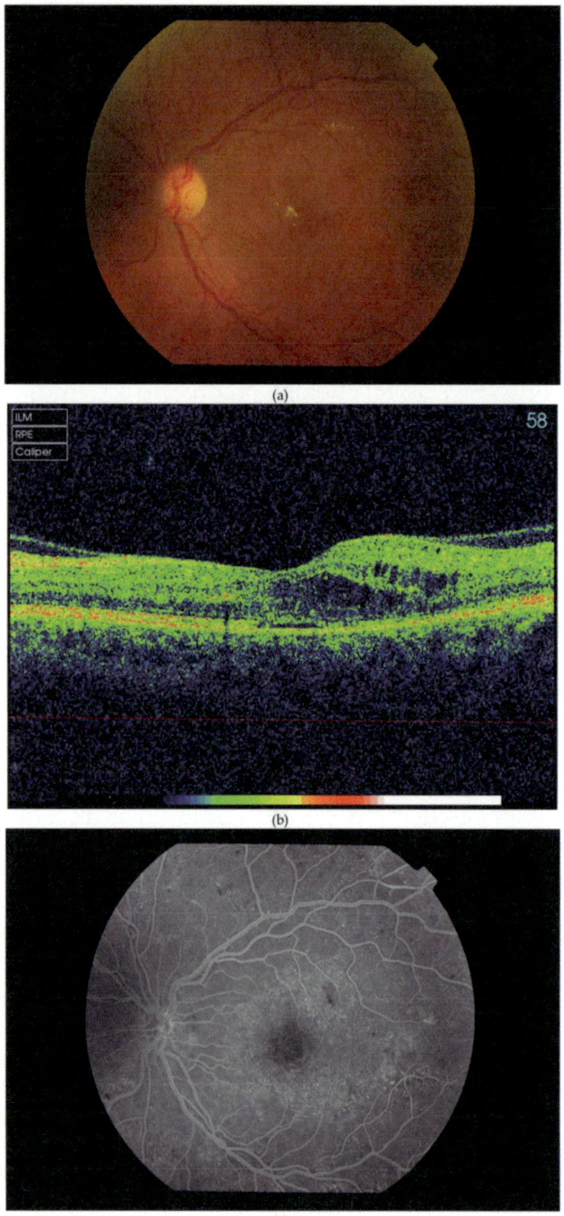

Figure 5. a. Fundus photograph of Diabetic Maculopathy (Circinate hard exudates, haemorrhages) **b.** Optical Coherence Tomography of Diabetic Maculopathy (Intraretinal cystic thickening) **c.** Fundus Fluorescein Angiogram of Diabetic Maculopathy

Normally 10-15 seconds elapse between dye injection and arrival of the dye in the short ciliary arteries. Choroidal circulation precedes retinal circulation by 1 second. Transit of dye through the retinal circulation takes approximately 15 to 20 seconds.

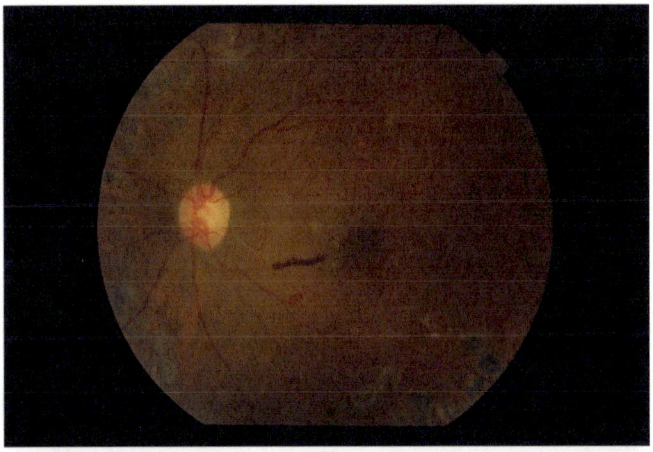

(a)

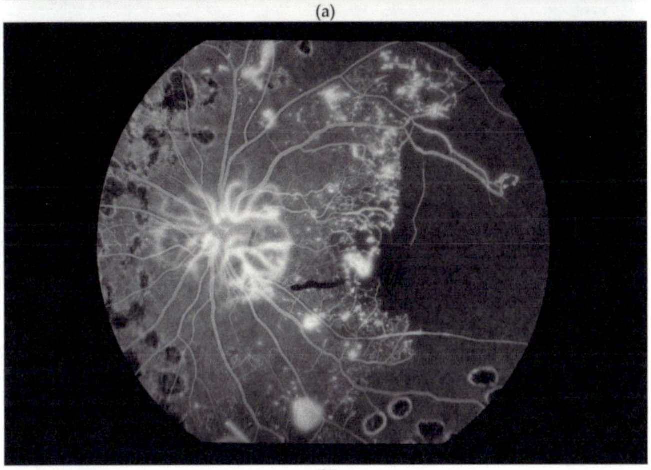

(b)

Figure 6. a. Fundus Photograph of New Vessel at Disc (NVD). Note PRP laser scars **b.** Fundus Fluorescein Angiogram of New Vessel at Disc (NVD) with evidence of peripheral ischaemia

The normal angiogram can be divided into five phases

1. **Choroidal phase**: The choroid is filled by the short ciliary arteries resulting in initial patching filling of lobules, quickly followed by a diffuse blush as dye leaks out of the choroidocapillaris.

2. **Arterial phase**: The central retinal artery fills about 1 second after choroidal filling

3. **Capillary phase**: The capillaries quickly fill following the arterial phase. The perifoveal capillary network is particularly prominent, as the underlying choroidal circulation is

masked by luteal pigment in the retina and melanin pigment in theretinal pigment epithelium (RPE). At the centre of this capillary ring is the foveal avascular zone 500um in diameter.

4. **Venous phase:** Early filling of the veins is from tributaries joining their margins, resulting in a tramline effect. Later the whole diameter of the veins is filled.

5. **Late (recirculation) phase:** 10 to 15 minutes later only a little dye remains within the blood circulation. Dye which has left the blood to ocular structures is particularly visible during this phase.

Below images are taken from clinical practice for common diabetic pathology (Images kindly provided by Mr Jignesh Patel, Essex County Hospital, Colchester).

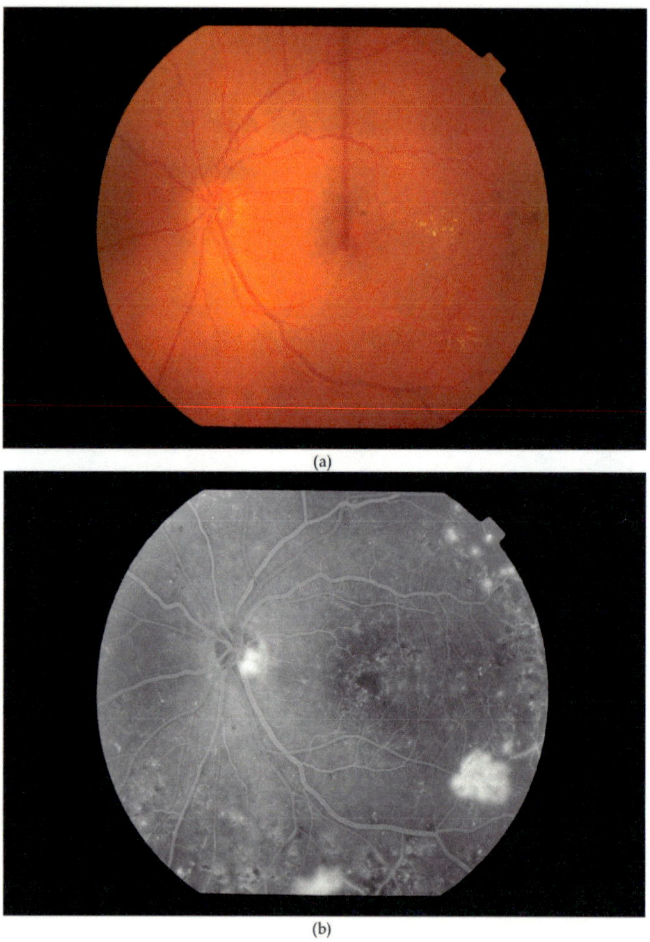

Figure 7. a. Fundus Photograph of New Vessels Elsewhere (NVE). **b.** Fundus Fluorescein Angiogram of New Vessels Elsewhere (NVE)

http://dx.doi.org/10.5772/58567

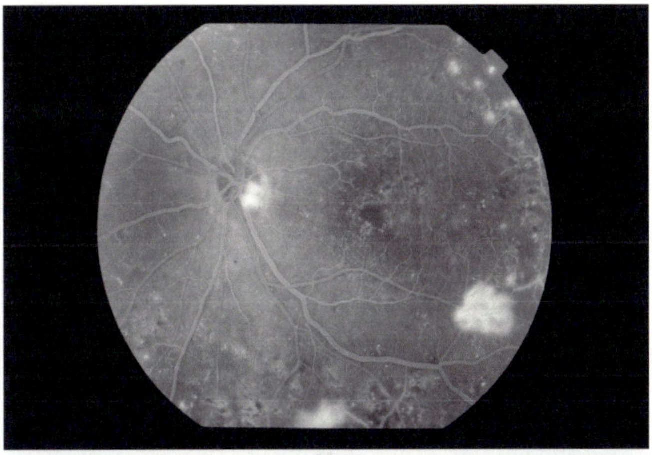

(a)

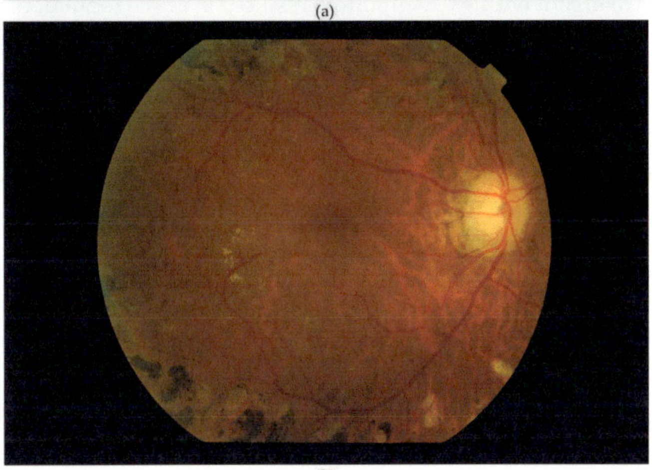

(b)

Figure 8. a. Fundus Photograph demonstrating PRP laser burns **b.** Fundus Fluorescein Angiogram of the above patient showing laser scars

8. Management of diabetic retinopathy

The management of diabetic retinopathy involves a multidisciplinary approach with involvement of the ophthalmologist, physician and dietician. The underlying diabetes and risk factors should be managed concurrently with the ocular complications of diabetes.

8.1. Medical management

8.1.1. Blood glucose control

Tight glycaemic control reduces the incidence and progression of diabetic retinopathy. The Diabetes Control and Complications Trial (DCCT)[131] showed that in type 1 diabetics effective glycaemic control reduced the incidence of diabetic retinopathy by 76% and progression of diabetic retinopathy by 54%. Similarly the United Kingdom Prospective Diabetes Study (UKPDS)[132] reported reduced microvascular complication, by 25% and the need for laser photocoagulation by 29% in type 2 diabetics.

8.1.2. Blood pressure control

The current British Hypertension Society guidelines define hypertension as systolic blood pressure ≥ 140mmHg and/ or diastolic blood pressure ≥ to 90mmHg [133]. In diabetes treatment targets should be systolic level <130 mm Hg and diastolic <80 mm Hg. Lower levels may be required for younger patients with Type 1 diabetes and microvascular complications. In this group of patients treatment with ACE inhibitors resulted in a 50% reduction in the progression of retinopathy and progression to proliferative diabetic retinopathy by 80% in the EURODIAB Controlled Trial of Lisinopril in Insulin Dependent Diabetes Mellitus (EUCLID) trial [134]. Type 2 diabetics in the UKPDS study showed that tight BP control prevented the progression of retinopathy. The beneficial effects of anti-hypertensive medication are immediate on commencing treatment, however the effects wear off as soon as control is lost. It is imperative therefore that blood pressure is measured at every clinical visit.

8.1.3. Lipid control

Observational studies suggest that dyslipideamia increases the risk of diabetic retinopathy particularly diabetic macula oedema[135, 136].

In the Fenofibrate Intervention and Event Lowering in Diabetes (FIELD) study [137], type 2 diabetic patients were treated with fenofibrate. Those patients treated with fenofibrate were less likely than controls to need laser treatment (5.2% vs 3.6%, $p<0.001$).

8.1.4. Cigarette smoking

In type 1 diabetes smoking increases the risk of diabetic retinopathy, nephropathy and neuropathy. Discontinuation of smoking is recommended for reducing the development of other complications of diabetes especially cardiovascular disease.

8.1.5. Management of macula oedema

Diabetic macula oedema is the most common cause for visual impairment particularly in type 2 diabetic patients. The management of clinically significant macula oedema depends on whether there is evidence of central macular thickening or vitreomacular traction. There are a wide variety of new treatments available currently some licensed and some unlicensed. A

http://dx.doi.org/10.5772/58567

summary guideline as to the use of these treatments and their indications are summarized in Table 3.

Is the centre involved?	Visual Acuity	Phakic/ Pseudophakic	OCT- central retinal thickness	Treatment options
No		Either		Focal/Grid laser
Yes	Normal or "/>78 letters	Either		Focal/Grid laser/Observation if lesions too close to fovea
Yes	78-24 letters or symptomatic	Phakic	≥ 250 microns	Intravitreal anti- VEGF with or without laser. If unresponsive consider flucinolone implant.
Yes	78-24 letters	Pseudophakic	≥250 microns	Intravitreal anti- VEGF or intravitreal triamcinolone preservative free with or without laser. If unresponsive consider flucinolone implant.
Yes	<24 letters	Pseudophakic	≥250 microns	Observation especially if long standing or unrepsonsive to laser. Consider macula ischaemia. Otherwise consider anti-VEGF or intravitreal steroid
Yes		Either	Vitreomacular traction	Consider vitrectomy with or without adjunctive intravitreal anti-VEGF or steroid treatment

Management of diabetic maculopathy. Adapted from Royal College of Ophthalmologists. Diabetic Retinopathy Guidelines December 2012 (19)

Table 3. Table for management of CMO in Royal College of Ophthalmology

8.1.6. Laser photocoagulation

There is a strong evidence from the Early treatment of Diabetic retinopathy Study that focal and grid laser photocoagulation for clinically significant macula oedema reduces the chance of moderate vision loss (3 ETDRS lines) by 50%, (from 24% for the control group to 12% for the treatment group) at 3 years [19].

It is important to perform a fundus fluorescein angiography prior to treatment to delineate the area of leakage and identify areas of macula ischaemia. In focal maculopathy, focal laser treatment burns are applied directly to microaneurysms and and microvascular lesions in the centre of rings of exudates located 500-3000 microns from the centre of the macula. The spot size is 50-100 microns and exposure time 0.1 second with sufficient power to obtain gentle whitening or darkening of the microaneurysm. In macula grid laser treatment burns are applied to areas of diffuse retinal thickening more than 500 microns from the centre of the macula and 500 microns from the temporal margin of the optic disc. The spot size is 100 microns and exposure time 0.1 sec giving a very light intensity burn. Treatment should be lighter if significant macular ischaemia is present.

In addition to argon laser treatment two other forms of laser treatment frequency-doubled Nd:YAG laser and micropulse laser are available for the treatment of macula oedema which reduce the degree of retinal collateral thermal damage. The 'Pattern Scan Laser' (Pascal) uses frequency –doubled micropulse YAG in single shot mode or in a predetermined array of upto 56 shots applied in less than a second. This not only reduces the potential destructive retinal effect but allows the operator to apply multiple spots simultaneously with a single foot pedal depression.

Using a micropulse mode laser, energy is delivered with a train of repetitive short pulses, micropulse power as low as 10%-25% of the visible threshold power has been demonstrated to be sufficient to show RPE-confined photothermal effect.

8.1.7. Intravitreal anti-vascular endothelial growth factors (anti-VEGF) agents

Multiple studies have demonstrated the benefit of the anti-VEGF agents including pegaptanib, ranibizumab and bevacizumab for the treatment of central involving diabetic macula oedema. A large multicenter trial DRCRnet(The Diabetic Retinopathy Research Network Laser-Ranibizumab-Triamcinolone Study)[138] showed that intravitreal injection of 0.5mg ranibizumab initially given monthly for 3 months with prompt or deferred (≥ 24 weeks) macular laser had significantly superior visual and OCT outcomes to laser alone in eyes with diabetic macula oedema involving the fovea.

The READ-2 (Ranibizumab for oedema of macula in diabetes) [139], RESOLVE (Safety and Efficacy of Ranibizumab in diabetic macula oedema) [140], RESTORE (Ranibizumab monotherapy or combined with laser versus laser monotherapy for diabetic macula oedema) [141], and BOLT (Bevacizumab or Laser therapy)[142] studies have all demonstrated that centre-involving macula oedema should be considered for treatment with a VEGF inhibitor alone or in conjunction with focal laser.

Ranibizumab is now licensed for use in the European Union for the treatment of centre involving diabetic macula oedema and NICE have approved its use in patients with a central retinal thickness of ≥ 400 microns on OCT.

The Da VINCI trial (14) evaluated the safety and efficacy of intravitreal aflibercept for diabetic macula oedema. Four treatment regimes were studied versus laser positive results have been reported at 1 year with aflibercept. The maximum letters gain with aflibercept has been 13.1 letters vs 1.3 letters in the laser treated group. It is expected that this treatment will be licensed for Diabetic retinopathy in 2014.

8.1.8. Intraocular steroid

DRCRnet[138] study found that in pseudophakic eyes intravitreal triamcinolone injection followed by prompt laser may be as effective as ranibizumab at improving vision and reducing retinal thickening. However, there was a significant risk of an elevation of intraocular pressure. No corresponding visual benefit above laser was shown for phakic eyes, which also has had a substantially increased rate of cataract surgery by two years.

Flucinolone acetonide is a non-biodegradable intravitreal insert (Illuvein) with sustained release flucinolone and is licensed for use in the UK for chronic diabetic macula oedema unresponsive to other treatment options but it is not yet approved by NICE. Studies have shown that Illuvein can provide treatment benefit for three years-the best corrected visual acuity showed an improvement of 15 or more letters in 28.7% of the low dose group vs 16.2% in controls[144]. The longer acting nature is advantageous in that the patient would not require monthly injections as is the case with the anti-VEGFs. However there is a greater chance of development of cataract and raised intraocular pressure.

8.1.9. Pars plana vitrectomy

A vitrectomy with or without ILM peel may be indicated when macular oedema with or without ischaemia is associated with tangential traction from a thickened and taut posterior hyaloid. Often the oedema is unresponsive to laser and optical coherence tomography scanning may show vitreomacular traction.

8.2. Management of Proliferative Diabetic Retinopathy (PDR)

8.2.1. Pan retinal photocoagulation

This is indicated in the presence of new vessels at the optic disc, iris, angle or elsewhere with or without associated vitreous haemorrhage. Where possible PRP laser treatment should be initiated on the same day and maximum within 2 weeks.

PRP laser treatment should be applied as far peripheral as possible using the laser contact lens up to the ora serrata as the main areas of retinal ischaemia exist in the far peripheral retina. The laser settings depend on the type of lens that is used. With a Goldmann lens the spot size is set at 200-500 microns but with a panfundsocopic-type lens it is set at 100-300 microns. The burn duration should be set between 0.05-0.1 seconds and the power should be sufficient to produce only a light intensity burn.

Initial treatment involves 1500-2000 burns in a scatter pattern extending from the posterior fundus to cover the peripheral retina in one or more sessions. PRP completed in one session carries a higher risk of complications and therefore treatment should be staggered. The number of burns recommended is dependent on the stage of PDR ; early PDR 1200-1800 burns, in moderate PDR 2000-2500 burns and in severe PDR 3000 burns.

The Diabetic Retinopathy Study[145] found that the risk of severe visual loss (5/200) was reduced by 50% in the "high-risk" group treated with PRP. Patients with early proliferative diabetic retinopathy were evaluated in the ETDRS study. In this group PRP decreased the risk of patients developing high risk characteristics by 50%.

The main side effects of PRP laser treatment is the progression or development of diabetic macula oedema, vitreous haemorrhage, tractional retinal detachment, loss of night vision and constricted peripheral visual fields. Vision loss within 6 weeks of treatment has also been reported in 10-23% of patients compared with 6 % of controls.

8.2.2. VEGF inhibitors

VEGF is implicated in the development of retinal neovascularization. Intravitreal anti-VEGF is likely to have an increasing role in the treatment of proliferative diabetic retinopathy, probably as an adjunct to laser. Anti-VEGFS can also be used in the setting of proliferative diabetic retinopathy and vitreous haemorrhage to facilitate sufficient clearing of the haemorrhage and allow administration of PRP.

8.2.3. Vitrectomy

Indications for pars plana vitrectomy are listed below:

1. Severe persistent vitreous haemorrhage

The surgical goal is to remove the vitreous opacity through a 3 port pars plana vitrectomy. The posterior hyaloid face should be removed as this provides a scaffold for fibrovascular proliferation. The Diabetic Retinopathy Vitrectomy Study (DRVS)[146] 2 year results demonstrate that in eyes with central vitreous haemorrhage that reduced acuity to 50/200 or less for at least a month, vitrectomy carried out before 6 months resulted in an increase in the number of eyes achieving 20/40 or better acuity compared with eyes in which vitrectomy was deferred to a year. Patients with vitreous haemorrhage should be monitored weekly to ensure early detection of retinal detachment.

Type 2 diabetics are less likely to have severe proliferative retinopathy, however there is a growing trend to operate within 3 months as opposed to deferred surgery in both type 1 and type 2 diabetics.

2. Tractional retinal detachment

Tractional retinal detachment recently involving or imminently threatening the fovea is another common indication for surgery. Progressive traction produces a retinal break usually posterior to the equator and near an area of fibrous proliferation. These detachments progress quickly and usually result in a worse prognosis. Fibrovascular tissue proliferation and contraction attached to multiple retinal foci results in macular distortion (heterotropia) or tractional detachment.

3. Combined tractional/rhegmatogenous retinal detachments

These should be treated urgently even if the macula is not involved as subretinal fluid is likely to spread quickly and involve the macula.

4. Premacular subhyaloid haemorrhage

If dense and persistent should be considered for vitrectomy because if untreated the internal limiting membrane or posterior hyaloid face may serve as a scaffold for subsequent fibrovascular proliferation and consequent tractional macular detachment or macular epiretinal membrane formation.

5. Ghost Cell Glaucoma

Vitrectomy has also been shown in case series to be of benefit when there is ghost cell glaucoma [147]. Raised intraocular pressure may be caused by partially lysed red cells (erthyroclasts) particularly in eyes with a disrupted anterior hyaloid face after previous vitrectomy for vitreous haemorrhage or in aphakic eyes with vitreous haemorrhage.

8.2.4. Management of Rubeosis Iridis

This occurs in eyes with severe retinal ischaemia or persistent retinal detachment. New vessels on the iris should be treated with PRP laser to induce regression of these vessels.

Current practice for new vessels on the iris and at the angle includes full PRP and an intravitreal anti-VEGF injection to prevent the progression to neovascular glaucoma. Treatment for neovascular glaucoma include cycloablative procedures, trabeculectomy with anti-proliferatives and implantation of a drainage tube.

Eyes that have become blind from neovascular glaucoma should be kept comfortable with topical steroids and atropine.

9. Conclusion

The global pandemic of diabetes means that retinopathy and associated visual difficulties are an ongoing problem. Further research is needed into the impact of diabetes on the neurovascular unit to facilitate greater understanding of pathophysiology. Improved screening and outcomes of treatment in developed countries mean vision can be maintained for longer. Ideally however, socioeconomic barriers need to be overcome to facilitate translational research to all parts of the world, including poorer areas. Most importantly, education on risk factors and tight glycaemic control are paramount to help prevent visual problems occurring.

Author details

Vikas Tah[1,3], Sonia Mall[2], James Myerscough[4], Kamran Saha[3], Elizabeth Emsley[5], Andrew Swampillai[6], Ganeshan Ramsamy[1], Daren Hanumunthadu[3] and Mandeep Bindra[1]

1 Stoke Mandeville Hospital, UK

2 Oxford Eye Hospital, UK

3 Moorfields Eye Hospital, UK

4 Colchester Hospital University Foundation Trust, UK

5 Imperial College London, UK

6 Barts and The London, School of Medicine and Dentistry, UK

References

[1] Diabetes in the UK 2010: Key statistics on diabetes. Diabetes UK. 2010.

[2] American Diabetes Association. Diabetes Basics. Available from: http://www.diabetes.org/diabetes-basics/diabetes-statistics/ (accessed 27th July 2013)

[3] Quality and Outcomes Framework (QOF) 2009:England: http://www.ic.nhs.uk/statistics-and-data-collections/supporting-information/audits-andperformance/the-quality-and-outcomes-framework/qof-2008/09/data-tables/prevalence-data-tablesScotland:http://www.isdscotland.org/isd/servlet/FileBuffer?namedFile=QOF_Scot_200809_Boards_all_prevalence.xls&pContentDisposition-Type=attachment

[4] Figures based on PBS diabetes prevalence model phase 3: key findings, Yorkshire and Humber Public Health Observatory, May 2008. The PBS model estimates that by 2025 there will be 3.6 million people with diabetes in England and that the diabetes prevalence will be 6.48 per cent of the population in England. The total UK figures have been calculated by including forecasts for the population of Wales, Scotland and Northern Ireland which gives a total of 4.2 million people with diabetes by 2025.

[5] Figures based on PBS diabetes prevalence model phase 3: key findings, Yorkshire and Humber Public Health Observatory, May 2008. The PBS model estimates that by 2025 there will be 3.6 million people with diabetes in England and that the diabetes prevalence will be 6.48 per cent of the population in England. The total UK figures have been calculated by including forecasts for the population of Wales, Scotland and Northern Ireland which gives a total of 4.2 million people with diabetes by 2025.

[6] Department of Health (2007). About diabetes www.dh.gov.uk/en/Healthcare/NationalServiceFrameworks/Diabetes/DH_074762

[7] Stratton IM, Adler AI, Neil HAW et al (2000). Association of glycaemia with macrovascular and microvascular complications of Type 2 diabetes (UKPDS 35): prospective observational study. BMJ 321;405–412

[8] Stratton IM, Adler AI, Neil HAW et al (2000). Association of glycaemia with macrovascular and microvascular complications of Type 2 diabetes (UKPDS 35): prospective observational study. BMJ 321;405–412

[9] Harris MI, Klein R, Welborn TA et al (1992). Onset of NIDDM occurs at least 4-7 years before clinical diagnosis. Diabetes Care 15 (7); 815–819

[10] Stitt A, Lois N, Medina R, et al. Advances in our understanding of diabetic retinopathy. Clinical Science. 2013;125;1-17

[11] Hamilton AMP, Ulbig MW, Polkinghorne P (1996). Management of diabetic retinopathy, London:BMJ Publishing

[12] Williams R, Airey M, Baxter H. Epidemiology of diabetic retinopathy and macular oedema: A systematic review. Eye. 2004;18;963-83.

[13] Malone J, Morrison A, Pavan P, et al. Diabetic Control and Complications Trial: Prevalence and significance of retinopathy in subjects with type 1 diabetes of less than 5 years duration screened for the diabetes control and complications trial. Diabetes Care. 200;124;522-6.

[14] Kohner E, Aldington S, Stratton I. United Kingdom Prospective Diabetes Study, 30: Diabetic retinopathy at diagnosis of non-insulin-dependent diabetes mellitus and associated risk factors. Arch Ophthalmol. 1998;116;297-303.

[15] Klein R, Klein B, Moss S. Visual impairment in diabetes. Ophthalmology. 1984;91;1-9.

[16] Moss S, Klein R, Klein B. Ten-year incidence of visual loss in a diabetic population. Ophthalmology. 1994; 101(6); 1061-70.

[17] Forlenza G, Stewart M. Diabetic retinopathy in children. Pediatr Endocrinol Rev. 2012-13; 10(2);217-26.

[18] Photocoagulation treatment of proliferative diabetic retinopathy: the second report of Diabetic Retinopathy Study findings. Ophthalmology. 1978;85;82-105.

[19] Photocoagulation for diabetic macular oedema: Early Treatment Diabetic Retinopathy Study report number 1. Arch Ophthalmology. 1985;103;1796-806.

[20] Antonetti D, Klein R, Gardner T. Diabetic retinopathy. NEJM. 2012;366;1227-39.

[21] Klein R, Lee K, Gangnon R, et al. The 25-year incidence of visual impairment in type 1 diabetes mellitus: the Wisconsin Epidemiologic Study of Diabetic Retinopathy. Ophthalmology. 2010;117;63-70.

[22] Hovind P, Tarnow L, Rossing K, et al. Decreasing incidence of severe diabetic microangiopathy in type 1 diabetes. Diabetes care. 2003;26;1258-64.

[23] Nordwall M, Bojestig M, Arnqvist H, et al. Declining incidence of severe retinopathy and persisting decrease of nephropathy in an unselected population of Type 1 diabetes – the Linkoping Diabetes Complications Study. Diabetologia. 2004;47;1266-72.

[24] Kempen J, O'Colmain B, Leske M, et al. The prevalence of diabetic retinopathy among adults in the United States. Arch Ophthalmol. 2004;122;552-63.

[25] Sloan F, Belsky D, Ruiz D, et al. Changes in incidence of diabetes mellitus-related eye disease among US elderly persons 1994-2005. Arch Ophthalmol. 2008;126;1548-53.

[26] Klein R, Klein B. Are individuals with diabetes seeing better? A long term epidemiological perspective. Diabetes. 2010;59;1853-60.

[27] Wild S, Roglic G, Green A, et al. Global prevalence of diabetes: estimates for the year 2000 and projections for 2030. Diabetes Care. 2004;27;1047-53.

[28] Al-Rubeaan K. Type 2 diabetes mellitus red zone. Int J Diabetes Mellitus. 2010;2(1); 1-2.

[29] Rema M, Premkumar S, Anitha B, et al. Prevalence of diabetic retinopathy in urban India: the Chennai Urban Rural Epidemiology Study (CURES) eye study. Invest Ophthalmol Vis Sci. 2005;46;2328-33.

[30] Targher G, Bertolini L, Chonchol M, et al. Non-alcoholic fatty liver disease is independently associated with an increased prevalence of chronic kidney disease and retinopathy in type 1 diabetic patients. Diabetologia. 2010;53;1341-8.

[31] Nguyen T, Alibrahim E, Islam F, et al. Inflammatory, haemostatic and other novel biomarkers for diabetic retinopathy: the multi-ethnic study of atherosclerosis. Diabetes Care. 2009;32;1704-9.

[32] West S, Groves D, Lipinski H, et al. The prevalence of retinopathy in men with Type 2 diabetes and obstructive sleep apnoea. Diabet Med. 2010;27;423-30

[33] Arnold E, Rivera J, Thebault S, et al. High levels of serum prolactin protect against diabetic retinopathy by increasing ocular vasoinhibins. Diabetes. 2010;59;3192-7.

[34] Zietz B, Buechler C, Kobuch K, et al. Serum levels of adiponectin are associated with diabetic retinopathy and with adiponectin gene mutations in Caucasian patients with diabetes mellitus type 2. Exp Clin Endocrinol Diabetes. 2008;116;532-6.

[35] Nathan D, Zinman B, Cleary P et al. Modern day clinical course of type 1 diabetes mellitus after 30 years' duration: the Diabetes Control and Complications Trial/ Epidemiology of Diabetes Interventions and Complications and Pittsburgh Epidemiology of Diabetes Complications experience (1983-2005). Arch Intern Med. 2009;169; 1307-16.

[36] Matthews D, Stratton S, Aldington S, et al. Risks of progression of retinopathy and vision loss related to tight blood pressure control in type 2 diabetes mellitus: UKPDS 69. Archives of Ophthalmology. 2004; 122 (11); 1631-1640.

[37] White N, Cleary P, Dahms W, et al. Beneficial effects of intensive therapy of diabetes during adolescence: outcomes after the conclusion of the Diabetes Control and Complications Trial (DCCT). The Journal of Paediatrics. 139 (6); 804-812.

[38] Tarr J, Kaul K, Chopra M, et al. Pathophysiology of Diabetic Retinopathy. ISRN Ophthalmology. 2013;343560.

[39] Singh R, Ramasamy K, Abraham C, et al. Diabetic retinopathy: an update. Indian Journal of Ophthalmology. 2008;56(3);179-188.

[40] Gabbay K. Hyperglycaemia, polyol metabolism and complications of diabetes mellitus. Annual Review of Medicine. 1975;26;521-536.

[41] Gabbay K. The sorbitol pathway and the complications of diabetes. The New England Journal of Medicine. 1973;288(16);831-836.

[42] Szwergold B, Kappler F, Brown T. Identification of fructose 3-phosphate in the lens of diabetic rats. Science. 1990;247(4941);451-454.

[43] Barnett P, Gonzalez R, Chylack L, et al. The effect of oxidation on sorbitol pathway kinetics. Diabetes. 1986;35(4);426-432.

[44] Hohman T, Nishimura C, Robison E. Aldose reductase and polyol cultured pericytes of human retinal capillaries. Experimental Eye Research. 1989;48 (1);55-60.

[45] Chakrabarti S, Sima A, Nakajima T. Aldose reductase in the BB rat: isolation, immunological identification and localisation in the retina and peripheral nerve. Diabetologia. 1987;30(4);244-251.

[46] Cheung A, Fung M, Lo A, et al. Aldose reductase deficiency prevents diabetes-induced blood-retinal barrier breakdown, apoptosis and glial reactivation in the retina of db/db mice. Diabetes. 2005;54(11);3119-3125.

[47] Dagher Z, Park Y, Asnaghi V, et al. Studies of rat and human retinas predict a role for the polyol pathway in human diabetic retinopathy. Diabetes. 2004;53(9); 2404-2411.

[48] Kuwabara T, Cogan D. Retinal vascular patterns. VI. Mural cells of the retinal capillaries. Arch Ophthalmol. 1963; 69; 492-502.

[49] Roy S, Lorenzi M. Early biosynthetic changes in the diabetic-like retinopathy of galactose-fed rats. Diabetologia. 1996;39(6);735-738.

[50] Glover J, Jacot J, Basso M, et al. Retinal capillary dilation: early diabetic-like retinopathy in the galactose-fed rate model. Journal of Ocular Pharmacology and Therapeutics. 2000;16(2);167-172.

[51] 51. Hattori T, Matsubara A, Taniguchi K, et al. Aldose reductase inhibitor fidarestat attenuates leukocyte-endothelial interactions in experimental diabetic rat retina in vivo. Current Eye Research. 2010;35(2);146-154.

[52] Chung S, Chung S. Genetic analysis of aldose reductase in diabetic complications. Current Medicinal Chemistry. 2003;10(15);1375-1387.

[53] Hammes H, Martin S, Federlin K, et al. Aminoguanidine treatment inhibits the development of experimental diabetic retinopathy. Proceedings of the National Academy of Sciences of the United States of America. 1991;88(24);11555-11558.

[54] Peppa M, Uribarri J, Vlassara H. Advanced glycation end products and diabetes complications: what is new and what works. Clinical Diabetes. 2003;21(4)186-187.

[55] Zong H, Ward M, Stitt A. AGEs, RAGE and diabetic retinopathy. Current Diabetes Reports. 2011;11(4);244-252.

[56] Stitt A, Gardiner T, Anderson N, et al. The AGE inhibitor pyridoxamine inhibits development of retinopathy in experimental diabetes. Diabetes. 2002;51(9);2826-2832.

[57] Hammes H, Weiss A, Fuhrer D, et al. Acceleration of experimental diabetic retinopathy in the rat by omega-3 fatty acids. Diabetologia. 1996; 39(3); 251-255.

[58] Williamson J, Kilo C. Extracellular matrix changes in diabetes mellitus. In: Scarpelli D, Migahi D, editors. Comparative pathobiology of major age-related diseases. New York: Liss, 1984. Pp 269-88.

[59] Koya D, King G. Protein kinase C activation and the development of diabetic complications. Diabetes. 1998;47(6);859-866.

[60] Wang Q. PKD at the crossroads of DAG and PKC signaling. Trends in pharmacological sciences. 2006;27(6);317-323.

[61] Aiello L, Bursell S, Clermont A, et al. Vascular endothelial growth factor-induced retinal permeability is mediated by protein kinase C in vivo and suppressed by an orally effective beta-isoform-selective inhibitor. Diabetes. 1997;46(9);1473-1480.

[62] Aiello L, Clermont A, Arora V, et al. Inhibition of PKC beta by oral administration of ruboxistaurin is well tolerated and ameliorates diabetes-induced retinal haemodynamic abnormalities in patients. Investigative Ophthalmology and Visual Science.

[63] Joy S, Scates S, Bearelly S, et al. Ruboxistaurin, a protein kinase C Beta inhibitor, as an emerging treatment for diabetes microvascular complications. Annals of Pharmacotherapy. 2005;39(10);1693-1699.

[64] Clarke M, Dodson P. PKC inhibition and diabetic microvascular complications. Best practice and research: clinical endocrinology and metabolism. 2007;21(4);573-586.

[65] Kohner E. The retinal blood flow in diabetes. Diabete et Metabolisme. 1993;19(5); 401-404.

[66] Wilkinson-Berka J. Angiotensin and diabetic retinopathy. International Journal of Biochemistry and Cell Biology. 2006;38(5-6);757-765.

[67] Funatsu H, Yamashita H, Nakanishi Y, et al. Angiotensin II and vascular endothelial growth factor in the vitreous fluid of patients with proliferative diabetic retinopathy. British Journal of Ophthalmology. 2002;86(3);311-315.

[68] Sjolie A, Klein R, Porta M, et al. Effect of candesartan on progression and regression of retinopathy in type 2 diabetes (DIRECT-Protect 2): a randomised placebo-controlled trial. The Lancet. 2008;372(9647);1385-1393.

[69] Chaturvedi N, Porta M, Klein R, et al. Effect of candesartan on prevention (DIRECT-Prevent 1) and progression (DIRECT-Protect 1) of retinopathy in type 1 diabetes: randomised, placebo-controlled trials. The Lancet. 2008;372(9647);1394-1402.

[70] Mauer M, Ziman B, Gardiner R, et al. Renal and retinal effects of enalapril and losartan in type 1 diabetes. The New England Journal of Medicine. 2009;361(1);40-51.

[71] Otani A, Takagi H, Suzuma K,et al. Angiotensin II potentiates vascular endothelial growth-factor induced angiogenic activity in retinal microcapillary endothelial cells. Circulation Research. 1998;82(5);619-628.

[72] Schroder S, Palinksi W, Schmid-Schonbein G. Activated monocytes and granulocytes, capillary nonperfusion and neovascularization in diabetic retinopathy. American Journal of Pathology.

[73] Lutty G, Cao J, McLeod D. Relationship of polymorphonuclear leukocytes to capillary dropout in the human diabetic choroid. American Journal of Pathology. 1997; 151(3);707-714.

[74] Chibber R, Ben-Mahmud M, Coppini D, et al. Activity of the glycosylating enzyme, core 2 GlcNAc (Beta1,6) transferase, is higher in polymorphonuclear leukocytes from diabetic patients compared with age-matched control subjects: relevance to capillary occlusion in diabetic retinopathy. Diabetes. 2000;49(10);1724-1730.

[75] Chibber R, Ben-Mahmud B, Mann G, et al. Protein kinase C Beta2-dependent phosphorylation of core 2 GlcNAc-T promotes leukocyte-endothelial cell adhesion: a mechanism underlying capillary occlusion in diabetic retinopathy. Diabetes. 2003;52(6);1519-1527.

[76] Kaul K, Hodgkinson A, Tarr J, et al. Is inflammation a common retinal-renal-nerve pathogenic link in diabetes? Current Diabetes Reviews. 2010;6(5);294-303.

[77] Hernandez C, Segura R, Fonollosa A, et al. Interleukin-8, monocyte chemoattractant protein01 and IL-10 in the vitreous fluid of patients with proliferative diabetic retinopathy. Diabetic Medicine. 2005;22(6);719-225.

[78] Doganay S, Evereklioglu C, Er H, et al. Comparison of serum NO, TNF-alpha, IL-1beta, SIL-2R, IL-6 and IL-8 levels with grades of retinopathy in patients with diabetes mellitus. Eye. 2002; 16(2);163-170.

[79] Takami S, Yamashita S, Kihara S, et al. High concentration of glucose induces the expression of intercellular adhesion molecule-1 in human umbilical vein endothelial cells. Atherosclerosis. 1998;138(1);35-41.

[80] Larson E, Springer T. Structure and function of leukocyte integrins. Immunological Reviews. 1990;114;181-217.

[81] Sfikakis P, Grigoropoulos V, Emfietzoglou I, et al. Infliximab for diabetic macular edema refractory to laser photocoagulation: a randomized, double-blind, placebo-controlled, crossover, 32-week study. Diabetes Care. 2010;33(7);1523-1528.

[82] Baynes J. Role of oxidative stress in development of complications in diabetes. Diabetes. 1991;40(4);405-412.

[83] Cui Y, Xu X, Bi H, et al. Expression modification of uncoupling proteins and MnSOD in retinal endothelial cells and pericytes induced by high glucose: the role of reactive oxygen species in diabetic retinopathy. Experimental Eye Research. 2006; 83(4); 807-816.

[84] Kowluru R, Chan P. Oxidative stress and diabetic retinopathy. Experimental Diabesity Research. 2007;43603.

[85] 85. El-Remessy A, Bartoli M, Platt D, et al. Oxidative stress inactivates VEGF survival signaling in retinal endothelial cells via PI 3-kinase tyrosine nitration. Journal of Cell Science. 2005;118(1);243-252.

[86] Hartnett M, Stratton R, Browne R, et al. Serum markers of oxidative stress and severity of diabetic retinopathy. Diabetes Care. 2000;23(2);234-240.

[87] Brownlee M. The pathobiology of diabetic complications: a unifying mechanism. Diabetes. 2005;54(6);1615-1625.

[88] Grant M, Mames R, Fitzgerald C, et al. The efficacy of octreotide in the therapy of severe nonproliferative and early proliferative diabetic retinopathy: a randomised controlled study. Diabetes Care. 2000;23(4);504-509.

[89] Zimmerman B, Molnar G. Prolonged follow up in diabetic retinopathy treated by sectioning the pituitary stalk. Mayo Clinic Proceedings. 1977;52(4);233-237.

[90] Comer G, Ciulla T. Pharmacotherapy for diabetic retinopathy. Current Opinion in Ophthalmology. 2004;15(6);508-518.

[91] Ishida S, Usui T, Yamashiro K, et al. VEGF164 is proinflammatory in the diabetic retina. Investigative Ophthalmology and Visual Science. 2003;44(5);2155-2162.

[92] Zhang X, Wen L, Chen Y et al. Vascular endothelial growth factor upregulates the expression of intracellular adhesion molecule-1 in retinal endothelial cells via reac-

tive oxygen species, but not nitric oxide. Chinese Medical Journal. 2009;122(3); 338-343.

[93] Adamis A, Shima D, Yeo K, et al. Synthesis and secretion of vascular permeability factor/vascular endothelial growth factor by human retinal pigment epithelial cells. Biochemical and Biophysical Research Communications. 1993;193(2);631-638.

[94] Wirostko B, Wong T,Simo R. Vascular endothelial growth factor and diabetic complications. Progress in Retinal and Eye Research. 2008;27(6);608-621.

[95] Gao B, Clermont A, Rook S, et al. Extracellular carbonic anhydrase mediates haemorrhagic retinal and cerebral vascular permeability through prekallikrein activation. 2007;13(2);181-188.

[96] Weiwei Z, Hu R. Targeting carbonic anhydrase to treat diabetic retinopathy: emerging evidences and encouraging results. Biochemical and Biophysical Research Communications. 2009;390(3);368-371.

[97] Park S, Park J, Park S, et al. Apoptotic death of photoreceptors in the streptozotocin-induced diabetic rat retina. Diabetologia. 2003;46(9);1260-1268.

[98] West SD, Groves DC, Lipinski HJ, et al. The prevalence of retinopathy in men with Type 2 diabetes and obstructive sleep apnoea. Diabet Med 2010;27:423-430

[99] Tong Z, Yang Z, Patel S, et al. Promoter polymorphism of the erythropoietin gene in severe diabetic eye and kidney complications. Proc Natl Acad Sci U S A 2008;105:6998-7003

[100] Klein R, Klein BE, Moss SE, Davis MD, DeMets DL. The Wisconsin epidemiologic study of diabetic retinopathy. II. Prevalence and risk of diabetic retinopathy when age at diagnosis is less than 30 years. Arch. Ophthalmol 1984; 102(4), 520–526

[101] Roy MS. Diabetic retinopathy in African Americans with type 1 diabetes: The New Jersey 725: I. Methodology, population, frequency of retinopathy, and visual impairment. Arch Ophthalmol 2000;118:97–104

[102] Klein R, Klein BE, Moss SE, Davis MD, DeMets DL. The Wisconsin epidemiologic study of diabetic retinopathy. III.

[103] Harvey JN. The influence of sex and puberty on the progression of diabetic nephropathy and retinopathy. *Diabetologia* 2011;54(8), 1943–1945

[104] Klein BE, Moss SE, Klein R. Is menarche associated with diabetic retinopathy? *Diabetes Care 1990*; 13(10), 1034–1038

[105] EDIC research group. Retinopathy and nephropathy in type 1 diabetes patients four years after trial of intensive therapy. N Engl J Med. 2000;342:381–9

[106] The Diabetes Control and Complications Trial Research Group. The effect of intensive treatment of diabetes on the development and progression of long-term complications in insulin-dependent diabetes mellitus. N Engl J Med. 1993;329:977–86

[107] Hirsch IB, Brownlee M. Beyond hemoglobin A1c — need for additional markers of risk for diabetic microvascular complications. JAMA 2010;303:2291-2

[108] Kern PA. Lipid disorders in diabetes mellitus. Mt Sinai J Med 1987-54: 245-252.

[109] Ferris III FL, Chew KY, Hoogwerf HJ. Serum lipids and diabetic retinopathy. Early treatment diabetic retinopathy study research group. Diabetes Care 1996; 19: 1291

[110] Chew EY. Diabetic retinopathy and lipid abnormalities. Curr Opin Ophtthal. 1997; 8: 59-62

[111] Hypertension in Diabetes Study (HDS). II. Increased risk of cardiovascular complications in hypertensive type 2 diabetic patients. J Hypertens 1993;11:319-25

[112] Patel V, Rassam S, Newsom R, Wiek J, Kohner EM. Retinal blood flow in diabetic retinopathy. BMJ. 1992;305678-683

[113] Rassam SMB, Patel V, Kohner EM. The effect of experimental hypertension on retinal autoregulation in humans: a mechanism for the progression of diabetic retinopathy. Exp Physiol. 1995;8053-68

[114] Hogeboom van Buggenum IM, Polak BC, Reichert-Thoen JW, et al. Angiotensin converting enzyme inhibiting therapy is associated with lower vitreous vascular endothelial growth factor concentrations in patients with proliferative diabetic retinopathy. Diabetologia. 2002;45:203-209

[115] UK Prospective Diabetes Study Group: Efficacy of atenolol and captopril in reducing risk of macrovascular and microvascular complications in Type 2 diabetes. UKPDS 39. Br Med J 1998;317:713-20.

[116] The Diabetes Control, Complications Trial Research Group. Effect of pregnancy on microvascular complications in the Diabetes Control and Complications Trial. Diabetes Care 2000; 23: 1084–1091

[117] Klein BE, Moss SE, Klein R. Effect of pregnancy on progression of diabetic retinopathy. Diabetes Care 1990; 13: 34–40

[118] Axer-Siegel R, Hod M, Fink-Cohen S, Kramer M, Weinberger D, Schindel B, Yassur Y. Diabetic retinopathy during pregnancy. Ophthalmology 1996; 103(11): 1815-1819

[119] Phelps RL, Sakol P, Metzger BE, Jampol LM, Frienkel N. Changes in diabetic retinopathy during pregnancy. Correlations with regulation of hyperglycaemia. Arch Ophthalmol 1986; 104: 1806–1810

[120] Diabetes in Early Pregnancy Study. Metabolic control and progression of retinopathy. Diabetes Care 1995; 18: 631–637

[121] Chew EY, Mills JL, Metzger BE, Remaley NA, Jovanovich-Peterson L, Knopp RH. Metabolic control and the progression of retinopathy. The diabetes in Early Pregnancy Study. Diabetes Care 1995; 18: 631–637

[122] Harding, S., R. Greenwood, S. Aldington, J. Gibson, D. Owens, R. Taylor, E. Kohner, P. Scanlon, and G. Leese. 2003. Grading and disease management in national screening for diabetic retinopathy in England and Wales. Diabet Med 20:965.

[123] Diabetic Retinopathy Study Research Group. Report 7. A modification of the Airlie House classification of diabetic retinopathy. Invest Ophthalmol Vis Sci 1981;21:210–26.

[124] Wilkinson, C. P., F. L. Ferris, 3rd, R. E. Klein, P. P. Lee, C. D. Agardh, M. Davis, D. Dills, A. Kampik, R. Pararajasegaram, and J. T. Verdaguer. 2003. Proposed international clinical diabetic retinopathy and diabetic macular edema disease severity scales. Ophthalmology 110:1677.

[125] Grading diabetic retinopathy from stereoscopic colour fundus photographs--an extension of the modified Airlie House classification. ETDRS report number 10. Early Treatment Diabetic Retinopathy Study Research Group. Ophthalmology 1991. 98:786.

[126] The Diabetes Control and Complications Trial Research Group (1997) Clustering of long-term complications in families with diabetes in the diabetes control and complications trial. The Diabetes Control and Complications Trial Research Group. Diabetes 46: 1829–1839.

[127] Chew, E., Klein, M., Ferris, F., III, Remaley, N., Murphy, R., Chantry, K. et al. (1996) Association of elevated serum lipid levels with retinal hard exudate in diabetic retinopathy. early treatment diabetic retinopathy study (ETDRS) report 22. Arch Ophthalmol 114: 1079–1084

[128] Keech, A., Mitchell, P., Summanen, P., O'Day, J., Davis, T., Moffitt, M. et al. (2007) Effect of fenofibrate on the need for laser treatment for diabetic retinopathy (FIELD study): a randomised controlled trial. Lancet 370: 1687–1697

[129] Gaede, P., Lund-Andersen, H., Parving, H. and Pedersen, O. (2008) Effect of a multifactorial intervention on mortality in type 2 diabetes. N Engl J Med 358: 580–591.

[130] Images courtesy of Mr Jignesh Patel, Essex County Hospital, Colchester.

[131] Diabetes Control and Complications Trial/Epidemiology of Diabetes Interventions and Complications Research Group. Retinopathy and nephropathy in patients with type 1 diabetes mellitus four years after a trial of intensive therapy. N Eng J Med. 2000;342:381-9

[132] UK Prospective Diabetes Study (UKPDS) Group. Intensive blood-glucose control with sulphonylureas or insulin compared with conventional treatment and risk of complications in patients with type 2 diabetes (UKPDS 33). Lancet.1998;352:837-53.

[133] Guidelines from the British Hypertensive Society. BMJ. 2004;328:593-4.

[134] Chaturvedi N, Sjolie AK, Stephenson JM et al; EUCLID Study Group. Effect of lisinopril on progression of retinopathy in normotensive people with type 1 diabetes. Lancet. 1998;351 (9095):28-31

[135] Van Leiden HA, Dekker HA, Moll AC, et al. Blood pressure, lipids, and obesity are associated with retinopathy: the Hoorn study. Diabetes Care. 2002;25:1320-5.

[136] Klein R, Sharrett AR, Klein BE, et al. The association of atherosclerosis, vascular risk factors, and retinopathy in adults with diabetes: the atherosclerosis risk in communities study. Ophthalmology.2002;109:1225-34

[137] Keech A, Simes RJ, Barter P, et al. Effects of long term fenofibrate therapy on cardiovascular events in 9795 people with type 2 diabetes mellitus (the FIELD study): randomized controlled trial. Lancet. 2005; 366:1849-61

[138] Diabetic Retinopathy Clinical Research Network. A randomized trial comparing intravitreal triamcinolone acetonide and focal/grid photocoagulation for diabetic macular oedema. Ophthalmology. 2008;115:1447-59.

[139] Nguyen QD, Shah SM, Khwaja AA, et al. Two year outcomes of ranibizumab for oedema of the macula in diabetes (READ-2) study. Ophthalmology. 2010;117:2146-51.

[140] Massin P, Bandello F, Garweg JG, et al. Safety and efficacy of ranibizumab in diabetic macula oedema (RESOLVE Study): a 12 month, randomized, controlled, double-masked multicenter phase II study. Diabetes Care. 2010;33:2399-405.

[141] Mitchell P, Bandello F, Schmidt-Erfurth U et al. The RESTORE study: ranibizumab monotherapy or combined with laser versus laser monotherapy for diabetic macular edema. Ophthalmology. 2011;118:615-25.

[142] Michaelides M, Kaines A, Hamilton RD, Fraser-Bell S, et al. A prospective randomized trial of intravitreal bevacizumab or laser therapy in the management of diabetic macula edema (BOLT study) 12-month data: report 2. Ophthalmology. 2010;117:1078-86.

[143] Do DV, Nguyen QD, Boyer D, Schmidt-Erfurth U, Brown DM, Vitti R, Berliner AJ, Gao B, Zeitz O, Ruckert R, Schmelter T, Sandbrink R, Heier JS; DAVINCI Study Group. One-Year Outcomes of the DA VINCI Study Group of VEGF Trap-Eye in Eyes with Diabetic Macula Edema. Ophthalmology 2012. April 24 epub ahead of print.

[144] Campochiaro PA, Brown DM, Pearson A, et al. FAME Study Group Susutained Delivery Fluocinolone Acetonide Vitreous Inserts Provide Benefit for at Least 3 years in Patients with Diabetic Macula Edema, Ophthalmology 2012 Jun 21 (epub ahead of print)

[145] The Diabetic Retinopathy Research Group. Indications for photocoagulation treatment of diabetic retinopathy: Diabetic Retinopathy Study No.14 Int Ophthal Clin 1987;27:239-252.

[146] Diabetic Retinopathy Vitrectomy Study Research Group. Early Vitrectomy for severe vitreous haemorrhage in diabetic retinopathy. Two year results of a randomized trial. DRVS report No 2. Archives of Ophthalmology. 1985103:1644

[147] Brucker AJ, Michels RG, Green WR. Pars plana vitrectomy in the management of blood-induced glaucoma with vitreous haemorrhage. Ann Ophthalmol. 1978;10:1427-37

[148] Royal College of Ophthalmologists. Diabetic Retinopathy Guidelines December 2012 http://www.rcophth.ac.uk/page.asp?section=451&sectionTitle=Clinical+Guidelines

Chapter 12

Retinopathy of Prematurity

Vikas Tah, Walid Sharif, Imran Yusuf,
Marcus Posner, Louise Ramskold, Farihah Tariq,
Dev Mukhey and Zuhair Sharif

Additional information is available at the end of the chapter

http://dx.doi.org/10.5772/58585

1. Introduction

Retinopathy of prematurity (ROP) is a disease of premature infants and a leading worldwide cause of child blindness [1]. An epidemic of ROP occurred between 1941 and 1953, when an estimated 12,000 infants in affluent countries suffered visual loss from ROP. The first case of ROP, known then as retrolental fibroplasia (RLF), was identified in 1942 [2] with likely total retinal detachment [1]. However, RLF is currently applied to describe later stage cicatricial (severe retinal scarring) disease with retinal detachment and formation of retrolental fibroplastic membrane [2]. It is likely that the severe, advanced disease stage of RLF would have been more readily identifiable in 1942, in the absence of technological advancements that have added precision and clarity to ophthalmic diagnosis· Cases of ROP were reported throughout the developed world over the following decade. Intensive oxygen therapy as the key determinant of ROP was not known until the early 1950s when the suggestion of oxygen toxicity in ROP was made.

ROP is a biphasic condition comprising an initial phase of vessel growth retardation followed by a second phase of vessel proliferation characterised by abnormal retinal vasculature development [2]. Broadly it is thought to be caused by disorganised blood vessel growth that may result in scarring of the retina and retinal detachment.

The precise aetiology of ROP remains unclear [1]. Onset is associated with immaturity. The three factors that have shown a consistently significant association with retinopathy of prematurity are low birth weight, low gestational age and prolonged supplementary oxygen exposure after delivery [3].

The pathological process includes several risk factors that impact on each other. These include premature birth, multiple gestation, prenatal complications, genetic factors, immature pulmonary function, intraventricular haemorrhage, sepis, anaemia, patent ductus arteriosus, growth factors, prostaglandin synthetase inhibitors, vitamin E deficiency, lactic acidosis [1,23], vasoactive substances development of retinal vessels, maturation of retinal cells with subsequent growth of metabolic demands and the state of the antioxidant system. The exact role of these remains undetermined [3].

ROP is one of the few preventable causes of childhood visual impairment [5]. Early identification and treatment prevent blindness and offer the affected child better visual development [6]. Thus, new, innovative evidence-based approaches to the investigation, screening, prevention and treatment of ROP are still required [1].

2. Epidemiology

Increases in the incidence and prevalence of ROP became recognised as specialists began to theorise that oxygen toxicity might be a contributory factor in pathology among premature babies [1,23] this leading to a perceived 'epidemic' of ROP. Two epidemics of ROP have occurred in the last 70 years in the developed world. The first occurred in 1941-53. This was thought to be related to hyperoxia from incubators[7].

Subsequent research has confirmed that high blood level oxygen causes obliteration of retinal vessels [24-26]. Based on this, recommendations to lower oxygen supply were undertaken and the levels of ROP declined dramatically. Consequently, incubator oxygen concentrations, frequency of administration and duration of oxygen therapy became reduced in many neonatal units throughout the developed world [31].

In the 1970-80s, despite closer oxygen supply monitoring, a second epidemic was recorded, with more extreme low birth weight infants surviving in developed countries [8].

Currently it is thought a possible third epidemic is occurring in industrial medium-developed countries, with several explanations attributable [9-10]. Firstly, there is a higher ratio of premature born to newborns owing to progress in neonatology. The survival of extremely low birth weight infants has increased from 5% to 65% in the last 40 years. Whilst compulsory screening is available in some countries like those of the UK, this is no longer the case in other western countries owing to lack of resources and adequate training. This means that there are a higher number of advanced ROP cases in immature and mature children.

The incidence of the disease was first reviewed in the Cryotherapy for Retinopathy of Prematurity Cooperative Group (CRYO-ROP) study, based on a multicentre trial in the United States. 9751 infants from 23 centres were recruited, and 65.8% of those premature babies with a birthweight less than 1251 grams were noted to have some form of ROP. 18% developed stage 3 disease and 6% were treated [11].

The Early Treatment of ROP study (ET-ROP) study [12] looked at 317 newborns from 26 different centres with birth weight less than 1251 grams. The incidence was very similar at

http://dx.doi.org/10.5772/58585

68%, and was noted to decrease sharply with increasing birth weight and gestational age. Other trials have been undertaken, but have used different criteria (notable birth weight) to these trials listed, meaning a direct comparison is futile. These trials are listed in the table 1 below [13-19].

author	age (weeks of gestation)	weight (grams)	incidence %
Al Amro2003	<37	<2000	3.4
Hussan1999		<1500	21.3
Fortes, 2007	<36	<1000	48.9
		<1500	16.2
Good 2005		<1251	68
Shah 2005		<1500	29.2
Martin Begué 2003		<1501	29.2
Rehka, 1996	<34	<1500	46%

Table 1. Trials undertaken for incidence retinopathy of prematurity looking at the gestational age and weight

3. Classification

The International Classification of Retinopathy of Prematurity (ICROP) was devised by expert ophthalmologists in the field from 11 countries to help more suitably describe the observations of the disease. This was designed to help clarify what stage of disease was being treated, and to help audit results of treatment. The original ICROP was devised in 1984 [20], with subsequent minor revision in 1987 [21] and with enhanced imaging techniques further modification in 2005 [22].

The classification system has always been based on 3 basic paradigms; *location*, *extent* and *staging* of the disease.

3.1. Location

The original classification in 1984 describes 3 concentric zones of retinal involvement to define the antero-posterior location of the retinopathy. Each zone is centered on the optic disc rather than the macula, since normal retinal growth proceeds forward from the optic disc towards the ora serrata in a systematic fashion (although it is observed that the extent of retinal vascularisation and ROP may be observed closer to the optic disc nasally than temporally).

Zone I (posterior pole or inner zone consists of a circle), the radius of which extends from the centre of the optic disc to twice the distance from the centre of the optic disc to the centre of the macula. The radius of this zone subtends an angle of 30 degrees. The limits of the zone are consequently defined as twice the disc-foveal distance in all directions from the optic disc; an arc of 60 degrees.

Zone II is the area extending from the edge of zone I peripherally to a point tangential to the nasal ora serrata (at the 3 o clock position in the right eye and the 9 o clock position in the left eye. The temporal edge of zone II cannot be more accurately defined as the anatomic landmarks needed to identify the equator in premature infants are obscured.

Zone III is the residual crescent of retina anterior to zone II. By convention zones I and II are considered mutually exclusive. Retinopathy of prematurity should be considered in zone II until it can be confirmed that the nasal most 2 clock hours are vascularised to the ora serrata.

For the clinician as a practical approach, using a 25D or 28 diopter (D) condensing lens can help to determine the approximate temporal extent of zone I. The limit of zone I is at the temporal field of view by placing the nasal edge of the optic disc at one edge of the field of view.

3.2. Extent

The extent of the disease specified as the hours of the clock or as 30 degree sectors. As the observer looks at each eye, the 3o'clock position is to the right and nasal in the right eye and temporal in the left eye. The 9 o'clock position is to the left and temporal in the right eye and nasal in the right eye.

3.3. Staging of the disease

This refers to the amount of abnormal vascular response observed. Prior to ROP development in the premature infant, vascularisation of the retina is incomplete. There are now 5 stages used to describe the abnormal vascular response at the junction of the vascularised and avascular retina. Initially the ICROP had 4 stages, but this has been modified to 5 stages for the eye as a whole, based on the most severe manifestation present since more than one ROP stage may be present in the same eye. For the purpose of recording the examination, each stage is defined and the extent of clock hours is recorded.

Stage 1: Demarcation line

This is a thin but destructive structure separating the avascular anteriorly and vascular retina posteriorly. There is abnormal arcading or branching of vessels leading up to the demarcation line that is relatively flat, white, and lies within the plane of the retina. Vascular changes can be apparent prior to the development of the demarcation line, such as dilatation rather than tapering of the peripheral retinal vessels, but these changes are subtle and different to quantify, inadequate for diagnosing early ROP.

Stage 2: Ridge

This is the hallmark of stage 2 ROP. It arises in the region of the demarcation line that has now grown, has height and width, and extends above the plane of the retina. The ridge may change colour from white to pink and vessels may leave the plane of the retina to enter it. Small isolated tufts of new vessels lying on the surface of the retina may be seen posterior to this ridge structure. They do not make part of the growth necessary for stage 3. These small isolated tufts are commonly referred to as 'popcorn'.

http://dx.doi.org/10.5772/58585

Stage 3: Extraretinal fibrovascular proliferation

In stage 3 extraretinal fibrovascular retinal proliferation tissue develops from the ridge and extends into the vitreous. This extraretinal proliferating tissue is has 3 characteristics; first it is continuous with the posterior aspect of the ridge, causing a ragged appearance as the proliferation becomes more extensive. Second, it is immediately posterior to the ridge but not always appearing to be connected with it. Third it projects theinto the vitreous perpendicular to the retinal plane. The severity of a stage 3 disease can be subdivided into mild, moderate or severe depending on the extent of the extraretinal fibrovascular tissue infiltrating the vitreous.

Stage 4: Partial Retinal Detachment

Stage 4 is divided into extrafoveal (stage 4A) and foveal (stage 4B) partial retinal detachments. This may be caused by exudative effusion of fluid, traction or both. These are generally concave and most tend to be circumferentially orientated. The extent of retinal detachment depends on the number of clock hours of fibrovascular traction and their degree of contraction. Typically, retinal detachments begin at the point of fibrovacular attachment to the vascularised retina. In progressive cases, the fibrous tissue continues to contract and the tractional retinal detachment increases in height, extending both anteriorly and posteriorly. Radial detachments and more complex configurations of retinal detachments are less common.

Stage 5: Total Retinal Detachment

Typically retinal detachments are tractional, but may occasionally be exudative. They are usually funnel shaped. Funnel configuration permits a subdivision of this stage. The funnel is divided into anterior and posterior parts. When open, both anteriorly and posteriorly the detachment often has a concave configuration to the optic disc. A second frequent configuration is one where the funnel is narrow in both the anterior and posterior aspects, and the detached retina is located just behind the lens. A third less common type is where the funnel is open anteriorly but narrowed posteriorly. Least common is a funnel that is narrow anteriorly and open posteriorly.

'Threshold' and 'Pre-threshold' categories of ROP severity were also developed as a result of the CRY-ROP findings [35,36]. 'Threshold ROP', as a subdivision of ROP Stage 3, was associated with an approximate 50% risk of blindness if untreated. These definitions have prognostic importance, as 47% of threshold ROP categorisations culminated in retinal detachment [37].

3.4. "Plus" and "Pre-Plus" disease

The terms 'Pre-plus and Plus disease' denote increased venous dilation and arteriolar tortuosity of the posterior retinal vessels, which often lead to increased ROP severity [35-38]. These may be accompanied by vitreous haze, iris vascular engorgement and inadequate dilation of pupils

3.4.1. "Plus" disease

Progressive vascular incompetence occurring along with the change at the edge of the abnormally developing retinal vasculature may have additional signs indicating the severity of active ROP that can occur. These include venous dilatation and arteriolar tortuosity of the posterior retinal vessels and may later increase in severity to include iris vascular engorgement, poor papillary dilatation and vitreous haze. This group of supplementary signs was referred to as 'plus' disease in the ICROP original classification. Subsequent refinement from clinical trials has resulted in diagnosis of plus disease that can be made if sufficient vascular dilatation and tortuosity are present in at least 2 quadrants of the eye. A+sign is added to the ROP stage number where there is plus disease present. For example stage 3 ROP combined with posterior vascular dilatation is written as 'stage 3+ROP'. Progression may be rapid where ROP is located in zone I or posterior zone II with plus disease present.

In the CRY-ROP study, significant retinal venous dilation and arteriolar tortuosity in all 4 vascular arcade quadrants served as diagnostic criteria for 'Plus disease'[35-38]. However. currently, changes in at least 2 quadrants are required for the diagnosis of 'plus disease' [51] representing a terminological modification with implications for screening and treatment decisions.

3.4.2. "Pre-Plus" disease

This has been a more recent addition to classification. Abnormal dilatation and tortuosity of posterior pole vessels that demonstrate more than normal arterial and venous tortuosity, but are insufficient for the diagnosis of plus disease is termed 'preplus' disease [8,51]. These changes may over time progress to plus disease as vessels dilate and become more tortuous.

Despite absence of simultaneous manifestation, these symptoms are likely indicators of ROP progression and the 'Pre-plus disease' category may be a useful indicator of sudden increases in ROP activity.

3.5. Aggressive Posterior ROP (AP-ROP)

This is an uncommon rapidly progressing severe form of ROP, termed AP-ROP. Not included in the original ICROP classification, it has recently been defined by ICROP revisited as aggressive posterior ROP and is noted for its rapid progression to stage 5 ROP if not treated [34]. It has been referred to as type II ROP and Rush disease. The characteristic features of this type of ROP are the posterior location, prominence of plus disease and ill defined nature of the retinopathy.

AP-ROP is observed most commonly in zone I, but can occur in posterior zone II. Early in the development of AP-ROP, the posterior pole vessels show increased vascular dilatation and tortuosity in all 4 quadrants that is out of proportion to the degree of retinopathy peripherally. These changes progess rapidly. Shunting does not occur soley at the junction of the avascular and vascular retina but occurs from vessel to vessel within the retina. This can make AP-ROP difficult to distinguish arterioles and venules owing to significant dilatation of both vessel types. There may also be haemorrhages at the junction of the vascular and avascular retina.

AP-ROP is deceptively featureless and does not usually progress through the classic stages 1-3 [40,9], appearing as a flat network of neovascularisation at the junction between the vascularisaed and nonvascularised retina. It typically extends circumferentially and is often accompanied by a circuimferential vessel. The use of a 20-D condensing lens instead of a 25-D lens in indirect ophthalmoscopy may help distinguish the featureless neovascularisation.

On the basis of this evidence it was concluded that when the characteristics of rapidly progressing disease are observed, or when aggressive posterior ROP is present, the baby should be monitored closely and screening should be undertaken at least weekly [39].

4. Investigations of retinopathy of prematurity: A chronological overview of change, development and future directions

Effective investigation of ROP is dependent on reliable classification. However, as we have mentioned, ROP classification is not a static entity and is subject to evolutionary change resulting from research findings, modifications to practice, technological advances and terminological refinements. Accordingly, standard screening should be performed more frequently, perhaps on a weekly basis [8,39].

Determining and maintaining optimal oxygen saturation levels in preterm infants has remained something of a challenge because data regarding early mortality and long-term neuro-developmental outcomes resulting from effects of different oxygen saturation ranges are lacking [23,33]. The CRYO-ROP study found that the rate of progression of ROP (mean ± standard error) was faster in eyes with an unfavourable outcome (8.2 ± 1.2 days between first observation of ROP to pre-threshold) compared with those with a favourable outcome (12.3 ± 1.2 days), suggesting that in some situations even twice-weekly examinations are not frequent enough [36,37].

The findings from a meta-analysis of infants with postmenstrual ages of < or=32 week published in 2010 indicated an association between early low levels of oxygen saturation and reduced risk for severe ROP among and late high oxygen saturation the effect of oxygen on the development and progression of ROP is not straight forward. Ongoing investigation is necessary to understand the relationships among oxygen concentration, variability in oxygen concentration, and timing of oxygen delivery. Low oxygen saturation appears to decrease the risk of severe ROP in preterm newborns when administered during the first few weeks after birth. High oxygen saturation seems to reduce the risk at later postmenstrual ages [32]. However, individual clinical studies have not been conclusive.

A recent study by the Benefits of Oxygen Saturation Targeting (BOOST) Collaborative Group, evaluated the effects of targeting an oxygen saturation of 85 to 89%, as compared with a range of 91 to 95%, on disability-free survival at 2 years in 2,448 infants born before 28 weeks' gestation in three international randomized, controlled trials [8]. Halfway through the trials, the oximeter-calibration algorithm was revised. Recruitment was stopped early when an interim analysis showed an increased rate of death at 36 weeks in the group with a lower oxygen saturation [8]. The rate of death was significantly higher in the lower-target group than in the higher-target group (23.1% vs. 15.9%; relative risk in the lower-target group, 1.45; 95%

confidence interval (CI), 1.15 to 1.84; P=0.002) [8]. Oxygen saturation levels below 90% in extremely preterm infants was associated with an increased risk of death [8]. Although the lower targeted saturation group had a significantly reduced incidence of ROP, the infants also had a significant increase in the rate of developing necrotizing enterocolitis [8].

5. Evidence to inform investigations

The first evidence of successful treatment came from the multi-centre CRYO-ROP study reported in 1988 [35]. The CRYO-ROP study reported findings after 3 months, then at 1, 3.5, 5.5, 10 and 15 years. Unfavourable outcomes (defined by ROP in the posterior retina and retinal detachment) were less in the treated group than in the untreated group at every time point [35-38].

The percentage of eyes with unfavourable outcomes increased over time in both groups from 25.1% at one year to 30.0% at 15 years for treated eyes, compared with 44.7% vs 51.9% for untreated eyes [35-38]. CRYO-OP study data, describing the natural history of ROP, are probably the most comprehensive, with current understanding of ROP based largely on the findings of this study. Indeed, it is apparent that the CRYO-ROP study findings have influenced redefinition of ROP classification and as noted, this has implications for investigations, screening and treatment as well as identification of risk factors, clinical course of ROP and outcomes.

However, while outcomes of treatment in the CRYO-ROP study were superior to the untreated controls, they are perceived less than ideal [42]. Outcomes among treated patients were frequently poor, with 21.8% progression to macular distortion or retinal detachment and long-term loss of vision. Cryotherapy did not benefit neonates with stage 4 ROP with partial retinal detachment [42]. Over the longer term, even eyes with favorable anatomic outcomes still had poor vision. ROP located in Zone 1, young gestational age, multiple births, birth outside hospital, low birth weight, white race, plus disease (based on 4 affected eye quadrants), stage 3, >6 clock hour stage 3, and iris vessel dilatation were associated with an unfavorable anatomic outcome [42].

Subsequent to the theory that supplemental oxygen therapy was an important factor in the causal chain of ROP, randomized controlled trial findings indicated that restricting oxygen might result in a lower incidence of severe ROP [43,44], but at a cost of increased mortality [41]. Indeed, current evidence suggests that it is unadvisable to target oxygen-saturation concentrations below 90% in infants born prior to 28 weeks' gestation [46]. However, after seven decades of investigation, knowledge regarding optimal concentrations of oxygen required to balance risk in favor of avoiding adverse effects of both hyperoxia and hypoxia remains inadequate with no 'safe' level of supplementation identified [1] the clinically appropriate range for oxygen saturation in preterm infants remains unknown. In the absence of complete consensus over the oxygen issue, including a definition of optimal oxygen concentration' [39], it is apparent that new approaches to the investigation and prevention of ROP are required [45-48].

http://dx.doi.org/10.5772/58585

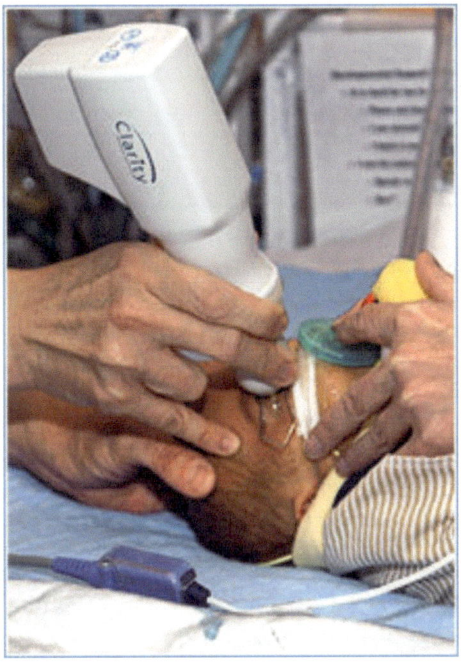

Figure 1. Courtesy of Hoag Levins. Clarity Medical Solutions. [72]

6. Current screening for ROP

An audit of UK ophthalmologists in 1999 established that although many of the 1995 Guideline recommendations were followed, practice varied in relation to when screening should stop and at what stage ROP should be treated [49]. Concerns were also expressed that the recommendations in the 1995 Guideline resulted in too many babies being screened, causing a heavy workload for ophthalmologists and distress to babies receiving unnecessary retinal examinations [33-35].

Key recommendations for good practice in the UK were published in 2008 by the Royal College of Paediatrics and Child Health and Royal College of Ophthalmologists [49].These were based largely on ICROP revisited publication [34], findings from the CRY-OP study [38] and the Early Treatment for Retinopathy of Prematurity study [53].

Babies of less than 32 weeks gestational age (up to 31 weeks and 6 days) or less than 1501g birth weight should be screened for ROP [49]. One criterion to be met for inclusion [49]: Babies of less than 31 weeks gestational age (up to 30 weeks and 6 days) or less than 1251g birth weight must be screened for ROP. Ophthalmological notes should be made after each ROP examination, detailing zone, stage, and extent in terms of clock hours of any ROP and the presence of any pre-plus or plus disease [49]. These notes should include a recommendation for the timing of the next examination (if any) and be kept with the baby's medical record [32]. Comfort care techniques (e.g. administering sucrose solution, nesting, swaddling and use of a pacifier) during the screening examination may be considered [49]. Babies with aggressive ROP (as defined in ICROP revisited) should be treated as soon as possible and within 48 hours. ROP requiring treatment but which is not aggressive posterior ROP should normally be treated within 48-72 hours [49].

The current screening guideline of ROP in the United States calls for dilated fundus examination by indirect ophthalmoscopy for all premature infants below 30 week gestational age or less than 1500g birth weight with the first examination performed by 31 week postmenstrual age or by 4 weeks chronologic age, with additional examinations performed repeatedly thereafter to detect late stage ROP requiring treatment [54]. Additional screening for older or larger babies is recommended at the discretion of the attending neonatologist [54].

Risk of sight-threatening ROP developing is considered to be minimal beyond 37 weeks postmenstrual age although any decision to cease screening certain babies before this point in time must be considered with caution. Examination of data from the CRYO-ROP study indicated that babies developing stage 1 or 2 ROP in zone III were at very low risk of developing sight-threatening ROP [55,56]. Investigations for serious ROP should be between 33 and 39 weeks post-conceptional age, while realizing that there is a degree of individual variability in the development of retinal vasculature [56].

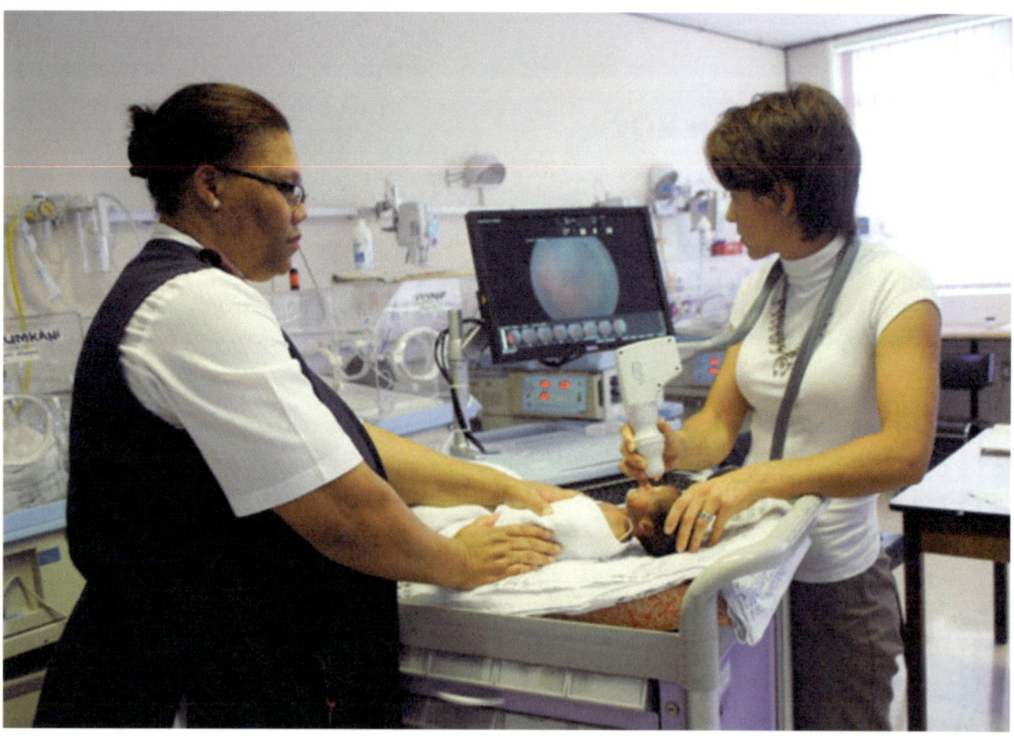

Figure 2. Courtesy of Tygerberg Children's Hospital. [71]

Risk of sight defect is regarded as minimal when regression occurs in babies with moderate ROP, with vascularisation of the retina spreading into zone III. However, it was shown that in 3% of babies, regression and zone III vascularisation had still not occurred by 3 months post term [56]. Therefore, the UK Guideline Development Group decided criteria for termination of screening should be when signs of regression of active ROP are apparent as opposed to vascularisation [49]. Signs of ROP regression have been defined by the ICROP revisited publication as lack of increase in severity, complete or partial resolution, reduction of pre-plus/plus disease, transgression of vessels through the demarcation line and the commencement of the process of replacement of active ROP lesions by scar tissue [51]. The signs of regression should be confirmed by at least two examinations [49]. In babies without ROP, eye examinations may be stopped when vascularisation has extended into zone III, usually after 36 weeks post-conceptional age [57].

Babies with ROP that did not require treatment can have screening stopped when clear regression is seen on 2 successive examinations [57]. Babies that required treatment for ROP and babies diagnosed with stage 3 ROP, which resolved spontaneously, require ophthalmic review at least until 5 years of age [57]. Babies with stages 1 or 2 ROP can have routine vision screening, unless there is specific concern [49]. It should be noted that the process of regression may differ between individuals and ophthalmologists should err on the side of caution when they believe that there is still the possibility of sight-threatening ROP [49].

Until recently, universally accepted treatment criteria of 'threshold' ROP have been used and there is a requirement for new studies using pre-threshold treatment criteria [49]. The UK recommendations were drawn up with the intention not to negate use of clinical judgment by experienced and competent ophthalmologists [49].

As with the classification, the screening for ROP is constantly evolving. Screening investigations include frequent retinal examinations of at-risk preterm infants [57]. Delaying or postponing a screening examination could mean that the window of opportunity for treatment is missed [58,62].

7. Future screening

Newly developed ROP screening and prediction methods based on post-natal weight gain and IGF-1 levels can predict infants who are at high risk for ROP. These infants may be monitored more closely while those identified to be at low risk may be spared unnecessary diagnostic procedures. ROP evaluations and weekly weight measurements from birth to postmenstrual week 36 were entered into a computer-based surveillance system.

A prospective study of 50 preterm infants with a mean gestational age of 26 weeks was conducted to validate a surveillance algorithm for detecting infants at risk for proliferative ROP [59]. Weekly measures of body weight and (IGF-I) level from birth until postmenstrual age 36 weeks were compared using the Weight, insulin like growth factor I (IGF-1), Neonatal Retinopathy of Prematurity (WINROP) algorithm [59]. Gestational age, birth weight, and IGF

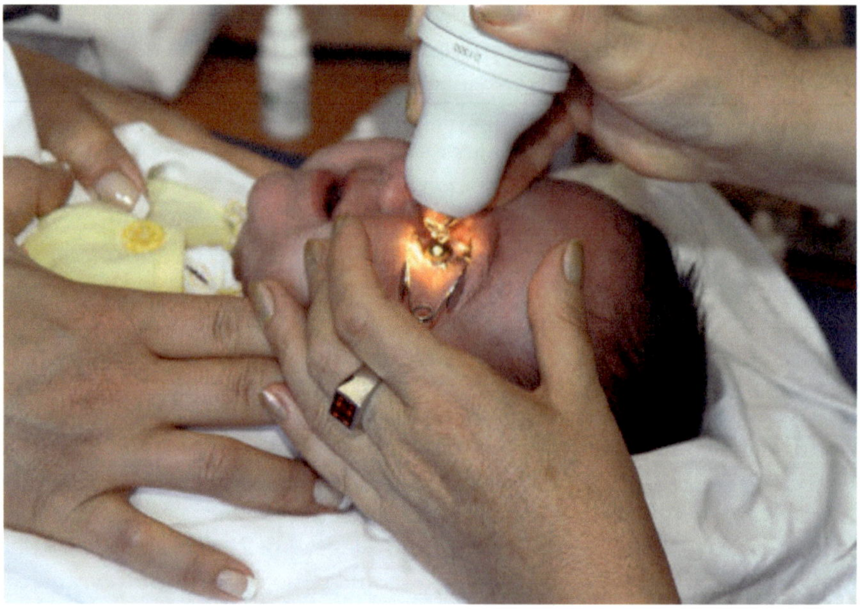

Figure 3. Courtesy of Minas Hambardzumyan. [73]

binding protein 3 level are entered. An alarm is raised if any of the variables indicate a certain degree of negative deviation [59]. The WINROP algorithm identified all infants (100% sensitivity) who were diagnosed with proliferative ROP 1. No infants with no alarm or with alarm at low risk developed proliferative ROP. Alarm at high risk before postmenstrual age 32 weeks was raised for 22 of 50 infants (44%); 9 of these infants developed proliferative ROP (54% specificity), of whom 8 were treated [60]. It was concluded that the WINROP algorithm may be a useful modification for ROP screening [59].

In another study using WINROP a total of 1706 infants with a median gestational age of 28 weeks (range, 22-31 weeks) and median birth weight of 1016 g (range, 378-2240 g) were included in the study analysis [60]. An alarm occurred in 1101 infants (64.5%), with a median time from birth to alarm of 3 weeks (range, 0-12 weeks) and from alarm to treatment of 8 weeks (range, 1 day to 22 weeks). The sensitivity of WINROP was 98.6% and the negative predictive value was 99.7%. Two infants with type 1 ROP requiring treatment after 40 weeks' postmenstrual age did not receive an alarm [60].

In a Mexican patient population, the WINROP algorithm correctly predicted severe retinopathy of prematurity in 84.7% of extremely preterm infants and correctly identified only 26.6% of infants in whom severe retinopathy of prematurity did not develop [61]. These findings suggest that potential differences exist among preterm infants with retinopathy of prematurity in different regions of the world.

The WINROP algorithm was recently tested using a retrospective cohort study in the South East of Scotland [63]. Anonymised clinical data were uploaded to the online WINROP site, and infants at risk of developing severe ROP were identified. The results using WINROP were compared with the actual ROP screening outcomes. Infants with incomplete weight data were included in the whole group, but were excluded from a subgroup analysis of infants with complete weight data. In addition, data were manipulated to test whether missing weight data points in the early neonatal period would lead to loss of sensitivity of the algorithm. The WINROP algorithm had 73% sensitivity for detecting infants at risk of severe ROP when all infants were included and 87% when the complete weight data subgroup was analysed. Manipulation of data from the complete weight data subgroup demonstrated that one or two missing weight data points in the early postnatal period lead to loss of sensitivity performance by WINROP [63]. It was concluded that the WINROP program offers a non-invasive method of identifying infants at high risk of severe ROP and also identifying those not at risk. However, for WINROP to function optimally, it has to be used as recommended and designed, namely weekly body weight measurements are required [63].

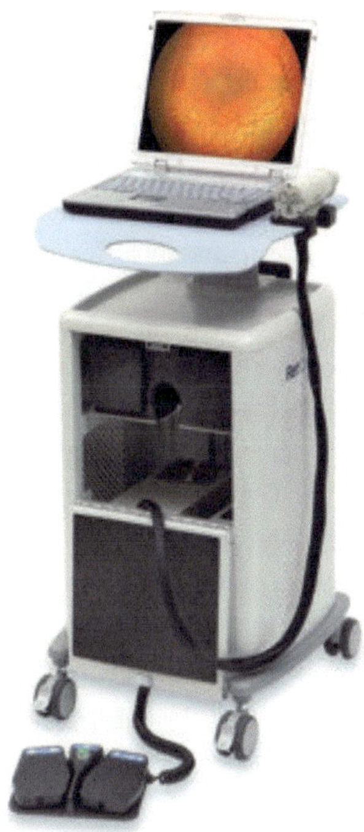

Figure 4. Courtesy of BIOPHOTONICS [74].

8. Digital imaging

Interpretation of digital images have been found to have good inter/intra-reader reliability [64,65] which enhances its potential for use in what is termed 'telemedicine' [49]. The use of digital photographic retinal images that are captured and sent for remote interpretation is a developing approach to ROP screening however, outcomes comparison between large-scale operational digital-imaging systems with remote interpretation versus binocular indirect ophthalmoscopy have not been published.

While there is not sufficient research evidence to demonstrate that wide field digital fundus photography is as effective as the indirect ophthalmoscope for ROP screening, some UK screeners already the technique 'RetCam' is of choice although the cost is likely to remain a deterrent for many units [49]. However, training of operators is an important issue and no studies have yet demonstrated that cameras operated by non-ophthalmologists are as sensitive at detecting ROP as the indirect ophthalmoscope in the hands of a skilled ophthalmologist [66].

Accurate assessment of ROP is essential in ensuring correct and timely treatment of this potentially blinding condition [67,68]. Current modes of assessment are based upon clinical grading by expert examination of retinal changes. However, this may be subjective, unreliable and difficult and there has been significant interest in alternative means of measurement. These have been made possible through technological advancements in image capture and analysis as well as progress in clinical research, highlighting the specific importance of the plus disease category in ROP [68]. Progress in these two fields has highlighted the potential for digital image analysis of plus disease to be used as an objective, reliable and valid measurement of ROP. However, with the potential benefits, there are significant challenges such as in image capture, segmentation, measurement of vessel width and tortuosity [68].

The standard method for diagnosis of ROP has been bedside indirect ophthalmoscopy for both routine clinical care and clinical trials. With this approach, the examiner's interpretations of the clinical findings are transcribed onto grading sheets, rather than a photographic record of the actual retinal features. One limitation to this approach is that the examiner's interpretation of fundus findings is presumed to be correct without opportunity for review. Photographic documentation would serve to confirm diagnosis and distinguish true therapeutic failure from poor outcome caused by incomplete treatment [68]. Thus, telemedicine may offer a solution to many of the current geographic and resource problems preventing a comprehensive ROP screening program throughout the world. Future additions to telemedicine could comprise weight-gain algorithms combined with other reliable quantitative data such as IGF-1 levels.

Furthermore, computer-based image analysis using quantitative methods has the potential to improve the objectivity of plus disease diagnosis [69]. Plus disease diagnosis is critical for decision-making in ROP, as it is necessary for threshold disease and sufficient for type 1 ROP. Plus disease is defined as abnormal arteriolar tortuorsity and venular dilation in the posterior pole greater than that of a standard published photograph, which was selected by expert consensus for the CRYO-ROP study and is still widely used [69]. During the past 10 years, several computer-based systems have been developed for ROP, particularly for detection of plus disease. This has potential to improve clinical ROP management [69,70]. However, more large-scale, robust clinical trials are still required to provide the necessary evidence to inform optimum investigation and screening for all aspects of ROP.

http://dx.doi.org/10.5772/58585

RISA analysis:

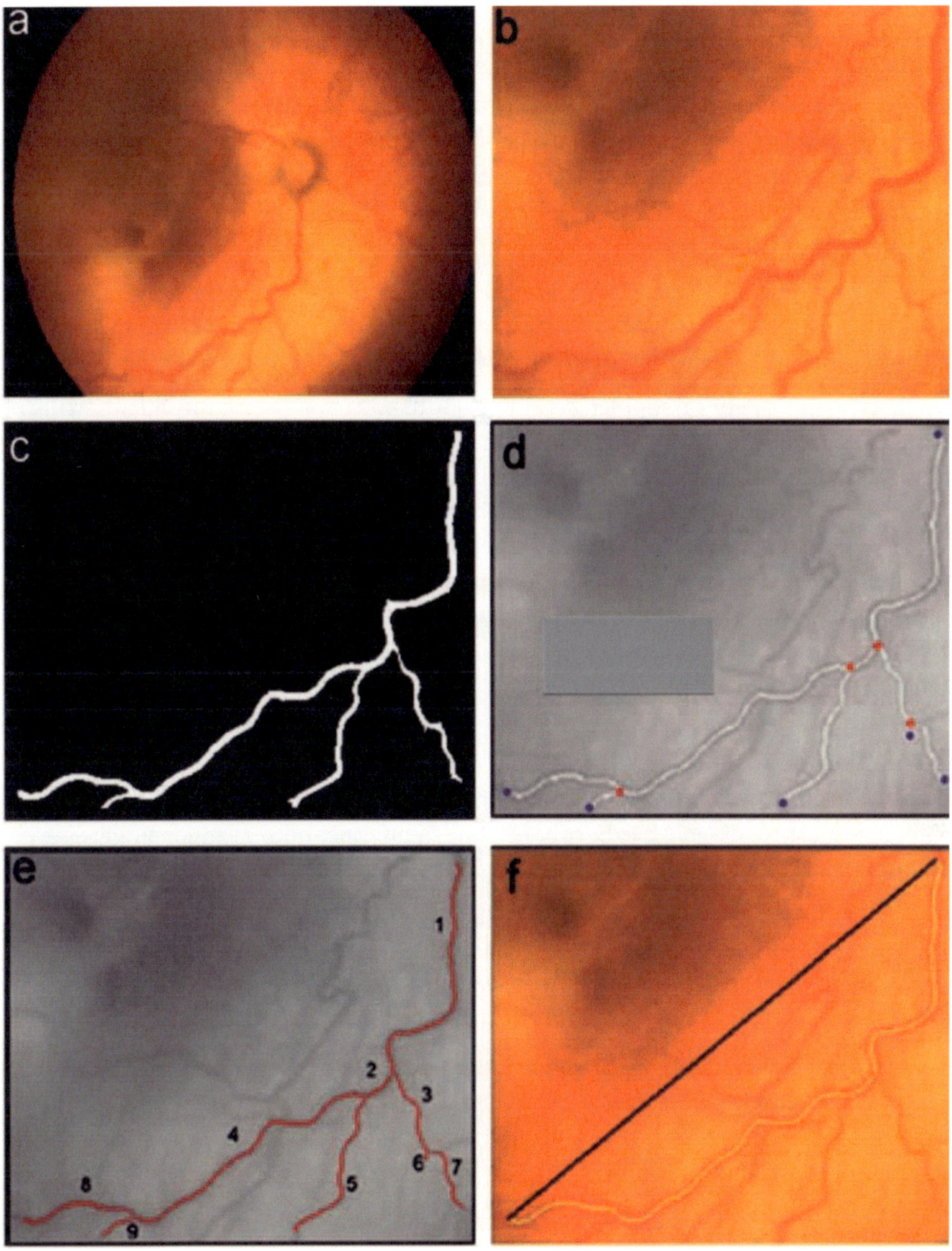

Figure 5. Image documented via RETCAM from (*Gelman et al., 2005*) [70] : a).(a) Retina (b) Choose the vessel. (c) Highlight the vessel. (d) & (e) Mark the vessel. (f) Tortuosity index :Measure actual vessel length, measure the length of point 1 to point 9, divide actual length by length of points 1&9

9. Management of retinopathy of prematurity medical management

9.1. Optimising oxygen therapy

Although incubators for infants had been developed around the mid-nineteenth century, it was not until the 1920s that neonates were grouped together for specialist care in early neonatal intensive care units. Special Care Baby Units became established in many hospitals in the 1940s, although incubators were expensive, oxygen, heat, humidity were considered desirable but influence of such parameters on clinical outcomes were anecdotal – hard clinical data were lacking.

The development of neonatal care, technology and research has reduced gestational age compatible with life to less than 24 weeks with additional challenges in the prevention of ROP. Identifying a safe level of oxygen therapy to prevent the development of ROP in such babies without increasing mortality has been the subject of numerous clinical trials [45, 76-82].

The efficacy and safety of supplemental oxygen therapy for premature infants with pre-threshold ROP was evaluated in the STOP-ROP trial [43]. Infants with oxygen saturations maintained at less than 94% with pre-threshold ROP were assigned to conventional oxygen of 89-94%, or supplemental oxygen with target saturations 96-99%. Supplemental oxygen did not increase progression to threshold ROP or reduce the numbers of infants requiring laser photocoagulation or cryotherapy. There was some suggestion in post-hoc subgroup analysis that infants without plus disease may be more responsive to supplemental oxygen therapy [43].

The HOPE study analysed data from the STOP-ROP trial, including infants who were excluded from STOP ROP with oxygen saturations >94% prior to enrolment [83]. The HOPE-ROP cohort were of a higher gestational age, progressing to threshold ROP in 25% of cases, compared to 46% of the STOP-ROP cohort. Logistic regression analysis identified oxygen saturation at the time of pre-threshold diagnosis to be of borderline significance once gestational age, race, post-menstrual age at diagnosis, zone I disease, and plus disease had been accounted for [83].

The NeOProM study is a prospective meta-analysis collaboration seeking to recruit 5,000 extremely premature neonates to detect rates of death and disability, including visual outcomes from ROP measured at 18 months gestation [85]. Results are expected from this study in 2014.

Increasing neonatal mortality with oxygen restriction suggests that ROP cannot be prevented by oxygen restriction alone in premature infants.

9.2. ROP: When to treat

The "ET-ROP" was a landmark study evaluating the *timing* of treatment of ROP [86], with some concern that a proportion of neonates would receive treatment for ROP that would regress spontaneously and therefore carry an excess risk of surgical complications. The ET-ROP trial was a nationally funded, prospective, randomized, controlled clinical trial that sought to identify clinical criteria to predict those neonates who had the highest risk for an adverse visual or structural outcome [86], and evaluate the implications for timing of ablative treatment for ROP. Natural history data of ROP from the CRYO-ROP study was used to formulate an algorithm, randomization occurred when the risk was calculated to be 15% or greater (high risk pre-threshold), either to early ablative treatment or observation until threshold or regression. Functional outcomes were assessed by grating visual acuity at 9 months gestation, and structural outcomes were evaluated through fundus examination with unfavourable outcome defined as retinal fold involving the macula, retinal detachment involving the macula, retrolental tissue obscuring posterior pole.

499 high risk pre-threshold neonates with ROP were randomized. The ET-ROP study identified that peripheral retinal ablation should be considered in any eye with zone I ROP with plus disease (any stage), zone I ROP stage 3 with or without plus, or zone II stage 2 or 3 ROP with plus disease (two quadrants, or six clock hours). Those neonates with type II ROP should be considered for treatment when progression to threshold or any of the above criteria are met. These treatment criteria have been influential and are incorporated into many national standards for ROP screening, defining thresholds for treatment [86,87].

9.3. ROP: How to treat

9.3.1. Cryotherapy

Reduction of VEGF production may be achieved with peripheral retinal ablation using cryotherapy. The (CRYO-ROP) studies evaluated the safety and efficacy of cryotherapy for stage 3 ROP. A randomised, controlled clinical trial evaluated 9,751 neonates, 291 of whom developed severe ROP. Cryotherapy reduced the incidence of unfavourable outcomes and improved functional outcomes in neonates with threshold ROP [88]. No intraoperative, or immediate post-operative complications were identified, and no deaths were attributed to cryotherapy treatment [89]. Risk reduction was found to be around 50% [35,36], and consequently recommendations were made for cryotherapy treatment to both eyes of neonates with stage 3 ROP in zone I [36]. The CRYO-ROP study was terminated prematurely due to significant treatment benefit with cryotherapy at the 3 month interim analysis [89,90]. A structural and functional benefit of cryotherapy was demonstrated after evaluation 3 years post-intervention [91]. 10 year follow-up revealed a clear protective effect of cryotherapy in ROP in the long-term in neonates with ROP [92]. New retinal detachments were identified in 15 year follow up [93].

The CRYO-ROP study provided numerous insights into the natural history of ROP, risk factors [94] and racial predilection [95], predictors of disease severity [96], prognosis [37,56,97], symmetry or concordance of disease between eyes [98], functional outcomes [99-101], involutional change [56], myopia [102], strabismus [103] and ocular comesis [104]. Cryotherapy did not benefit neonates with stage 4 ROP with partial retinal detachment [105]. The CRYO-ROP study identified a small loss of peripheral field around 6.4 degrees compared to controls [106] in eyes with severe ROP [107], and an increased incidence of myopia [108].

9.3.2. *Laser photocoagulation*

9.3.2.1. *Anterior to the ridge laser photocoagulation (Avascular retina)*

Zone I ROP owing to posterior location and area of ischaemic or avascular retina cannot be treated with cryotherapy alone. Diode laser photocoagulation anterior to the neovascular ridge in neonates with threshold zone I ROP has been demonstrated effective treatment, in contrast to cryoablation [109]. Further studies have demonstrated diode laser photocoagulation for stage 3 ROP to be at least as effective as cryotherapy treatment, with 40 of 42 eyes of eyes regressing after a single laser treatment; only 1 eye progressed to stage 4 ROP.

A study of 48 eyes found argon laser photocoagulation to be effective in the management of threshold ROP in zone I or posterior zone II with confluent laser to the avascular retina, with only 7 eyes progressing to stage 4A retina or beyond, without any recorded complications attributable to laser itself [110]. The mechanism of argon laser photocoagulation in stage 3 ROP is thought to be through reduced peripheral retinal oxygen consumption and reduction of VEGF.

Laser photocoagulation may be achieved with scattered laser; near-confluent [111] or confluent laser burns [112]. Confluent laser burns anterior to the ridge through 360 degrees in threshold ROP demonstrated low rates of progression to stage 4 or 5 ROP (6%), with mean spherical equivalent of-3.80DS in infants [112]. Near confluent laser photocoagulation anterior to the neovascular ridge prevented progression in 4 of 7 eyes with zone I ROP, and all with zone II ROP [111]. A larger combined retrospective and prospective study evaluated 107 neonates with threshold ROP compared near-confluent with scatter diode laser, finding that near-confluent laser photocoagulation was superior to scatter laser in reducing progression in eyes with both zone I and zone 2 ROP [113]. However, randomized trials of anterior to the ridge laser photocoagulation have not been conducted to evaluate the relative efficacy of burn distribution; it is likely that large studies are required to detect a difference as rate of progression to stage 4 and 5 ROP are low.

9.3.2.2. *Ridge laser photocoagulation*

A randomized, interventional comparative study evaluated the efficacy of argon laser photocoagulation to the neovascular ridge and anterior avascular retina versus laser to the avascular retina only [114] in neonates with threshold ROP. No immediate benefit of ridge laser photocoagulation was apparent, but longterm analysis is awaited. A retrospective study of anterior and ridge laser photocoagulation for threshold ROP with a favourable anatomical outcome in 96% of eyes, although long-term sequalae were not reported [115]. No vitreous haemorrhage was reported in this series. The additional benefit of direct laser photocoagulation of the neovascular ridge in ROP remains unproven [116].

9.3.2.3. *Posterior to the ridge laser (Vascular retina)*

Posterior to the ridge argon laser photocoagulation is a surgical approach that considers the presence of ischaemic retina posterior to the neovascular ridge, with or without confirmation

http://dx.doi.org/10.5772/58585

of ischaemia with fluorescein angiography. Posterior to the ridge laser has been demonstrated in a non-comparative case series (no control arm) to be effective in the management of stage 3 ROP in zone II, where only 2 of 18 eyes progressed to stage 4A ROP. None developed stage 4B [117]. Aggressive posterior ROP (AP-ROP) may benefit from posterior argon laser photocoagulation in neonates with late stage 3 or stage 4A ROP following unsuccessful treatment to the avascular retina in threshold stage 3 disease [109]. The benefit of FFA guided posterior to the ridge laser has not been evaluated.

9.3.3. Anti-VEGF agents

9.3.3.1. Bevacizumab

Bevacizumab (Avastin) is a humanized monoclonal antibody raised against vascular endothelial growth factor (VEGF) isoform A, directly inhibiting angiogenesis. Avastin was originally developed and licensed for treatment of metastatic colorectal cancer, non-small cell lung cancer, renal carcinoma and glioblastoma multiforme. Avastin has been used off-label for the treatment of choroidal neovascularisation secondary to age-related macular degeneration, degenerative myopia, retinal vein occlusion, diabetic macular oedema and other disorders characterised by retinal or choroidal vascular abnormalities.

Retinopathy of prematurity is associated with high levels of VEGF within the vitreous and the rationale of administering intravitreal biologic drugs to inactivate it was considered as early as 2008. Avastin for stage 3 ROP with plus disease in zone I or posterior zone II was shown in a limited, non-comparative series to prevent progression of ROP with a single intravitreal injection of Avastin [118]. The BEAT-ROP study was the first prospective, randomized controlled trial comparing laser photocoagulation with intravitreal Avastin for zone I or posterior zone II stage 3+ROP, finding a significant benefit for zone I disease with Avastin, with continued vascularisation compared with conventional laser photocoagulation [119]. Laser photocoagulation for Zone I ROP involves extensive retinal ablation, with increased risk of visual field loss and secondary myopia.

Some studies have evaluated the outcome of combined laser and bevacizumab (0.25mg) for zone I ROP, finding all 18 study eyes demonstrated regression of plus disease without recurrence and vascularisation retina in zone I in all patients. The authors argue that a lower dose of bevacizumab may be used if combined with laser photocoagulation, reduced recurrence than with monotherapy and preservation of central field [120]. Others demonstrate the use bevacizumab as monotherapy (0.625mg), demonstrating efficacy in zone I stage 3 ROP [119,121]. Other groups demonstrate efficacy with rescue intravitreal bevacizumab following laser photocoagulation in aggressive posterior ROP [122]. The optimal dosage for ROP remains to be determined [123]. Late recurrence of ROP in has been reported with subsequent late tractional retinal detachment following initial regression of ROP [124]. Bevacizumab is associated with less significant myopia and astigmatism compared to laser [125].

Systemic absorption of bevacizumab is of concern, and although short-term follow-up studies and surveillance has not demonstrated any attributable systemic morbidity or mortality, this remains unproven. Fellow eyes demonstrate response to contralateral bevacizumab in ROP, suggesting significant systemic absorption of the drug [126].

9.3.3.2. Ranibizumab

Ranibizumab (Lucentis) is a monoclonal antibody directed against all isoforms of VEGF. It has been used off-label in retinopathy of prematurity, although data is more limited compared to that of bevacizumab. Experience from studies with ranibizumab in adult disorders, particularly neovascular age-related macular degeneration, has demonstrated fractionally increased systemic risk with bevacizumab versus ranibizumab but not enough to reach statistical significance. Logic would therefore consider ranibizumab in the treatment of ROP, particularly zone I ROP in which the ETROP study demonstrated a 55% treatment failure rate.

Combined laser-ranibizumab in this patient group has demonstrated promising control of stage 3 zone I ROP with regression in all cases, in a non-comparative series of 34 eyes [127]. Combination laser-ranibizumab has been demonstrated effective in the treatment of aggressive, posterior ROP, although this was a limited series of two neonates [128]. Three year outcomes with ranibizumab monotherapy in a series of six eyes with high-risk pre-threshold or threshold ROP with plus disease demonstrated complete regression of neovascularisation with a single treatment and continued vascularisation [129]. No attributable ocular or systemic side-effects were recorded [129]. Single case series of efficacy add limited evidence in favour of ranibizumab in ROP [130] Late retinal detachment in stage 3 zone I ROP has been reported similar to bevacizumab after initial neovascular regression [131].

Different pharmacokinetic and pharmacodynamic properties of ranibizumab and bevacizumab require randomized clinical studies to compare the efficacy in AP-ROP, threshold ROP. Ocular effects and systemic absorption, and non-inferiority demonstrated between ranibizumab and bevacizumab in neovascular AMD cannot be extrapolated to neonates with ROP. Long-term surveillance is required to document systemic outcomes in neonates treated with anti-VEGF agents for ROP to detect late adverse effects not currently encompassed in short-term published trial data.

9.3.3.3. Pegaptinib

Pegaptinib (Macugen, 0.3mg in 0.02mls) has been evaluated for stage 3+ROP with adjunctive laser photocoagulation in a randomized controlled clinical trial found to be more efficacious than laser alone [132]. Recurrence of neovascularisation was noted at 14.4 weeks with bevacizumab, at 15.1 weeks with pegaptinib with laser, and 5.9 weeks with laser alone [133]. Risk factors for recurrence, the interval for follow-up examination, and length of time required for follow-up is unknown [133].

10. Surgical management

Surgical intervention is necessary for patient with stage 4 partial retinal detachments, which may or may not involve the fovea, or those with open or closed funnel retinal detachments. Surgical approaches include scleral buckle, vitrectomy and combined vitrectomy-lensectomy.

Factors affecting surgical outcome of stage 4 and 5 ROP have been examined and a poorer surgical outcome may be associated with vitreous haze, active neovascularisation and plus disease [134]. Plus disease was identified as the most significant factor associated with failed retinal reattachment; additional surgery or intravitreal anti-VEGF agents may be considered pre-operatively to improve outcome in this group [134].

Outcomes from neonates from the ET-ROP study who stage 4 or 5 ROP were generally poor. Vitreoretinal surgery was associated with macular attachment in 16 of 48 eyes (33%). Normal acuity was maintained in 21% of eyes after 4a retinal detachment. Stage 5 ROP was associated with good anatomical but poor functional outcome [135].

10.1. Scleral buckling

Stage 4 ROP, partial retinal detachment with or without foveal involvement (stage 4a/ stage 4b respectively) may be treated with lens-sparing vitrectomy with or without the use of external tamponade with a scleral buckle. Studies on the outcome of scleral buckles for stage 4 ROP are limited, and limited study numbers, without randomization make conclusions on the efficacy of scleral buckles difficult. Variability in surgical experience and expertise with scleral buckles in stage 4 ROP makes comparison between studies difficult. Long-term outcome in patients from the ETROP trial with retinal detachments (stage 4a/4b/5 ROP) were reported [87]. Vitrectomy with or without scleral buckle resulted in macular attachment in 17 of 50 eyes, scleral buckle only achieved macular attachment in 6 of 9 eyes after 7 years. This data was from multiple centres and surgeons, and not randomized making cross comparison difficult. A high proportion of retinal detachments (20%) were not classified [87].

A small retrospective interventional case series identified 21 eyes with stage 4 ROP, comparing anatomical outcomes of lens-sparing vitrectomy versus combined lens-sparing vitrectomy and scleral buckle [135]; 12 undergoing combined LSV and SB, and 9 LSV alone. The authors conclude that scleral buckle adds little to the success or failure of LSV with similar outcomes in each group [135], but this small series may not have been adequately powered to detect a difference in treatment outcome. Another retrospective series of 16 eyes who underwent scleral buckling for stage 4 ROP reported anatomical success of 100% in stage 4a and 50% in stage 4b ROP [136]. The buckle was removed in 11 of 12 infants, and mean refraction was-8.68 diopters. There was no control group in this study, but evidence was offered of reducing progression to stage 5 ROP [136].

A further single-surgeon series of 8 neonates who underwent scleral buckling for stage 4a ROP conclude efficacy in preventing progression of retinal detachment, although this study was non-comparative [137].

Scleral buckling requires further procedures under general anaesthetic to reduce the tension of the buckle, or remove it altogether. The tension created by the buckle causes axial myopia (reduced by 5.5 dioptres after division of the buckle), and removal or adjustment of tension necessitates repeat refraction to prevent ametropic amblyopia [138]. Removal of scleral buckle has been demonstrated without resulting retinal detachment or vitreous traction [139].

Anatomical success in patients with repair of stage 4 or 5 ROP may not equate simply to visual improvement in such studies [134]. This is supported by evidence from a systematic review of outcomes of surgical intervention for ROP [140], which demonstrated poor vision in many patients regardless of retinal attachment status. There is difficulty in many studies of measuring low visual acuity in infants; this may not be achieved by grating acuity that is often used as an output in many ROP series.

Large, multicentre, long term studies with randomization are required to determine the efficacy of scleral buckling, but variations in surgical expertise and preference may be prohibitive. It is unlikely that meta-analysis will be valid for this reason. A systematic review of anatomical and visual function outcomes in ROP with vitrectomy and scleral buckle identified a wide variation of retinal reattachment rates between centres of 0.8 to 90% [140]. Earlier surgery was associated with a superior retinal reattachment rate, although longer follow-up was associated with increasing anatomical failure [140].

10.2. Vitrectomy

Evaluating surgical outcomes in ROP is difficult due to the long interval between intervention and reliable recording of monocular visual acuities, variability in surgical technique and experience, and the effect of neurological co-morbidity in clinical evaluation. Many studies are retrospective case series with non-standardised follow-up intervals, and no control arms which limits inferences of efficacy.

Early data from the CRYO-ROP study evaluated the functional outcome of neonates with stage 5 ROP (total retinal detachment) who underwent lensectomy-vitrectomy procedures before one year of age, comparing this cohort with infants who did not. Almost all infants had visual acuity of light perception or worse at 5 years [141].

Further studies demonstrate more promising results. A single-centre retrospective case series reported 37 eyes treated with LSV for stage 4A and 4B ROP, with follow up of 5 years. 63% had measureable visual acuity, 18% had form vision, and 19% had light perception vision or worse [142]. Further similar series evaluated LSV in the setting of progressive posterior-type stage 4A ROP with plus disease, documenting low anatomical success of LSV in progressive posterior stage 4A ROP, particularly associated with plus disease [143].

A consecutive, non-randomized, retrospective series comparing outcomes patients with stage 4 ROP treated with scleral buckle or lens-sparing vitrectomy found that LSV was associated with retinal reattachment in 72% of patients versus 31% of SB patients. At final follow-up, after further procedures, LSV and SB were found comparable in outcome as a first procedure. LSV was favoured in this study as more effective as a single procedure to stop stage 4 ROP [144].

The advent of anti-VEGF agents has led to widespread adjuvant use prior to vitrectomy in vasoproliferative disease to augment surgical outcome. Stage 4A ROP with plus disease has poorer surgical outcomes, and many reports have evaluated the benefit of bevacizumab prior to vitrectomy in these patients [145-148]. Several reports have documented the apparent pro-fibrotic effect of bevacizumab with contraction of fibrovascular membranes which may increased tractional retinal detachment [149] and require surgical treatment. Case reports document acute retinal fibrosis 1 day following bevacizumab despite acute resolution of the vascular component, with centripetal contraction of fibrovascular tissue and retinal detachment [150]. One series evaluated the efficacy of intravitreal bevacizumab 72 hour prior to vitrectomy or laser, finding improved visualisation in high risk ROP [151]. This finding has been demonstrated in other series [87,154], with no adverse effects attributable to bevacizumab in the short-term [152].

Author details

Vikas Tah[1], Walid Sharif[2], Imran Yusuf[5], Marcus Posner[4], Louise Ramskold[3], Farihah Tariq[1], Dev Mukhey[2] and Zuhair Sharif[2]

1 Stoke Mandeville Hospital, UK

2 UCL Institute of Ophthalmology, UK

3 East and North Hertfordshire NHS Trust, UK

4 Royal Free Hospital, UK

5 Oxford, UK

References

[1] Hartnett ME, Penn JS. Mechanisms and management of retinopathy of prematurity. *New England Journal of Medicine*. 2012; 367:2515-2526.

[2] Terry TL. Extreme prematurity and fibroblastic overgrowth of persistent vascular sheath behind each crystalline lens. *Am J Ophthalmol*. 1942;25:203-4

[3] Akkoyun I, Oto S, Yilmaz G, Gurakan B, Tarcan A, Anuk D, Akgun S, Akova YA. Risk factors in the development of mild and severe retinopathy of prematurity. *J AAPOS*. 2006 Oct; 10(5):449-53

[4] Kim TI, Sohn J, Pi SY, Yoon YH. Postnatal risk factors of retinopathy of prematurity. *Paediatr Perinat Epidemiol*. 2004 Mar; 18(2):130-4.

[5] Coats DK, Aaron MM, Mohamed AH. Involution of retinopathy of prematurity after laser treatment: Factors associated with development of retinal detachment. *Am J Ophthalmol.* 2005;140:214–22

[6] Fanaroff AA, Martin RJ, editors. Neonatal perinatal medicine. 7th ed. *Louis: Mosby;* 2002. pp. 676–74

[7] Saugstad OD. Is oxygen more toxic than currently believed? *Pediatrics.* 2001; 108:1203-1205

[8] Gilbert C. Retinopathy of prematurity ; a global perspective of the epidemics, population of babies at risk and implications for control. *Early Hum Dev.* 2008; 84;77-82

[9] Bouzas L, Bauer G, Novali L et al. Retinopathy of prematurity in the XXI century in a developing country; an emergency that should be resolved. *Annals de paediatrica.*2007; 66: 551-8

[10] Chen Y, Li X. Characteristics of severe retinopathy of prematurity patients in China: a repeat of the first epidemic? *Br J Ophthal.* 2006; 90: 268-271

[11] Palmer EA, Flynn JT, Hardy RJ et al. The cryotherapy for retinopathy cooperative study group. Incidence and early course of ROP. *Ophthalmology.* 1991; 98: 1628-1640

[12] Good VW, Hardy RJ, Dobson V et al. Early Treatment for Retinopathy of Prematurity Cooperative Study Group. The incidence and course of retinopathy of prematurity; findings from the early treatment for retinopathy of prematurity study. *Pediatrics.* 2005; 116: 15-23 (http://pediatrics.aappublications.org/cgi/content/full/116/1/15)

[13] Al-Amro SA, Al-Kharfi TM, Thabit AA et al. Retinopathy of prematurity at a university hospital in Riyadh, Saudi Arabia. *Saudi Medical Journal Online.* 2002. (http://www.smj.org.sa/DetailArticle.asp?ArticleId=862)

[14] Hussan N, Clive J, Bhandari V. Current incidence of retinopathy of prematurity 1989-97. *Pediatrics.* 1999 Sep;104(3):e26 (http://pediatrics.aappublications.org/cgi/content/full/104/e26)

[15] Fortes Filho JB, Eckert GU, Procianoy L. Incidence of retinopathy of prematurity in very low and in extremely low birthweight infants in a unit based approach in Brazil. *EYE(Lon).* Jan 2009; 23(1): 25-30 (http:/nature.com/eye//journal/v23/n/full/6702924a.html)

[16] Good WV. Screening for retinopathy of prematurity; no ophthalmologist required? *Brit Ophthal.* 2000; 84: 124-7

[17] Shah VA, Yeo CL, LingYL et al. Incidence, risk factors of retinopathy of prematurity among very low birthweight infants in Singapore. *Annals Academy of Medicine.* 2005; 34: 169-178 (http://annals.edu.sg/pdf//34vol200501/V34N2p169.pdf)

[18] M Begué N, Perapoch Lopez J. Retinopathy of prematurity; incidence, severity and outcome. *Anales de Pediatria.* 2003: 58; 156-61

[19] Rekha S, Battu RR; Retinopathy of prematurity; incidence and risk factors. *Indian Pediatr.* 1996; 33(12): 999-1003 (http://indianpediatrics.net/dec1996/999.pdf)

[20] The International Committee for the Classification of Retinopathy of Prematurity. An International Classification of Retinopathy of Prematurity.. *Arch Ophthalmol.* 1984;102: 1130-1134

[21] An International Classification of Retinopathy of Prematurity. The International Committee for the Classification of Retinopathy of Prematurity. *Arch Ophthalol. 1987;* 105

[22] The International Classification of Retinopathy of Prematurity revisited. The International Committee for the Classification of Retinopathy of Prematurity. *Arch Ophthalmol.* 2005;123.

[23] Lucey JF, Dangman B. A re-examination of the role of oxygen in retrolental fibroplasia. *Pediatrics*.1984;73(1):82-96.

[24] Michaelson IC. The mode of development of the vascular system of the retina with some observations on its significance for certain retinal diseases. *Trans Ophthalmol Soc.* 1948; 68:137–180.

[25] Ashton N, Ward B, Serpell G. Effect of oxygen on developing retinal vessels with particular reference to the problem of retrolental fibroplasia. *Br J Ophthalmol.* 1954; 38:397–432.

[26] Patz A, Eastham A, Higginbotham DH, Kleh T. Oxygen studies in retrolental fibroplasia. *Am J Ophthalmol.* 1953;36:1511–1522.

[27] Kinsey VE, Arnold HJ, Kalina RE, et al. PaO2 levels and retrolental fibroplasia: a report of the cooperative study. *Pediatrics*. 1977;60(5):655–668.

[28] Flynn JT. Acute proliferative retrolental fibroplasia: multivariate risk analysis. *Trans Am Ophthalmol Soc*. 1983; 81:549–591.

[29] Smith LE. Pathogenesis of retinopathy of prematurity. *Semin Neonatol.* 2003;8(6):469–473.

[30] Tasman W, Patz A, McNamara JA, Kaiser RS, Trese MT, Smith BT. Retinopathy of prematurity: the life of a lifetime disease. *Am J Ophthalmol*. 2006;141(1):167–174.

[31] Lutty GA, Chan-Ling T, Phelps DL, et al. Proceedings of the Third International Symposium on Retinopathy of Prematurity: an update on ROP from the lab to the nursery (November 2003, Anaheim, California) *Mol Vis.* 2006;12:532–580.

[32] Silverman W. Retrolental fibroplasia: a modern parable. New York: *Grune and Stratton*.1980.

[33] Askie, LM. Optimal oxygen saturations in preterm infants: a moving target. *Current Opinion in Pediatrics*. 2013; 25: 2:188–192.

[34] Palmer EA, Hardy RJ, Dobson V, Phelps DL, Quinn GE, Summers CG et al. International Committee for the Classification of Retinopathy of Prematurity. The International Classification of Retinopathy of Prematurity Revisited. *Arch Ophthalmol.* 2005;123:991-999.

[35] Cryotherapy for Retinopathy of Prematurity Cooperative Group. Multicentre trial of cryotherapy for retinopathy of prematurity: Preliminary results. *Arch Ophthalmol.* 1988;106: 471-479.

[36] Cryotherapy for Retinopathy of Prematurity Cooperative group. Multicentric trial of cryotherapy for retinopathy of prematurity. Three-month outcome. *Arch Ophthalmol* 1990;108: 195-204.

[37] Cryotherapy for Retinopathy of Prematurity Cooperative Group. The natural ocular outcome of premature birth and retinopathy status at 1 year. *Arch Ophthalmol.* 1994; 112(7):903-912.

[38] Cryotherapy for Retinopathy of Prematurity Cooperative group. Multicentric trial of cryotherapy for retinopathy of prematurity: natural history ROP: ocular outcome at 5 ½ years in premature infants with birth weight less than 1251 g. *Arch Ophthalmol.* 2002;120: 595-599.

[39] Ellsbury, D, Ursprung, R. Comprehensive Oxygen Management for the Prevention of Retinopathy of Prematurity: The Pediatrix Experience. *Clinics in Perinatology.* 2010; 37:1: 203–215.

[40] Flynn JT, Chan-Ling T. Retinopathy of prematurity: two distinct mechanisms that underlie zone 1 and zone 2 disease. *Am J Ophthalmol.* 2006; 142(1):46-59.

[41] Stenson BJ, Tarnow-Mordi WO, Darlow Ba, et al. Oxygen Saturation and Outcomes in Pre-term Infants. *N Engl J Med.* 2013; 368:2094-2104.

[42] Mills, MD. Evaluating the Cryotherapy for Retinopathy of Prematurity Study (CRYO-ROP). *Arch Ophthalmol.* 2007;125 (9):1276-1281.

[43] The STOP-ROP Multi-center Study Group. Supplemental Therapeutic Oxygen for Pre-threshold Retinopathy of Prematurity (STOP-ROP), a randomized, controlled trial. I: primary outcomes. *Pediatrics.* 2000;105:295–310.

[44] Chow, LC. et al. Can Changes in Clinical Practice Decrease the Incidence of Severe Retinopathy of Prematurity in Very Low Birth Weight Infants? *Pediatrics.* 2003;111:1:339-345.

[45] Chen ML, Guo L, Smith LE, Dammann CE, Dammann O. High or low oxygen saturation and severe retinopathy of prematurity: a meta-analysis. *Pediatrics.* 2010;125:6: e1483-1492.

http://dx.doi.org/10.5772/58585

[46] Fleck BW, Stenson, BJ. Retinopathy of Prematurity and the Oxygen Conundrum: Lessons Learned from Recent Randomized Trials. *Clinics in Perinatology*. 2013; 40: 2229–2240.

[47] Wilson CM, Ells AL, Fielder AR. The Challenge of Screening for Retinopathy of Prematurity. *Royal College of Paediatrics and Child Health, Royal College of Ophthalmologists and British Association of Perinatal Medicine*. 2007.

[48] Blakeman, TC. Evidence for Oxygen Use in the Hospitalized Patient: Is More Really the Enemy of Good? *Respiratory Care*. 2013;58 :10: 1679-169.

[49] Guideline for the Screening and Treatment of Retinopathy of Prematurity. Royal College of Paediatrics and Child Health, Royal College of Ophthalmologists and British Association of Perinatal Medicine. 2008.

[50] Fielder AR, Haines L, Scrivener R, Wilkinson AR, Pollock JI on behalf of the Royal Colleges of Ophthalmologists and Paediatrics and Child Health and the British Association of Perinatal Medicine. Retinopathy of prematurity in the UK II: audit of national guidelines for screening and treatment. *Eye*. 2002; 16(3):285-291.

[51] Goble RR, Jones HS, Fielder AR. Are we screening too many babies for retinopathy of prematurity? *Eye*.1997; 11(Pt 4):509-514.

[52] Mathew MR, Fern AI, Hill R. Retinopathy of prematurity: are we screening too many babies? *Eye*. 2002; 16(5):538-542.

[53] Early Treatment for Retinopathy of Prematurity Cooperative Group. Revised indications for the treatment of retinopathy of prematurity: results of the early treatment for retinopathy of prematurity randomized trial. *Arch Ophthalmol*. 2003; 121(12): 1684-1694.

[54] AMERICAN ACADEMY OF OPHTHALMOLOGY, AMERICAN ASSOCIATION FOR PEDIATRIC OPHTHALMOLOGY AND STRABISMUS, AMERICAN ASSOCIATION OF CERTIFIED ORTHOPTISTS. Policy Statement: Screening Examination of Premature Infants for Retinopathy of Prematurity. *Pediatrics*. 2013;l: 131:89-195.

[55] Reynolds JD, Dobson V, Quinn GE, Fielder AR, Palmer EA, Saunders RA et al. Evidence-based screening criteria for retinopathy of prematurity: natural history data from the CRYO-ROP and LIGHT-ROP studies. *Arch Ophthalmol* 2002; 120(11): 1470-1476.

[56] Repka MX, Palmer EA, Tung B. Cryotherapy for Retinopathy of Prematurity Cooperative Group. Involution of retinopathy of prematurity. *Arch Ophthalmol* 2000; 118(5): 645-649.

[57] Kanski J. Clinical Ophthalmology; A Systematic Approach (7th Ed) Butterworth Heinemann 2011.

[58] Chen, J, Stahl, A, Hellstrom, A, Smith, LE. Current update on retinopathy of prematurity: screening and treatment. *Curr Opin Pediatr*. 2011; 23(2): 173–178.

[59] Löfqvist C, Hansen-Pupp I, Andersson E, et al. Validation of a new retinopathy of prematurity screening method monitoring longitudinal postnatal weight and insulin like growth factor I. *Arch Ophthalmol* 2009;127:622-627.

[60] Wu C, Löfqvist C, Smith LH, VanderVeen DK, Hellström A. Importance of early postnatal weight gain for normal retinal angiogenesis in very preterm infants: a multicenter study analyzing weight velocity deviations for the prediction of retinopathy of prematurity. *Arch Ophthalmol*. 2012;130:992–999.

[61] Zepeda-Romero LC, Hård AL, Gomez-Ruiz LM, et al. Prediction of retinopathy of prematurity using the screening algorithm WINROP in a Mexican population of preterm infants. *Arch Ophthalmol* 2012; 130:720-3.

[62] Mohamed, S, Murray, JC, Dagle, JM, Colaizy, T. Hyperglycemia as a risk factor for the development of retinopathy of prematurity. *BMC Pediatr*. 2013; 13

[63] Piyasena C, Dhaliwal C, et al. Prediction of severe retinopathy of prematurity using the WINROP algorithm in a birth cohort in South East Scotland. *Archives of Disease in Childhood Fetal and Neonatal Edition*. 2014; 99:1 29-33.

[64] Chiang MF, Keenan JD, Starren JB, Du YE, Schiff WM, Barile GR et al. Accuracy and reliability of remote retinopathy of prematurity diagnosis. *Arch Ophthalmol*. 2006; 124:322-327.

[65] Chiang MF, Starren JB, Du YE, Keenan JD, Schiff WM, Barile GR et al. Remote image based retinopathy of prematurity diagnosis: a receiver operating characteristic analysis of accuracy. *Br J Ophthalmol*. 2006; 90(10):1292-1296.

[66] Roth DB, Morales D, Feuer WJ, Hess D, Johnson RA, Flynn JT et al. Screening for retinopathy of prematurity employing the Retcam 120: sensitivity and specificity. *Arch Ophthalmol*. 2001; 119(2):268-272.

[67] Capone, A. The Photographic Screening for Retinopathy of Prematurity Study Group. The Photographic Screening for Retinopathy of Prematurity Study (Photo-ROP): Study design and baseline characteristics of enrolled patients. *Retina*. 2006; 26(7 Suppl):S4-S10.

[68] Aslam T, Fleck B, Patton N, Trucco M, Azegrouz H. Digital image analysis of plus disease in retinopathy of prematurity. *Acta Ophthalmologica*. 2009;87:4: 368–377.

[69] Wittenberg LA, Jonsson L, Chan RVP, Chiang, MF. Computer-Based Image Analysis for Plus Disease Diagnosis in Retinopathy of Prematurity. *Journal of Pediatric Ophthalmology and Strabismus*. 2012;49 :1: 11-19.

[70] Gelman R, Martinez-Perez M, Vanderveen D, Moskowitz A, Fulton A. Diagnosis of Plus Disease in Retinopathy of Prematurity using Retinal Image multiscale Analysis. *Invest Ophthalmol Vis Sci*. 2005;46(12):4734-4738

[71] Courtesy of Tygerberg Children's Hospital. From: http://www.tch-trust.org.za/improve-the-care-of-children-and-babies-by-acquiring-the-most-modern-technology/. (Accessed : 28/12/13)

[72] Courtesy of Hoag Levins. Clarity Medical Solutions. From: http://ldihealtheconomist.com/he000017.shtml. (Accessed:24/12/14)

[73] Courtesy of Minas Hambardzumyan.. From: https://picasaweb.google.com/lh/photo/47DVdk1Ed1eD6wmgEtcVyw (Accessed: 28/12/14)

[74] Courtesy of BIOPHOTONICS. From: http://photonics.com/Product.aspx?PRID=38590 (Accessed: 28/12/13)

[75] Kinsey VE. Retrolental fibroplasia; cooperative study of retrolental fibroplasia and the use of oxygen. *AMA Arch Ophthalmol* 1956;56:481-543.

[76] Higgins RD, Bancalari E, Willinger M, et al. Executive summary of the workshop on oxygen in neonatal therapies: controversies and opportunities for research. *Pediatrics* 2007;119:790-6.

[77] Kirchner L, Weninger M, Unterasinger L, et al. Is the use of early nasal CPAP associated with lower rates of chronic lung disease and retinopathy of prematurity? Nine years of experience with the Vermont Oxford Neonatal Network. *J Perinat Med* 2005;33:60-6.

[78] Flynn JT, Bancalari E, Bawol R, et al. Retinopathy of prematurity. A randomized, prospective trial of transcutaneous oxygen monitoring. *Ophthalmology* 1987;94:630-8.

[79] Berkowitz BA, Berlin ES, Zhang W. Variable supplemental oxygen during recovery does not reduce retinal neovascular severity in experimental ROP. *Curr Eye Res* 2001;22:401-4.

[80] Mills MD. STOP-ROP results suggest selective use of supplemental oxygen for prethreshold ROP. *Arch Ophthalmol* 2000;118:1121-2.

[81] Flynn JT, Bancalari E. Supplemental therapeutic oxygen for prethreshold retinopathy of prematurity (STOP-ROP), a randomized, controlled trial. I: Primary outcomes. *J Aapos* 2000;4:65-6.

[82] Hay WW, Jr., Bell EF. Oxygen therapy, oxygen toxicity, and the STOP-ROP trial. *Pediatrics* 2000;105:424-5.

[83] McGregor ML, Bremer DL, Cole C, et al. Retinopathy of prematurity outcome in infants with prethreshold retinopathy of prematurity and oxygen saturation >94% in room air: the high oxygen percentage in retinopathy of prematurity study. *Pediatrics* 2002;110:540-4.

[84] Askie LM, Henderson-Smart DJ, Irwig L, et al. Oxygen-saturation targets and outcomes in extremely preterm infants. *N Engl J Med* 2003;349:959-67.

[85] Askie LM, Brocklehurst P, Darlow BA, et al. NeOProM: Neonatal Oxygenation Prospective Meta-analysis Collaboration study protocol. *BMC Pediatr* 2011;11:6.

[86] Good WV. Final results of the Early Treatment for Retinopathy of Prematurity (ETROP) randomized trial. *Trans Am Ophthalmol Soc* 2004;102:233-48; discussion 248-50.

[87] Repka MX, Tung B, Good WV, et al. Outcome of eyes developing retinal detachment during the Early Treatment for Retinopathy of Prematurity Study (ETROP). *Arch Ophthalmol* 2006;124:24-30.

[88] Multicenter trial of cryotherapy for retinopathy of prematurity. One-year outcome--structure and function. Cryotherapy for Retinopathy of Prematurity Cooperative Group. *Arch Ophthalmol* 1990;108:1408-16.

[89] Palmer EA, Hardy RJ, Davis BR, et al. Operational aspects of terminating randomization in the Multicenter Trial of Cryotherapy for Retinopathy of Prematurity. Cryotherapy for Retinopathy of Prematurity Cooperative Group. *Control Clin Trials* 1991;12:277-92.

[90] Hardy RJ, Davis BR, Palmer EA, et al. Statistical considerations in terminating randomization in the Multicenter Trial of Cryotherapy for Retinopathy of Prematurity. Cryotherapy for Retinopathy of Prematurity Cooperative Group. *Control Clin Trials* 1991;12:293-303.

[91] Multicenter trial of cryotherapy for retinopathy of prematurity. 3 1/2-year outcome--structure and function. Cryotherapy for Retinopathy of Prematurity Cooperative Group. *Arch Ophthalmol* 1993;111:339-44.

[92] Multicenter Trial of Cryotherapy for Retinopathy of Prematurity: ophthalmological outcomes at 10 years. *Arch Ophthalmol* 2001;119:1110-8.

[93] Palmer EA, Hardy RJ, Dobson V, et al. 15-year outcomes following threshold retinopathy of prematurity: final results from the multicenter trial of cryotherapy for retinopathy of prematurity. *Arch Ophthalmol* 2005;123:311-8.

[94] Hardy RJ, Palmer EA, Dobson V, et al. Risk analysis of prethreshold retinopathy of prematurity. *Arch Ophthalmol* 2003;121:1697-701.

[95] Saunders RA, Donahue ML, Christmann LM, et al. Racial variation in retinopathy of prematurity. The Cryotherapy for Retinopathy of Prematurity Cooperative Group. *Arch Ophthalmol* 1997;115:604-8.

[96] Kivlin JD, Biglan AW, Gordon RA, et al. Early retinal vessel development and iris vessel dilatation as factors in retinopathy of prematurity. Cryotherapy for Retinop-

athy of Prematurity (CRYO-ROP) Cooperative Group. *Arch Ophthalmol* 1996;114:150-4.

[97] Schaffer DB, Palmer EA, Plotsky DF, et al. Prognostic factors in the natural course of retinopathy of prematurity. The Cryotherapy for Retinopathy of Prematurity Cooperative Group. *Ophthalmology* 1993;100:230-7.

[98] Quinn GE, Dobson V, Biglan A, et al. Correlation of retinopathy of prematurity in fellow eyes in the cryotherapy for retinopathy of prematurity study. The Cryotherapy for Retinopathy of Prematurity Cooperative Group. *Arch Ophthalmol* 1995;113:469-73.

[99] Dobson V, Quinn GE, Tung B, et al. Comparison of recognition and grating acuities in very-low-birth-weight children with and without retinal residua of retinopathy of prematurity. Cryotherapy for Retinopathy of Prematurity Cooperative Group. *Invest Ophthalmol Vis Sci* 1995;36:692-702.

[100] Dobson V, Quinn GE, Summers CG, et al. Effect of acute-phase retinopathy of prematurity on grating acuity development in the very low birth weight infant. The Cryotherapy for Retinopathy of Prematurity Cooperative Group. *Invest Ophthalmol Vis Sci* 1994;35:4236-44.

[101] Reynolds J, Dobson V, Quinn GE, et al. Prediction of visual function in eyes with mild to moderate posterior pole residua of retinopathy of prematurity. Cryotherapy for Retinopathy of Prematurity Cooperative Group. *Arch Ophthalmol* 1993;111:1050-6.

[102] Quinn GE, Dobson V, Repka MX, et al. Development of myopia in infants with birth weights less than 1251 grams. The Cryotherapy for Retinopathy of Prematurity Cooperative Group. *Ophthalmology* 1992;99:329-40.

[103] Bremer DL, Palmer EA, Fellows RR, et al. Strabismus in premature infants in the first year of life. Cryotherapy for Retinopathy of Prematurity Cooperative Group. *Arch Ophthalmol* 1998;116:329-33.

[104] Summers G, Phelps DL, Tung B, et al. Ocular cosmesis in retinopathy of prematurity. The Cryotherapy for Retinopathy of Prematurity Cooperative Group. *Arch Ophthalmol* 1992;110:1092-7.

[105] Gilbert WS, Quinn GE, Dobson V, et al. Partial retinal detachment at 3 months after threshold retinopathy of prematurity. Long-term structural and functional outcome. Multicenter Trial of Cryotherapy for Retinopathy of Prematurity Cooperative Group. *Arch Ophthalmol* 1996;114:1085-91.

[106] Quinn GE, Dobson V, Hardy RJ, et al. Visual fields measured with double-arc perimetry in eyes with threshold retinopathy of prematurity from the cryotherapy for retinopathy of prematurity trial. The CRYO-Retinopathy of Prematurity Cooperative Group. *Ophthalmology* 1996;103:1432-7.

[107] Quinn GE, Dobson V, Hardy RJ, et al. Effect of retinal ablative therapy for threshold retinopathy of prematurity: results of Goldmann perimetry at the age of 10 years. *Arch Ophthalmol* 2001;119:1120-5.

[108] Quinn GE, Dobson V, Siatkowski R, et al. Does cryotherapy affect refractive error? Results from treated versus control eyes in the cryotherapy for retinopathy of prematurity trial. *Ophthalmology* 2001;108:343-7.

[109] O'Keefe M, Burke J, Algawi K, et al. Diode laser photocoagulation to the vascular retina for progressively advancing retinopathy of prematurity. *Br J Ophthalmol* 1995;79:1012-4.

[110] Axer-Siegel R, Snir M, Cotlear D, et al. Diode laser treatment of posterior retinopathy of prematurity. *Br J Ophthalmol* 2000;84:1383-6.

[111] Rezai KA, Eliott D, Ferrone PJ, et al. Near confluent laser photocoagulation for the treatment of threshold retinopathy of prematurity. *Arch Ophthalmol* 2005;123:621-6.

[112] Gonzalez VH, Giuliari GP, Banda RM, et al. Confluent laser photocoagulation for the treatment of retinopathy of prematurity. *J Pediatr Ophthalmol Strabismus* 2010;47:81-5; quiz 86-7.

[113] Banach MJ, Ferrone PJ, Trese MT. A comparison of dense versus less dense diode laser photocoagulation patterns for threshold retinopathy of prematurity. *Ophthalmology* 2000;107:324-7; discussion 328.

[114] Uparkar M, Sen P, Rawal A, et al. Laser photocoagulation (810 nm diode) for threshold retinopathy of prematurity: a prospective randomized pilot study of treatment to ridge and avascular retina versus avascular retina alone. *Int Ophthalmol* 2011;31:3-8.

[115] Steinmetz RL, Brooks HL, Jr. Diode laser photocoagulation to the ridge and avascular retina in threshold retinopathy of prematurity. *Retina* 2002;22:48-52.

[116] Tasman W. To laser the ridge or not laser the ridge, that is the question. *Retina* 2002;22:4-5.

[117] Ells AL, Gole GA, Lloyd Hildebrand P, et al. Posterior to the ridge laser treatment for severe stage 3 retinopathy of prematurity. *Eye (Lond)* 2013;27:525-30.

[118] Mintz-Hittner HA, Kuffel RR, Jr. Intravitreal injection of bevacizumab (avastin) for treatment of stage 3 retinopathy of prematurity in zone I or posterior zone II. *Retina* 2008;28:831-8.

[119] Mintz-Hittner HA, Kennedy KA, Chuang AZ. Efficacy of intravitreal bevacizumab for stage 3+retinopathy of prematurity. *N Engl J Med* 2011;364:603-15.

[120] Kim J, Kim SJ, Chang YS, et al. Combined Intravitreal Bevacizumab Injection and Zone I Sparing Laser Photocoagulation in Patients with Zone I Retinopathy of Prematurity. *Retina* 2013.

[121] Sahin A, Sahin M, Cingu AK, et al. Intravitreal bevacizumab monotherapy for retinopathy of prematurity. *Pediatr Int.*

[122] Dani C, Frosini S, Fortunato P, et al. Intravitreal bevacizumab for retinopathy of prematurity as first line or rescue therapy with focal laser treatment. A case series. *J Matern Fetal Neonatal Med* 2012;25:2194-7.

[123] Spandau U. What is the optimal dosage for intravitreal bevacizumab for retinopathy of prematurity? *Acta Ophthalmol* 2013;91:e154.

[124] Mireskandari K, Adams GG, Tehrani NN. Recurrence of retinopathy of prematurity following bevacizumab monotherapy: is it only the tip of the iceberg? *JAMA Ophthalmol* 2013;131:544-5.

[125] Harder BC, Schlichtenbrede FC, von Baltz S, et al. Intravitreal bevacizumab for retinopathy of prematurity: refractive error results. *Am J Ophthalmol* 2013;155:1119-1124 e1.

[126] Karaca C, Oner AO, Mirza E, et al. Bilateral effect of unilateral bevacizumab injection in retinopathy of prematurity. *JAMA Ophthalmol* 2013;131:1099-101.

[127] Orozco-Gomez LP, Hernandez-Salazar L, Moguel-Ancheita S, et al. Laser-ranibizumab treatment for retinopathy of prematurity in umbral-preumbral disease. Three years of experience. *Cir Cir* 2011;79:207-214, 225-32.

[128] Mota A, Carneiro A, Breda J, et al. Combination of intravitreal ranibizumab and laser photocoagulation for aggressive posterior retinopathy of prematurity. *Case Rep Ophthalmol* 2011;3:136-41.

[129] Castellanos MA, Schwartz S, Garcia-Aguirre G, et al. Short-term outcome after intravitreal ranibizumab injections for the treatment of retinopathy of prematurity. *Br J Ophthalmol* 2013;97:816-9.

[130] Lin CJ, Chen SN, Hwang JF. Intravitreal ranibizumab as salvage therapy in an extremely low-birth-weight infant with rush type retinopathy of prematurity. *Oman J Ophthalmol*;5:184-6.

[131] Jang SY, Choi KS, Lee SJ. Delayed-onset retinal detachment after an intravitreal injection of ranibizumab for zone I plus retinopathy of prematurity. *J Aapos* 2010;14:457-9.

[132] Autrata R, Krejcirova I, Senkova K, et al. Intravitreal pegaptanib combined with diode laser therapy for stage 3+retinopathy of prematurity in zone I and posterior zone II. *Eur J Ophthalmol* 2012;22:687-94.

[133] Mintz-Hittner HA. Intravitreal pegaptanib as adjunctive treatment for stage 3+ROP shown to be effective in a prospective, randomized, controlled multicenter clinical trial. *Eur J Ophthalmol* 2012;22:685-6.

[134] Hartnett ME. Features associated with surgical outcome in patients with stages 4 and 5 retinopathy of prematurity. *Retina* 2003;23:322-9.

[135] Sears JE, Sonnie C. Anatomic success of lens-sparing vitrectomy with and without scleral buckle for stage 4 retinopathy of prematurity. *Am J Ophthalmol* 2007;143:810-3.

[136] Ratanasukon M, Visaetsilpanonta S, Tengtrisorn S, et al. Outcomes of scleral buckling for stage 4 retinopathy of prematurity in Thai children. *J Med Assoc Thai* 2006;89:1659-64.

[137] Hinz BJ, de Juan E, Jr., Repka MX. Scleral buckling surgery for active stage 4A retinopathy of prematurity. *Ophthalmology* 1998;105:1827-30.

[138] Chow DR, Ferrone PJ, Trese MT. Refractive changes associated with scleral buckling and division in retinopathy of prematurity. *Arch Ophthalmol* 1998;116:1446-8.

[139] Choi MY, Yu YS. Efficacy of removal of buckle after scleral buckling surgery for retinopathy of prematurity. *J Aapos* 2000;4:362-5.

[140] Ertzbischoff LM. A systematic review of anatomical and visual function outcomes in preterm infants after scleral buckle and vitrectomy for retinal detachment. *Adv Neonatal Care* 2004;4:10-9.

[141] Quinn GE, Dobson V, Barr CC, et al. Visual acuity of eyes after vitrectomy for retinopathy of prematurity: follow-up at 5 1/2 years. The Cryotherapy for Retinopathy of Prematurity Cooperative Group. *Ophthalmology* 1996;103:595-600.

[142] Singh R, Reddy DM, Barkmeier AJ, et al. Long-term visual outcomes following lens-sparing vitrectomy for retinopathy of prematurity. *Br J Ophthalmol* 2012;96:1395-8.

[143] Choi J, Kim JH, Kim SJ, et al. Long-term results of lens-sparing vitrectomy for progressive posterior-type stage 4A retinopathy of prematurity. *Korean J Ophthalmol* 2012;26:277-84.

[144] Hartnett ME, Maguluri S, Thompson HW, et al. Comparison of retinal outcomes after scleral buckle or lens-sparing vitrectomy for stage 4 retinopathy of prematurity. *Retina* 2004;24:753-7.

[145] Kychenthal A, Dorta P. Vitrectomy after intravitreal bevacizumab (Avastin) for retinal detachment in retinopathy of prematurity. *Retina*;30:S32-6.

[146] Xu Y, Zhang Q, Kang X, et al. Early vitreoretinal surgery on vascularly active stage 4 retinopathy of prematurity through the preoperative intravitreal bevacizumab injection. *Acta Ophthalmol*;91:e304-10.

[147] Axer-Siegel R, Snir M, Ron Y, et al. Intravitreal bevacizumab as supplemental treatment or monotherapy for severe retinopathy of prematurity. *Retina*;31:1239-47.

[148] Wu WC, Yeh PT, Chen SN, et al. Effects and complications of bevacizumab use in patients with retinopathy of prematurity: a multicenter study in taiwan. *Ophthalmology*;118:176-83.

[149] Sun HJ, Choi KS, Lee SJ. Adjunctive effect of intravitreal bevacizumab prior to lens-sparing vitrectomy in aggressive posterior retinopathy of prematurity: a case report. *Jpn J Ophthalmol* 2012;56:476-80.

[150] Honda S, Hirabayashi H, Tsukahara Y, et al. Acute contraction of the proliferative membrane after an intravitreal injection of bevacizumab for advanced retinopathy of prematurity. *Graefes Arch Clin Exp Ophthalmol* 2008;246:1061-3.

[151] Law JC, Recchia FM, Morrison DG, et al. Intravitreal bevacizumab as adjunctive treatment for retinopathy of prematurity. *J Aapos* 2010;14:6-10.

[152] Kychenthal A, Dorta P. Vitrectomy after intravitreal bevacizumab (Avastin) for retinal detachment in retinopathy of prematurity. *Retina* 2010;30:S32-6.

[153] Xu Y, Zhang Q, Kang X, et al. Early vitreoretinal surgery on vascularly active stage 4 retinopathy of prematurity through the preoperative intravitreal bevacizumab injection. *Acta Ophthalmol* 2013;91:e304-10.

[154] Ittiara S, Blair MP, Shapiro MJ, et al. Exudative retinopathy and detachment: a late reactivation of retinopathy of prematurity after intravitreal bevacizumab. *J Aapos* 2013;17:323-5

Chapter 13

Disorders of Optic Nerve and Visual Pathways

Ipek Midi

Additional information is available at the end of the chapter

http://dx.doi.org/10.5772/58312

1. Introduction

The evaluation of a patient with visual acuity and visual field defect depends on a detailed history, careful examination and knowledge of anatomic pathways. The structures which are responsible for these pathologies include the retina, optic nerve, optic chiasm, optic tract, optic radiation and visual cortex of the occipital lobe. These structures are called the afferent systems of visual pathways.

Multiple aetiologies can affect and cause different disorders. The history gives the information about the possible aetiologies of the optic neuropathy. There are simple and advanced investigation methods that can support the diagnosis of optic neuropathy. Visual field testing by either manual kinetic or automated static perimetry, cranial and orbital MR, visually evoked potentials and optic coherence tomography are the investigation methods that help in diagnosis. In this chapter optic nerve and visual pathway disorders will be discussed.

1.1. The anatomy of optic nerve and the visual pathways

The visual pathway begins from the globes and extends to the visual cortex in the occipital lobe [1]. The optic nerve (cranial nerve II) leaves the orbit; it reaches to the optic chiasm, which is located besides the pituitary gland. The optic nerve fibres originate from the nasal half of each retina decussate at the optic chiasm level and form an X-shaped structure; on the other hand the nerve fibres of the temporal retina continue their way without crossing [1-3]. From there, most of the axons of the nerve fibres terminate in the lateral geniculate nucleus of the thalamus which is called the **optic tract**, while the other axons terminate in the pretectal nucleus which is responsible for pupillary reflex movements. In its course from the lateral geniculate nucleus to the striate cortex, **optic radiation** fans out under the temporal and parietal lobes. Some of the optic radiation axons run out into the temporal lobe called Meyer's loop. Meyer's loop carries information from the superior portion of the contralateral visual field. More medial parts of the optic radiation, which pass under the cortex of the parietal lobe, carry information from the inferior portion of the contralateral visual field. Damage to parts of the temporal lobe results in a superior homonymous quadrantanopsia; damage to the optic radiation underlying the parietal cortex results in an inferior homonymous quadrantanopsia type in the visual field. Then the fibres from both the temporal and parietal lobe reach the visual cortex in the occipital lobe [1-3].

Signs of optic nerve dysfunction

1. Reduced visual acuity
2. Afferent pupillary defect
3. Dyschromatopsia (impairment of colour vision)
4. Diminished light brightness sensitivity
5. Diminished contrast sensitivity
6. Visual field defect

1.2. Examination of visual field

Confrontation technique is used to examine the central or peripheral visual dysfunction. The examiner asks the patient to cover one eye and the examiner also covers the opposite eye at the same time. The examiner moves a colourful object in his hand out of the patient's visual field and then brings it centrally. He has to tell the examiner when he notices the object. The same examination must be done for the opposite side [4].

1.3. Clinical features of visual field defect

Damage to the optic nerve causes permanent and severe loss of vision and pupillary reflex abnormalities. According to the localization of lesion, different type of visual field defect can occur. In general [1, 5]:

- If the optic nerve is damaged anterior to the optic chiasm, it causes loss of vision on the same side as the damage
- If the optic nerve is damaged in the optic chiasm level, it causes bitemporal hemianopia. This may occur in expanding pituitary adenoma (Figure 1).
- If optic nerve is damaged posterior to the optic chiasm (optic tract, optic radiation), it causes a visual field defect on the opposite side to the damage [5-7].

The main symptom is vision loss, frequently maximal within one or two days and varying from a small central or paracentral scotoma to complete blindness. Most patients complain of mild eye pain, which often feels worse with eye movements [3, 8].

Optic neuropathy describes abnormalities of the optic nerve [8].This may occur as a result of ischaemia, vascular and blood pressure abnormalities, toxins, compression, infiltrations and trauma [9,10]. Optic neuropathy is divided into anterior and posterior types: anterior optic

http://dx.doi.org/10.5772/58312

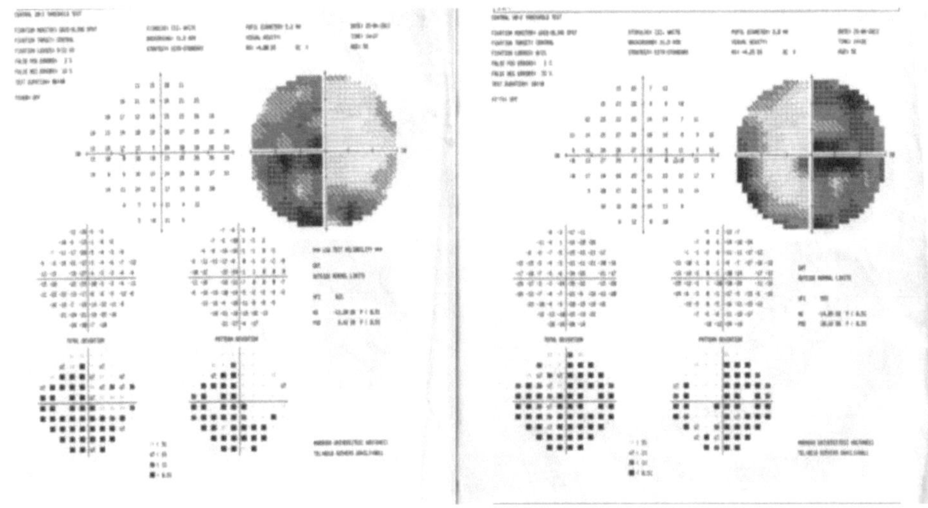

Figure 1. Visual field analysis shows bitemporal hemianophia in a patient with pituitary adenoma.

neuropathy, which causes a pale oedema of the optic disc; and posterior, in which the optic disc is not swollen and the abnormality occurs between the globe and the optic chiasm [3, 4, 8].

1.4. Optic disc oedema and papilloedema

Optic disc oedema is the swelling and elevation of the disc. It can be caused by a number of conditions. Papilloedema relates more specifically to optic nerve head swelling secondary to raised intracranial pressure (Table 1). Disc swelling is distinct from disc atrophy which refers to a loss of nerve fibres at the optic nerve head [2, 3, 11]. There are various signs visible during fundoscopic evaluation. These are: optic disc swelling, unclearness around the margin of the disc, optic disc hyperaemia, venous dilatation, peripapillary haemorrhages, disc exuda or exuda in peripapillar area and cotton wood spots [11].

The pathogenesis of optic disc oedema is mostly related to inhibition of axoplasmic flow. Although histopathological and ophthalmoscopic findings are similar, it is important for treatment approaches to find the causes of optic disc swelling. Often, the cause remains obscure despite undergoing a thorough evaluation [3-11].

Papilloedema is swelling of the optic nerve head, secondary to raised intracranial pressure. This may be due to obstruction of the ventricular system, space-occupying lesion, impairment of cerebro-spinal fluid (CSF) absorption, diffuse cerebral oedema or idiopathic (benign/ essential) intracranial hypertension. The patient complains of headache (worse on waking and when coughing) and may have nausea/vomiting. There may be diplopia if there is a VI cranial nerve palsy [3].

In papilloedema, disc swelling is nearly always bilateral (it may be asymmetrical in the early phase) and may be hyperaemic; dilatation of veins and loss of spontaneous venous pulsation

Optic nerve lesions	Tumour (optic nerve sheath meningioma, glioma)
	Infiltrative lesions (leukaemia, lymphoma)
	Inflammatory lesions (sarcoidosis)
	Anterior ischemic optic neuropathy (hypertension, diabetes)
	Parainfectious and infectious optic neuropathy
	Trauma
Orbital lesions	Tumour
	Carotid-cavernous fistula
	Thyroid ophthalmopathy
	Trauma or surgery related
Intraocular events	Central retinal vein occlusion
	Uveitis
	Ocular hypotonia
	Papillophelibitis (optic disc vasculitis)
Systemic disease	Hypertension
	Anaemia
	Diabetes Mellitus
Leber's optic neuropathy	
Raised intracranial pressure: papilloedema	

Table 1. Causes of optic disc swelling

are the findings of fundoscopic examination. All other causes of disc oedema in the absence of raised intracranial pressure are referred to as disc swelling. But not all patients who have raised intracranial pressure will necessarily develop papilloedema [3]. Visual acuity (VA) is normal in the early stage and will be reduced in the late stage. Colour vision is impaired and there may have a relative afferent pupillary defect (RAPD). Transient obscurations are frequently seen. VI cranial nerve palsy and diplopia are the others clinical features of raised intracranial pressure. In some cases chronic papilloedema can progress to chronic atrophic papilloedema and in this situation visual loss develops [3, 8].

Papilloedema is a neurological emergency. The underlying cause needs to be investigated. After taking a detailed history and physical examination, Cranial CT or MRI has to be evaluated. If there is no space-occupying lesion on Cranial CT or MRI, lumbar puncture decreases the pressure.

2. Disorders of optic nerve (clinical symptoms/ diagnosis/ treatment/ imagings)

2.1. Arteritic ischemic optic neuropathy

Ischemic optic neuropathy is the most commonly seen neuropathy in elderly. Ischemic neuropathy is divided into two parts: 1) Anterior and 2) Posterior. (Both of them are also divided arteritic and non-arteritic forms.)

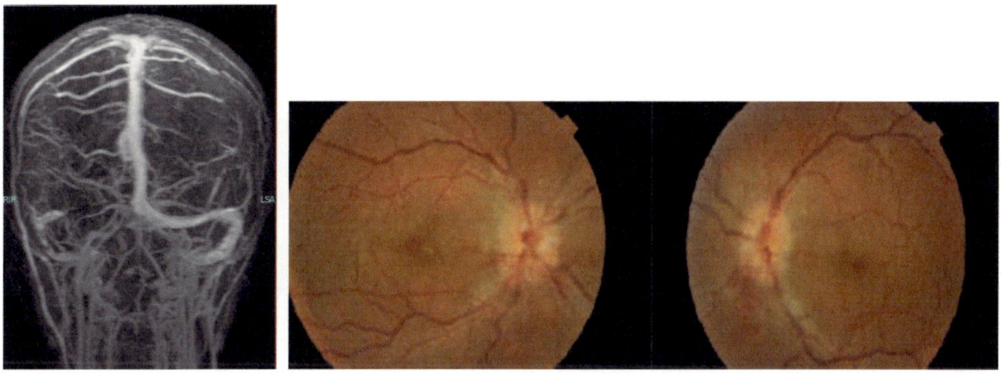

Figure 2. 37 year-old man with venous sinus thrombosis. Papilloedema in early phase is seen. The boundaries of the optic disc are not seen clearly. We do not observe vascular tortuousity (With the permission of Marmara University Dept. of Ophthalmology).

2.1.1. Non-Arteritic Anterior Ischemic Optic Neuropathy (NAAION)

Non-arteritic anterior ischemic optic neuropathy is the most common form of ischemic optic neuropathy. The underlying mechanism of **anterior ischemic optic neuropathy** is the interruption of the blood flow in the short posterior ciliary arteries that supply the optic nerve head. It generally occurs between the ages of 55 and 70 years old. The non-arteritic type involves mainly vascular occlusive disease or disorders that reduce the circulation of blood in the short posterior ciliary arteries. Predisposing systemic conditions include hypertension, diabetes mellitus, hypercholesterolaemia and collagen vascular disease (Table 2).

Visual loss may be sudden or occur over several days. Most of the patients complain of painless *monocular visual loss*. Visual acuity may be normal in about 30% of patients. Impairment of visual acuity in ischemic optic neuropathy may vary from moderate to severe with no light perception. Fundoscopic examination shows a pale, swollen optic disk, with peripapillary haemorrhages noticeable (Figure 3). Inferior altitudinal visual field defects are typical findings but other defects may also be seen. An afferent pupillary defect is present [3, 8, 12, 13].

Investigations: Fasting lipid profile and blood glucose, serological analysis, vasculitis markers, investigations of the carotid artery [3].

Treatment: There is no definite treatment to reverse the damage. Aspirin treatment is effective in reducing systemic vascular events but it does not appear to prevent the involvement of the other eye [3]. However, a recent large study has shown that if patients are treated with large doses of corticosteroid therapy during the early stages of NAION, there was visual acuity improvement in 70% of the treated group compared to 41% in the untreated group (odds ratio of improvement: 3.39; 95% CI:1.62, 7.11; $p < 0.001$) [14]. That study and a natural history study on NAION [15] showed that visual acuity can improve for up to six months.To minimize the risk of further visual loss in the other eye or the same eye, it is essential to reduce the risk factors.

Prognosis: In most patients, there is no further loss of vision but vision loss continues for six weeks in a small percentage of patients. Recurrence rate in the same eye occur is about 6% of patients. Bilateral visual loss may be seen in non-arteritic anterior ischemic optic neuropathy and it usually occurs sequentially instead of simultaneously [16].The second eye involvement occurs in about 10% of patients after two years and 15% after five years. When the second eye becomes involved, optic atrophy in one eye and disc oedema in the other eye gives the definition of "pseudo-Foster Kennedy Syndrome" [3].

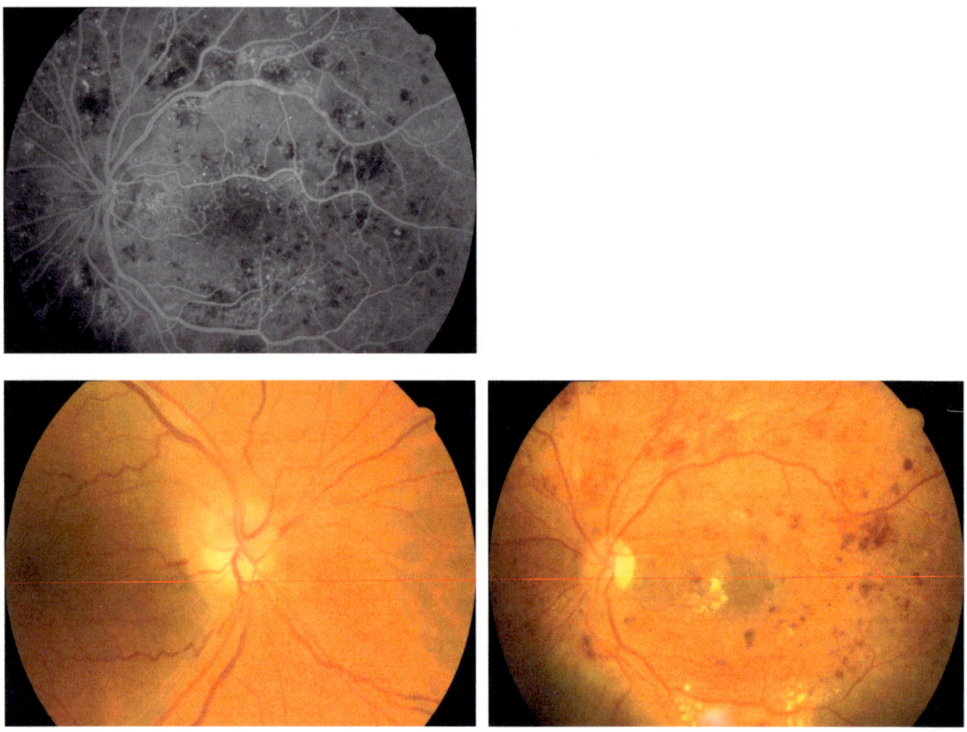

Figure 3. Non-arteritic anterior ischemic optic neuropathy: FFA shows hypofluorescence area caused by diffuse haemorrhage; diffuse microaneurysms, ischemic hypofluorescence area related to peripheric capillary blockages (right eye); crowded optic disc; oedema especially on the upper side; and boundaries on the nasal and temporal side show haemorrhages (left eye) diffuse haemorrhages, exudates and microvascular abnormalities in intraretinal segments (With the permission of Bezmialem University Dept. of Ophthalmology).

2.1.2. Arteritic Anterior Ischemic Optic Neuropathy (AAION)

The arteritic type is less common (25 %). Arteritic anterior ischemic optic neuropathy (AAION) is an acute ischaemia of the posterior ciliary arteries and/or ophthalmic artery due to inflammation. It is also known as giant cell arteritis. The ischaemia of the posterior ciliary arteries and/or the ophthalmic artery is caused by a granulomatous vasculitis of the vessel walls. Therapy is immediate intervention with systemic steroids, especially to protect against vision loss in the other eye [17-19].

The visual loss is sudden and unilateral, but if the treatment is delayed, bilateral visual loss may be seen. Patients with arteritic anterior ischemic optic neuropathy (AION) often have symptoms other than visual loss, such as malaise, weight loss, headache, scalp tenderness and loss of pulsation of one or both temporal arteries, jaw pain on mastication (jaw claudication), generalized muscle aches and swelling. [3, 20]

Investigations: ESR and CRP should be evaluated and they are usually raised. Temporal artery biopsy is the gold standard for diagnosis and should be performed within seven days of starting treatment. But the treatment should never be delayed while waiting for biopsy.

Treatment: Most patients' treatment continues for one or two years. a) Intravenous methylprednisolone: 1 gr/day for three days and oral prednisolone 80 mg/daily. The treatment regime continues by tapering the oral doses.

CRP is a sensitive marker in monitoring disease activity.

Prognosis: The course of the illness results in poor prognosis. Visual loss is generally permanent; partial visual recovery can be achieved by steroid therapy [3].

Posterior ischemic optic neuropathy is a rare type of neuropathy and diagnosis depends largely upon exclusion of other causes, such as stroke and brain tumour. Decreased visual acuity and altitudinal visual field defects are present. Decreased blood flow in the pial capillary plexus supplying the nerve, connective tissue disorders, diabetes mellitus, trauma and radiotherapy to the orbit have all been described as causes. It is also divided into two types; arteritic and non-arteritic [3, 12] (Table 2).

NON-ARTERITIC	ARTERITIC
Hypertension	Takayasu arteritis
Diabetes Mellitus	Romatoid arterid
Hypercholesterolaemia	Poliarteritis nodusa
Cardiac disease	Behçet's Disease
Anaemia, hypotension	Crohn's Disease
Cataract surgery	
Coagulopathies	
Collagen vascular disease	
Hyperhomocysteinaemia	
Antiphospholipid antibody synd.	
Sleep apnoea synd.	

Table 2. Anterior ischemic optic neuropathy

2.2. Inflammatory optic neuropathy

The dysfunction of the optic nerve due to inflammation is called optic neuritis. The acute demyelinating optic neuropathy is the most common type of inflammatory optic neuropathy. Systemic or local inflammations and infections can cause inflammatory optic neuropathy other than acute optic neurolopathy [21].

Symptoms are usually unilateral, with eye pain and partial or complete vision loss. Diagnosis is primarily clinical. Treatment is directed at the underlying condition; most cases resolve spontaneously [3, 8].

Optic neuritis: Optic neuritis is an inflammatory, demyelinating condition occurring in 50% of individuals at some point in the course of their illness [21]. Optic neuritis is highly associated with multiple sclerosis (MS), approximately 15-20% of MS patients attend hospital with optic neuritis and optic neuritis occurs in 50% of patients with established MS [3]. The ages of the patients are generally between 18 and 40 years. Symptoms develop over a few to several days, reaching maximum severity within two weeks. Fundoscopic examination shows that the appearance of optic disc is normal because the illness enhances the optic nerves of the retrobulber type. Ninety-five percent of patients demonstrate an optic nerve enhancement in Gadolinium-enhanced magnetic resonance imaging (MRI).

Patients typically present with subacute, monocular visual loss. The patients complain of pain in or around the eye which increases with ocular movement. Characteristic findings other than visual loss include a visual field deficit (usually central scotoma type), disturbed colour vision, an afferent pupillary defect, diminished light brightness and impairment contrast sensitivity. The Optic disc is normal in about two thirds of patients (inflammation is entirely retrobulbar).The rest show disc hyperaemia, oedema in or around the disk and vessel engorgement. A few exudates and haemorrhages may be present. Visual recovery is common and often complete; most patients achieve better vision over 6-12 months [3]. Despite the return of visual acuity, colour vision, contrast sensitivity and light brightness often remain abnormal [3]. Recurrent attacks may cause optic atrophy.

The Optic Neuritis Study Group published their findings in 2003 [22]. The aim of the study was to identify the factors associated with a high and low risk of developing multiple sclerosis after an initial episode of optic neuritis. Three hundred and eighty-eight patients who had acute optic neuritis were included the study and were followed up for the development of multiple sclerosis after an initial episode of acute optic neuritis for a 10 year risk. The 10-year risk of multiple sclerosis was 38% (95% confidence interval, 33%-43%). Patients (160) who had one or more typical lesions on baseline T2 weighted magnetic resonance imaging (MRI) scan of the brain had a 56% ; those with no lesions (191) had a 22% risk ($P<.001$, log rank test).

Diagnosis: Optic neuritis is suspected in patients with characteristic pain and vision loss. Gadolinium-enhanced orbital MRI may show an enlarged, enhanced optic nerve. Typical demyelinating lesions in a periventricular location in cranial MRI especially T2 or FLAIR weighed imaging may also help the diagnosis of multiple sclerosis (Figure 4).

Prognosis: Prognosis depends on the underlying condition. Most episodes resolve spontaneously, but > 25% have a recurrence in the same eye or in the other eye.

http://dx.doi.org/10.5772/58312

Treatment: Corticosteroids are an option, especially if multiple sclerosis is suspected. Treatment with methylprednisolone (1 gr /day) for five to seven days may speed recovery, but ultimate visual recovery is no different from those with observation alone.

Final visual outcomes are not influenced by treatment, but recovery can be reached quickly by intravenous methylprednisolone. Oral prednisone therapy alone is contraindicated because it is associated with a significantly higher recurrence rate. Patients at high risk for multiple sclerosis, assessed on the basis of MRI, may benefit from immunomodulatory therapy [3].

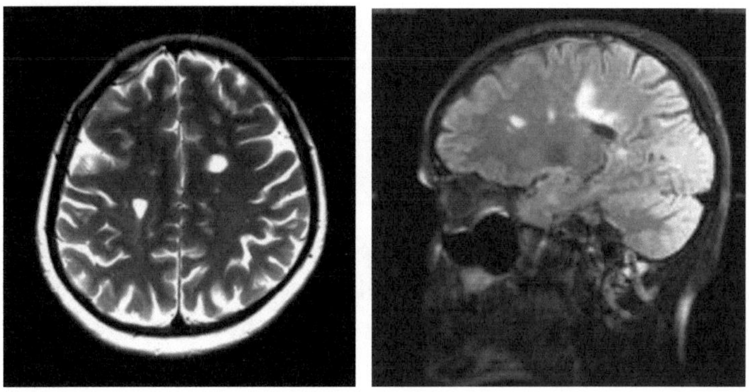

Figure 4. The hyperintense lesion on T2-and FLAIR weighted images. Corpus callosum involvement is noted on the sagittal T2WI.

2.3. Traumatic Optic Neuropathy (TON)

TON refers to the direct or indirect injury of the optic nerve secondary to trauma. The optic nerve runs in the optic canal and can be affected indirectly from blunt head trauma. The visual loss may be partial or complete and generally causes severe and permanent visual defects.

The incidence of traumatic optic neuropathy in a closed traumatic head injury ranges from 0.5-5%. The International Optic Nerve Trauma Study revealed that it was much more common in males (up to 85%) and that the average age of patients was 34 years old [23]. The most common causes were motor vehicle and bicycle accidents, followed by falls and assaults. Loss of consciousness can accompany 40-72% of cases. The diagnosis of TON is difficult and can be delayed when life-threatening systemic symptoms are present.

Direct optic nerve injury is generally rare because of the protecting effect of the orbital bones. It is caused by trauma to the head or orbit. In direct trauma, the anatomy and function of the optic nerve are disrupted. Penetrating injury to the orbit and bony fragments in the optic canal or orbit can result in optic nerve piercing. Orbital haemorrhage and optic nerve sheath haematoma can also cause TON by direct compression. The diagnosis of TON depends on the clinical signs. The cases of TON are generally of monocular involvement. Visual acuity is generally below 0.1. Visual defect is often seen in the acute phase. But delayed visual loss can develop in 10% of cases. The diagnosis of it is important because of the possibility of surgical intervention. Colour vision dysfunction, visual field defect and visual evoked potential are established.

Indirect injuries transmit force to the optic nerve without transgressing tissue planes. This type of injury is most common in the intracanalicular portion of the nerve. Direct optic nerve injuries crosses normal tissue planes and disrupts the anatomy and function of the optic nerve; e.g., a bullet or forceps that physically injures the optic nerve. Indirect injuries, like blunt trauma to the forehead during a motor vehicle accident, transmit force to the optic nerve without transgressing tissue planes. This type of force causes the optic nerve to absorb excess energy at the time of impact. The most common site of injury is the intracanalicular portion of the nerve. Optic neuropathy is most commonly seen in patients in an unconsciousness state associated with a fall [3, 8, 24, 25].

2.4. Compressive optic neuropathy (CON)

CON is the result of compression of the optic nerve. The optic nerve can be pressed in the orbit, the optic canal and the intracranial levels. But it is much more strongly related to orbital pathologies. The optic nerve is most vulnerable to injury by a compressive force in the orbital apex or optic canal [26]. The optic nerve is resistant to force in other parts of the orbita and intracranial level. The most common causes of compressive optic neuropathy in the orbit are inflammatory disease (thyroid orbitopathy, pseudotumour orbita, orbiata cellulitis), tumours and orbital traumas. A variety of tumours can produce optic nerve compression. Sellar and parasellar masses (craniopharyngioma, meningioma, or pituitary adenoma), optic nerve sheath meningiomas and metastatic lesions are included in the differential diagnosis. The other causes related to intracranial pathologies include hypophysis tumours, meningiomas, craniopharyngiomas and aneurisms [3, 8, 27].

Tumours can also infiltrate the optic nerve, particularly optic nerve gliomas (in neurofibromatosis), also lymphoma and other hematologic malignancies. These pathologies can also infiltrate rather than compress the optic nerve [28, 29].

Cranial computerized tomography is preferred as a means to detect orbital lesions and MRI is a useful technique to find out intracranial pathologies [3, 27].

Tumours and thyroid orbitopathy cause slowly progressive visual loss in the course of the disease [27, 30]. But in the situations like orbital trauma, hematoma and cellulitis cause acute vision loss. If compressive optic neuropathy cannot be treated, the results will be optic atrophy and blindness. Pain is variable in these cases.

2.5. Toxic and nutritional optic neuropathy

The causes of these disorders are various. A lot of drugs may cause toxic optic neuropathy; alcohol and tobacco have also a greater risk of causing toxic neuropathy [31-38].

http://dx.doi.org/10.5772/58312

2.6. Nutritional optic neuropathy

The predominant cause of nutritional optic neuropathy is thought to be a deficiency of B-complex vitamins while folic acid also seems to play a role. The toxic agents are summarized in Table 3.

Signs and symptoms: vision loss in toxic and nutritional optic neuropathy is bilateral, usually symmetric, painless, onset may be abrupt or gradual and progressive [3, 8, 32] (Figure 5).

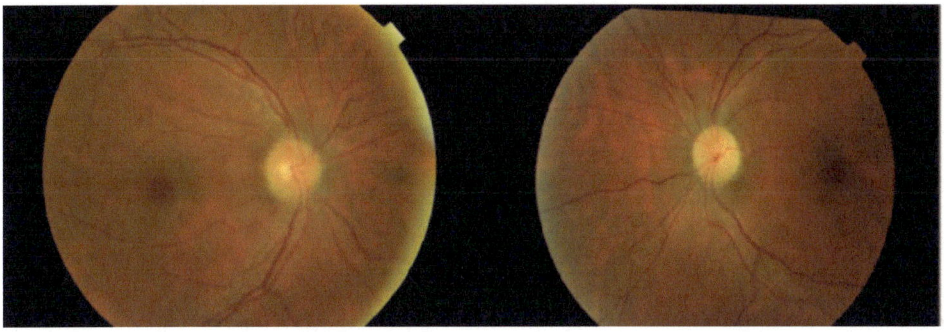

Figure 5. 56 year-old man who has a diagnosis of gastric cancer and is being treated with chemotherapy. Optic atrophy on the right eye and oedema of the optic nerve head on the left eye. The boundary of the optic disc is not seen clearly (With the permission of Marmara University Dept. of Ophthalmology).

DRUGS	Antibiotics: Chloramphenicol, linezolid, sulphonamides
	Antitubercular drugs: Ethambutol, isoniazid, streptomycin
	Antimalarials: Quinine, chloroquine
	Antiarrhytmic drugs: Amiodarone, digitals
	Anticancer drugs: Methotrexate, vincristine, 5FU, carboblastine
	Immune modulators and suppressants: Cyclosporine, tacrolimus, α interferon-2b
	Other: Sildenafil, cimetidine, infliximab, melatonin, sertraline hydrochloride (Zoloft)
ALCOHOLS	Alcohols derives: Methanol, ethylene glycol (antifreeze), toluen
METALS	Heavy metals: Lead, mercury, thallium
OTHERS	Carbon monoxide, tobacco, radiation (unshielded exposure to >3,000 rads)
NUTRITIONALS	Vitamin B1 (tiamin), vitamin B2 (riboflavin), vitamin B3 (niacin), vitamin B6 (pyridoxine), vitamin B12 (cyanocobalamin), folic acid

Table 3. Common causes of toxic and nutritional optic neuropathy

Management: The first step in the treatment of toxic optic neuropathy is to remove the offending agent. The prognosis is variable and dependent upon the affected individual, the nature of the agent, the total exposure duration and doses before the removal of agent and the degree of vision loss at diagnosis.

Patients with toxic/nutritional optic neuropathy should be observed initially every four to six weeks and then, depending on their recovery, every six to 12 months. The patient's visual acuity, pupils, optic nerves, colour vision and visual fields should be checked at each visit. Vision gradually recovers to normal over several weeks, though it may take months for full recovery. Some patients have a risk of permanent residual vision deficit. Visual acuity usually recovers before colour vision [30].

2.7. Hereditary optic neuropathy

Hereditary optic neuropathies are divided into two types. Primary hereditary optic neuropathy refers to cases in which optic nerve pathology is the only sign. On the other hand there are also other groups of hereditary diseases which include various neurological and systemic abnormalities other than optic nerve abnormalities. [(These include: autosomal recessive and maternal inheritance forms of optic atrophy with diabetes incipidus, diabetes mellitus and deafness (Wolfram syndrome, DIDMOAD); autosomal recessive bilateral optic atrophy with spastic paraparesia, chorea and cognitive impairment (Costeff syndrome)]. The most common of these disorders are autosomal dominant optic atrophy (Kjer's disease) and maternally-inherited Leber's hereditary optic neuropathy (Table 4) and these will be discussed in this chapter. However autosomal recessive and X-recessive pattern have been shown in very rare cases [3, 8, 39, 40].

Autosomal Dominant Optic Atrophy (OPA1, Kjer's type)
Leber's Hereditary Optic Neuropathy (LHON)

Table 4. Primary hereditary optic neuropathies

With the remarkable advances in genetic science, the locus of the chromosome was defined and localized in optic neuropathies related to hereditary origin. Despite their genetic origin, these two hereditary optic neuropathies have a pathophysiology reflecting a common pathway in mitochondrial dysfunction. (LHON is a result of point mutations in the mitochondrial DNA and Dominant Optic Atrophy (DOA) is a consequence of mutations in nuclear chromosomes).

Kjer's type autosomal dominant optic atrophy: This is the most commonly seen hereditary optic neuropathy. The incidence of dominant optic atrophy has been estimated to be 1:50000 with a prevalence of 1:10000 in the Danish population. This entity primarily affects children in the first decade of life. But in some cases the beginning of the disease is delayed to 60-70 years of age. Bilateral visual acuity loss is commonly present and relatively symmetrical. Most patients cannot identify a precise onset and the illness usually shows mild, slow and gradual progression. More than 80% of patients maintain better than 20/200 vision, but interfamilial and intrafamilial variation in visual acuity can be seen [41]. There is pallor of the optic disc, cecocentral scotoma and colour vision loss also accompanies the visual acuity [42-43].

Kjer et al. have examined 62 patients from three large Danish families with autosomal dominant optic atrophy and followed up 30 patients retrospectively. They found great inter-

http://dx.doi.org/10.5772/58312

and intrafamiliar variation in visual acuity and visual decline. They analysed 175 chromosomal markers in 118 family members. All markers are located on chromosome 3q in the telomeric area. They found the most probable location for the OPA1 gene was D3S1601-OPA1-D3S1265. Using data from the Danish Family Register of Hereditary Eye Diseases, the minimum prevalence rate was estimated to be 1:12.301. With the results of this investigation, DOA has become the most common hereditary optic atrophy [44].

Leber's hereditary optic neuropathy (LHON): this is a rare disease when compared to Kjer's. Maternal inheritance is present. So this disorder affects young males predominantly (80 to 90% of patients) between the ages of 15 and 35 years. It is inherited through a mitochondrial DNA mutation. More than 90% of all cases have three mutations at positions 11778, 3460 and 14484 [45]. These genes are involved in the Complex I enzyme subunit in the mitochondrial respiratory chain [39].

The vision loss in patients with LHON is subacute and painless, severe, with sequential involvement of both eyes over a period of weeks to months. Fundoscopic examination usually shows circumpapillary telangiectasia, but up to 30% of patients can have normal disc appearance. Nerve fibre layer swelling around the disc can be seen; leakage from the disc or papillary area is not present in the fluorescein angiography [46]. Central vision is affected more severely. With the progression of the disease, telangiectasia vessels and pseudopapilloedema of the disc disappears and optic atrophy takes place. Optic nerve abnormality can be shown in MRI, but enhancement usually does not occur [47, 48]. LHON shows varying penetration and the prognosis for recovery depends on the mutation [45]. The 11778 mutation carries the worst prognosis.

Management: Therapies for mitochondrial disorders are very limited. Currently there is no effective therapy for dominant optic atrophy. Children of patients should be screened regularly for visual changes related to dominant optic atrophy. Nutritional supplements such as vitamin B12 and C, Coenzyme-Q10 and lutein have been suggested [49, 50].

2.8. Parainfectious optic neuritis

Optic neuropathy may be associated with postviral infections and occur as a post vaccination phenomenon [3, 8].Underlying mechanisms may be related to immune mediated process. Children are affected more frequently than adults and this may occur after immunizations [51].

Presentation: Severe acute visual loss, usually bilateral and occurs one to three weeks following a viral infection (e.g., measles, mumps, chickenpox, whooping cough, glandular fever). Other neurological features such as headache, seizure or ataxia may also be seen. There may also be a meningoencephalitis. Bilateral optic neuritis can also occur in Guillain-Barré syndrome [52, 53].

Ocular findings: The optic disc frequently shows bilateral papillitis or may be normal.

Treatment: Treatment is not necessary in the majority of patients. Spontaneous visual recovery is very good [3]. However when visual loss is severe and bilateral, intravenous steroids should be considered.

2.9. Infectious optic neuritis

Meningitis or encephalitis may cause optic neuritis, either as a direct effect of the infectious organism or from secondary vasculitis [51]. Signs and symptoms related to infection, MRI and CSF findings carry some information about causative agents [54-62]. When the meningitis is more indolent, as in some cases of tuberculosis and cryptococcus, optic nerve involvement may be a primary manifestation.

Sinus infections: Sinus related optic neuritis is a rare condition. It may occur following spheno-ethmoidal sinusitis. The underlying mechanisms include spread of infection directly, occlusive vasculitis and pressure by a mucocele. Patients complain of severe headaches and recurrent episodes of unilateral visual loss. Treatment with systemic antibiotics is necessary but surgical drainage of the sinus may also be needed.

Acute viral infections, as well as cat scratch disease and toxoplasmosis and others, can cause an isolated infection of the eye. Inflammation of the retina associated with the optic disc is called neuroretinitis. Neuroretinitis is another finding of ophthalmoscopic investigation. Fundoscopic examination usually reveals macular oedema, in addition to optic disc swelling. Corticosteroids and systemic antibiotics can be used for treatment. The West Nile virus in particular has been reported to produce optic neuritis in association with meningitis. Syphilitic optic neuritis may be monocular or binocular and is associated with vitreal inflammation; acute optic neuritis may occur both in the primary or secondary stages. Antibiotic therapy may improve the symptoms, but relapse may be seen. Lyme disease may cause acute retrobulbar optic neuritis and neuroretinitis. It may mimic multiple sclerosis symptoms. The treatment includes intravenous ceftriaxone [3].

Varicella-zoster virus: primary optic neuritis is uncommon unless the patient is immuno-compromised. Secondary optic neuritis arises from viruses spread from contiguous retinitis. Treatment is with intravenous (IV) antivirals. Cat-scratch fever: this self-limiting infection has a good prognosis with visual recovery. Treatment is with antimicrobial agents.

2.10. Infiltrative optic neuropathy

The optic nerve can be infiltrated by a variety of factors, including tumours, inflammation and infections [63].

The optic nerve has three parts as described by anatomic localization: intraocular, intraorbital and intracranial. The tumours which originate in these locations can expand to the optic nerve. Optic neuropathy related to tumours is generally of the compressive type, but the tumour cells can also infiltrate directly into the optic nerve, which cause infiltrative optic neuropathy. The difference between these two entities is important because removing the compression is the only solution in compressive neuropathy whereas in infiltrative neuropathy the eradication of tumour is the treatment. Tumours that infiltrate the optic nerve can be primary (optic gliomas, capillary haemangioma and cavernous haemangioma) or secondary (metastatic carcinoma, nasopharyngeal carcinoma, lymphoma and leukaemia). The underlying mechanism of paraneoplastic optic neuropathy is related to the development of autoantibodies (ex:anti-CV2) (Figure 6).

http://dx.doi.org/10.5772/58312

Infections, which include viruses, bacteria and opportunistic fungi, may also infiltrate the optic nerve. The appearance of the nerve on examination depends on the portion of the nerve that is affected. If the infiltration occurs in the proximal portion of the nerve, the optic nerve may be elevated. The optic nerve can be affected by a variety of systemic, auto-immune and infectious disorders such as sarcoidosis, systemic lupus erythematosus, Behçet's disease, inflammation, bowel disease, Sjogren's syndrome, Wegener's granulomatosis, syphilis, Lyme disease and cat-scratch disease. [8, 64, 65] (Figure 7).

Sarcoidosis is the most common inflammatory disorder that infiltrates the optic nerve. One to 5% of patients with neurosarcoid develop optic neuritis. Optic nerve head exhibits a characteristic lumpy appearance. Steroid treatment is effective and rapid, but some patients require long term low dose steroid therapy. In addition to steroids, some patients may also be given methotrexate treatment and methotrexate is an alternative to steroids for intolerant patients [3].

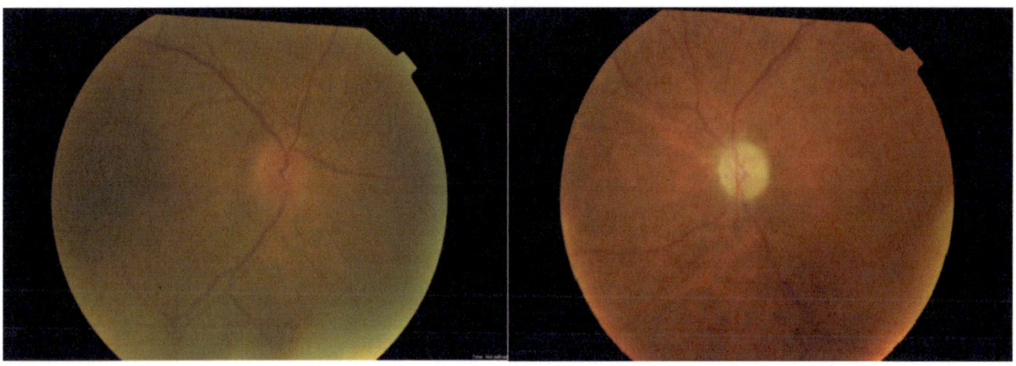

Figure 6. Optic neuropathy with underlying paraneoplastic aetiology (With the permission of Marmara University Dept. of Ophthalmology).

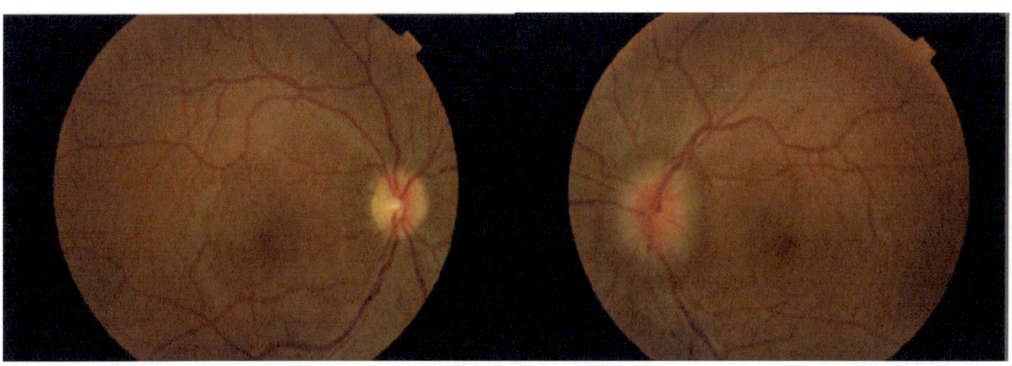

Figure 7. 43 year-old female patient using plaquenil (hydroxychloroquine) following diagnosis SLE. (With the permission of Marmara University Dept.Of Neurology)

2.11. Idiopathic intracranial hypertension *(pseudotumour cerebri, benign intracranial hypertension)*

Idiopathic intracranial hypertension (IIH) is known by raised intracranial pressure in the absence of a mass lesion or of hydrocephalus. It is mostly related to impaired cerebrospinal fluid (CSF) absorption from the subarachnoid space. It is common in obese woman of 20-40 years of age. The female to male ratio is between 3:1 and 8:1. Up to 90% of patients are overweight. IIH may result in permanent visual loss due to papilloedema (Figure 8). The clinical signs and symptoms are summarized in Table 5 (66). IIH may also be caused by drugs. Lumbar puncture (LP) is one of the treatment methods and is also useful for the diagnosis. If the opening pressure is >250 mm $H2O$ and LP shows no inflammatory cells with normal CSF protein and glucose levels, the diagnosis will be achieved. Cranial MRI shows normal ventricles and often an empty sellar. Venous sinus thrombosis should be excluded by the cranial MR venography. Other secondary causes are summarized in Table 6. Regular perimetric examination is important to follow the progression of the disease [3].

Medical and lifestyle treatment: 1) weight loss, 2) Asetozolamide, 3) Furosemide, 4) Topiramate.

Surgical treatment: 1) repeated lumbar puncture, 2) optic nerve sheath decompressions, 3) ventriculoperitoneal shunt placements, 4) lumboperitoneal shunt placement [3]

Symptoms (68)	*Signs*
Headache (92%)	Papilloedema
Transient visual obscurations (72%)	Visual fields deficit
Pulsatil tinnitus (60%)	Contrast sensitivity loss
Photopsia (54%)	Decrease in visual acuity
Retrobulbar pain (44%)	Problems in colour vision
Diplopia (38%)	Relative afferent pupillary defect
Sustained visual loss (26%)	VI nerve paralysis (transient)

Table 5. Signs and symptoms in intracranial hypertension

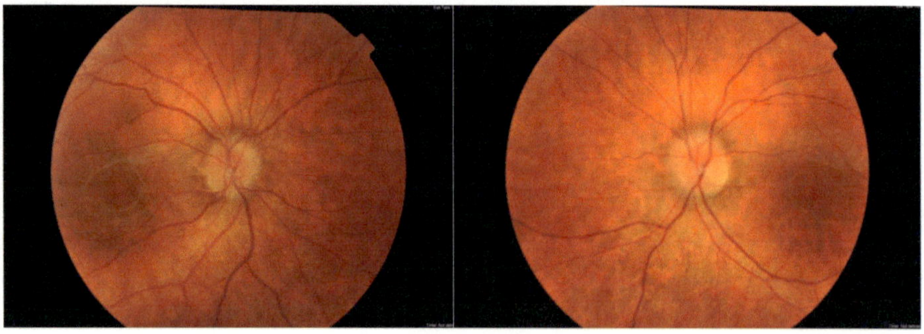

Figure 8. Early papilloedema (With the permission of Marmara University Dept. of Ophthalmology).

http://dx.doi.org/10.5772/58312

Endocrine	Addison disease, Cushing disease, puerpurium, polycystic ovarian syndrome, hyper and hypothyroidism, hypoparathyroidism
Venous hypertension	Venous sinus thrombosis
Metabolic disease	Renal insufficiency, Diabetes mellitus, iron deficiency, pernicious anaemia, hypercapnia, Addison disease, Cushing disease, puerpurium, polycystic over syndrome, hyper and hypothyroidism, hypoparathyroidism
Cranial trauma	
Parainfectious and immunological states	Behçet's disease, systemic lupus erithomatosus, sarcoidosis, HIV, Lyme
Meningial carsinomatosus	
Gliomatosus cerebri	
Medication and vitamin	cimetidine, corticosteroids, levothyroxine, lithium, minocycline, nalidixic acid, nitrofurantoin, tamoxifen, tetracycline, ciclosporin, oral contraceptive, recombinant and natural human growth hormone, Hypervitaminosis A
Obstructive sleep apnoea syndrome	

Table 6. Causes of secondary intracranial hypertension

2.12. Pseudopapilloedema (Drusen)

Hyaline-like calcific material on the optic nerve head is the characteristic feature of optic disc drusen. They are generally bilateral. In early childhood, its diagnosis is difficult because they lie deep. They may mimic papilloedema. Hyperaemia is absent and the surface vessels are not obscured. Disc is elevated without a physiological cup [3].

Ultrasound B-scan is the most reliable method and calcific deposits are detected easily. CT also shows the disc calcification but it is less sensitive than ophthalmic ultrasound [3] (Figure 9).

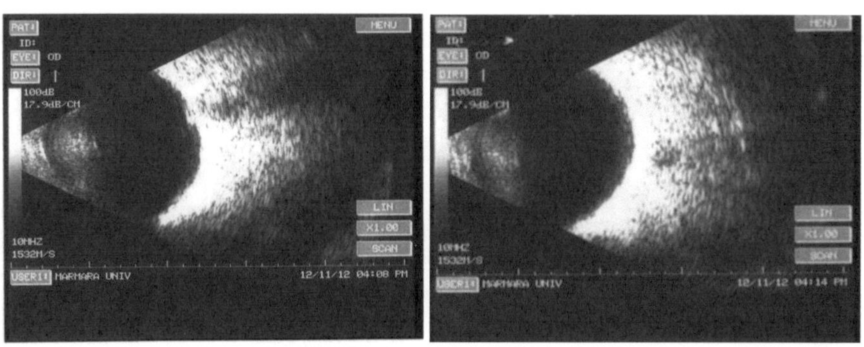

Figure 9. B-scan shows high acoustic reflectivity (With the permission of Marmara University Dept. of Ophthalmology).

In conclusion, disorders of the optic nerve may be related to congenital or acquired causes. There are many aetiologies that affect the optic nerve and according to the localization of lesion,

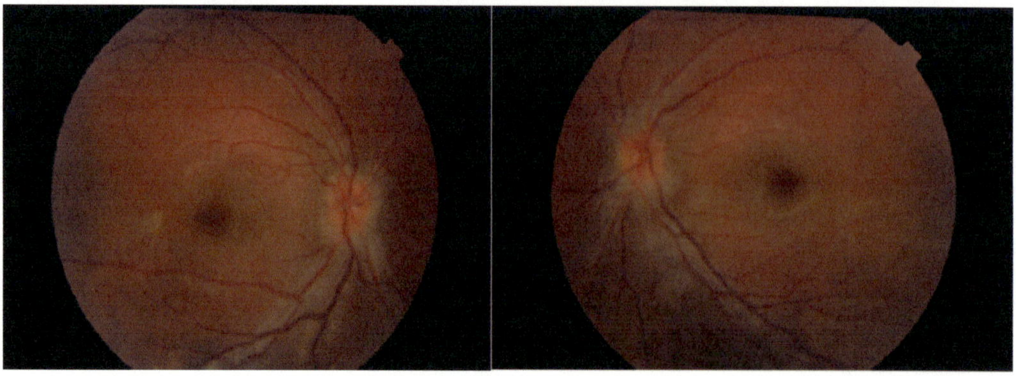

Figure 10. Optic disc drusen (With the permission of Marmara University Dept. of Ophthalmology).

different types of visual field defect can occur. The optic disc may show different abnormalities or may be of normal appearance on fundoscopic examination.

Acknowledgements

I greatly appreciate the Ophthalmology Department of Marmara University Hospital for supplying images for this chapter. I am very grateful to the following colleagues for their help Professor Dr. Ozlem Sahin, Assistant Dr. Umeyye Taka Aydin from Marmara University Dept. of Ophthalmology and Assistant Associate Professor Dr. Arif Koytak from Bezmialem University in the Dept. of Ophthalmology.

Author details

Ipek Midi*

Marmara University Pendik Research and Training Hospital, Department of Neurology, Istanbul, Turkey

References

[1] Smith MM, Strottmann JM. Imaging of the optic nerve and visual pathways. Semin Ultrasound CT MR. 2001; 22(6): 473-87.

[2] Anatomy and Physiology of the Retina and Optic Nerve. In Walsh & Hoyt's. Clinical Neuro-ophthalmology. 5th ed. The Essentials. Ed. NR Miller, NJ Newman. Williams & Wilkins. 1999: 59-86.

[3] Burton B. Chapter 21: Neuro-ophthalmology. In Clinical Ophthalmology A Systemic Approach. 6th ed. Ed. Kanski JJ. Butterworth Heinemann Elsevier 2007: 785-836.

[4] Kansu T. Chapter 2 (Section I): Afferent System (Examination and diagnosis) In Neuro-ophthalmology Handbook. 1st ed. Ed. O'Dwyer PA, Kansu T, Torun T. Güneş Medicine Publishing;2008: 9-17 (Turkish).

[5] Sadun AA. The afferent visual system: Anatomy and Physiology. In Ophthalmology, 2nd ed. Ed, Yanoff M, Duker JS. Mosby, St. Louis 2004: 186.

[6] Glaser JS. Topical diagnosis: Prechiasmal visual pathways. In Neuro-ophthalmology. Ed. Glaser JS. JB Lippincott, Philadelphia 1990: 83.

[7] Purves D, Augustine GJ, Fitzpatrick D, et al., Visual Field Deficits. In Neuroscience. 2nd ed. Ed. Sunderland (MA). Sinauer Associates; 2001.

[8] Osborne B, Balcer LJ. Optic Neuropathies. Section Ed: Brazis PW. Up to date 2013.

[9] Behbehani R. Clinical approach to optic neuropathies. Clin. Ophthalmol. 2007; 1(3): 233–46.

[10] Purvin VA. Optic neuropathies for the neurologist. Semin Neurol. 2000; 20(1): 97-110.

[11] Kadayifcilar S. Chapter 9 (Section II): Optic disc edema and papilloedema. In Neuro-ophthalmology Handbook. 1st ed. Ed. O'Dwyer PA, Kansu T, Torun T. Güneş Medicine Publishing;2008: 101-5. (Turkish).

[12] Bajin MS. Chapter 2 (Section II): Ischeic Optic Neuropathies. In Neuro-ophthalmology Handbook. 1st ed. Ed. O'Dwyer PA, Kansu T, Torun T. Güneş Medicine Publishing; 2008:51-8. (Turkish).

[13] Newman NJ, Scherer R, Langenberg P, Kelman S, Feldon S, Kaufman D, Dickersin K; Ischemic Optic Neuropathy Decompression Trial Research Group. "The fellow eye in NAION: report from the ischemic optic neuropathy decompression trial follow-up study." Am J Ophthalmol. 2002; 134(3): 317-28.

[14] Hayreh SS, Zimmerman MB. Non-arteritic anterior ischemic optic neuropathy: role of systemic corticosteroid therapy. Graefes Arch Clin Exp Ophthalmol. 2008; 246(7): 1029-46.

[15] Hayreh SS, Zimmerman MB. Non-arteritic anterior ischemic optic neuropathy: natural history of visual outcome. Ophthalmology 2008; 115:298–305.

[16] Anterior Ischemic Optic Neuropathy Author: Brian R Younge; Chief Editor: Hampton Roy Sr, et al. Medscape Jan 2012.

[17] Thorne JE, Jabs DA. Ocular manifestations of the rheumatic diseases. In: Duane's Clinical Ophthalmology. Ed. Tasman William. Vol. 5. Philadelphia: Lippincott Williams & Wilkins; 2005: 22–24.

[18] Hayreh SS, Zimmerman B, Kardon RH. Visual improvement with corticosteroid therapy in giant cell arteritis. Report of a large study and review of literature. Acta Ophthalmol Scand. 2002; 80:353–67.

[19] Foroozan R, Deramo VA, Buono LM, et al. Recovery of visual function in patients with biopsy-proven giant cell arteritis. Ophthalmology. 2003; 110: 539–42.

[20] Hayreh SS. Anterior ischaemic optic neuropathy, differentiation of arteritic from non-arteritic type and its management. Eye 1990; 4: 25–41;

[21] Acaroglu G. Chapter 1 (Section II): Inflammatory Optic Neuropathy. In Neuro-ophthalmology Handbook 1st ed. Ed. O'Dwyer PA, Kansu T, Torun T. Güneş Medicine Publishing;2008: 43-49 (Turkish)

[22] Beck RW, Trobe JD, Moke PS, GalRL, Xing D, BhattiMT, et al; Optic Neuritis Study Group. High-and low-risk profiles for the development of multiple sclerosis within 10 years after optic neuritis: experience of the optic neuritis treatment trial. Arch Ophthalmol.2003; 121(7): 944-9.

[23] Levin LA, et al., The treatment of traumatic optic neuropathy: the International Optic Nerve Trauma Study. Ophthalmology, 1999. 106(7): 1268-77.

[24] Steinsapir KD, Goldberg RA. Traumatic optic neuropathy: an evolving understanding. American Journal of Ophthalmology. 2011; 151: 928-933.

[25] Onder F. Chapter 3 (Section II): Afferent System (Examination and diagnosis). In Neuro-ophthalmology Handbook. 1st ed. Ed. O'Dwyer PA, Kansu T, Torun T. Güneş Medicine Publishing;2008: 59-64 (Turkish)

[26] Miller NR, Newman NJ, Biousse V. Walsh and Hoyt's Clinical Neuro-Ophthalmology. 6th ed. Lippincott, Williams & Wilkins; 2004.

[27] Yazici B. Chapter 4 (Section II): Compressive Optic Neuropathy. In Neuro-ophthalmology Handbook. 1st ed. Ed. O'Dwyer PA, Kansu T, Torun T. Güneş Medicine Publishing;2008: 65-71 (Turkish)

[28] Lee AG, Tang RA, Roberts D, et al. Primary central nervous system lymphoma involving the optic chiasm in AIDS. J Neuro-ophthalmol 2001; 21:95.

[29] Grimm SA, McCannel CA, Omuro AM, et al. Primary CNS lymphoma with intraocular involvement: International PCNSL Collaborative Group Report. Neurology 2008; 71:1355.

[30] Maheshwari R, Weis Ezekiel. Thyroid associated orbitopathy. Indian J Ophthalmol. 2012; 60(2): 87–93.

[31] Sharma P and Sharma R. Toxic optic neuropathy. Indian J Ophthalmol. 2011; 59(2): 137–141.

[32] Kargi SH. Chapter 6 (Section II): Toxic and Nutritional Optic Neuropathy. In Neuro-ophthalmology Handbook. 1st ed. Ed. O'Dwyer PA, Kansu T, Torun T. Güneş Medicine Publishing;2008: 81-88 (Turkish)

[33] Lim SA. Ethambutol-associated optic neuropathy. Ann Acad Med Singapore. 2006; 35(4): 274-8.

[34] Orssaud C, Roche O, Dufier JL. Nutritional optic neuropathies. J Neurol Sci. 2007; 262(1-2): 158-64.

[35] Murphy MA, Murphy JF. Amiodarone and optic neuropathy: the heart of the matter. J Neuroophthalmol. Sep 2005; 25(3): 232-6.

[36] Grzybowski A, Holder GE. Tobacco optic neuropathy (TON)-the historical and present concept of the disease. Acta Ophthalmol. 2011; 89(5): 495-9.

[37] Wilczynski M, Wilczynska O. Severe acute bilateral alcohol-induced toxic optic neuropathy-case report. Klin Oczna. 2012; 114(3): 208-12.

[38] Kerrison JB. Optic neuropathies caused by toxins and adverse drug reactions. Ophthalmol Clin North Am 2004: 17:481.

[39] Dogulu C. Chapter 7 (Section II): Hereditary Optic Neuropathy. In Neuro-ophthalmology Handbook. 1st ed. Ed. O'Dwyer PA, Kansu T, Torun T. Güneş Medicine Publishing;2008: 89-94 (Turkish).

[40] Newman NJ. Hereditary Optic Neuropathies: from the mitochondria to the optic nerve. Am J Ophthal. 2005; 140(3): 517-523.

[41] Votruba M, Fitzke FW, Holder CE, Carter A, Bhattacharya SS, Moore AT. Clinical features in affected individuals from 21 pedigrees with dominant optic atrophy. Arch Ophthalmol. 1998; 116(3): 353-358.

[42] Votruba M, Thiselton D, Bhattacharya SS.Optic disc morphology of patients with OPA1 autosomal dominant optic atrophy. Br J Ophthalmol 2003: 87:48.

[43] Alexander C, Votruba M, Pesch UE, et al. OPA1, encoding a dynamin-related GTPase, is mutated in autosomal dominant optic atrophy linked to chromosome 3q28. Nat Genet 2000: 26:211.

[44] Kjer B, Eiberg H, Kjer P, Rosenberg T. Dominant optic atrophy mapped to chromosome 3q region. II. Clinical and epidemiological aspects. Acta Ophthalmol Scand. 1996; 74(1): 3-7

[45] Howell N. LHON and other optic nerve atrophies: the mitochondrial connection. Dev Ophthalmol. 2003: 37:94.

[46] Smith JL, Hoyt WF, Susac JO. Ocular fundus in acute Leber optic neuropathy. Arch Ophthalmol 1973; 90:349.

[47] Kermode AG, Moseley IF, Kendall BE, et al. Magnetic resonance imaging in Leber's optic neuropathy. J Neurol Neurosurg Psychiatry 1989; 52:671.

[48] Lamirel C, Cassereau J, Cochereau I, et al. Papilloedema and MRI enhancement of the prechiasmal optic nerve at the acute stage of Leber hereditary optic neuropathy. J Neurol Neurosurg Psychiatry 2010; 81:578.

[49] Carelli V, La Morgia C, Sadun AA. Mitochondrial dysfunction in optic neuropathies: animal models and therapeutic options. Curr Opin Neurol. 2013; 26(1): 52-58.

[50] DiMauro S, Mancuso M. Mitochondrial diseases: therapeutic approaches. Biosci Rep. 2007; 27:125-3751-Golnik KC. Infectious optic neuropathy. Semin Ophthalmol 2002; 17:11.

[51] Ginestal RC, Plaza JF, Callejo JM, et al. Bilateral optic neuritis and Guillain-Barré syndrome following an acute Mycoplasma pneumoniae infection. J Neurol 2004; 251:767.

[52] Pfausler B, Engelhardt K, Kampfl A, et al. Post-infectious central and peripheral nervous system diseases complicating Mycoplasma pneumoniae infection. Report of three cases and review of the literature. Eur J Neurol 2002; 9:93.

[53] Venkatesh P, Garg SP, Verma L, et al. Combined optic neuropathy and central retinal artery occlusion in miliary tuberculosis. Retina 2001; 21:375.

[54] Rex JH, Larsen RA, Dismukes WE, et al. Catastrophic visual loss due to Cryptococcus neoformans meningitis. Medicine (Baltimore) 1993; 72:207.

[55] Fukushima A, Yasuoka M, Tsukahara M, Ueno H. A case of cat scratch disease neuroretinitis confirmed by polymerase chain reaction. Jpn J Ophthalmol 2003; 47:405.

[56] Gilden DH, Mahalingam R, Cohrs RJ, Tyler KL. Herpesvirus infections of the nervous system. Nat Clin Pract Neurol 2007; 3:82.

[57] Küçükerdönmez C, Akova YA, Yilmaz G. Ocular toxoplasmosis presenting as neuroretinitis: report of two cases. Ocul Immunol Inflamm 2002 10:229.

[58] Benz MS, Glaser JS, Davis JL. Progressive outer retinal necrosis in immunocompetent patients treated initially for optic neuropathy with systemic corticosteroids. Am J Ophthalmol 2003: 135:551.

[59] Ray S, Gragoudas E. Neuroretinitis. Int Ophthalmol Clin 2001: 41:83.

[60] Smith GT, Goldmeier D, Migdal C. Neurosyphilis with optic neuritis: an update. Postgrad Med J 2006: 82:36.

[61] Sibony P, Halperin J, Coyle PK, Patel K. Reactive Lyme serology in optic neuritis. J Neuroophthalmol 2005: 25:71.

[62] Tunc M. Chapter 5 (Section II): Inflammatory Optic Neuropathy. In Neuro-ophthalmology Handbooks. 1st ed. Ed. O'Dwyer PA, Kansu T, Torun T. Güneş Medicine Publishing;2008: 73-80 (Turkish)

[63] Jabs DA, Miller NR, Newman SA, et al. Optic neuropathy in systemic lupus erythematosus. Arch Ophthalmol 1986; 104:564.

[64] Kansu T, Kirkali P, Kansu E, Zileli T. Optic neuropathy in Behçet's disease. J Clin Neuroophthalmol 1989; 9:277.

[65] Wall M, George D. Idiopathic intracranial hypertension. A prospective study of 50 patients. Brain 1991; 114 (Pt 1A): 155.

Chapter 14

Low Vision Rehabilitation

Bennett McAllister and Rebecca Kammer

Additional information is available at the end of the chapter

http://dx.doi.org/10.5772/58436

1. Introduction

Low vision rehabilitation has developed along two approaches based on either the education/ vocational system or the medical model. In 1999, Massof and Lidoff [1] reviewed the issues in vision rehabilitation from a public policy, service delivery, and funding perspective. They delineate the evolution of services for persons with visual impairment as primarily originating within the education and vocational rehabilitation systems. The end goals from these perspectives would be educational achievement or vocational training and placement. Simultaneously, though, a medical model of low vision rehabilitation also existed within the United States' Veteran's Administration as it historically has provided military veterans comprehensive, in-patient rehabilitation services including visual aids or adaptive devices, instruction in living skills, communication, orientation & mobility (O&M) and more. The objective of the medical model of low vision rehabilitation is to restore function for improveddaily living skills. Although the strategies for rehabilitation within the education model and the medical model may be similar, the framework of this chapter is primarily based on principles of the medical model while borrowing valuable insight from the educational model.

Outside of the Veterans Administration but within health care professionals, some version of low vision rehabilitation has developed over the last several decades from a specialty or area of emphasis practiced by a few scattered experts in optometry, ophthalmology, and most recently nursing and occupational therapy. Entry-level skills in low vision rehabilitation have become a required competency for all optometry graduates [2]. It is also a requirement of all U.S. ophthalmology residencies to expose students to low vision rehabilitation.. Even so, low vision rehabilitation remains a field that is difficult to define precisely in that it still faces barriers within reimbursement structures and funding mechanisms [1].

In 2006, some progress in funding models was made as rehabilitation codes were designated by Medicare as applicable to vision rehabilitation. Occupational therapists with their training in aging and activities of daily living began offering low vision rehabilitation under the order or referral of a physician. Under Medicare definitions, this physician role in most cases is fulfilled by the low vision optometrist or ophthalmologist. Together with occupational therapy, a rehabilitation model similar to physical therapy rehabilitation models has emerged, however, the consensus and uniformity of low vision rehabilitation service provision in the U.S. remains inconsistent. In 2009, Cynthia Owsley [3] performed a large census of non-Veterans Affairs entities that performed low vision rehabilitation in the United States in an effort to describe the characteristics of services, types of providers and profile of patients. The result was the first large scale picture on the state of low vision rehabilitation. Among several findings were that 74.1% of patients had central vision loss with its attendant reading (85.9%) and driving (44.9%) problems. 67.1% were diagnosed with age related macular degeneration (AMD). Notably, the patient complaints were function related. This chapter presents an overview of the low vision rehabilitation field from a functional care perspective with the goal of enhancing the patient's quality of life. The emphasis is on a comprehensive, inclusive and interprofessional approach to the treatment and management of the whole patient related to their visual impairment and their specific functional goals.

2. Definitions and model

Every doctor who prescribes minus lenses to allow a myope to see distance objects, or vision therapy to relieve symptoms of convergence insufficiency or cataract surgery to give clearer vision is practicing vision rehabilitation even if not using the term. Indeed, most primary ophthalmic and optometric treatments are designed to restore visual system efficiency and patient functioning, and can surely be considered forms of vision rehabilitation in the broadest sense. Low Vision Rehabilitation, however, emphasizes care for people who have degraded visual function such as visual acuity, visual fields or contrast sensitivity to the point that restoration of previous visual abilities with standard optical corrective techniques like glasses and contact lenses or surgical procedures is no longer possible. The World Health Organization (WHO) provides two definitions for low vision:

1. Low vision is visual acuity less than 6/18 and equal to or better than 3/60 in the better eye with best correction.
2. A person with low vision is one who has impairment of visual functioning even after treatment and/or standard refractive correction, and has a visual acuity of less than 6/18 to light perception, or a visual field less than 10 degrees from the point of fixation, but who uses, or is potentially able to use, vision for the planning and/or execution of a task for which vision is essential.

These definitions are primarily based on measurement of visual abilities rather than the loss of function secondary to the loss of vision. This difference is crucial to the vision rehabilitation of the individual. What is important to one person may be inconsequential to another and treatments based on only visual acuity or visual field may prove unsatisfying for the patient. Therefore, our focus will be on the functional loss of independence when performing critical and desired activities of daily life (ADL). For our purposes in this chapter we will maintain the World Health Organization definitions and propose an additional definition:

3. Low Vision is *a loss of visual function (i.e.* Visual acuity, visual fields and/or contrast sensitivity) caused by an organic or non-organic mechanism resulting in a loss of functional ability and quality of life

Our emphasis in this chapter will be on people who developed as fully sighted then suffered an event or series of events that negatively impacted their visual systems. While it is true that infants with Retinopathy of Prematurity, inborn errors in metabolism, trauma, or other sight affecting conditions can be, and are, considered in the low vision field, and the principles in this chapter are applicable to them, the core view for this chapter will include rehabilitation approaches for those who have acquired vision loss in adulthood, rather than on congenital vision loss. With most visual impairment caused by conditions related to aging or present in aging adults, acquired vision loss in older adults presents the most challenge and burden from a social and economic perspective [4].

Low vision rehabilitation is presented as a three-part paradigm to provide a framework for the physician's evaluation and guided rehabilitation process within the medical model to the linking of services available outside of that model but within the valuable educational and vocational system.

Vision Rehabilitation secondary to our above definition is approached herein as a three part paradigm:

1. *Cause* Visual abilities loss and their measures
2. *Effect* How a person functions given their visual status
3. *Impact* How vision loss impacts quality of life (QOL) and the amelioration of Impact

Cause refers to the loss of visual ability in the key areas of visual acuity, visual fields and contrast sensitivity and how such losses operate to interfere with optimal eye and vision system performance.

Whereas *Cause* implies a vision dysfunction, *Effect* is related to the level of functional visual ability and performance independence given the associated *Cause. Effect* is addressed with standard health history questioning, symptom survey measures of functional independence and observational evaluation of the patient performing a task or series of tasks.

Lastly but quite important, we consider *Impact*, or how the loss of visual function contributes to the degradation of the person's quality of life. This is viewed from a patient reported, subjective evaluation of life status but it is addressed through referral and partnership with a number of providers that may be within or outside the medical system. Whereas the first two, *Cause* and *Effect*, can be addressed within the evaluation process of physician and therapist, the concept of *Impact* can be addressed in a broad fashion with appropriate referrals and education about resources. *Cause, Effect* and *Impact*, will be considered herein as overlapping and interconnected in order to effectively practice comprehensive, inclusive and interprofessional low vision rehabilitation.

It should be noted that health care has become increasingly divided into specialties in spite of a number of initiatives to integrate care across and among various disciplines. The sheer volume of knowledge necessary to become expert in just the various specialties of the eye and visual system, let alone the whole human body, strongly mitigate against the interprofessional efforts of universities, governments and non-government groups. As each provider's specific view of the patient becomes more and more limited to the aspect unique of their specialty, the overall view of the wellbeing of the patient can become more at risk of being diminished or lost. While the results of specialty treatments are separately efficacious to the parts they address, there is a danger in viewing the patient as an assemblage of parts. Many patients with low vision report hearing, "nothing more can be done" from the authority they trust when the authority means "I cannot do any more". The critical missing part of the conversation is: "but there may be someone who can." [5]

3. Chain of vision

One approach to moderating this potential point of patient vulnerability is by addressing it early in the exam process with the analogy that vision is like a chain. Each link in the chain is necessary for full visual functioning but none is sufficient alone. Therefore, repairing a single link does not make one see if there is more than one issue, but rather removes one barrier to vision. All link weaknesses must be ameliorated and all links must be whole for the chain of vision to be strong.

Chain Link One: Light
Chain Link Two : Clarity of Ocular Media
Chain Link Three: Optical Focus
Chain Link Four: Receptor Elements
Chain Link Five: Optic nerve and Pathways
Chain Link Six: Neural processing and brain associations

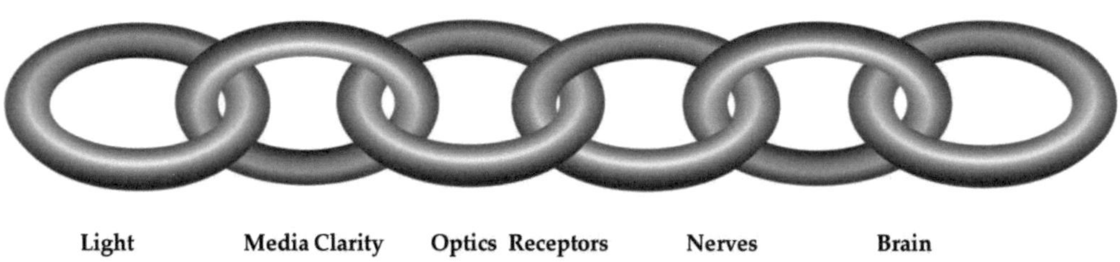

Figure 1. Chain of Vision

The first link is a sufficient amount of **light** to illuminate the object of regard and mitigation of glare.

The second link is **clear media** which can be compromised by cloudy corneas or lenses.

http://dx.doi.org/10.5772/58436

Third is the sharp **optical focus** of the image. This link is the only one impacted by glasses, contact lenses or refractive surgery.

Fourth are the **receptor elements** of the eye, or the retina which takes the "picture". Age related macular degeneration and diabetic retinopathy are primary diseases affecting this chain link.

Fifth we have transmission to the brain via the **optic nerve** and related pathways which can be compromised by atrophies, vascular accidents and trauma.

The sixth link is in the **brain** where **neural processing** takes place and associations occur. Stroke, aneurysms and accidents interfere with the chain of vision in this link.

While the Chain of Vision analogy sounds simplistic at first glance, it has proven memorable to patients who commonly believe it requires only glasses or surgery to make them see. Taking a few moments to introduce this model of Chain of Vision can yield multiple benefits downstream. Once the patient realizes all the links must work to see and once the specialist acts on the reality that their specialized treatment for one link is necessary but potentially insufficient for restoration of visual ability, we can work toward improving the patient's quality of life using the tools and techniques of the Low Vision Rehabilitation field.

Caution:

When considering the *Cause* of loss of vision ability, it is important to remember that the patient is not to be equated with their condition [6]. Regrettably, language frequently betrays a, perhaps unintended though nevertheless real, diminishment of our patients into a single category of disease through our labels. The adjective becomes the noun and the person becomes the condition. It is easy to think of a person as a "diabetic" or "albino" or "strabismic" but in so labeling them, we belittle, in a real way, the totality of the individual in our substitution of their wholeness into a single attribute. A person with diabetes or a person with albinism or a person with strabismus is first and foremost a person. A whole, complete person who has all the hopes, traits, abilities, talents, relationships and fears comparable to any other person. This clarity of differentiation is not trivial for many of our patients as it is language that shapes perception of reality and influences attitudes that direct care and treatment.

4. Cause

As Cause refers to the etiology and assessment of vision loss, the measure of that dysfunction on the patient's function will guide the low vision rehabilitation practitioner's approach to understanding the *Effect* and to ameliorate the *Impact* on the patient's quality of life. Although there are many visual capacities explored in a comprehensive low vision rehabilitation exam, this chapter will highlight the three key measurable attributes of (1) visual acuity, (2) visual fields and (3) contrast sensitivity. Visual acuity (VA), or sharpness of vision, is the primary vision attribute measured in assessing visual ability as it directly affects reading and driving. Visual fields and contrast sensitivity are reviewed later in this chapter as they have been demonstrated to correlate with particular patient complaints and functioning such as reading ability, facial recognition, mobility and fall risk.

The two most common causes of low vision in the U.S. are age related macular degeneration and diabetic retinopathy affect all three of the above visual functions [7-9]. Most commonly found in people over age 65, age related macular degeneration primarily disrupts visual acuity and central visual fields. The leading cause of vision loss for those under age 65 is diabetic retinopathy which similarly yields reduced visual acuity but generally with greater contrast sensitivity loss and varying amounts of visual field loss. Though visual acuity is typically easy to measure, the standard in-office charts have been designed for the fully sighted person and the design assumptions underlying them can lead to invalid outcomes when used to measure visual acuity in people with low vision.

4.1. *Cause* — Visual acuity

There are several types of visual acuity. Therefore, it might be more appropriate to speak of "the visual acuities" rather than just the singular "visual acuity" and review them sequentially to develop a common foundation that provides us good confidence in the validity of our clinical results. Measurements in one category do not necessarily correlate with those of another. Indeed, as there can be significant variances between and among the categories, it is important to identify the type of acuity one is assessing and not compare across psychometric boundaries. We will then examine these systems used to measure and record VA and investigate how the proper documentation can generate useful extrapolations regarding patient performance and treatment choices.

The first type of VA is **Detection Acuity**. This is the "ah-ha" acuity often expressed by subjects with the expression, "look, something is there!" Detection acuity is useful for safe ambulation, scanning for new information sources in the environment, and defense against approaching dangers. It is not, however, much use in the gathering of form details such as reading, driving or facial recognition.

The second category of VA on our list is **Resolution Acuity**, or the ability to differentiate (resolve) a gap or change in an object or image. This allows an observer to tell a letter "C" from an "O" and forms the basis for the Landolt C acuity charts. The patient is to tell which direction the opening is pointing. Multiple presentations of the Landolt C in various orientations quickly yield a high level of confidence in the final result if the patient gets them all correct. Resolution is useful when an observer knows something is there (detection) but cannot recognize any elements. Extracting some details from the image can generate knowledge of space, distance and, in unfamiliar areas, safety. Resolution acuity does not, however, allow the observer to gather detailed or coded (e.g. alphabet) information.

Vernier Acuity is generally of more interest to vision scientists than to the clinician. Still, it has found utility in geographic areas where it is important to triage patients with severe cataracts when there are not enough ophthalmic surgeons to meet the need. Screening with vernier acuity can help determine who has macular function sufficient to benefit from cataract removal.

Recognition Acuity is the standard of most distance visual acuity test charts. Being able to not only know something is there (detection) and that there are gaps or a space in the image

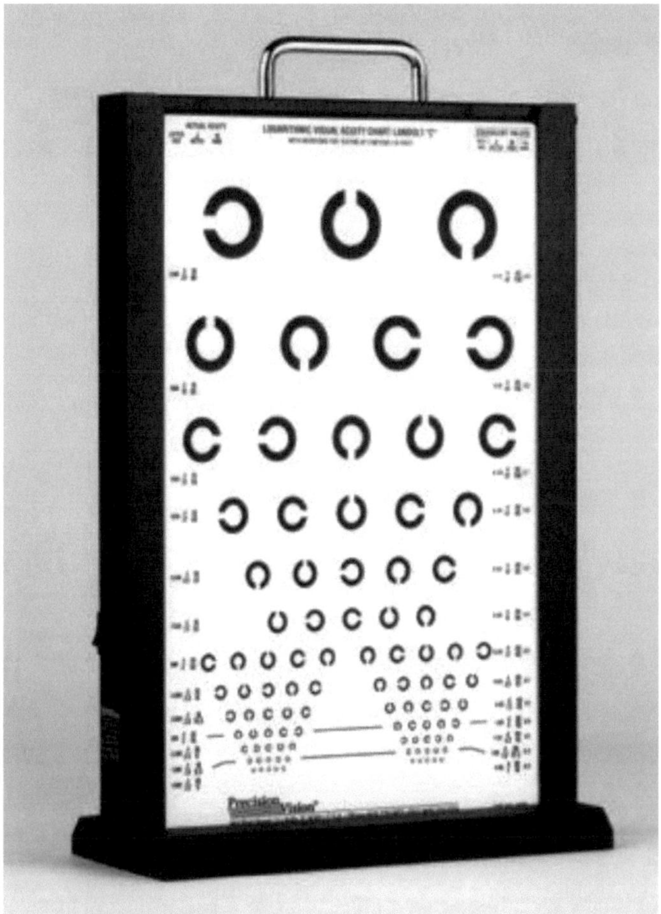

Figure 2. Landolt C Resolution Acuity Chart

(resolution), but to identify it with visual cues is the key to reading printed materials and language. This is the core issue for people with the central vision impairment caused by age related macular degeneration or diabetic retinopathy. Poor recognition acuity is the primary motivator for people with macular issues to present for a low vision rehabilitation evaluation. Inability to recognize faces and difficulty reading disempowers the individual leading to dependencies in the demands of modern daily life and, too frequently, less than optimal quality of life. The concept of recognition acuity, unfortunately, is so comfortably familiar to clinicians that its real meaning can become muddled when it is inappropriately used. Therefore, we need a psychometric standard for our results to have useful meaning in low vision rehabilitation.

The first chart incorporating the most significant psychometric principles was the Bailey-Lovie chart, first introduced in the late 1970s [10]. It was developed to address all the significant factors in the measurement of recognition acuity including equivalent readability of the letters, stroke height of letters, equal contour interaction both within and between rows of letters,

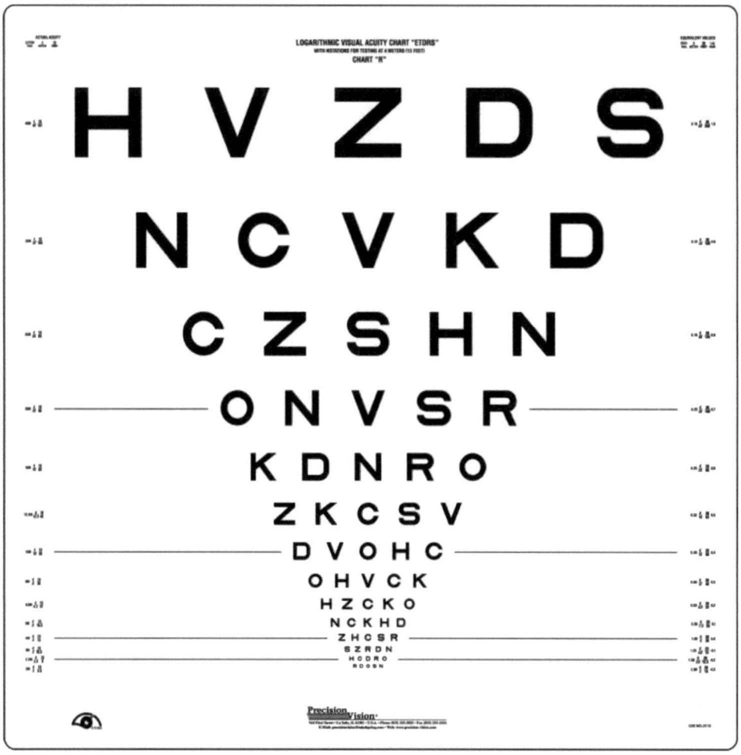

Figure 3. Recognition Acuity Chart ETDRS

equal numbers of single letters per row and logarithmic progression of test task within and between rows. This last aspect takes advantage of Weber's Law and yields valuable predictive power in choosing lenses, working distance, magnification and telescopes for patients' needs. In the early 1980s, the Early Treatment of Diabetic Retinopathy Study (ETDRS) test chart was developed, largely from the Bailey-Lovie design and has been the standard for Recognition visual acuity ever since. The standardizing of test task equivalence yielded by both these charts gives a high level of confidence in the validity and repeatability of measurements, allowing more accurate and consistent collection of data and a solid basis for comparison of past and future visual performance when tracking the course of the patient's condition and the success or lack thereof in treatment.

Recording recognition visual acuity is optimally done with the Snellen fraction, writing the numerator as the test distance, preferably in the logarithmic progression of distances and letter size read at threshold as the denominator, also in the logarithmic sequence of Just-Noticeable-Differences (JND) (both discussed more fully in the *Cause*-LogMAR section below) while always keeping the units in the same system (English or Metric). When visual acuity is always and only recorded as a fraction with actual test distance over actual letter size measured, all the pertinent visual acuity information is captured and available for use by the clinician.

http://dx.doi.org/10.5772/58436

Refraction is an aspect of visual acuity that requires addressing even if it is too large a topic to explore completely in our chapter context. The phoropter is the instrument developed for refraction of fully sighted patients and serves that purpose very well. It uses small steps of dioptric power to determine the patient's ametropia because the Just-Noticeable-Difference of fully sighted patients is roughly only a quarter of a diopter (0.25D) as found in the phoropter. Partially sighted patients, however, have variable Just-Noticeable-Differences depending on their level of acuity or sensitivity and therefore need an approach based on differential lens steps to accommodate the presenting Just-Noticeable-Difference. This is achieved by the use of a trial frame and trial lens set with techniques adapted to the sensitivity of the partially sighted patient. The whole range of visual acuities and Just-Noticeable-Difference variances can be addressed using the principles of LogMAR progression steps of significance.

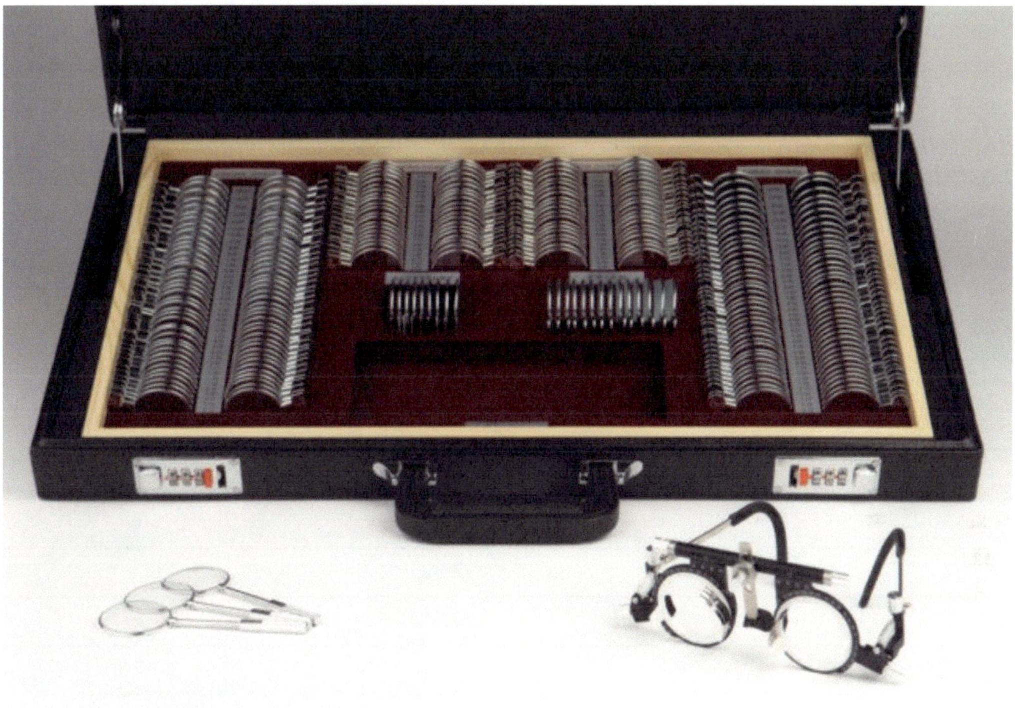

Figure 4. Trial Lens Set with Trial Frame and hand held Jackson Flip Cross Lenses

4.2. *Cause* — LogMAR

Weber's Law – The change in stimulus which is necessary to evoke a just-noticeable-difference (JND) in sensation bears a constant ratio to the original stimulus from which it was derived.

This broad law of human stimulus perception is deceptively simple in its presentation yet potentially powerful for predicting patient performance with induced changes in stimulus. While Weber's law is not immutable, especially with stimuli at the extremes of the spectrum, it does provide guidance with stimuli changes that are manifest in the activities of daily life. When considering formed image stimuli measurable by recognition acuity charts, the constant ratio, or logarithmic progression, of Just-Noticeable-Differences is remarkably consistent and reliable over the range of standard measures. Given this characteristic of Just-Noticeable-Differences being a constant ratio, and charts designed with the principles of psychometric integrity and test task equivalence, we have the foundation for using acuity measurements to predict visual performance when we introduce reading lens changes, working distance adjustments or telescopic power variations to the patient, other factors being equal. All that is missing for us to lever the potential power of Weber's Law in predicting patient performance is a starting "original stimulus." Fortunately, we have Robert Hooke, sometimes known as "England's DaVinci." We can thank him for developing an employment test aimed at potential astronomy assistants. Hooke had the assistant candidates count the stars in the Big Dipper. Since one "star" is really two stars (Alcor and Mizar) separated visually by approximately one minute of arc, he declared those that passed had good vision and the stage was set for one minute of arc to be the standard of visual acuity. However apocryphal the story might be, we have our "original stimulus" or minimum angle of resolution (MAR) from which to begin our logarithmic progression for charts, working distances, dioptric lens powers and telescopic magnification: one minute of arc.

Work in the late nineteenth century demonstrated the constant ratio for detecting visual change as 0.1 $\log_{10}$ units. From our starting point of a minimum angle of resolution of one minute of arc, and a Weber's Law constant of 0.1 log units we can build a table of significance for visual acuity:

LogMAR	MAR (′)	VA (English)	VA (Metric)
0.0	1.0	20/20	6/6
0.1	1.25	20/25	6/8
0.2	1.6	20/32	6/10
0.3	2.0	20/40	6/12.5
0.4	2.5	20/50	6/16
0.5	3.2	20/63	6/20
0.6	4.0	20/80	6/25
0.7	5.0	20/100	6/32
0.8	6.3	20/125	6/40
0.9	8.0	20/160	6/50
1.0	10.0	20/200	6/60

Table 1. MAR, LogMAR and Visual Acuity

http://dx.doi.org/10.5772/58436

This chart design enables thinking of the steps between the lines as "steps of significance". These steps can be Diopters (D), working distance, letter size when working at near, or telescopic magnification for distance. At near, a change in one step for diopters necessitates a change in one step of distance, resulting (all other variables being equal) of one step in letter size. As diopters add increases by a step, working distance decreases by a step as does letter size. In the above table, the MAR column can be thought of as the "Steps" column.

Steps	Diopters Add (D)	Working Distance (cm)	Letter Size (M)
Start	2.50	40	2.0
1	3.25	32	1.6
2	4.00	25	1.25
3	5.00	20	1.0
4	6.25	16	0.8
5	8.00	12.5	0.63
6	10.00	10	0.5

Table 2. LogMAR Reading Example

When working with telescopic powers, one always begins with best distance refraction and working distance is always infinity. Since the eye by definition has a magnification at distance of "1", all step changes start from there.

Steps	Telescope Power	Acuity
Start	1.0	20/200
1	1.25	20/160
2	1.6	20/125
3	2.0	20/100
4	2.5	20/80
5	3.25	20/63
6	4.0	20/50
7	5.0	20/40
8	6.3	20/32
9	8.0	20/25

Table 3. LogMAR telescope example

One can see the utility in charts built with LogMAR, but before using these steps of significance for treatment choices in the *Impact* section, it is important to examine near visual acuity and reading ability.

4.3. *Cause* — Reading

Near visual acuity and reading ability are different tasks yet sometimes conflated inappropriately thereby becoming a source of frustration for the doctor and patient when expectations of reading ability in the patient's life and near acuity measures from the doctor's office do not align.

Charts properly designed for near visual acuity give results strongly correlated with distance acuity. The rules of building significance for distance ETDRS charts apply for the near charts allowing maximum degrees of freedom in choosing working distance, add powers and magnification. Image 5 shows a single digit near visual acuity chart with a 40cm string that can be used to control working distance. The string can also be folded in half for a 20cm working distance but any distance on the LogMAR scale can reasonably be used.

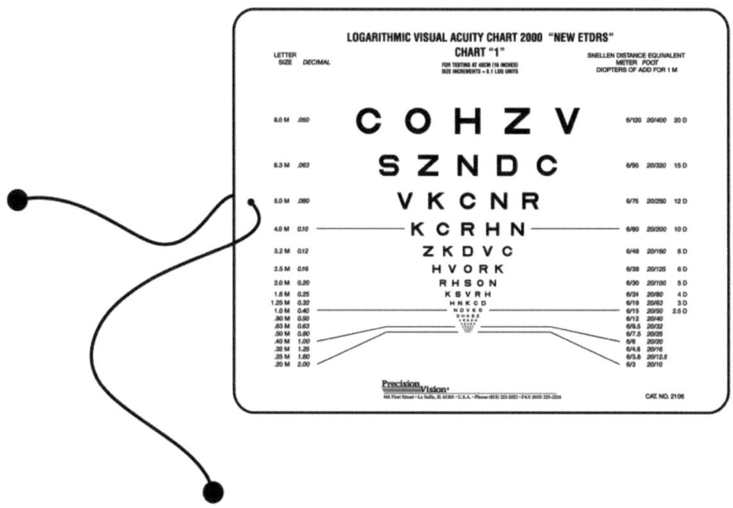

Figure 5. Single Digit near chart

Near Visual Acuity has four common systems of recording, only one of which has the psychometric integrity necessary for our purposes. (1) Reduced Snellen does not capture either letter size or working distance. (2) Point system (n-units) captures image size but not working distance in a useable format. (3) Jaeger or "J" size is not standardized among chart manufacturers and does not record working distance in a meaningful way. Only (4) M-Units recorded as a Snellen fraction of distance in meters over M size provides information in a fashion which can be used in calculating dioptric lens powers and working distances for low vision rehabilitation work.

http://dx.doi.org/10.5772/58436

Example of Recorded M-Unit acuity: 0.4/1.0M means at 40 cm, the patient was able to recognize a 1.0M letter

Once the near single digit visual acuity is determined and recorded in M-Unit fashion, variations in working distance and dioptric lens power can be manipulated to meet patient acuity goals using LogMAR principles discussed previously.

Reading for information, however, is a complex activity of which near Visual Acuity is only one part. Therefore, a reading task requires a more complete description than just acuity. One method that accounts for reading's complexity is the MN Read cards system which incorporates three factors affecting reading performance: (1) Reading Acuity, (2) Maximum Reading Speed and (3) Critical Print Size.

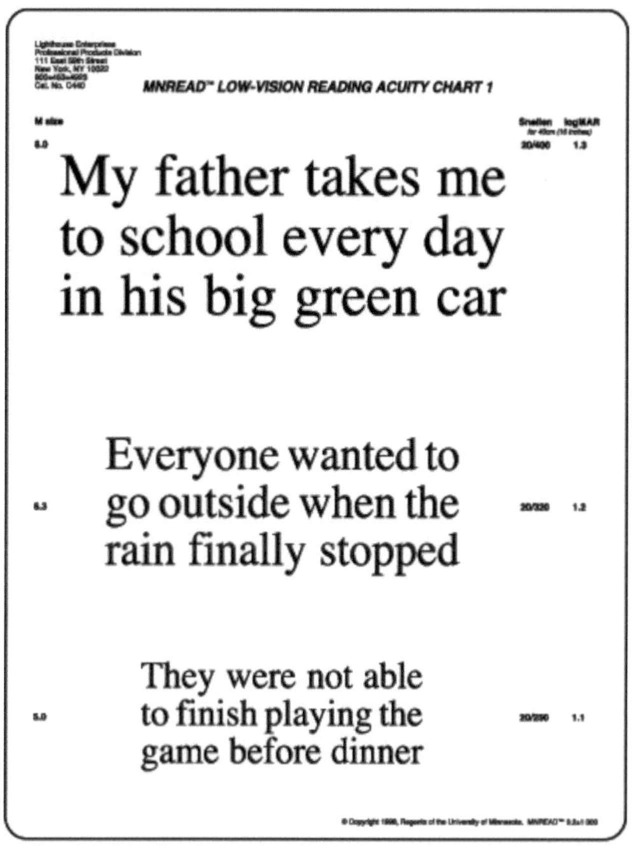
MNREAD™ LOW-VISION READING ACUITY CHART 1
My father takes me
to school every day
in his big green car
Everyone wanted to
go outside when the
rain finally stopped
They were not able
to finish playing the
game before dinner

Figure 6. MN Read Near Card

Reading acuity (1) is the smallest resolvable print size, similar to near visual acuity. Maximum Reading Speed (2) is the top rate at which a patient can read contextual words for information. Critical Print Size (3) is the smallest print size that the patient can read at maximum reading speed. Combining these three reading components allows a more thorough understanding of reading in patients with low vision. Additionally, it demonstrates to the patient how their reading is affected by the three factors and that it can be improved with changes in add, working distance and letter size.

A reading test developed primarily for the patient with the central field defects (scotomas) that are commonly found in age related macular degeneration is the Smith-Kettlewell Reading test (SK Read) by Don Fletcher. The test is different from the MN read as it uses words that when combined into a block of a particular size print, the block contains no contextual meaning. This means that reading errors caused by central field defects or scotomas and the corresponding preferred retinal locus (PRL) will be apparent as the patient cannot use context to guess words. Both the reading speed and number of errors are recorded which results in a reading error rate per block of text. The test instructions provide guidance for interpreting the locations of the errors as related to the location of the patient's scotoma relative to fixation. The test can also be used to educate the patient on the impact of central scotomas on reading so that when both magnification and fixation training are included in the final rehabilitation plan, the patient is aware of the complexities of their reading facility and the rehabilitation process.

4.4. *Cause* — Visual field

The low vision rehabilitation domain has traditionally divided visual field impairments into the two general areas of centralfields and peripheral fields. The type of loss in either area affects patient function in different ways. Peripheral field losses such as overall constriction and hemianopsias can affect mobility and activities of daily life but are a small percentage of total scotomas compared to acquired central field loss as found in age related macular degeneration. Therefore, the emphasis in low vision rehabilitation is properly on central and paracentral loss.

Although it has been well understood that scotomas or visual field defects occur in the progression of many visually debilitating conditions, the understanding of how to best measure the central and paracentral scotoma and relate that measurement to patient visual abilities and low rehabilitation strategies is a newer concept. Traditionally, a central automated visual field or an Amsler grid was considered the test of choice for evaluating the central visual field but both of these tests are problematic when applied to rehabilitation of a patient.

As early as 1987, Timberlake, Peli, and Augliere [12] used a Scanning LASER Ophthalmoscope (SLO) and derived the term preferred retinal locus (PRL) to describe a "single, idiosyncratic retinal area, immediately adjacent to the scotoma, for fixating, inspecting acuity targets, and scanning simple, nonsense-syllable text". They also determined the preferred retinal locus may not be the ideal location for reading text nor was it always situated as close to the fovea as possible. In 1999, Schuchard, Naseer and de Castro determined both that the location of the preferred retinal locus affects visual performance of the patient and the location may shift over the progression of the disease-true especially of patients with a ring scotoma [13]. Additional studies have suggested that the development of a preferred retinal locus occurs within 6 months of visual loss and that multiple fixation locations can be used depending on the visual task.

There are varying opinions about how the location of the scotoma relative to the preferred retinal locus impact reading rates and about how to best train patients to use their preferred retinal locus or to even use a new better positioned trained retinal locus (TRL). For example, Deruaz (2006) [14] asserted that reading requires two conditions (1) detailed discrimination and (2) global viewing (i.e. seeing the whole length or words). A natural preferred retinal locus may only provide detailed discrimination but might be in a location that prevents the second important reading criteria, global viewing (2006). Nillson (2003) [15] and Deruaz (2006) have successfully selected a new location for the patient, a trained retinal locus (TRL), typically above or below the scotoma for hopes of improving function. Although they achieved short term success in the use of a trained retinal locus or a combination of preferred retinal locus and trained retinal locus for reading, it is unclear how the patient may utilize the trained retinal locus alone or in combination with their preferred retinal locus for activities of daily life in the long term or for improved vision related quality of life (VRQOL).

Another rehabilitation approach, training with the existing preferred retinal locus for fixation stability, has been demonstrated to successfully improve reading speed. Most recent literature on scotomas and function support the use of strategies aimed at improving fixation stability with the natural preferred retinal locus strategies [16, 17].

Many clinicians, instead of using any type of perimetry with age related macular degeneration patients, employ techniques such as asking the patient to identify parts of the doctor's face that may be missing or numbers on a clock face that may be absent or difficult to view. These techniques suffer from subjectivity and poor quantification. The patient is an unreliable source to describe the presence of binocular scotomas and the "missing areas" that result. Fletcher found that out of 153 patients with age related macular degeneration who were asked if they were able to see or notice their blind spots, 56% were totally unaware of their presence, and of those patients who did notice something missing they were only able to vaguely describe how objects disappeared. Microperimetry and determination of the patients most commonly used preferred retinal locus is invaluable for modern rehabilitation methods that incorporate training strategies teaching steady eye fixation. [18]

According to Markowitz (2013), the three parameters of macular function that should be assessed during a low vision rehabilitation evaluation are (1) scotoma characteristics, (2) preferred retinal loci and (3) oculomotor control [19]. This can be done through the use of microperimeter or scanning LASER ophthalmoscope to view the fundus while simultaneous projecting viewing targets directly on areas of the retina. Although microperimetry is used extensively in research settings and in a few comprehensive low vision clinics, the cost and time to perform such testing limits their current use in low vision rehabilitation clinics. Until more widespread adoption of microperimetry in low vision clinics occurs, less expensive and time intensive strategies have been recommended such tests as the California Central Visual Field Test (CCVFT) by Fletcher, Cole, and Kammer [20]. The California Central Visual Field Test utilizes three different modified LASER pointers with varying output and beam diameters as visual stimulation. The fixation target is in the center of series of rings printed on letter size paper. The test is positioned at a near distance that allows for simple determination of size of the scotoma in degrees with simultaneous recording of scotoma boundaries directly on the test. The test is similar to a tangent screen in the utilization of both static and kinetic target presentations and does require the clinician to simultaneously observe both the patient's fixation and record the boundaries of the scotoma.

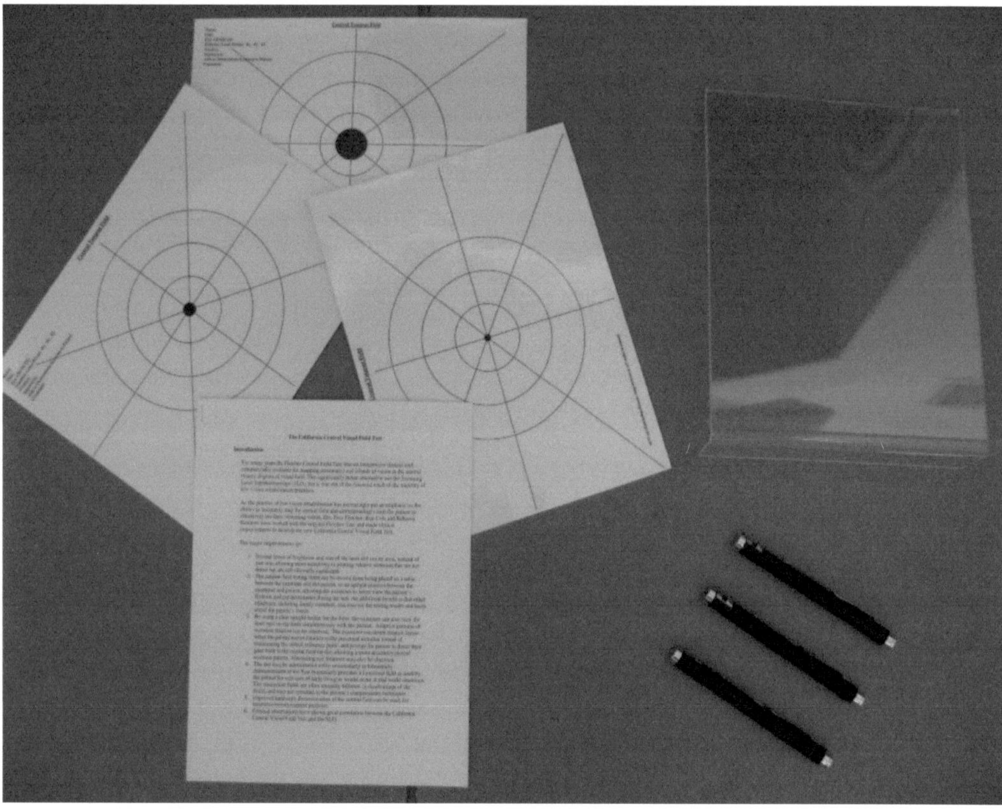

Figure 7. California Central Visual Field Test (CCVFT)

4.5. *Cause* — Contrast sensitivity

Contrast Sensitivity Function is the third important attribute of visual ability quantified in a low vision rehabilitation exam. The term "Contrast" refers to the difference between the highest and lowest brightness levels of a target. A person's ability to detect the minimum difference in contrast for a particular size image is designated "Contrast Sensitivity" and the plot of Contrast Sensitivity to object (letter) size is called the "Contrast Sensitivity Function". Contrast Sensitivity is affected primarily by optics, retinal function and neural processing. Since the most common conditions that cause visual impairment are age related macular degeneration and diabetic retinopathy, poor retinal function is the predominant cause of contrast sensitivity loss in this population.

http://dx.doi.org/10.5772/58436

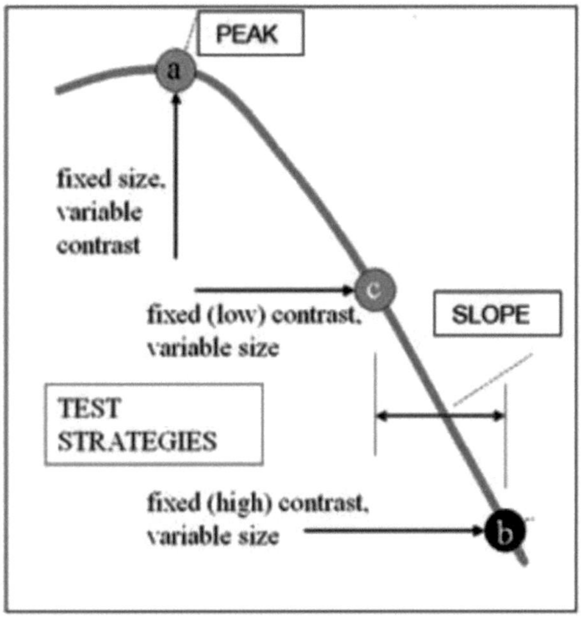

Figure 8. Contrast Sensitivity Curve

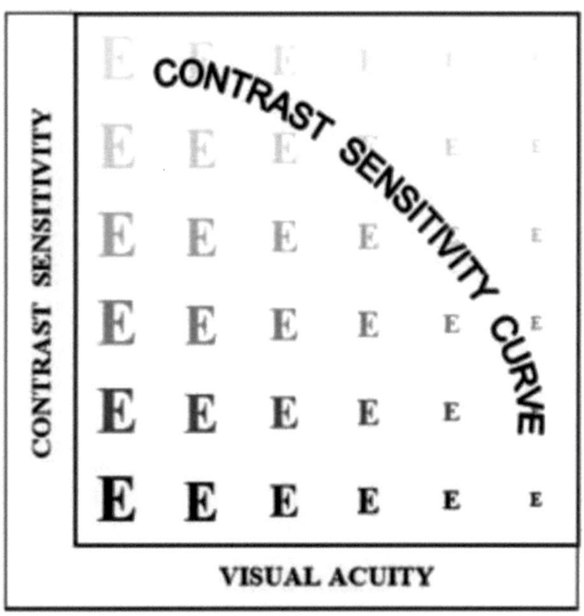

Figure 9. Contrast Sensitivity Curve Illustration

Threshold visual acuity is actually measured on a CSF graph being, in essence, the single point farthest to the right.

Reasonably, therefore, Contrast Sensitivity Function has not been shown to add any prescriptive value beyond standard visual acuity in measures of reading function when using high contrast materials. Activities of daily living such as walking, cooking, and grooming, however, often consist of visual cues with less than optimum contrast that present as various sizes and can cause functional visual difficulties for patients with low vision. In particular, mobility speed and safety are correlated with Contrast Sensitivity Function [21].

In examining the CSF, where visual acuity is along the X-axis and contrast sensitivity along the Y-axis, we find the peak contrast sensitivity for fully sighted people at mid-sized objects. As objects get smaller or larger, contrast sensitivity performance drops off. The CSF curve deviates differentially when retinal function is negatively affected by a condition or disease. Typical contrast measurements might be obtained with high contrast, small letter objects even while the ability to detect larger, lower contrast objects declines. This would be manifest by the ability to read standard vision charts well but subjective patient reports of significant issues in mobility such as not being able to see a curb or step. Functionally, this can lead to increased fall risk. When only considering visual acuity, these functional complaints seem to be out of proportion to the measured acuity, and indeed they are. Only when Contrast Sensitivity Function is considered are the subjective complaints accounted for.

There are several tests to evaluate CSF including sine wave gratings of variable contrast and size, Pelli-Robson or MARS letter triplets of varying contrast, and ETDRS or Text charts at distance or near with varying levels of contrast between presented charts. Each test has its own scoring which makes cross test extrapolation less than satisfactory, but each type of testing yields results that characterize patient complaints unaccounted for by acuity and visual field tests. Loss of Contrast in the higher spatial frequencies (small letters) usually signifies threshold visual acuity loss, while Contrast loss in lower spatial frequencies (large letters) could indicate poor ability to detect large, low contrast items in a path and lead to increased trip hazard and fall risk. Since visual acuity can be a good predictor of higher spatial frequency losses, particular attention regarding CSF should be paid to loss of contrast in lower spatial frequencies. In the past, contrast sensitivity testing was often left to the vision researchers and less commonly addressed in clinical vision examinations. This could be due to the complexity and the time required to complete and interpret testing. New types of charts that enable a quick screening of CSF loss such as the Mixed Contrast Chart by Gus Colenbrander [22] could be used to identify significant defects as well as educate patients and caregivers about the impact of loss.

Losses in the lower spatial frequencies are not generally improved by optical devices, but the attendant functional losses can be ameliorated with techniques and training by qualified professionals such as Orientation and Mobility (O&M) instructors and Occupational Therapists (OT).

http://dx.doi.org/10.5772/58436

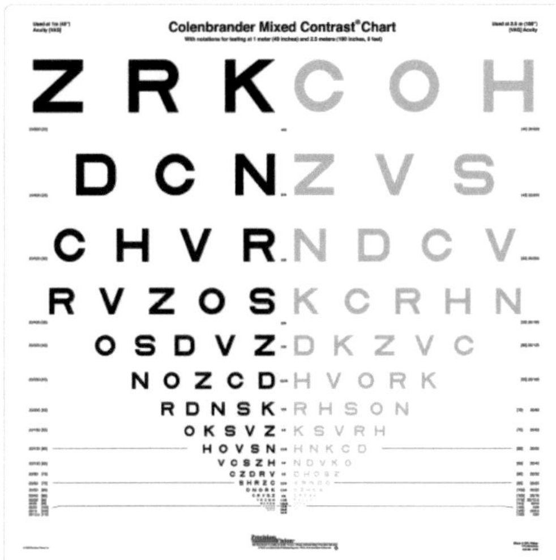

Figure 10. Colenbrander Mixed Contrast Chart

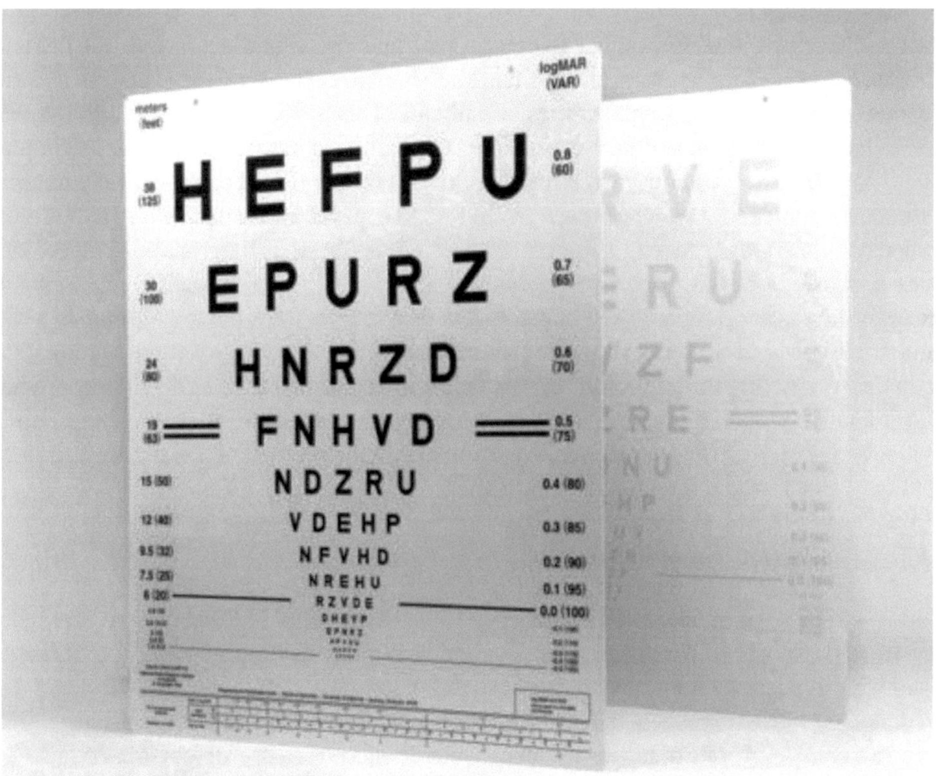

Figure 11. ETDRS Two Contrast Charts

4.6. *Cause* — Lighting

Lighting is more problematic to quantify than visual acuity, visual fields and contrast sensitivity function, and although it is not a measure of visual dysfunction directly, understanding how it may change the assessment of the other deficits is important. Lighting or illumination is a potentially key factor in ameliorating the *Effect* of the visual condition on function and its *Impact* on quality of life. For patients with significant contrast sensitivity loss, illumination can improve function and effectively decrease the amount of magnification needed to achieve the patients reading goals [23]. In addition, Schuchard and Lei discovered that in patients with relative central scotomas, some patients use different preferred retinal loci locations in high illumination settings for different visual and reading tasks [24]. Compounding contrast sensitivity loss with central scotomas can result in reading impairment to a much greater degree than would predicted by single optotype acuity testing under optimum office conditions. Therefore, evaluating the patient's response to lighting during the low vision rehabilitation exam process is necessary if both contrast sensitivity and the central visual field have been found to be compromised during standard testing of visual acuity, visual field and contrast sensitivity testing.

4.7. *Effect* — Functional sequelae of cause

Once the *Cause* of the vision deficit is determined and the visual acuity, visual fields and contrast sensitivity parameters measured, it is important to define how the visual deficit affects the patient's function regarding activities of daily life. This is done initially with the standard vision exam history. In a primary care exam, the standard measures of Chief Complaint, Review of Systems (ROS) and Past, Family & Social History (PFSH) are generally adequate. For the patient with low vision, however, these three standard history categories are often insufficient. Vision loss can affect the patient in such a way that they adapt by avoiding an activity and may not even recognize they can no longer perform it or that they even want to. Once accommodation is made, the specific loss of function may not be elicited in a Chief Complaint, Review of Systems, Past Family and Social History profile of questioning. Therefore, in a low vision rehabilitation history it is important to probe in a more comprehensive and systematic manner. Symptom surveys of independence and third party observations of activities of daily living can provide a more complete picture of the *Effect* and give us guidance for effective low vision rehabilitation treatment.

4.8. *Effect* — Directed symptom survey

Vision specific questions alone do not always address the totality of *Effect* on activities of daily living for the person with a vision loss. A more complete system needs to be utilized for evaluating the patient's level of ability and independence. The Functional Independence Measures (FIM) structure meets these requirements [25, 26]. FIM separately evaluates thirteen tasks on a seven point scale of Independence – Dependence. It is a useful tool to ascertain where a patient is having difficulty performing common activities of daily living, identify those activities a patient has given up on or is avoiding, and to direct the rehabilitation team's ongoing efforts. Functional independence measures can also be used to monitor progress of the patient's treatment regimen and evaluate care goals. While functional independence measure scaling is necessarily subjective, it is rubric driven around specified criteria to improve validity. Limiting the number of questions and the number of associated scaled responses to each question allows us to glean valuable information regarding activities of daily life objectives in a short time.

The following is a list of thirteen categories for the functional tasks that have been selected to be each graded using a seven point scale of perceived independence/dependence.

1. Cooking
2. Cleaning
3. Grooming
4. Finances
5. Self-Care
6. Ambulating Home
7. Ambulating Out
8. Reading Sustained
9. Reading Spot
10. Other Near Tasks
11. Intermediate Tasks
12. Distance Tasks
13. Technology

These thirteen functional task categories are reasonably self-explanatory and understandable for the patient who ranks each task on a seven point scale with a score of seven being completely independent and a score of one being total dependence. A measure of independence with no helper is only possible at the level of six or seven. Dependence levels are ranked from five to one with subscales for modified dependence and complete dependence. Details for scaling independence are described in Table 4.

After the level of Dependency is established for each of the thirteen categories, we can direct our rehabilitation efforts more rationally in mitigating the *Effect* of the vision deficit on the patient's life. For example, a patient with scores of six and seven in all categories except Sustained Reading needs little attention to distance rehabilitation devices or activities of daily living training. Rather, we should concentrate on reading devices, training and techniques. Similarly, a patient with scores of six and seven in all categories except Ambulating Out will need a referral to the Orientation and Mobility (O&M) member of the rehabilitation team, not new magnifiers. Processing functioning scores at the entrance testing level of our low vision rehabilitation evaluation not only directs the doctor toward the most efficacious avenue to proceed in the exam, but makes the patient aware there might be possibilities for them in

INDEPENDENT Another person is not required for the activity (NO HELPER).	
	7 Complete Independence - All of the tasks described as making up the activity are typically performed safely without modification, assistive devices (other than standard glasses or contact lenses) and within a reasonable time frame.
	6 Modified Independence - Activity requires any one or more of the following: An assistive device beyond standard glasses or contact lenses, more than reasonable time, or there are safety (risk) considerations.
DEPENDENT Another person is required for either supervision or physical assistance in order for the activity to be performed, or it is not performed (REQUIRES HELPER).	
	MODIFIED DEPENDENCE - The subject expends 50% or more of the needed effort to perform the task. The levels of assistance required are:
	5 Supervision or Setup - Subject requires no more help than standby, cueing or coaxing, without physical contact. Or, helper sets up needed items.
	4 Minimal Contact Assistance - With physical contact the subject requires no more help than touching, and subject expends 75% or more of the effort.
	3 Moderate Assistance - Subject requires more help than touching, or expends between 50% and 75% of the effort required to perform the task.
	COMPLETE DEPENDENCE - The subject expends less than 50% of the effort, maximal or total assistance is required, or the activity is not performed. The levels of assistance required are:
	2 Maximal Assistance - Subject expends between 25% and 50% of effort for task
	1 Total Assistance - Subject expends less than 25% of the effort.

Table 4. FIM Independence Rubric

categories on which they had given up or are avoiding. This sets functional scoring apart from standard history taking of Chief Complaint, Review of Systems and Past, Family and Social History and opens up options for addressing aspects in the life of the patient with low vision that are never manifest in fully sighted patients and hence have never become a part of standard history taking in a primary care vision exam. Asking the patient their Chief Complaint or reason for presenting is necessary yet many times inadequate for those with vision impairment. Directed probing at the beginning of the low vision rehabilitation evaluation rationalizes the process for the doctor, opens up the patient to possibilities they might not have considered and prepares the patient for thinking beyond just glasses and magnifiers. As the *Effect* on the low vision patient is qualitatively different from the fully sighted patient, so must the history be.

4.9. *Impact* — Quality of life

Impact in our paradigm of low vision rehabilitation refers to how the how the loss of vision and vision related function (*Cause* and *Effect*) contribute to the degradation of the individual's quality of life. Whereas *Cause* and *Effect* can be addressed within the evaluation process of physician and therapist, the concept of *Impact* may need to be additionally addressed in a broader fashion beyond low vision rehabilitation optical devices with appropriate referrals and education about resources.

Quality of life is a common phrase, but as a precisely definable concept remains elusive. The various conceptualizations of quality of life do, however, generally tend to include objective and subjective measures in a multi-dimensional manner while recognizing individual, societal and economic values. Though details do vary between the various instruments of quality of life measures, the categories essentially overlap and usually include aspects of a person's physical, material, social and emotional well-being. Therefore, rather than a blueprint of precision, quality of life definitions and measurement tools present a more general framework of reference. They are not typically used clinically on every low vision rehabilitation patient due to the time limitations for their administration, but have been used to validate the efficacy of treatment models.

Patient Reported Outcomes (PRO) are being increasingly used by third party and government regulators to assess care quality from the viewpoint of the patient and society. Among these are a number of quality of life surveys that seek to validate treatment efficacy. Khadka, McAlinden, and Pesudovs [27] conducted a comprehensive survey of the field in 2013 and found 121 vision related patient reported outcomes with 48 meeting the quality inclusion criteria for question unidimensionality and interval-level measurement. Of those, only six were related to low vision rehabilitation and one, the Veteran Affairs Low-Vision Functioning Questionnaire was considered highest quality. This patient reported outcome structure was validated in the Veteran Affairs Low Vision Intervention Trial (LOVIT) which reported significant improvement in every facet of visual function outcomes for patients who received low vision rehabilitation treatment. Even so, with 48 questions, it involved a significant time commitment to administer. While the outcomes of low vision rehabilitation have been shown to be positive, the studies point to time constraints as one of the main difficulties in performing current quality of life surveys on every patient. In addition, the current state of quality of life surveys is limited by the fixed question format which does not provide for adaptive questions based on preceding answers, thus limiting the comprehensiveness and individuality of the results.

The World Health Organization [28] broadly defines quality of life as "an individual's perception of their position in life in the context of the culture and value systems in which they live and in relation to their goals, expectations, standards and concerns. It is a broad ranging concept affected in a complex way by the person's physical health, psychological state, personal beliefs, social relationships and their relationship to salient features of their environment."

The Center for Disease Control [29] subsequently added the concept of health related quality of life (HRQOL) in order to parse out those aspects of overall quality of life pertaining particularly to health. Defining, measuring and tracking health related quality of life is intended to be used to improve public health decision-making and allocation of resources.

Vision Related Quality of Life (VRQOL) [30] is a term referring to those parts of quality of life affected by vision. Instruments have been developed that seek to provide guidance in making economic health evaluations of eye care and rehabilitation programs. These instruments have currently not received widespread clinical acceptance.

A factor impacting quality of life that is commonly seen in low vision rehabilitation practice is that of depression. Renaud and Bedard (2013) completed a review of the literature of studies linking the relationship between quality of life and depression in elders with visual impairment and, as is expected, their findings indicate that better quality of life is strongly related to less severe depressive symptoms. The complexity of psychological evaluation makes it difficult to deconstruct out the exact link with vision loss in seniors, but Eramudugolla, Wood and Anstey [31] showed a significant association between objective indices of visual impairment (visual acuity, contrast sensitivity, visual fields) and functional vision with depressive and anxiety symptoms. This would lead us to encourage primary care practitioners to consider deeper evaluation of depression and anxiety in adults with age related eye disease. Several studies have demonstrated a lack of appropriate screening methods among practitioners while also calling for methods to train low vision rehabilitation practitioners in screening and referral methods [32, 33]. Some leaders have been successful in developing a training program to assist health professionals and rehabilitation professionals in detection but the program has not been adopted in widespread use in the U.S [34].

Another impacting phenomenon for people with low vision is Charles Bonnet Syndrome (CBS). This involves visual hallucinations that many people with binocular vision loss experience, many times, on a regular basis. Some scholars suggest that 30% of persons with ARMD and binocular vision loss experience these [35]. Commonly described as colorful and sometimes dynamic scenes, they do not usually induce an unpleasant experience. The symptoms may decrease over time but in some patients it is an ongoing phenomenon. The exact process causing the hallucinations is unknown but thought by some to be similar to the mechanisms of "phantom limb syndrome". Others based their theories on functional MRI studies suggesting Charles Bonnet Syndrome results from increased function in certain pathways other than those caused by external visual stimulus [36]. Regardless of the cause, doctors may reassure patients of the benign nature of these hallucinations and that they are unrelated to cognitive decline.

5. Interventions and management

5.1. *Impact* — Vision enhancement — Optical

Vision enhancement by optical and electronic devices have been a mainstay of low vision rehabilitation but modern low vision approaches and advancement in knowledge have supported the evolution of prescribing to include more factors for enabling patients to use the devices and incorporate them in daily life. For example, rather than prescribing optical or electronic devices after an evaluation with a low vision physician, many rehabilitation teams provide basic tools but incorporate rehabilitation methods such as teaching stable fixation with a preferred retinal locus (PRL) in patients with age related macular degeneration prior to

http://dx.doi.org/10.5772/58436

prescribing final devices. This allows for an evaluation of activities of daily life, lifestyle, and cognitive dimensions alongside the low vision physician that supports an integration of the devices by the rehabilitation therapist into daily life. Rehabilitation then becomes an ongoing process where the patient is encouraged to develop lifestyle adaptations over the course of rehabilitation. After several sessions with the therapist, the low vision physician would re-evaluate the patient's progress and prescribe additional devices as needed. In the U.S. a growing trend is for the low vision physician (optometrist or ophthalmologist) to refer to a low vision experienced occupational therapist (OT) who can be supported within the medical model by the Center for Medicare and Medicaid Services (CMS). [37].

Optical vision enhancement devices encompass high dioptric add powers, single vision near point glasses, magnifiers of various types (hand held, stand, illuminated) and telescopes. Unfortunately for our model of psychometric integrity, these devices can be variously labeled with non-standard power and/or magnification descriptors leading to confusion and frustration when attempting to compare patient performance and response. Magnification nomenclature is not homogeneous between companies that manufacture low vision rehabilitation devices and, in addition, are based on different assumptions of working distance. The assumptions are limiting and the various magnification formulae confusing.

The power of lenses and lens systems is most correctly defined with diopters and Equivalent Power (F_e) is the standard by which they are most properly described. Eyeglasses for the fully sighted are generally such low power that thin lens formulae give good approximations of Equivalent power (F_e). Therefore, office lensometers which measure back vertex power (F_v) give results which can be considered correspondent with F_e when used for the most common eyeglass powers. As lens powers increase to the ranges often used in low vision rehabilitation, the thin lens calculations generate measurement errors that become significant. Using F_e rationalizes observed lens effects on performance and makes treatment decisions on lens more systematic and rational. Consequently, describing the power of low vision rehabilitation optical devices with F_e is desirable.

The logarithmic progression of steps of significance in the ETDRS chart design in combination with the standardization of F_e for describing the power of low vision rehabilitation optical devices means predictions of patient near point performance can be made with good levels of confidence. Since each step on the LogMAR scale is a Just Noticeable Difference (JND), the steps can be thought of as either dioptric power steps, working distance steps or M-Unit size steps. Following is a four stage procedure that leads to performance predictions with changes in working distance, letter size and lens power for near acuity:

Stage 1-Measure and Record Visual Acuity in M-Units

Stage 2-Set letter size Goal for Performance Improvement

Stage 3-Count steps from Measurement to Goal

Stage 4-Implement counted steps for both working distance and F_e

0.4	0.5	0.63	0.8	1.0	1.25	1.6	2.0	2.5	3.2	4.0	5.0	6.3	8.0	10.0	12.5	16.0	20.0

Table 5. LogMAR steps of significance in JND increments of Diopters, Working Distance and M-Units

Once the Equivalent power needed to attain the patient's goal has been determined, the manner of delivery is chosen. Given that the important factor is the angular subtense of the image on the retina, the dioptric power can be supplied to the patient by single vision glasses, bifocal add, hand held magnifier, stand magnifier or telescope. In choosing between the various power delivery methods, factors other than diopters come into play. These factors include the particular task logistics, the ability of the patient to hold magnifiers steady, spot vs. sustained reading and others.

Low vision rehabilitation single vision glasses and bifocals delivery equivalent power to the eye by traditional means but with much higher dioptric power. The advantage to the patient is both hands are free to manipulate books and objects. The disadvantage is the close working distance. Since the working distance is the reciprocal in meters of the dioptric power and powers over+4.00D make binocular fusion problematic with high convergence demands, low vision rehabilitation glasses tend to be reserved for monocular use. This is in keeping with the common asymmetry in visual acuity found in patients with age related macular degeneration and diabetic retinopathy. Monocular spectacle powers in low vision rehabilitation glasses are prescribed in powers as high as+48.00D

Hand held magnifiers are the traditional means of delivering power for spot reading mail, prices in stores and other time limited near visual tasks. They can be lens power alone with a handle or in combination with illumination. Their advantage is easy portability and general inexpensiveness. The chief disadvantage is the necessity to reserve one hand for manipulation of the device while attempting to hold the object of regard with the other. This makes sustained reading difficult.

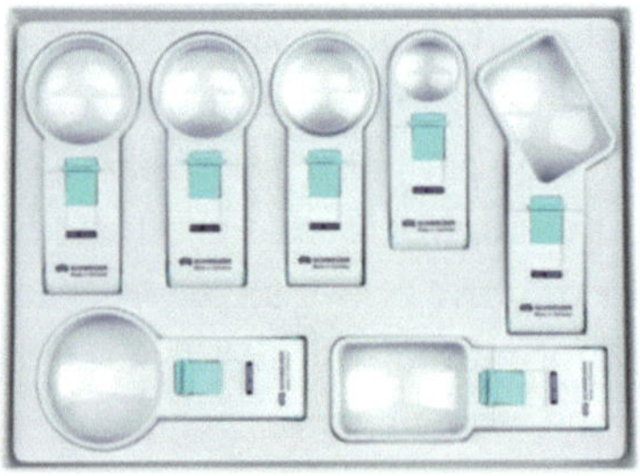

Figure 12. Hand Held Magnifier Set

Stand magnifiers were developed from hand held magnifiers in order to provide an optimal lens placement from the object of regard. While helping to alleviate the issue of managing lens to object distance, stand devices are bulkier and less portable. They can be found with handles

http://dx.doi.org/10.5772/58436

and illumination, no handles with open plastic stands or in domes. In any form, spot reading is the primary task for which they are used.

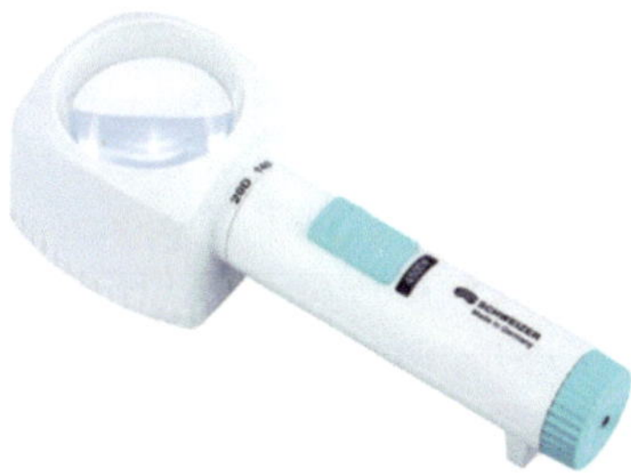

Figure 13. Stand Magnifier with Illumination

Telescopes have traditionally been prescribed for distance tasks such as reading street signs, taking notes from the board or spotting for mobility. New, closer focusing monocular or binocular telescopes allow television watching, computer viewing and even near point reading with extended length or reading caps on the telescope's objective lens. Telescopes can be hand held for spot use as needed or spectacle mounted for more continuous use. The tradeoff for improving distance visual acuity with any telescope is visual field restriction.

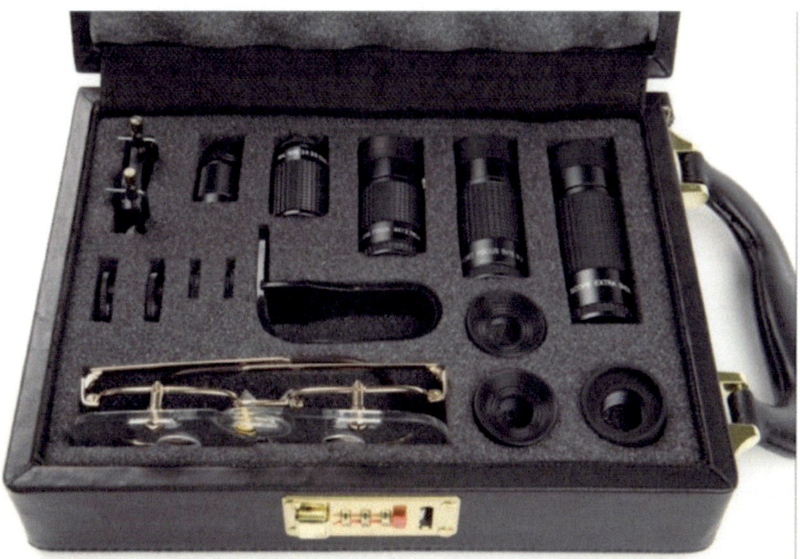

Figure 14. Telescope Set

Although all low vision optical and electronic magnification devices have until recently been extraocular, three intraocular devices have recently been developed; (1) the Implantable

Miniature Telescope (IMT, VisionCare OphthalmicTechnologies,Saratoga,CA), (2) Intraocular Lens for Visually Impaired People (IOL-VIP,IOL-VIP System, Soleko, Pontecorvo, Italy), and (3) Lipschitz Mirror Implant (LMI, Optolight Vision Technology, Herzlia, Israel). The IMT is the only device approved for commercial use in the US. It is implanted in one eye only and it enables patients with end-stage age related macular degeneration to see enlarged views at both distance and near. The internal design allows for a larger field of view than external telescopic devices and the rehabilitation program accompanying the implant supports patients' perceptual adaptation to the 2.7x magnified view. The IMT process requires bi-ocular viewing with the non-implant eye used for wide angle general mobility and the IMT implanted eye used for more detailed activities of daily living such as seeing faces, participating in hobbies, and viewing large print on labels. An increased quality of life score at 6 months post implantation compared to baseline has been demonstrated with the IMT. [38]

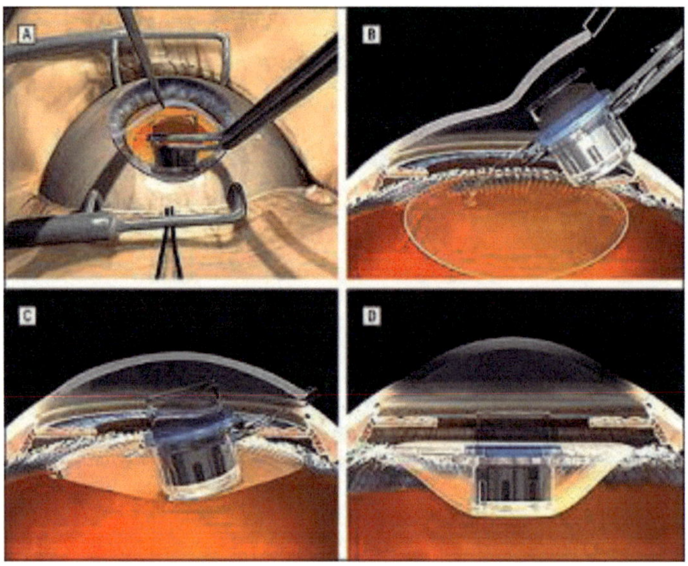

Figure 15. IMT surgical insertion sequence

5.2. *Impact* — Vision enhancement — Non optical

Non-optical vision enhancement has traditionally meant lighting and glare control devices and techniques. These entailed dark glasses, hats with brims, and typoscopes or line guides to cut white page glare while giving peripheral clues to maintain position on the line of letters. The benefits of these devices were subjective and their prescription was done symptomatically with no significant psychometric measure beyond observation of improved performance. This does not diminish their utility, however and a good Occupational Therapist (OT) or low vision trainer can identify useful non-optical devices and teach the techniques of their use in short order with good outcomes.

http://dx.doi.org/10.5772/58436

In recent years, the electronic miniaturization revolution which has given the world cell coverage, smart phones, GPS and mobile connectivity tablets for the fully sighted, has also added a great depth to the armamentarium of the low vision rehabilitation practitioner and opened up a whole world of possibilities to partially sighted and blind patients. Accessibility features are imbedded into every smart phone and tablet that allows many more degrees of freedom in accessing information. Global Positioning System (GPS) and mapping programs inform the patient who cannot see street signs or read storefronts just where they are and what businesses are nearby. Directions for walking routes are a few screen swipes away. A quick picture of an approaching bus and a finger gesture that magnifies the photo enables the person to identify the bus number and route. Similarly, menu items can be read independently and people far away recognized unobtrusively. Specialized apps for the patient with low vision are legion, so many in fact that the Braille Institute [39] has an app just to help organize, categorize and find those apps designed for the visually impaired. Some companies have dedicated their whole enterprise to providing tools and devices for these patients. However, the field of electronic accessibility for the partially sighted changes almost daily so any attempt at detailing it is futile. Suffice it to say that annual meetings for doctors and providers for the visually impaired invariably have sessions on the latest advances and the reader should make the effort to keep abreast of the changes in the field in order to provide the best information and treatment to their patients.

5.3. *Impact* — Vision substitution

When the patient's vision has been reduced to the point that some or all of the functional independence measures are no longer positively impacted by vision enhancement devices, techniques or training, there are still avenues of patient benefit open to the low vision rehabilitation practitioner. That is the field of vision substitution where functional independence can be achieved with devices, techniques and training that do not rely on vision. Some of the more common components of vision substitution are Braille, orientation and mobility (O&M) instruction and audible books. Vision substitution and vision enhancement, however, are not mutually exclusive. In some aspects of functional independence, the patient may perform satisfactorily with vision enhancement while in other functional independence categories they may require vision substitution. An example may be someone who is able to read their mail with high dioptric power devices (vision enhancement) yet is unable to enjoy sustained reading. For them, audible books (vision substitution) are a reasonable accommodation. Additionally, there are devices that provide text to speech or to a file form that allows large viewing on a computer monitor or to a refreshable Braille display. GPS devices without a touch screen empower the functionally blind person with the option of safe, extended and independent travel. Students can quickly receive their assignments electronically rather than having to wait for a Braille transcription. Vision loss no longer has to mean functionality loss when the tools and interprofessional resources of vision substitution are employed by the low vision rehabilitation practitioner. However, this remains an area that has potential not yet fully realized.

6. Conclusion

Low vision rehabilitation is a field which is optimally practiced with a comprehensive, inclusive and interprofessional approach involving optometrists, ophthalmologists, occupational therapists, orientation and mobility specialists, social or rehabilitation workers and teachers of the visually impaired. In our paradigm of *Cause*, *Effect* and *Impact*, diagnosing and treating in the traditional medical model is shown to be frequently inadequate. We need to also look at incorporating the vocational and rehabilitation model. Determining visual ability in *Cause* by measuring visual acuity, visual fields and contrast sensitivity may not sufficiently take into consideration the functional *Effect* upon the patient's independence in their varied activities of daily life. Therefore, the patient history needs to go beyond the standard queries about chief complaint, review of systems and past, family and social history to a more directed functional survey as seen with quantified functional independence measures (FIM). Early interprofessional referrals thus generated can provide crucial input to the development of a rehabilitation plan that is comprehensive and inclusive addressing the *Effect* through activities of daily life and ultimately *Impact* the patient's qualify of life. Even when the options for vision enhancement are no longer sufficient for the patient, independence can be achieved through interdisciplinary referrals for vision substitution devices, techniques and training. It is incumbent upon the eye doctor to either provide low vision rehabilitation services or refer to those who can.

Acronyms and abbreviations

ADL	Activities of Daily Life
AMD	Age-Related Macular Degeneration
CBS	Charles Bonnet Syndrome
CMS	Center for Medicare & Medicaid Services
DM	Diabetes Mellitus
DR	Diabetic Retinopathy
ETDRS	Early Treatment of Diabetic Retinopathy Study
FIM	Functional Independence Measure
GPS	Global Positioning System
HPI	History of Present Illness
HRQOL	Health Related Quality of Life
IMT	Implantable Miniature Telescope
JND	Just Noticeable Difference
LASER	Light Amplification by the Stimulated Emission of Radiation

http://dx.doi.org/10.5772/58436

LogMAR	Logarithm (base 10) of Minimum Angle of Resolution
LOVIT	Low Vision Intervention Trial
LV	Low Vision
LVR	Low Vision Rehabilitation
MAR	Minimum Angle of Resolution
MN Read	Minnesota Reading Charts
NEI-VFQ	National Eye Institute Vision Function Quality
O&M	Orientation and Mobility
OD	Doctor of Optometry
OT	Occupational Therapist
PFSH	Past, Family and Social History
PRL	Preferred Retinal Locus
QOL	Quality of Life
ROS	Review of Systems
SK Read	Smith-Kettlewell Reading Test
SLO	Scanning LASER Ophthalmoscope
TRL	Trained Retinal Locus
TVI	Teacher of the Visually Impaired
VA	Visual Acuity
VRQOL	Vision Related Quality of Life
WHO	World Health Organization

Acknowledgements

The authors would like to thank Precision Vision of La Salle, Illinois for their generous contribution of images used in this chapter.

Author details

Bennett McAllister[1,2] and Rebecca Kammer[1]

1 Low Vision, American Academy of Optometry, USA

2 Primary Care Service, College of Optometry, Western University of Health Sciences, Pomona, California, USA

References

[1] edited by Robert W. Massof, Lorraine Lidoff Issues in Low Vision Rehabilitation: Service Delivery, Policy, and Funding 2001, AFB Press, NY http://books.google.com/books?hl=en&lr=&id=qm3KCDWxougC&oi=fnd&pg=PR7&dq=Massof,+low+vision+rehabilitation,+book&ots=q82s6fsQUT&sig=lFM6GuU_5R-xXYjKM803ZhaOJN0#v=onepage&q=Massof%2C%20low%20vision%20rehabilitation%2C%20book&f=false

[2] Association of Schools and Colleges of Optometry. http://www.opted.org/files/Entry-LevelCompetencies_LowVision.pdf

[3] Owsley C, McGwin G Jr, Lee PP, Wasserman N, Searcey K Characteristics of low-vision rehabilitation services in the United States. Arch Ophthalmol. 2009 May;127(5): 681-9. doi: 10.1001/archophthalmol.2009.55.

[4] WHO. Main Causes of Vision Impairment. http://www.who.int.blindness/causes/priority/en/indes.html

[5] Tranton JH. Nothing More Can Be Done…A Fable for our Times. Ophthalmology Clinics of North America. June 1994 Volume 7 Number 2

[6] Chous AP. Those who aren't what we call them. doi: 10.1016/j.optm.2008.10.009

[7] CDC. Statement on Vision Loss in America. http://www.cdc.gov/visionhealth/data/national.htm

[8] NIH. NEI. Statement on Age-Related Macular Degeneration. http://www.nei,nih.gov/eyedata/amd.asp

[9] CDC. Statement on Diabetes. http://www.cdc.gov/diabetes/statistics/prev/national/figbyage.htm

[10] Bailey IL, Lovie-Kitchin JE. Visual Acuity Testing. From the Laboratory to the Clinic. Vision Research, Volume 90, September 2013 pages 2-9.

[11] Lovie-Kitchin J Reading with low vision: the impact of research on clinical management. Clin Exp Optom. 2011 Mar;94(2):121-32. doi: 10.1111/j.1444-0938.2010.00565.x. Epub 2011 Jan 26

[12] G T Timberlake, E Peli, E A Essock and R A Augliere. Abstract Reading with a macular scotoma. II. Retinal locus for scanning text.Invest. Ophthalmol. Vis. Sci. August 1987 vol. 28 no. 8 1268-1274

[13] Ronald A. Schuchard, PhD Preferred retinal loci and macular scotoma characteristics in patients with age-related macular degeneration *Canadian Journal of Ophthalmology / Journal Canadien d'Ophtalmologie, Volume 40, Issue 3, June 2005, Pages 303-312*

[14] Déruaz A, Goldschmidt M, Whatham AR, Mermoud C, Lorincz EN, Schnider A, Safran AB. A technique to train new oculomotor behavior in patients with central mac-

ular scotomas during reading related tasks using scanning laser ophthalmoscopy: immediate functional benefits and gains retention. BMC Ophthalmol. 2006 Nov 23;6:35.

[15] Nilsson U, Frennesson C, Nilsson S. Patients with AMD and a large absolute central scotoma can be trained successfully to use eccentric viewing, as demonstrated in a scanning laser ophthalmoscope. *Vision Research* [serial online]. July 2003;43(16): 1777-1787.

[16] Helle K. Falkenberg[a], Gary S. Rubin[b], Peter J. Bex[c]. Acuity, crowding, reading and fixation stability Vision Research Volume 47, Issue 1, January 2007, Pages 126–135

[17] Mandelcorn MS, Podbielski DW, Mandelcorn ED. Fixation stability as a goal in the treatment of macular disease. Can J Ophthalmol. 2013 Oct;48(5):364-7. doi: 10.1016/j.jcjo.2013.05.006. Epub 2013 Sep 2.

[18] Ronald A. Schuchard, PhD Preferred retinal loci and macular scotoma characteristics in patients with age-related macular degeneration *Canadian Journal of Ophthalmology / Journal Canadien d'Ophtalmologie, Volume 40, Issue 3, June 2005, Pages 303-312*

[19] Markowitz S, Reyes S. Microperimetry and clinical practice: an evidence-based review. *Canadian Journal Of Ophthalmology. Journal Canadien D'ophtalmologie* [serial online]. October 2013;48(5):350-357

[20] Kammer R., Poulter C, Clark J. *The Effect of Altered Stimulus Luminance on the Size of Scotomas Mapped with the Fletcher Central Visual Field Test*. ARVO, Florida, May 2009; poster

[21] Pelli DG, Bex P. Testing Vision: From Laboratory Psychophysical Tests to Clinical Evaluation-Measuring Contrast Sensitivity. Vision Research, Volume 90, September 2013 pages 10-14

[22] Colenbrander A, Fletcher D C. The Mixed Contrast Reading card, a new screening test for contrast sensitivity. In: Jones S, Rubin G, Hamlin D, eds. Vision 2005International Congress Series. London, 2006

[23] Book: Low Vision: Research and New Developments in Rehabilitation edited by A. C. Kooijman, IOS press 1994 Chapter: Optimizing illumination for visually impaired persons; comparing subjective and objective criteria. Ch authors: Cornelissen, Kooijman, Schoot, Bootsma, and Wildt

[24] H Lei and R A Schuchard Using two preferred retinal loci for different lighting conditions in patients with central scotomas. Invest. Ophthalmol. Vis. Sci. August 1997 vol. 38 no. 9 1812-1818

[25] Granger CV, Deutsch A, Linn RT. Rasch analysis of the Functional Independence Measure (FIM) Mastery Test. Arch Phys Med Rehabil. 1998 Jan;79(1):52-7.

[26] Young Y, Fan MY, Hebel JR, Boult C. Concurrent validity of administering the functional independence measure (FIM) instrument by interview. Am J Phys Med Rehabil. 2009 Sep;88(9):766-70. doi: 10.1097/PHM.0b013e3181a9f1d6.

[27] [27]Khadka J, McAlinden C, Pesudovs K. Quality assessment of ophthalmic questionnaires: review and recommendations. Optom Vis Sci. 2013 Aug;90(8):720-44. doi: 10.1097/OPX.0000000000000001.

[28] (no authors listed) The World Health Organization Quality of Life Assessment (WHOQOL): Position paper from the World Health Organization. Soc Sci Med. 1995 Nov;41(10):1403-9

[29] http://www.cdc.gov/hrqol/concept.htm

[30] de Boer MR, Moll AC, de Vet HC, Terwee CB, Volker-Dieben HJ, van Rens GH. Psychometric Properties of Vision-Related Quality of Life Questionnaires: a Systematic Review. Ophthalmic Physician Opt. 2004 Jul;24(4):257-73

[31] Eramudugolla R, Wood J, Anstery KJ. Co-Morbidity of Depression and Anxiety in Common Age-Related Eye Diseases. Frontiers in Aging Neuroscience. October 2013 doi: 10.3389/fnagi.2013.00056

[32] Owsley C. Aging and vision. Vision Res. 2011 Jul 1;51(13):1610-22. doi: 10.1016/j.visres.2010.10.020. Epub 2010 Oct 23.

[33] Renaud J, Bédard E Depression in the elderly with visual impairment and its association with quality of life. Clin Interv Aging. 2013;8:931-43. doi: 10.2147/CIA.S27717. Epub 2013 Jul 19.

[34] Rees G, Mellor D, Heenan M, Fenwick E, Keeffe JE, Marella M, Lamoureux EL. Depression training program for eye health and rehabilitation professionals. Optom Vis Sci. 2010 Jul;87(7):494-500. doi: 10.1097/OPX.0b013e3181df5286.

[35] [35] Khan JC, Shahid H, Thurlby DA, Yates JRW, and Moore AT. Charles Bonnet Syndrome in Age-Related Macular Degeneration: The Nature and Frequency of Images in Subjects with End-Stage Disease. *Ophthalmic Epidemiology*, 15:202–208ISSN: 0928-6586 print / 1744-5086 online Copyright c 2008 Informa Healthcare USA, Inc. DOI: 10.1080/09286580801939320 p.202-208

[36] [36] Ffytche DH, Howard RJ, Brammer MJ, David A, Woodruff P, Williams S. The anatomy of conscious vision: An fMRI study of visual hallucinations. *Nat Neurosci.* 1998;1:738–42.

[37] Liu CJ, Brost MA, Horton VE, Kenyon SB, Mears KE. Occupational therapy interventions to improve performance of daily activities at home for older adults with low vision: a systematic review. Am J Occup Ther. 2013 May-Jun;67(3):279-87. doi: 10.5014/ajot.2013.005512.

http://dx.doi.org/10.5772/58436

[38] Singer A, Amir N., Herro A., Porbandarwalla S., Pollard J. Improving quality of life in patients wit end-stage age-related macular degeneration: focus on miniature ocular implants. Clinical Ophthalmology 2012:6 33–39

[39] Braille Institute. Visually Impaired Apps. https://itunes.apple.com/us/app/via-by-braille-institute/id528499232?mt=8 http://www.who.int/blindness/causes/priority/en/index5.html

Section 4

Updates in Research in Ophthalmology, Optometry and Vision Science

Chapter 15

Fabry Disease – Ocular Manifestations and Visual Symptoms

Pinakin Gunvant Davey

Additional information is available at the end of the chapter

http://dx.doi.org/10.5772/58677

1. Introduction

Fabry disease is a rare lysosomal disorder that has a prevalence of 1 in 40,000 males.[1] This disease follows x-linked inheritance and the individuals affected with the disease show multi system disorders that are present at birth and signs and symptoms worsen with time. The *GLA* gene mutation leads to the deficiency of an enzyme alpha galactidose A which leads to the progressive accumulation of globotriacylceramide (GB3) deposits in a variety of cells including those in kidneys, and the autonomic the cardiovascular systems.[2-4]

The ocular manifestations of Fabry disease includes a cornea verticillata which is a "vortex whorl" like corneal opacity. It is the most common finding and is seen in all hemizygotes and majority (up to 70%) of hetrozygotes.[5] The cornea verticillata is the outcome of the deposit of GB3 in the basal layer of the corneal epithelium. The cornea verticillata is visible using a slitlamp biomicroscope and in-vivo confocal microscopic studies have shown that even when the cornea verticillata may not be visible using a slitlamp there are intracellular inclusion bodies in the basal epithelial cells.[6] To a lesser degree and fewer Fabry disease patients have subtle lenticular deposits which is the Fabry cataract.[7] The Fabry cataract tends to be off axis dendritic or subcapsular opacities along the posterior suture lines. It is believed that patients with cornea verticillata will not have any visual symptoms due to the deposits. [7-9]

The role of the cornea and the crystalline lens is to provide the eye with necessary refractive power and unhindered path to the light rays that pass through them. To this accord the corneal physiology is finely tuned and causes the least amount of scatter of light rays in ocular healthy individuals. It can be hypothesized that individuals with Fabry disease could have problems with visual function given that both the cornea and the crystalline lens have deposits of GB3 and opacities. It can further be hypothesized that the vision problems would be present and will be worst at night time when compared to the day time, with patients with Fabry disease having additional problems of glare, blurry vision or dim vision (contrast sensitivity issues).

The patients with Fabry disease also experience anhydrosis or hypohydrosis as one of the symptom. This is due to the neurological manifestations of the disease. Prior reports have suggested that patients with Fabry disease may have deposits of GB3 in the ganglia or the lacrimal gland itself.[10-12] It can be hypothesized that patients with Fabry disease could also have symptoms of dry eyes.

The present study utilized an ocular symptom survey instrument to evaluate for the symptoms of general ocular problems like itching, tearing, dryness, burning sensation, sensation of foreign body or difficulty in vision or asthenopic symptoms in patients with Fabry disease and compared the findings to healthy controls.

2. Materials and methods

2.1. Study participants

A total of 95 individuals (75 patients with Fabry disease and 20 healthy controls) completed the survey. The mean age and standard deviation (SD) of the patients in the Fabry group and the control group was 32.5 and SD 19.1 years and 42.6 SD 14.7 years respectively. Ninety six percent of the participants completed all the survey questions, with 4 individuals not answering the question about "soreness and fatigue" of eyes.

The survey was administered live at the conferences for lysosomal disease storage which was conducted by the Fabry Support and Information Group in San Diego California, USA and the National Fabry Disease Foundation in Greensboro, North Carolina, USA. These events were attended by individuals that had a confirmed case of Fabry disease or by a family member who were tested and confirmed of being healthy and did not have Fabry disease or healthy spouse. The participants were instructed to answer the survey questions with regards to their self-perceived ocular and vision status when they were wearing optimal refractive correction. Data was collated and analyzed in a masked fashion with the data entry performed by a separate individual and the statistical analysis performed by the author.

2.2. Survey instrument

A modified survey instrument that was utilized by Lee et al [13] to investigate the ocular and visual symptoms in glaucoma patients was utilized in the present study. The survey instrument proposed by Lee et al[13] was called the Glaucoma Symptom Scale (GSS) and is a simple 10 question survey that was developed by modifying the survey used in the Ocular Hypertension Treatment Study. The GSS was tested and validated on a group of glaucoma patients in four tertiary care glaucoma centers. This survey instrument was administered to both patients with Fabry disease and their healthy family members (controls).

The survey administered in the present study is shown in Figure 1. The major difference between the GSS and the survey administered in the present study is the scale of the symptoms.

The GSS graded the symptoms in 4 point scale whereas the present study utilized a 6 point scale. The larger scale in the present survey allowed evaluating a wide range of symptom level as it was likely that the ocular symptoms in patients with the ocular manifestations of Fabry disease could be mild or minimal. The GSS survey instrument mainly evaluated for dryness and tear film and ocular surface issues in questions 1 to 4 and 7, whereas question 4 is designed to evaluate for general fatigue or asthenopic symptoms. The survey instruments question number 6, 8-10 were designed to evaluate vision related problems primarily the difficulty in contrast sensitivity issues, day time night time vision and glare respectively.

Almost Never Almost Always

1	Burning /stinging	1	2	3	4	5	6
2	Tearing	1	2	3	4	5	6
3	Dryness	1	2	3	4	5	6
4	Itching	1	2	3	4	5	6
5	Soreness/tiredness	1	2	3	4	5	6
6	Blurry/Dim vision	1	2	3	4	5	6
7	Feeling of something in your eyes	1	2	3	4	5	6
8	Hard to see in daylight; I need to wear sunglasses	1	2	3	4	5	6
9	Hard to see in dark places	1	2	3	4	5	6
10	Halos around light	1	2	3	4	5	6

Figure 1. Survey instrument administered to the study participants; Survey instrument used in the study was developed by Lee et al [13]. The only modification made to the survey was the scale. The present study used a 6 point scale where as the survey instrument used by Lee et al had a 4 point scale.

2.3. Statistical analysis

The difference in the mean age between the groups was analyzed using a one–way analysis of variance (ANOVA). The severity for each variable was graded in an ordinal scale with 1 being "almost never" and 6 as "almost always". A Mann-Whitney test was performed to evaluate the median difference between the Fabry group and the healthy control for each symptom survey question. A p-value of <0.05 was considered to be significant.

3. Results

The mean age of the control group was greater than the mean age of the Fabry group (ANOVA $F=4.75$; $p=0.03$). The table-1 provides the mean symptom severity score for the Fabry group and the control group and the p-value obtained using the Mann-Whitney test.

	Symptom	Mean Severity Score		p-value
		Fabry group	Control group	
1	Burning /stinging	1.9	1.5	0.06
2	Tearing	2.0	1.9	0.2
3	Dryness	2.3	1.5	**0.02**
4	Itching	2.0	1.8	0.3
5	Soreness/tiredness	2.4	1.7	***0.009***
6	Blurry/Dim vision	2.2	1.6	**0.02**
7	Feeling of something in your eyes	2.0	1.5	0.07
8	Hard to see in daylight; I need to wear sunglasses	2.4	1.7	0.15
9	Hard to see in dark places	2.6	1.6	**0.01**
10	Halos around light	2.4	1.7	**0.01**

p-value in bold are significant at p<0.05 and in bold and italics are significant p <0.01

Table 1. Symptoms surveys and the median severity of groups and statistical significance

Of the survey instruments items, it was found that patients in the Fabry group had more complaints of "dryness" of eyes (p=0.02). The Fabry group also showed significantly greater symptom severity score and complained of "Blurry/Dim vision", "hard to see in dark places" and "halos around light" (p=0,02, 0.01 and 0.01 respectively). The Fabry group also had a mean severity score for "soreness/tiredness" significantly higher than the control group (p=0.009). The tally of number of participants with symptoms and without symptoms is given in Table 2

4. Discussion

The survey instrument (GSS) utilized in this study was designed by Lee et al [13] to study the ocular and vision issues in glaucoma patients with the purpose of surveying daytime and night time vision, contrast sensitivity, glare, dryness and tear film related problems. The present study utilized the GSS survey instrument to identify ocular and visual symptoms in the Fabry disease and ocular healthy controls. The study results indicate that compared to healthy controls, the patients with Fabry disease had greater ocular symptom severity score in particularly areas related to night vision, contrast sensitivity and glare. Further they also have greater symptom severity score and complaint of soreness/tiredness and dry eyes.

Prior reports have indicated that patients with Fabry disease do not have any visual problems due to the cornea verticillata. [7-9] This is perhaps true to the point that the cornea verticillata may not cause a decline in Snellen visual acuity charts that uses 100% contrast optotypes (black letters on white background) as long as the patients wear appropriate refractive error correction. The findings of this study indicate that the symptoms of "dim vision", "hard to see in dark places" perhaps indicates decrease in contrast sensitivity or difficulty in identifying targets in day to day life that are in shades of grey not of 100% contrast.. The Fabry group also had a symptom severity score significantly higher for the survey item seeing "Halo around lights" which is perhaps a result due to the scatter or glare problems that patients experience. This problem may perhaps be further exaggerated at night time.

Symptoms		Problem	No Problem
Burning and stinging	Disease	38	37
	No disease	5	15
Tearing	Disease	44	31
	No disease	11	9
Dryness*	Disease	44	31
	No disease	7	13
Itching	Disease	44	31
	No disease	9	11
Soreness tiredness*	Disease	52	23
	No disease	6	14
Blurry, Dim vision*	Disease	48	27
	No disease	7	13
Feeling something in your eyes	Disease	40	35
	No disease	6	14
Hard to see in daylight, I need sunglasses	Disease	39	36
	No disease	7	13
Hard to see in dark places*	Disease	45	30
	No disease	7	13
Halos around light*	Disease	44	31
	No disease	6	14

* indicates symptoms that was statistically significant greater severity score between the groups

Table 2. The tally of study participants that reported experiencing symptoms in the Fabry group and the control group

The vision problems related to scotopic (night) vision, contrast sensitivity and glare are most likely due to the deposits of GB3 in corneal epithelium and lens which causes increased scatter of light rays and decreased transmittance of light (See figures 2 A-C). The confocal microscopic studies have revealed that even when there is no clinically visible cornea verticillata the basal layer of the epithelium show hyper reflectivity due to the intracellular inclusion bodies. Thus although one can expect the symptom severity score to be related to the amount of corneal deposits visible, the patients that do not have visible deposits or cornea verticillata may still have some visual problems given that have the intracellular inclusion bodies in the corneal epithelial cells.

The Fabry group also had greater complaints of "dryness" compared to the control group. This could be due to the fact that GB3 gets deposited both in the ganglia and the lacrimal gland. [10-12] Prior researchers have also suggested that patients with Fabry disease can have a dry

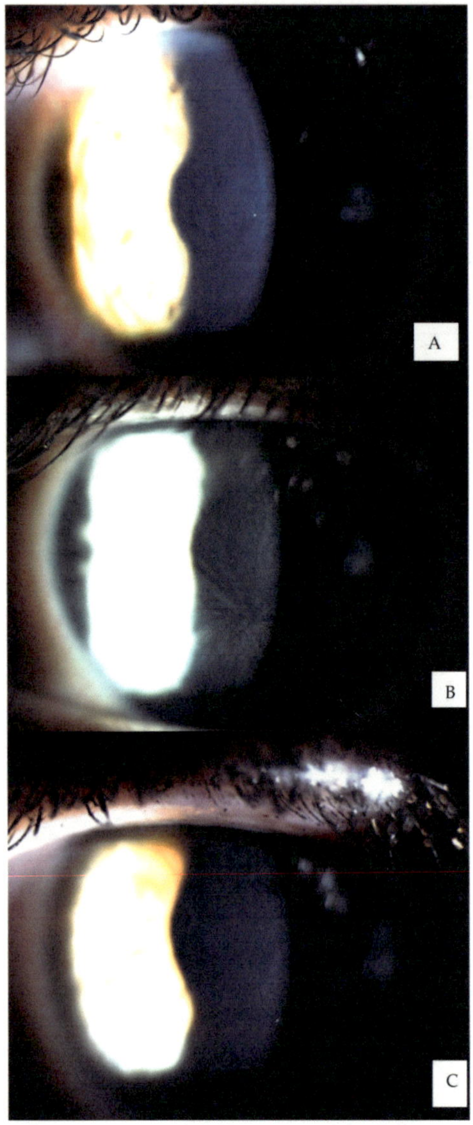

Figure 2. Cornea verticillata in patients with Fabry disease A: Top panel: Cornea verticillata giving a even spread of smear of deposits throughout the cornea. B: Middle panel: A vortex like deposits. C: Bottom panel: A subtle verticillata in a patient with Fabry disease

eye syndrome.[9] The report of this survey quantifies that patients may have a subtle yet clinically significant dry eye.

The patients with Fabry disease also complain of lack of energy or chronic fatigue. [14] It is intriguing to note that symptom survey score for "soreness/tiredness of eyes was significantly greater than the control group. This could have multiple reasons. The simplest explanation is they experience chronic fatigue of their body and thus also experience "soreness/tiredness" with eyes. Although it is possible that dry eye, dim vision may contribute to some of these asthenopic problems. It will be interesting to see if this symptom severity score would decrease if appropriate therapy using glare filters, contrast enhancing filters or treatment for dry eyes was administered.

The cornea verticillata in patients with Fabry disease can vary significantly; they can be absent, subtle, or dramatic in appearance. The figures 2 A-C provide slit lamp photographs of cornea verticillata in patients with known Fabry disease. The figures 3 A B provide images of of conjunctival vascular findings in patients with Fabry disease. It should be noted that the cornea verticillata is not limited to Fabry disease and patients on medication like amiodorone or aminoquinolones on chronic use can have similar corneal appearance.[7] It can be postulated that any person with cornea verticillata can have vision problems pertaining to night time, contrast discrimination and glare.

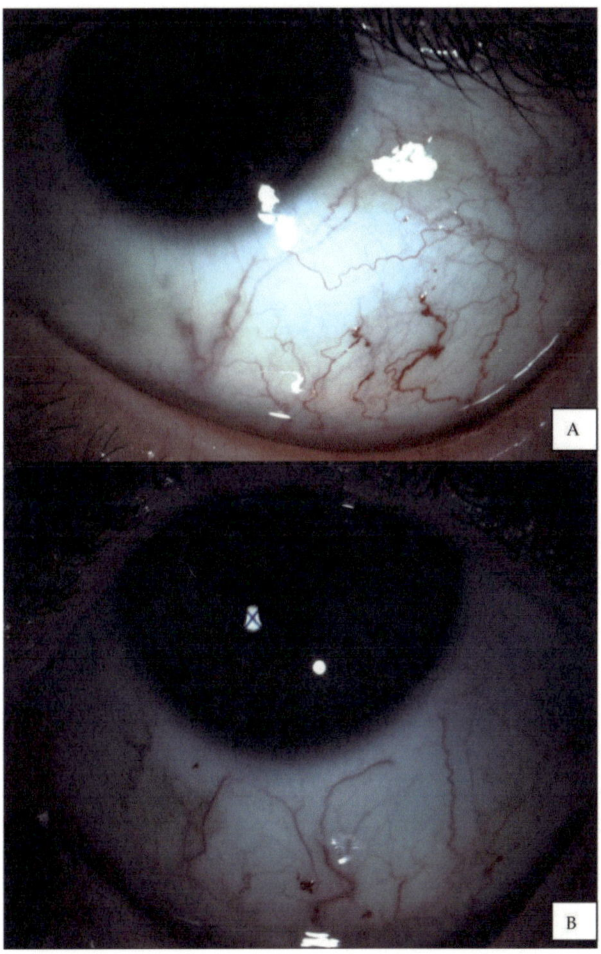

Figure 3. Conjunctival tortousity with aneurysms like out pouching (A: Top and B: Bottom panel)

This is first report to my knowledge that has evaluated the ocular symptom severity survey in patients with Fabry disease. Future studies are needed and should look at quantifying the problems and symptoms with contrast sensitivity function testing, glare testing and investigate tear function tests to evaluate the vision related difficulty and dry eye problems.

Acknowledgements

I would like to thank Mr. Jerry Walter Founder and President National Fabry Disease Foundation (NFDF) and Mr. Jack Johnson Executive Director Fabry Support & Information Group for their kind help in administering the survey to Fabry patients I would like to thank Mr. Nate Klingensmith of Haag Striet USA for his assistance in ocular imaging of Fabry group and Mr. Jack Greenan for the data entry related to the study. A special thank you to Dr. Rebecca Kammer for interesting discussion on ocular survey instruments and all the study participants for their time and efforts in completing the survey.

Author details

Pinakin Gunvant Davey

Western University of Health Sciences, College of Optometry, Pomona CA, USA

References

[1] Meikle PJ, Hopwood JJ, Clague AE, et al. Prevalence of lysosomal storage disorders. JAMA 1999;281:249-54.

[2] MacDermot KD, Holmes A, Miners AH. AndersoneFabry disease: clinical manifestations and impact of disease in a cohort of 98 hemizygous males. J Med Genet 2001;38:750-60.

[3] MacDermot KD, Holmes A, Miners AH. AndersoneFabry disease: clinical manifestations and impact of disease in a cohort of 60 obligate carrier females. J Med Genet 2001;38:769-75

[4] Branton MH, Schiffmann R, Sabnis SG, et al. Natural history of Fabry renal disease: influence of a-galactosidase A activity and genetic mutations on clinical course. Medicine 2002;81:122-38

[5] Desnick RJ, Brady RO. Fabry disease in childhood. J Pediatr 2004;144:20-26.

[6] Wasielica-Poslednik J, Pfeiffer N, Reinke J, Pitz S Confocal laser-scanning microscopy allows differentiation between Fabry disease and amiodarone-induced keratopathy Graefes Arch Clin Exp Ophthalmol (2011) 249:1689–1696

[7] Samiy N: Ocular Features of Fabry Disease: Diagnosis of a Treatable Life-threatening Disorder Surv Ophthalmol 53:416--423, 2008.

[8] Sodi A, Ioannidis A, Pitz S. Ophthalmological manifestations of Fabry disease. In: Metha A, Beck M, Sunder-Plassmann G, eds. Fabry disease. Perspectives from 5 years of FOS. Oxford, UK: Oxford Pharmagenesis Ltd, 2006:249-61.

[9] Sivley MD Fabry Disease: A Review of Ophthalmic and Systemic Manifestations Optom Vis Sci 2013;90:e63-e78

[10] Cable WJ, Kolodny EH, Adams RD. Fabry disease: impaired autonomicfunction. Neurology 1982;32:498-502.

[11] Hilz MJ. Evaluation of peripheral and autonomic nerve function in Fabry disease. Acta Paediatr Suppl 2002;91:38-42.

[12] Kolodny EH, Pastores GM. Anderson-Fabry disease: extrarenal, neurologic manifestations. J Am Soc Nephrol 2002;13(Suppl. 2):S150-3.

[13] Lee BL, Gutierrez P, Gordon M, Wilson MR, Cioffi GA, Ritch R, Sherwood M, MangioneCM The Glaucoma Symptom Scale. A brief index of glaucoma-specific symptoms. Arch Ophthalmol. 1998 Jul;116(7):861-6

[14] Zarate YA, Hopkin RJ Fabry's disease. Lancet. 2008 Oct 18;372(9647):1427-35

Applications of Perceptual Learning to Ophthalmology

Jenni Deveau, Gary Lovcik and Aaron R. Seitz

Additional information is available at the end of the chapter

http://dx.doi.org/10.5772/58364

1. Introduction

Our knowledge of the world is derived from our perceptions, and an individual's ability to navigate his/her surroundings or engage in activities of daily living such as walking, reading, watching TV, and driving, naturally relies on his/her ability to process sensory information. Thus deficits in visual abilities, due to disease, injury, stroke or aging, can have significant negative impacts on all aspects of an individual's life. Likewise, an enhancement of visual abilities can have substantial positive benefits to one's lifestyle. While a central concern of Ophthalmology is to address diseases of the eye (e.g. ocular impairments), an equally important component of vision is how the brain processes information that is received from the eye.

Vision is a synergistic effect of eye sensing and brain processing mechanisms. Vision can be compared to a satellite dish with the eye representing the dish or the sensor receiving aspect of the system. The eye/sensor captures light signals and transfers these signals to the brain, which is our visual processor. Through a series of brain processing stages, the image is processed by perceptual, higher order cognitive, and then motor systems resulting in decisions and responses. Thus, vision deficits can be due to eye mechanics, brain processing problems or both. Research of Perceptual Learning provides some answers and solutions for brain processing issues. This research demonstrates that the adult visual system is sufficiently plastic to ameliorate effects of low vision, including amblyopia [1], presbyopia [2], macular degeneration [3], stroke [4, 5], and late-life recovery of visual function [6]. Likewise, normal sighted individuals have the potential to further improve their vision through Perceptual Learning. These visual gains are related to brain function improvement (plasticity).

In this chapter we review the field of Perceptual Learning and its promise to achieve better outcomes in clinical practice. The significance of the development of effective, low-cost therapies to treat brain-based low vision can be life-altering for millions of people worldwide.

2. Perceptual Learning

Perceptual Learning (PL) refers to a long lasting improvement in perceptual abilities as a result of experience. Research of this topic has undergone tremendous development over the last 30 years. Plasticity in the sensory systems was previously thought to occur only in early development. This view has been substantiated by studies of a "critical period". The concept of a critical period states some processes develop early in life, and do not develop, or develop to a lesser degree, later in life. For example, classic experiments done in kittens demonstrate a critical period for ocular dominance where early patching enables inputs from the open eye to take over much of primary visual cortex, however, in adult cats patching has little impact on connectivity [7, 8]. This data was used to support the hypothesis that the low-level sensory stages need to consistently process primitive sensory features; such as in vision, orientation, spatial frequency, and local motion. However, studies of perceptual learning show that even in adults, perceptual abilities can be sharpened with repeated exposure or training. For example, perceptual abilities, including elementary processes (e.g., contrast sensitivity [9] and visual acuity [1, 2, 10, 11]) can be strengthened through appropriate training approaches.

Perceptual Learning is exemplified by long-lasting improvement on simple but difficult perceptual tasks. The effects of perceptual learning have been shown to last months, even years [12-14]. The field of perceptual learning is one of growing interest largely due to the fact training on visual perception can be highly specific to the trained visual features and can give clues into the stages of processing at which learning occurs. For example, a series of studies conducted by Schoups and colleagues [15, 16] showed that training subjects (human and monkey) on an orientation discrimination task around a particular reference orientation yielded learning effects that failed to transfer to other stimulus orientations at the trained location or that same orientation at a different retinotopic location. They postulated that these learning effects were consistent with plasticity in neurons residing in primary visual cortex, which show a high degree of both retinotopic and orientation specificity. Physiological studies by this group confirmed these predictions with the demonstration of plasticity of orientation tuning across early visual cortex [15, 17]. Consistent with this, numerous behavioral studies show perceptual learning can be highly specific to a wide range of trained stimulus features including retinotopic location [18, 19], visual orientation [15, 20] and direction [12, 19], among others. Likewise, many neuroscientific studies provide evidence of sensory plasticity in all stages of visual processing through single-unit recording in monkeys [15, 21-23] and fMRI signal changes in humans [24-26].

An important caveat is that psychophysical studies of perceptual learning are only a rough tool for making inferences of the underlying neural structures. Accordingly, physiological studies demonstrating low-level perceptual learning typically fail to explain the magnitude of the behavioral changes [27] and some models of perceptual learning demonstrate that channel reweighting in the readout of sensory areas can account for some aspects of perceptual learning specificity without requiring plasticity in primary sensory areas [28-31]. Other studies have found plasticity in higher-level visual areas that were originally hypothesized to be lower level features [14, 32-34]. For instance, Law and Gold [33] failed to find plasticity in monkey area middle temporal cortex (MT), but found learning effects in a later area (lateral intraparietal cortex; LIP) that largely explained behavioral changes after training in a visual motion task. Likewise, learning in visual area V4 has been found to be more robust than that in V1 [17, 22, 32, 35, 36]. Also, some aspects of learning could be taking place in other brain regions, an interesting case was recently found in which the superior colliculus [37, 38] and frontal brain areas [39] develop tuning to motion directions after extensive training. While the exact locus of visual plasticity in a given study is often an issue of significant controversy, as a whole these studies give indication that plasticity is likely occurring at all stages of visual processing; although with a distribution that varies across tasks and training paradigms.

3. Perceptual Learning as a method to improve vision

Software programs integrating perceptual learning are being utilized more frequently to optimize outcomes in specific visual conditions, both in research/clinical studies and commercially. Using computer generated visual stimuli presented in repetitive patterns, users interact with visual stimuli and the training process induces neurological visual system plasticity and patient benefits. The observed benefits can include increased neuro-adaptation to new visual environments, improved contrast sensitivity and increases in spatial or visual acuity. Recent research provides examples of perceptual learning techniques that result in visual improvements for a variety of visual conditions.

4. Amblyopia

Amblyopia results in a lack of stereovision and poor vision in the amblyopic eye (even after the optics of the eye, and misalignment between the eyes, are corrected). Amblyopia impacts 2-3% of the population and is conventionally considered untreatable in adults. The gold standard for treating amblyopia is to restore stereovision. To accomplish this, (1) cortical processing of the amblyopic eye needs to be strengthened, (2) suppression from the non-amblyopic eye needs to be lessened, and (3) binocular integration needs to process correctly in the visual system. Amblyopia is typically treated only children, where traditional approaches focusing on patching or the use of atropine in the non-amblyopic eye, with no treatment attempted in adults due to a believed lack of plasticity.

However, recently perceptual learning paradigms have been found to be effective in improving acuity and stereopsis in adults, and in children where traditional patching was unsuccessful [40-42]. More recently there has been focus on binocular interactions in amblyopia with push-pull trainings that put the eyes in competition successfully lessening suppression in the amblyopic eye [43, 44], or binocular integration, which trains the two eyes to work better together [45]. Perceptual learning techniques, or more recently commercial video games [46], have also been found to reduce crowding [47], and improve spatial frequency and contrast discrimination, which also transferred to untrained spatial frequencies in adults with amblyopia [48]. Together these approaches have led to numerous examples which demonstrate substantial benefits in vision in the amblyopic eye and provide great promise for future perceptual learning based treatment approaches.

5. Age-related Macular Degeneration (AMD)

Age-related Macular Degeneration (AMD) is the leading cause of central low vision in adults. The prevalence of AMD increases after age 50, and is expected to affect nearly three million Americans by 2020 (*The Eye Diseases Prevalence Research Group, 2004*). AMD patients suffer a retinal disorder in which photoreceptors are damaged or displaced, resulting in visual field loss, spatial distortions to the visual field, and impairments of acuity and contrast sensitivity. Despite a range of treatments to arrest the progress of AMD, damage to the retina cannot be reversed, resulting in a need for effective visual training therapies. There are a number of studies that show both functional learning in the development of preferred looking points [49-51] and cortical reorganization in foveal responses to peripheral stimuli [3, 52]. Difficulty reading is a common complaint in AMD patients due to the central vision loss. Recently, Chung [53] demonstrated that perceptual learning could improve reading speed in these patients after training. Additionally, Liu et al [54] trained profoundly visually impaired individuals (including AMD, glaucoma, retinitis pigmentosa, and other conditions) on a visual search task. Search speed and accuracy improved after training, effects that remained for at least one month.

While, there are limited perceptual-learning studies in AMD patients and it is unclear the extent to which normally occurring reorganizations are driven through use-dependent mechanisms [55], there is significant potential benefit to applications of perceptual learning in AMD.

6. Age related visual decline

It is well documented that vision declines with age [56]. Deficits are seen in many aspects of vision including eye optics, luminance, contrast, orientation, motion processing, form, scene and depth perception, and optical flow. Recent research has found perceptual learning can improve visual performance in older individuals. For example, after training on a visual discrimination task older participants improved up to the same performance level of untrained college age participants, with improvements lasting at least 3 months after training [57]. Additionally, older individuals improved on a motion detection task (either drifting sine wave gratings or random dot motion), and learning transferred to the untrained motion type [58].

The most common age related visual deficit is presbyopia. Presbyopia is a progressive normal aging process where the elasticity of the lens of the eye is reduced [59]. Although the decrease in elasticity of lens starts at birth, this condition, noticed by most people in their early 40's, manifests as a reduced ability to focus on nearby stimuli and a reduction of contrast sensitivity

http://dx.doi.org/10.5772/58364

[2]. There is no cure for presbyopia. Typical treatments are reading glasses or multifocal lenses, contact lenses or more recently, surgery like the Laser-Assisted in Situ Keratomileusis (LASIK). While treatments do exist, their use can be inconvenient for some as many treatments are not ideal for all daily activities, or can represent a significant challenge to others. All treatment options of presbyopia induce further reduction in optical contrast [60, 61]. Additionally, the use of multifocal lenses (common form of therapy) introduces unnatural viewing conditions where the point of focus depends upon gaze angle and optical aberration in transition regions. Of note, encouraging research from Polat and colleagues [62] suggest perceptual learning can ameliorate the effects of presbyopia, and in some cases, enable mild presbyopes to read without glasses. After training on a contrast detection task using Gabor patches of a range of spatial frequencies participants improved near vision acuity, reading speed, contrast detection and discrimination without changing the optics of the eye.

In general, perceptual learning also shows great promise for conditions for which there are no standard treatments. These include the conditions mentioned above as well as other low-vision conditions such as glaucoma, night vision deficits, retinitis pigmentosa, low myopia, diabetes, etc., as well as a complement to medical technologies such as LASIK, intraocular lens implantations, retinal implants, and other treatments that yield improvements in vision but for which suboptimal cortical processing leaves patients without the full potential benefit of the optical improvements that they've gained.

7. Applying Perceptual Learning in ophthalmology practice

As eyecare technology advances, so do patient expectations. Optimizing outcomes and managing expectations is a consistent challenge in clinical practice. Eye practitioners agree that good vision promotes healthier lifestyles [63], aids educational processes [64] and visual impairment is detrimental to life itself [65, 66]. An international online survey sponsored by Bausch and Lomb called NSIGHT (Needs, Symptoms, Incidence, Global Eye Health Trends) found that "seeing better" was the most important consideration for choosing vision products. Patients prefer vision related products that emphasize vision improvement, therefore therapy goals need to involve products and methods to improve vision to a maximum. Clinicians pay tremendous attention to the "eye side" of the visual system but emerging research shows that we need to pay more attention to the neurological or brain processing aspect of vision which lies outside of conventional treatments.

Vision training is not a new phenomenon in Ophthalmology, eye exercises have been used for hundreds of years. The most common vision training procedures, currently and traditionally, focus on exercising the optics of the eye (e.g. flippers, prisms, and alternating fixation between distances). However these techniques lack reliable evidence of success [67]. Alternatively, recent perceptual learning based software intervention programs for eye related disorders have shown great promise and there is increasing evidence of their efficacy. Historically reserved for database and assessment tool functions, eyecare software is expanding rapidly into therapeutic interventions and treatment. Computer software is now finding real world use in the visual world of binocular disorders, amblyopia, neuro-rehabilitation and visual enhancement. Researchers and software developers are encouraged by research showing that specific software use actualizes the potential of the visual system and translates into real life gains. Therefore, the science of improving brain processing is not only relevant but utilizing these tools to treat these disorders can prove life changing. With that said, not all computer programs produce positive visual benefits and the results derived from training can vary from individual to individual. In other words, a simple software program may create entertainment but does not necessarily create real world vision improvement.

Here, we highlight a few perceptual training products currently on the market that doctors are using to help patients.

GlassesOff is an iOS app that enhances contrast sensitivity. Studies have found that contrast sensitivity decreases in disease states but also diminishes with age [68, 69]. Therefore, presbyopia is a combination of both decreased accommodation but also decreased contrast sensitivity. GlassesOff reports several studies on their website related to their product. A recent study found acuity and contrast sensitivity improved in presbyopes after using GlassesOff for approximately 3 months [62]. A perceptual learning technique called "collinear facilitation" is utilized to strengthen neural connections and reduce visual noise. The reduction of visual noise then increases visual clarity. It claims a 90% success rate for dismissing glasses for reading. For more information see glassesoff.com.

Nova Vision is a home computer training program used to reduce visual field deficits and provide visual benefits to patients suffering from the effects of stroke and traumatic brain injury. Nova studies show that visual field can be expanded an additional 5% over time [70]. According to another study, 75% of the trainees reported improved mobility after training [71]. Ideal training consists of using the technology twice daily for 30 minutes a session for approximately 6 months. One can find more information at Novavision.com.

RevitalVision/NeuroVision was developed to aid doctors in the treatment of amblyopia, presbyopia and cataract surgery. RevitalVision has also been used to enhance the vision of sports athletes. Depending on the visual condition, the program requires 40 training sessions for the treatment of amblyopia and 20 sessions for other conditions. Three sessions are recommended weekly and each session lasts up to 30 minutes. Stated benefits include increased contrast sensitivity, enhanced visual acuity, reduction in haloes and improved sense of night vision [72]. The program is used at home on a Windows PC. Some doctors are prescribing the technology to patients to accelerate adaptation to altered visual states due to cataract or LASIK surgery. For more information see Revitalvision.com

ULTIMEYES is a recent application that works on a home computer (Windows PC, Apple Mac) or iOS or Android to train vision. Implementing recent neuroscience advances, ULTIMEYES training combines paired visual and auditory stimuli and was designed in a videogame like way, to make the training more enjoyable for the patient. Benefits include improved contrast sensitivity, enhanced visual acuity, increased night vision and a reduction of haloes. Training time requires 4 weekly sessions for a total of 30 sessions, and each training session takes approximately 25 minutes to complete. A recent study found improved acuity and contrast sensitivity in normal sighted individuals after 2 months of ULTIMEYES training [10]. ULTIMEYES has also been used in the treatment of low vision conditions including presbyopia, amblyopia, post-LASIK rehabilitation, and post-cataract surgery rehabilitation (especially effective for multifocal patients), and with athletes for improved sports performance [11]. For more information see Ultimeyesvision.com.

This is not an exhaustive list of available technologies but gives the reader an idea of commercially available products using software technology to tune brain processing and create better visual performance.

8. Principles of Perceptual Learning

An important question in evaluating studies of PL, is how do we know *what* to learn? In other words, how does a neural system know which information is behaviorally relevant and which is not? Given that plasticity can occur in adult sensory systems, there must be some mechanism that gates what is learned (i.e. to control what aspects are allowed and what aspects are restricted). In the following sections, we review different mechanisms and approaches that help guide perceptual learning.

8.1. Attention

Attention refers to a set of fundamental mental process that selectively modulates the processing of relevant information over irrelevant information; it informs decisions, guides memory processes, and our executive control to direct resources to act upon the world. A common belief is that perceptual learning cannot occur without persistent and intensive attention to the feature to be learned [73]. Profound learning effects are often present for task-relevant features but are typically absent or very limited for the task-irrelevant and unattended features. For example, Ahissar and Hochstein [74] found no or little transfer of learning effects between two tasks that involved judgments on different stimulus attributes (either orientation of local elements or global shape) of the same stimuli. It was also reported that the ability of subjects to discriminate the orientation of a line did not improve when the brightness rather than orientation of the line was attended [75]. Additionally, a single-unit recording study in monkeys found neuronal plasticity manifested as a change in the orientation tuning curves of V1 cells with receptive fields overlapping the spatial location of the training task. No plasticity was found for cells with receptive fields overlapping the location of task-irrelevant stimuli presented at a different location from those relevant to the task [15]. While in the next section we'll discuss how attention to stimuli is not actually required to achieve on those stimuli, nonetheless attention plays an important role in selecting what we do (and do not) learn.

8.2. Reinforcement

Theories of reinforcement learning show that rewards and punishment sculpt when and what we learn. At these times reinforcement signals are released to better learn aspects of the environment (even those for which the organism is not consciously aware) that are predictive or co-vary with the event. For example, in a natural environment a target (e.g., a predator) to which one needs to direct attention is usually presented in the same or similar context. Thus, gaining higher sensitivity to features in such a context may lead one to more easily notice that he/she is in the environment in which a target tends to appear and to better recognize the target [e.g. 76].

Recent research demonstrates the fundamental importance of reinforcement processes in guiding perceptual learning. For example, the research paradigm of "task-irrelevant perceptual learning" shows that sensory plasticity occurs without attention being directed to the learned stimuli, and even for those that participants are not aware [19, 77-88]. Seitz and Watanabe [84] found that a sensitivity enhancement occurred as the result of temporal-pairing between the presentation of a subliminal, task-irrelevant, motion stimulus and a task-target. In this experiment, four different directions of motion were presented an equal number of times during the exposure stage, but a single direction of interest was consistently paired (temporally preceded and then overlapped) with the task-targets. Learning was found only for the motion-direction that was temporally-paired with the task-targets, not for the other motion-directions. Similar results were obtained when the luminance contrast of the dots (100% coherence) was made so low that the subjects did not notice the presentation of the motion stimuli [81]. These results suggest that task-irrelevant perceptual learning does not occur as a result of purely passive exposure, but that the irrelevant feature must be related to task performance. These results have led to the idea that plasticity is gated by confluence between a spatially diffusive task-related signal and a task-irrelevant feature signal [79]. Later research confirmed this idea by demonstrating that task-irrelevant perceptual learning can arise through pairing a stimulus with a liquid reward [80].

Seitz and Watanabe [79] suggested a model of perceptual learning where learning results from interactions between spatially diffusive task-driven signals and bottom-up stimulus signals. Namely, that learning is gated by behaviorally relevant events (rewards, punishment, novelty, etc). At these times reinforcement signals are released to better learn aspects of the environment (even those for which the organism is not consciously aware) that are predictive or co-vary with the event. By now, task-irrelevant perceptual learning has been shown to be a robust learning phenomenon that generalizes to a wide range of stimulus features, for example, motion processing [19], orientation processing [89], critical flicker fusion thresholds [82, 83], contour integration [90], auditory formant processing [91], and phonetic processing [92]. Importantly, task-irrelevant perceptual learning produces learning effects that are often as strong, and sometimes stronger, than learning effects produced through direct training [91, 93]. While the phenomenon of task-irrelevant perceptual learning has been studied in most detail in the case of low-level perceptual learning, recent research has identified a high-level, fast form, of task-irrelevant perceptual learning (fast-task-irrelevant perceptual learning) [94-101]. In this fast-task-irrelevant perceptual learning paradigm, participants conducted target detection tasks (looking for a target, letter, color, or word among a series of distractors), while also memorizing other stimuli (images, pictures) that were consistently paired with the stimuli of the target-detection task. Similar to task-irrelevant perceptual learning for low-level perceptual learning, visual memory was enhanced for stimuli that were paired with the targets of the target-detection task. Thus task-irrelevant perceptual learning is arguably a basic mechanism of learning in the brain that spans multiple levels of processing and sensory modalities.

While we have discussed attention and reinforcement as separate processes, this distinction may be overly simplistic (e.g. [79, 86]). For example, the orienting of attention, in the direction of the target-arrow, has been linked with the acetylcholine neuromodulatory system [102]. The same neuromodulatory system has been suggested to have an important role in learning: some studies indicate that a reduction of the cholinergic input reduces cortical plasticity [103] and impairs learning [104-106]. However, other neuromodulatory systems, such as dopamine and norepinephrine have also been linked to both attention [107, 108] and to learning [109, 110]. Indeed, these three neuromodulators (acetylcholine, norepinephrine, and dopamine) have been linked to the three attentional systems described by Posner and Petersen (1990): the alerting network that involves temporal cueing and the maintenance of an alert state (norepinephrine; [111-113]; the orienting network that spatially selects information from sensory input (acetylcholine; [102]; and the executive control network that resolves conflict among responses (dopamine; [114]). These studies indicate that attention and reinforcement are deeply interrelated and that a good training approach should aim to direct both attention and reinforcement in a manner to promote learning.

8.3. Applying rules of synaptic plasticity

At the cellular level, it is widely accepted that the process of synaptic plasticity underlies learning and memory. Synaptic plasticity is the ability of the strength of the connections between synapses to change, strengthening or weakening the connections of existing neurons to modulate the effectiveness of their communication. Bliss and Lomo discovered a method to experimentally induce a persistent synaptic plasticity termed long-term potentiation (LTP) [115]. By inducing brief high frequency electrical stimulation in the perforant pathway of anaesthetized rabbits and recording in the dentate gyrus they discovered an increase of excitatory post-synaptic potentials (EPSPs) over baseline response that lasted up to 10 hours. Conversely, long-term depression (LTD) is induced by persistent low frequency electrical stimulation, resulting in weakened synaptic connections.

Recent research has established that non-invasive exposure-based stimulation protocols can be applied to the sensory systems and result in plasticity of the corresponding sensory cortices. Passive high frequency stimulation (HFS) (20 Hz) of the fingertip resulted in the behavioral improvement of a 2-point discrimination task, and low frequency stimulation (LFS) (1 Hz) decreased performance on this task [116]. Additionally, improvements on the behavioral task after HFS was correlated with cortical reorganization as assessed by mapping somatosensory evoked potentials. This effect was abolished by oral application of an NMDA receptor antagonist, indicating this effect shares similar requirements to cellular LTP and long-term memory formation as identified in the animal model [117]. Using a visual stimulation protocol Beste and colleagues [118] demonstrated behavioral changes on a change-detection task. Here, two bars were presented where a change could occur in the luminance of one bar, the orientation of one bar, the luminance and orientation of the same bar, or the luminance of one bar and the orientation of the other bar. The participants had to report a change in luminance, and ignore a change in orientation. The orientation change in the last condition was highly distracting, and made the luminance detection more difficult. A visual stimulation protocol consisted of alternating black and white bars flashing at either a high (20 Hz) or low (1 Hz) frequency with the goal of increasing or decreasing luminance saliency. The authors found a high frequency visual stimulation protocol improved the behavioral outcome on the detection task tested up to 10 days after induction. Conversely, a low frequency LTD-like protocol impaired performance. These studies of exposure-based learning provide a clear connection between the animal model and the human system, and suggest that approaches based upon knowledge of synaptic plasticity can be applied to improved perception in humans.

8.4. Multisensory facilitation

The human brain has evolved to learn and operate optimally in natural environments in which behavior is guided by information integrated across multiple sensory modalities. Crossmodal interactions are ubiquitous in the nervous system and occur even at early stages of perceptual processing [119-123]. Until recently, however, all studies of perceptual learning focused on training with one sensory modality. This unisensory training fails to tap into natural learning mechanisms that have evolved to optimize behavior in a multisensory environment. Recent research shows that subjects trained with auditory-visual stimuli exhibit a faster rate of learning and a higher degree of improvement than found in subjects trained in silence [124, 125]. Critically, these benefits of multisensory training are even found for perceptual tests *without* auditory signals. In other words, *multisensory training facilitates unisensory learning*. While, to date, most vision training procedures either don't include sounds as part of the task (other than as feedback) or include sounds that are not coordinated with visual stimuli, the advantage of multisensory training over visual-alone training is substantial; reducing the number of sessions required to reach asymptote by ~60%, while also raising the maximum performance [126]. We suggest that having complementary information about the target objects come from different sensory modalities allows the senses to work together to facilitate learning.

8.5. Promoting transfer of learning

Classically, a translational barrier to perceptual learning has been its high degree of specificity to trained stimulus features [127]; such as orientation [20], retinal location [128] or even the eye of training [80, 129]. For example training with a single visual stimulus at a single screen location can result in learning that is specific to that situation. While such studies have been informative regarding the mechanisms of learning, specificity limits therapeutic benefits.

Recent research suggests methods of how this "curse of specificity" can be overcome. Approaches that depart from the most simple training approaches, such as those using multi-stimulus training [130, 131] and off-the-shelf video games [132, 133] show a greater generalization of learning. For example, the recently developed technique of 'double training' found that the specific learning effects found in their paradigms can show broad transfer when

http://dx.doi.org/10.5772/58364

more than one stimulus attribute is trained at a time. Xiao, Zhang [131] trained participants on the Vernier discrimination task at a specific orientation at a specific location in the visual field, which normally yields location and orientation specific learning effects [129]. But when they subsequently trained a second orientation at a different spatial location, they found that the training induced changes for the second orientation transferred to the first location. Such findings of broad location transfer undermine the argument that this learning is due to plasticity in retinotopic visual areas.

There exist a growing number of studies that address how specificity, or its opposite, transfer, is controlled by different factors. In a discrimination task, Jeter, Dosher, Petrov and Lu [134] showed that transfer was observed in low-precision transfer tasks while specificity was observed in high-precision transfer tasks. Then, Jeter, Dosher, Liu and Lu [135] showed that specificity was the result of an extensive training, confirming more classical results [20, 128, 136], while a substantial transfer was observed at early in the training. Interestingly, another study, reported by Aberg, Tartaglia and Herzog [137] presented a series of experiments showing, in one hand, that the number of trials per session influenced the overall improvement of the participant's performance, and in another hand, the transfer depended on the number of trials presented during each session, not the total number of trials. Zhang *et al.*, [138] showed a peripheral orientation discrimination task transferred to new locations only after a pre-test was given to participants. These studies add to the double-training studies that show transfer after training multiple features or at multiple locations [130, 131]. Together these studies show that many factors (extent of training, blocking of trials, precision of training stimuli, diversity of training set, etc), influence the transfer of learning.

9. Conclusion

While extant applications of perceptual learning to Ophthalmology show great promise, a limitation of modern perceptual learning research is that learning is studied in very specific ways, focusing on one particular stimulus or factor. This narrow focus has limited understanding of the multiple learning factors that are present in natural settings and how these factors interact to determine the speed and nature of learning. We suggest a new paradigm of integrating perceptual learning methodologies into a coordinated approach that achieves a more comprehensive form of perceptual learning than typically studied in the lab. For example the approach used in the ULTIMEYES program combines many factors that are known to promote neural plasticity and generalization of learning [10, 11]. Furthermore, findings that playing off-the-shelf video games can improve vision [132, 133, 139] suggests another avenue of research where principles derived from video games should be combined with those from the field of perceptual learning to create an enriching user experience that encourages compliance with treatment while effectively optimizing how the brain process its ocular inputs.

Author details

Jenni Deveau[1], Gary Lovcik[2] and Aaron R. Seitz[1]

*Address all correspondence to: aseitz@ucr.edu

1 Department of Psychology, University of California – Riverside, Riverside, CA, USA

2 Anaheim Hills Optometric Center, Anaheim, CA, USA

References

[1] Levi, D.M. and R.W. Li, *Perceptual learning as a potential treatment for amblyopia: a mini-review.* Vision Res, 2009. 49(21): p. 2535-49.

[2] Polat, U., *Making perceptual learning practical to improve visual functions.* Vision Res, 2009. 49(21): p. 2566-73.

[3] Baker, C.I., et al., *Reorganization of visual processing in macular degeneration.* J Neurosci, 2005. 25(3): p. 614-8.

[4] Huxlin, K.R., et al., *Perceptual relearning of complex visual motion after V1 damage in humans.* J Neurosci, 2009. 29(13): p. 3981-91.

[5] Vaina, L.M. and C.G. Gross, *Perceptual deficits in patients with impaired recognition of biological motion after temporal lobe lesions.* Proc Natl Acad Sci U S A, 2004. 101(48): p. 16947-51.

[6] Ostrovsky, Y., A. Andalman, and P. Sinha, *Vision following extended congenital blindness.* Psychol Sci, 2006. 17(12): p. 1009-14.

[7] Hubel, D.H. and T.N. Wiesel, *Effects of Monocular Deprivation in Kittens.* Naunyn Schmiedebergs Arch Pharmacol, 1964. 248: p. 492-7.

[8] Hubel, D.H. and T.N. Wiesel, *Binocular interaction in striate cortex of kittens reared with artificial squint.* J Neurophysiol, 1965. 28(6): p. 1041-59.

[9] Adini, Y., D. Sagi, and M. Tsodyks, *Context-enabled learning in the human visual system.* Nature, 2002. 415(6873): p. 790-3.

[10] Deveau, J., G. Lovcik, and A.R. Seitz, *Broad-based visual benefits from training with an integrated perceptual-learning video game.* Vision Res, 2014.

[11] Deveau, J., D.J. Ozer, and A.R. Seitz, *Improved vision and on field performance in baseball through perceptual learning.* Curr Biol, 2014. 24(4).

[12] Ball, K. and R. Sekuler, *Adaptive processing of visual motion.* J Exp Psychol Hum Percept Perform, 1981. 7(4): p. 780-94.

[13] Sagi, D. and D. Tanne, *Perceptual learning: learning to see.* Curr Opin Neurobiol, 1994. 4(2): p. 195-9.

[14] Crist, R.E., W. Li, and C.D. Gilbert, *Learning to see: experience and attention in primary visual cortex.* Nat Neurosci, 2001. 4(5): p. 519-25.

[15] Schoups, A., et al., *Practising orientation identification improves orientation coding in V1 neurons.PG-549-53.* Nature, 2001. 412(6846).

[16] Schoups, A.A., R. Vogels, and G.A. Orban, *Human perceptual learning in identifying the oblique orientation: retinotopy, orientation specificity and monocularity.* J Physiol, 1995. 483 (Pt 3): p. 797-810.

[17] Raiguel, S., et al., *Learning to see the difference specifically alters the most informative V4 neurons.* J Neurosci, 2006. 26(24): p. 6589-602.

[18] Crist, R.E., et al., *Perceptual learning of spatial localization: specificity for orientation, position, and context.* J Neurophysiol, 1997. 78(6): p. 2889-94.

[19] Watanabe, T., et al., *Greater plasticity in lower-level than higher-level visual motion processing in a passive perceptual learning task.* Nat Neurosci, 2002. 5(10): p. 1003-9.

[20] Fiorentini, A. and N. Berardi, *Perceptual learning specific for orientation and spatial frequency.* Nature, 1980. 287(5777): p. 43-4.

[21] Li, C.S., C. Padoa-Schioppa, and E. Bizzi, *Neuronal correlates of motor performance and motor learning in the primary motor cortex of monkeys adapting to an external force field.* Neuron, 2001. 30(2): p. 593-607.

[22] Yang, T. and J.H. Maunsell, *The effect of perceptual learning on neuronal responses in monkey visual area V4.* J Neurosci, 2004. 24(7): p. 1617-26.

[23] Zohary, E., et al., *Neuronal plasticity that underlies improvement in perceptual performance.* Science, 1994. 263(5151): p. 1289-92.

[24] Furmanski, C.S., D. Schluppeck, and S.A. Engel, *Learning strengthens the response of primary visual cortex to simple patterns.* Curr Biol, 2004. 14(7): p. 573-8.

[25] Schwartz, S., P. Maquet, and C. Frith, *Neural correlates of perceptual learning: a functional MRI study of visual texture discrimination.* Proc Natl Acad Sci U S A, 2002. 99(26): p. 17137-42.

[26] Vaina, L.M., et al., *Neural systems underlying learning and representation of global motion.* Proc Natl Acad Sci U S A, 1998. 95(21): p. 12657-62.

[27] Roelfsema, P.R. and A. van Ooyen, *Attention-gated reinforcement learning of internal representations for classification.* Neural Comput, 2005. 17(10): p. 2176-214.

[28] Dosher, B.A. and Z.L. Lu, *Perceptual learning reflects external noise filtering and internal noise reduction through channel reweighting.* Proc Natl Acad Sci U S A, 1998. 95(23): p. 13988-93.

[29] Sotiropoulos, G., A.R. Seitz, and P. Series, *Perceptual learning in visual hyperacuity: A reweighting model.* Vision Res, 2011. 51(6): p. 585-99.

[30] Dosher, B.A. and Z.L. Lu, *Mechanisms of perceptual learning.* Vision Res, 1999. 39(19): p. 3197-221.

[31] Petrov, A., A. Dosher, and Z. Lu, *Perceptual learning without feedback in non-stationary contexts: data and model.* Vision Res, 2006. in press.

[32] Ghose, G.M., T. Yang, and J.H. Maunsell, *Physiological correlates of perceptual learning in monkey V1 and V2.* J Neurophysiol, 2002. 87(4): p. 1867-88.

[33] Law, C.T. and J.I. Gold, *Neural correlates of perceptual learning in a sensory-motor, but not a sensory, cortical area.* Nat Neurosci, 2008. 11(4): p. 505-13.

[34] Gu, Y., et al., *Perceptual learning reduces interneuronal correlations in macaque visual cortex.* Neuron, 2011. 71(4): p. 750-61.

[35] Rainer, G., H. Lee, and N.K. Logothetis, *The effect of learning on the function of monkey extrastriate visual cortex.* PLoS Biol, 2004. 2(2): p. E44.

[36] Ghose, G.M., *Learning in mammalian sensory cortex.* Curr Opin Neurobiol, 2004. 14(4): p. 513-8.

[37] Horwitz, G.D., A.P. Batista, and W.T. Newsome, *Direction-selective visual responses in macaque superior colliculus induced by behavioral training.* Neurosci Lett, 2004. 366(3): p. 315-9.

[38] Horwitz, G.D., A.P. Batista, and W.T. Newsome, *Representation of an abstract perceptual decision in macaque superior colliculus.* J Neurophysiol, 2004. 91(5): p. 2281-96.

[39] Zaksas, D. and T. Pasternak, *Directional signals in the prefrontal cortex and in area MT during a working memory for visual motion task.* J Neurosci, 2006. 26(45): p. 11726-42.

[40] Huang, C.B., Y. Zhou, and Z.L. Lu, *Broad bandwidth of perceptual learning in the visual system of adults with anisometropic amblyopia.* Proc Natl Acad Sci U S A, 2008. 105(10): p. 4068-73.

[41] Polat, U., et al., *Improving vision in adult amblyopia by perceptual learning.* Proc Natl Acad Sci U S A, 2004. 101(17): p. 6692-7.

[42] Polat, U., T. Ma-Naim, and A. Spierer, *Treatment of children with amblyopia by perceptual learning.* Vision Res, 2009. 49(21): p. 2599-603.

[43] Ooi, T.L., et al., *A push-pull treatment for strengthening the 'lazy eye' in amblyopia.* Curr Biol, 2013. 23(8): p. R309-10.

[44] Xu, J.P., Z.J. He, and T.L. Ooi, *Effectively reducing sensory eye dominance with a push-pull perceptual learning protocol.* Curr Biol, 2010. 20(20): p. 1864-8.

[45] Li, J., et al., *Dichoptic training enables the adult amblyopic brain to learn.* Curr Biol, 2013. 23(8): p. R308-9.

[46] Li, R.W., et al., *Video-game play induces plasticity in the visual system of adults with amblyopia.* PLoS Biol, 2011. 9(8): p. e1001135.

[47] Hussain, Z., et al., *Perceptual learning reduces crowding in amblyopia and in the normal periphery.* J Neurosci, 2012. 32(2): p. 474-80.

[48] Astle, A.T., B.S. Webb, and P.V. McGraw, *Spatial frequency discrimination learning in normal and developmentally impaired human vision.* Vision Res, 2010. 50(23): p. 2445-54.

[49] Fletcher, D.C. and R.A. Schuchard, *Preferred retinal loci relationship to macular scotomas in a low-vision population.* Ophthalmology, 1997. 104(4): p. 632-8.

[50] Kwon, M., A.S. Nandy, and B.S. Tjan, *Rapid and persistent adaptability of human oculomotor control in response to simulated central vision loss.* Curr Biol, 2013. 23(17): p. 1663-9.

[51] Kwon, M., et al., *Contour enhancement benefits older adults with simulated central field loss.* Optom Vis Sci, 2012. 89(9): p. 1374-84.

[52] Baker, C.I., et al., *Reorganization of visual processing in macular degeneration: replication and clues about the role of foveal loss.* Vision Res, 2008. 48(18): p. 1910-9.

[53] Chung, S.T., *Improving reading speed for people with central vision loss through perceptual learning.* Invest Ophthalmol Vis Sci, 2011. 52(2): p. 1164-70.

[54] Liu, L., T. Kuyk, and P. Fuhr, *Visual search training in subjects with severe to profound low vision.* Vision Res, 2007. 47(20): p. 2627-36.

[55] Dilks, D.D., et al., *Reorganization of visual processing in macular degeneration is not specific to the "preferred retinal locus".* J Neurosci, 2009. 29(9): p. 2768-73.

[56] Andersen, G.J., *Aging and Vision: Changes in Function and Performance from Optics to Perception.* Wiley Interdiscip Rev Cogn Sci, 2012. 3(3): p. 403-410.

[57] Andersen, G.J., et al., *Perceptual learning, aging, and improved visual performance in early stages of visual processing.* J Vis, 2010. 10(13): p. 4.

[58] Lu, Z.L. and B.A. Dosher, *Characterizing observers using external noise and observer models: assessing internal representations with external noise.* Psychol Rev, 2008. 115(1): p. 44-82.

[59] Koretz, J.F., et al., *Accommodation and presbyopia in the human eye--aging of the anterior segment.* Vision Res, 1989. 29(12): p. 1685-92.

[60] Llorente-Guillemot, A., et al., *Visual performance with simultaneous vision multifocal contact lenses.* Clin Exp Optom, 2012. 95(1): p. 54-9.

[61] Alarcon, A., et al., *Visual quality after monovision correction by laser in situ keratomileusis in presbyopic patients.* J Cataract Refract Surg, 2011. 37(9): p. 1629-35.

[62] Polat, U., et al., *Training the brain to overcome the effect of aging on the human eye.* Sci Rep, 2012. 2: p. 278.

[63] Fong, C.S., et al., *Correction of visual impairment by cataract surgery and improved survival in older persons: the Blue Mountains Eye Study cohort.* Ophthalmology, 2013. 120(9): p. 1720-7.

[64] Basch, C.E., *Healthier students are better learners: a missing link in school reforms to close the achievement gap.* J Sch Health, 2011. 81(10): p. 593-8.

[65] De Leo, D., et al., *Blindness, fear of sight loss, and suicide.* Psychosomatics, 1999. 40(4): p. 339-44.

[66] CDC. *The State of Vision, Aging, and Public Health in America.* 2013; Available from: cdc.gov/visionhealth/pdf/vision.pdf.

[67] Helveston, E.M., *Visual training: current status in ophthalmology.* Am J Ophthalmol, 2005. 140(5): p. 903-10.

[68] McKendrick, A.M., et al., *Contrast sensitivity changes due to glaucoma and normal aging: Low-spatial-frequency losses in both magnocellular and parvocellular pathways.* Investigative Ophthalmology & Visual Science, 2007. 48(5): p. 2115-2122.

[69] Ross, J.E., D.D. Clarke, and A.J. Bron, *Effect of age on contrast sensitivity function: uniocular and binocular findings.* Br J Ophthalmol, 1985. 69(1): p. 51-6.

[70] Kasten, E., et al., *Computer-based training for the treatment of partial blindness.* Nat Med, 1998. 4(9): p. 1083-7.

[71] Mueller, I.P., D.A.; Kenkel, S.; Kasten, E. and Sabel, B.A., *Vision Restoration Therapy after brain damage; subjective improvements of activities of daily life and their relationship to visual field enlargements.* Vision Impairment Research, 2003(5): p. 157-178.

[72] Revitalvision.com. *Amblyopia Effectiveness* 2013; Available from: Revitalvision.com/amblyopia/effectiveness.

[73] Ahissar, M. and S. Hochstein, *Attentional control of early perceptual learning.* Proc Natl Acad Sci U S A, 1993. 90(12): p. 5718-22.

[74] Ahissar, M. and S. Hochstein, *Task difficulty and the specificity of perceptual learning.* Nature, 1997. 387(6631): p. 401-6.

[75] Shiu, L.P. and H. Pashler, *Improvement in line orientation discrimination is retinally local but dependent on cognitive set.* Percept Psychophys, 1992. 52(5): p. 582-8.

[76] Chun, M.M., *Contextual cueing of visual attention.* Trends Cogn Sci, 2000. 4(5): p. 170-178.

[77] Nishina, S., et al. *The spatial spread of task-irrelevant perceptual learning.* in *Society for Neuroscience 35th Annual Meeting*. 2005. Washington, D.C.

[78] Seitz, A., et al., *Requirement for high-level processing in subliminal learning.* Curr Biol, 2005. 15(18): p. R753-5.

[79] Seitz, A. and T. Watanabe, *A unified model for perceptual learning.* Trends Cogn Sci, 2005. 9(7): p. 329-34.

[80] Seitz, A.R., D. Kim, and T. Watanabe, *Rewards evoke learning of unconsciously processed visual stimuli in adult humans.* Neuron, 2009. 61(5): p. 700-7.

[81] Seitz, A.R., et al., *Seeing what is not there shows the costs of perceptual learning.* Proc Natl Acad Sci U S A, 2005. 102(25): p. 9080-5.

[82] Seitz, A.R., et al., *Visual experience can substantially alter critical flicker fusion thresholds.* Hum Psychopharmacol, 2005. 20(1): p. 55-60.

[83] Seitz, A.R., et al., *Perceptual learning of motion leads to faster flicker perception.* PLoS ONE, 2006. 1: p. e28.

[84] Seitz, A.R. and T. Watanabe, *Psychophysics: Is subliminal learning really passive?* Nature, 2003. 422(6927): p. 36.

[85] Seitz, A.R. and T. Watanabe, *Is task-irrelevant learning really task-irrelevant?* PLoS ONE, 2008. 3(11): p. e3792.

[86] Seitz, A.R. and T. Watanabe, *The phenomenon of task-irrelevant perceptual learning.* Vision Res, 2009. 49(21): p. 2604-10.

[87] Tsushima, Y., A.R. Seitz, and T. Watanabe, *Task-irrelevant learning occurs only when the irrelevant feature is weak.* Curr Biol, 2008. 18(12): p. R516-7.

[88] Watanabe, T., J.E. Nanez, and Y. Sasaki, *Perceptual learning without perception.* Nature, 2001. 413(6858): p. 844-8.

[89] Nishina, S., et al., *Effect of spatial distance to the task stimulus on task-irrelevant perceptual learning of static Gabors.* Journal of Vision, 2007. 7(13): p. 1-10.

[90] Rosenthal, O. and G.W. Humphreys, *Perceptual organization without perception: the subliminal learning of global contour.* Psychol Sci, 2010. 21(12): p. 1751-8.

[91] Seitz, A.R., et al., *Unattended exposure to components of speech sounds yields same benefits as explicit auditory training.* Cognition, 2010. 115(3): p. 435-43.

[92] Vlahou, E., A.R. Seitz, and A. Protopapas. *Implicit learning of non-native speech stimuli.* in *Acoustical Society of America*. 2009. Portland, OR.

[93] Vlahou, E.L., A. Protopapas, and A.R. Seitz, *Implicit training of nonnative speech stimuli.* J Exp Psychol Gen, 2012. 141(2): p. 363-81.

[94] Swallow, K.M. and Y.V. Jiang, *The Attentional Boost Effect: Transient increases in attention to one task enhance performance in a second task.* Cognition, 2010. 115(1): p. 118-32.

[95] Swallow, K.M. and Y.V. Jiang, *The role of timing in the attentional boost effect.* Atten Percept Psychophys, 2011. 73(2): p. 389-404.

[96] Lin, J.Y., et al., *Enhanced memory for scenes presented at behaviorally relevant points in time.* PLoS Biol, 2010. 8(3): p. e1000337.

[97] Leclercq, V. and A.R. Seitz, *Enhancement from targets and suppression from cues in fast task-irrelevant perceptual learning.* Acta Psychol (Amst), 2012. 141(1): p. 31-8.

[98] Leclercq, V. and A.R. Seitz, *Fast-TIPL occurs for salient images without a memorization requirement in men but not in women.* PLoS ONE, 2012. 7(4): p. e36228.

[99] Leclercq, V. and A.R. Seitz, *The impact of orienting attention in fast task-irrelevant perceptual learning.* Atten Percept Psychophys, 2012. 74(4): p. 648-60.

[100] Leclercq, V. and A.R. Seitz, *Fast task-irrelevant perceptual learning is disrupted by sudden onset of central task elements.* Vision Res, 2012. 61: p. 70-6.

[101] Leclercq, V., C.C. Le Dantec, and A.R. Seitz, *Encoding of episodic information through fast task-irrelevant perceptual learning.* Vision Res, 2013.

[102] Davidson, M.C. and R.T. Marrocco, *Local infusion of scopolamine into intraparietal cortex slows covert orienting in rhesus monkeys.* J Neurophysiol, 2000. 83(3): p. 1536-49.

[103] Juliano, S.L., W. Ma, and D. Eslin, *Cholinergic depletion prevents expansion of topographic maps in somatosensory cortex.* Proc Natl Acad Sci U S A, 1991. 88(3): p. 780-4.

[104] Easton, A., et al., *Unilateral lesions of the cholinergic basal forebrain and fornix in one hemisphere and inferior temporal cortex in the opposite hemisphere produce severe learning impairments in rhesus monkeys.* Cereb Cortex, 2002. 12(7): p. 729-36.

[105] Winkler, J., et al., *Essential role of neocortical acetylcholine in spatial memory.* Nature, 1995. 375(6531): p. 484-7.

[106] Warburton, E.C., et al., *Cholinergic neurotransmission is essential for perirhinal cortical plasticity and recognition memory.* Neuron, 2003. 38(6): p. 987-96.

[107] Fan, J., et al., *Mapping the genetic variation of executive attention onto brain activity.* Proc Natl Acad Sci U S A, 2003. 100(12): p. 7406-11.

[108] Posner, M.I. and S.E. Petersen, *The attention system of the human brain.* Annu Rev Neurosci, 1990. 13: p. 25-42.

[109] Dalley, J.W., et al., *Distinct changes in cortical acetylcholine and noradrenaline efflux during contingent and noncontingent performance of a visual attentional task.* J Neurosci, 2001. 21(13): p. 4908-14.

[110] Bao, S., V.T. Chan, and M.M. Merzenich, *Cortical remodelling induced by activity of ventral tegmental dopamine neurons.* Nature, 2001. 412(6842): p. 79-83.

[111] Witte, E.A. and R.T. Marrocco, *Alteration of brain noradrenergic activity in rhesus monkeys affects the alerting component of covert orienting.* Psychopharmacology (Berl), 1997. 132(4): p. 315-23.

[112] Coull, J.T., et al., *A fronto-parietal network for rapid visual information processing: a PET study of sustained attention and working memory.* Neuropsychologia, 1996. 34(11): p. 1085-95.

[113] Marrocco, R.T., E.A. Witte, and M.C. Davidson, *Arousal systems.* Curr Opin Neurobiol, 1994. 4(2): p. 166-70.

[114] Fossella, J., et al., *Assessing the molecular genetics of attention networks.* BMC Neurosci, 2002. 3(1): p. 14.

[115] Bliss, T.V. and T. Lomo, *Long-lasting potentiation of synaptic transmission in the dentate area of the anaesthetized rabbit following stimulation of the perforant path.* J Physiol, 1973. 232(2): p. 331-56.

[116] Ragert, P., et al., *Differential effects of tactile high-and low-frequency stimulation on tactile discrimination in human subjects.* BMC Neurosci, 2008. 9: p. 9.

[117] Dinse, H.R., et al., *Pharmacological modulation of perceptual learning and associated cortical reorganization.* Science, 2003. 301(5629): p. 91-4.

[118] Beste, C., et al., *Improvement and impairment of visually guided behavior through LTP-and LTD-like exposure-based visual learning.* Curr Biol, 2011. 21(10): p. 876-82.

[119] Calvert, G., C. Spence, and B.E. Stein, *The handbook of multisensory processes.* 2004: The MIT Press.

[120] Driver, J. and T. Noesselt, *Multisensory interplay reveals crossmodal influences on 'sensory-specific' brain regions, neural responses, and judgments.* Neuron, 2008. 57: p. 11-23.

[121] Ghazanfar, A. and C.E. Schroeder, *Is neocortex essentially multisensory?* Trends Cogn Sci, 2006. 10(6): p. 278-285.

[122] Shimojo, S. and L. Shams, *Sensory modalities are not separate modalities: plasticity and interactions.* Current Opinion in Neurobiology, 2001. 11: p. 505-509.

[123] Schroeder, C.E. and J. Foxe, *Multisensory contributions to low-level, 'unisensory' processing.* Current Opinion in Neurobiology, 2005. 15: p. 454-458.

[124] Kim, R.S., A.R. Seitz, and L. Shams, *Benefits of stimulus congruency for multisensory facilitation of visual learning.* PLoS ONE, 2008. 3(1): p. e1532.

[125] Seitz, A.R., R. Kim, and L. Shams, *Sound facilitates visual learning.* Current Biology, 2006. 16: p. 1422-1427.

[126] Seitz, A.R., R. Kim, and L. Shams, *Sound facilitates visual learning.* Curr Biol, 2006. 16(14): p. 1422-7.

[127] Fahle, M., *Perceptual learning: specificity versus generalization.* Curr Opin Neurobiol, 2005. 15(2): p. 154-60.

[128] Karni, A. and D. Sagi, *Where practice makes perfect in texture discrimination: evidence for primary visual cortex plasticity.* Proc Natl Acad Sci U S A, 1991. 88(11): p. 4966-70.

[129] Poggio, T., M. Fahle, and S. Edelman, *Fast perceptual learning in visual hyperacuity.* Science, 1992. 256(5059): p. 1018-21.

[130] Yu, C., et al., *Rule-Based Learning Explains Visual Perceptual Learning and Its Specificity and Transfer.* Journal of Neuroscience, 2010. 30(37): p. 12323-12328.

[131] Xiao, L.Q., et al., *Complete Transfer of Perceptual Learning across Retinal Locations Enabled by Double Training.* Curr Biol, 2008. 18(24): p. 1922-6.

[132] Green, C.S. and D. Bavelier, *Action video game modifies visual selective attention.* Nature, 2003. 423(6939): p. 534-537.

[133] Li, R., et al., *Enhancing the contrast sensitivity function through action video game training.* Nat Neurosci, 2009. 12(5): p. 549-51.

[134] Jeter, P.E., et al., *Task precision at transfer determines specificity of perceptual learning.* J Vis, 2009. 9(3): p. 1 1-13.

[135] Jeter, P.E., et al., *Specificity of perceptual learning increases with increased training.* Vision Res, 2010. 50(19): p. 1928-40.

[136] Ball, K. and R. Sekuler, *A specific and enduring improvement in visual motion discrimination.* Science, 1982. 218(4573): p. 697-8.

[137] Aberg, K.C., E.M. Tartaglia, and M.H. Herzog, *Perceptual learning with Chevrons requires a minimal number of trials, transfers to untrained directions, but does not require sleep.* Vision Res, 2009. 49(16): p. 2087-94.

[138] Zhang, T., et al., Decoupling location specificity from perceptual learning of orientation discrimination. Vision Res, 2010. 50(4): p. 368-74.

[139] Green, C.S. and D. Bavelier, Action-video-game experience alters the spatial resolution of vision. Psychol Sci, 2007. 18(1): p. 88-94.

Chapter 17

New Understandings on Pathogenesis of Dry Eye — From Animal Models to Clinical Therapy

Cintia S. de Paiva, Andrew J.W. Huang,
De-Quan Li and Stephen C. Pflugfelder

Additional information is available at the end of the chapter

http://dx.doi.org/10.5772/57585

1. Introduction

As defined by the International Dry Eye Workshop, dry eye is a multifactorial disease of the tears and ocular surface with symptoms of discomfort, visual disturbance, and tear film instability with potential damage to the ocular surface resulting in a dysfunctional lacrimal functional unit [1]. It is one of the most common medical problems that affects 6 to 44 million people in the United States based on reported prevalence figures of 4 to 33% from large epidemiological studies [2-4].

Dry eye affects quality of vision and quality of life. It is also associated with a significant financial burden to the individual and society [5, 6]. It has been shown that dry eye significantly decreases work productivity among office workers, by preventing them from performing at their full potential [7]. The cost of work performance loss associated with dry eye was estimated to be between $10-15 million/year in Japan [7].

The corneal surface irregularity in dry eye degrades visual function by decreasing contrast sensitivity and functional visual acuity [8]. Visual impairment is one of the 10 most common disabilities and vision impacts mobility, independence and quality of life. The presence of dry eye was found to significantly impact the ability to perform daily activities such as reading, using a computer and driving [9]. Visual impairments associated with dry eye disease have been associated with falls and hip fractures in the elderly [10], and complications from these falls is the leading cause of death from injury in men and women over the age of 65 [11]. As vision deteriorates, one's ability to perform activities of daily living becomes exceedingly more difficult. Using time trade off techniques, Schiffman and colleagues calculated that patients with severe dry eye expecting to live 10 years or more, were willing to give up 1.6 years of that time to be disease free [12], an amount similar to patients with moderate to severe angina [13]. Even though dry eye is a chronic disease, dry eye patients often complain about daily exacerbations. One frequent complaint is worsening of irritation symptoms and vision after prolonged use of a computer or grocery shopping.

While its pathogenesis has not been fully elucidated, it has been shown that changes in tear composition including increased proinflammatory cytokines, chemokines, metalloproteinases, increased expression of immune activation and adhesion molecules by the conjunctival epithelium and increased number of T lymphocytes in the conjunctiva play a pathogenic role in both dry eye patients and in animal models [14-21]. Increased knowledge has shown that inflammation is responsible in part for the irritation symptoms, ocular surface epithelial disease including loss of goblet cell, conjunctival metaplasia, and altered corneal epithelial barrier function in dry eye. This book chapter will discuss diverse pathogenic aspects of dry eye.

2. Experimental animal models of dry eye

There are several animal models of dry eye currently used throughout the world. They have been used to evaluate the natural history of the disease, to elucidate pathogenic mechanisms (risk factors and molecular mediators, pathways) and also to evaluate efficacy of therapeutic candidates. Models of dry eye rely on decreasing tear volume and production. To achieve that, surgical excision of the lacrimal gland, injection of pro-inflammatory cytokine IL-1 or isolated lymphocytes into the lacrimal gland, pharmacological blockade of lacrimal gland secretion have been used [22-24]. Autoimmune strains have also been studied. These strains have age-related lymphocytic infiltration of the lacrimal and salivary glands and ocular surface inflammation mimicking Sjögren's syndrome to a certain extent. These include the non-obese diabetic (NOD), MRL/Lpr, NZB/W F1 mouse, and TGF-β1, CD25 and Thrombospondin knock-out (KO) strains [25-32].

We have developed an inducible experimental murine dry eye model where wild-type mice are subjected to an environmental stress for five or ten days and lacrimal gland secretion is pharmacologically inhibited by administration of scopolamine. Mice are kept in an environmentally controlled room where relative humidity is kept below 30% at all times. Mice subjected to this experimental model develop conjunctival goblet cell (GC) loss and increased CD4+T cell infiltration in the conjunctival epithelium (Figure 1A) and increased expression of inflammatory mediators, corneal barrier disruption measured by a fluorescent dye (Figure 1B) similar to human dry eye patients (Figure 1C). Since the initial studies, this experimental model has been used extensively by us and other groups within the US but also worldwide. A significant body of evidence providing insight into the pathogenesis of dry eye has been derived from this animal model and will be discussed in more detailed in the sequential topics.

http://dx.doi.org/10.5772/57585

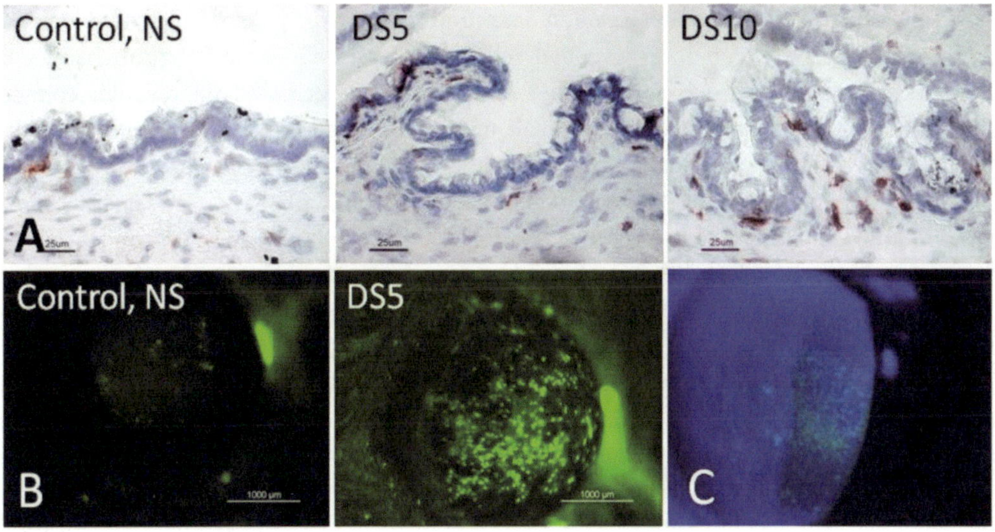

Figure 1. A. Representative images of immunohistochemical CD4⁺staining (red cells) in the goblet cell rich area of the conjunctiva of C57BL/6 mice without desiccating stress (control, non-stressed, NS) and with desiccating stress for 5 or 10 days (DS5 or DS10, respectively). **B.** Representative images of Oregon-Green-Dextran corneal staining in C57BL/6 mice without desiccating stress (control, non-stressed "NS") and with desiccating stress for 5 days (DS5). **C.** Representative image of human cornea stained with sodium fluorescein and visualized under a blue filter showing punctate dry spots in central cornea.

3. Role of tear hyperosmolarity

Hyperosmolarity has been shown to be a potent pro-inflammatory stimulus involved in the pathogenesis of the ocular surface disease of dry eye, termed keratoconjunctivitis sicca (KCS). Von Bahr was the first to suggest in 1941 that tear film osmolarity is dependent on tear secretion and evaporation, and that decreased secretion would lead to increased osmolarity [33]. Balik appears to have been the first to suggest in 1952 that the corneal and conjunctival changes in KCS could be explained on the basis of an increased "concentration of sodium chloride" in the tear film [34]. It would not be until two decades later that Mishima and colleagues were able to evaluate tear osmolarity and found an elevation of about 25 mOsm/liter in six eyes with KCS [35]. Subsequent studies reported significantly increased tear fluid osmolarity in patients with KCS, with the mean value 343 ± 32 (SD) mOsM, and the ranging up to 441 mOsM [36]. Based on its sensitivity and specificity, tear osmolarity was proposed as a gold standard diagnostic test for dry eye by Farris in 1992 [37], which was further evidenced by the fact that the use of sodium hyaluronate eye drops with pronounced hypotonicity showed greater therapeutic efficacy on the severity of Sjögren's syndrome associated KCS than isotonic solutions [38].

In rabbit dry eye models, the elevated tear film osmolarity caused decreased corneal glycogen and reduced conjunctival goblet cell density, as well as pathological changes in the corneal epithelium, such as increased desquamation, decreased intercellular connections, blunting and loss of microplicae, cell membrane disruptions and cellular swelling [39-41]. In mice following 2 days of DS, tear volume significantly decreased from 0.066ul to 0.026ul in C57BL/6J and 0.093ul to 0.028ul in BALB/c mice while tear osmolarity concomitantly and significantly increased from 177 to 300 mOsM in C57BL/6J mice, and nearly doubled from 285 to 559 mOsM in BALB/C mice. Topical treatment of ocular surface with hypertonic saline (500 mOsM) was found to stimulate expression and production of interleukin (IL)-1β, tumor necrosis factor (TNF) α and MMP-9 by the corneal and conjunctival epithelia, when compared with age matched controls and mice treated with iso-osmolar (305 mOsM) balanced salt solution [42, 43]. In our murine dry eye model [44], the stimulated expression of pro-inflammatory mediator, TNF-α, IL-1β and MMP-9 was observed [45]. The mitogen-activated protein kinases (MAPKs) are well conserved signaling pathways that include extracellular signal regulated kinases (ERK), c-Jun N-terminal kinases (JNK) and p38 MAPK [46-48]. Interestingly, the levels of phosphorylated JNK1/2, ERK1/2, and p38 MAPKs in the corneal and conjunctival epithelia were markedly increased in mice treated with hypertonic saline [45].

In human corneal epithelial cultures, the expression and production of a number of pro-inflammatory mediators, IL-1β, TNF-α, IL-8, and MMPs, including gelatinase MMP-9, collagenases MMP-1 and MMP-13, and stromelysin MMP-3 were progressively increased as the media osmolarity increased from 312 mOsM to 500 mOsM [49, 50]. Activated phospor (p)-JNK-1/p-JNK-2 and p-ERK-1/p-ERK-2 were also detected by Western blot and peaked at 60 minutes in cells exposed to hypertonic media. The levels of p-JNK-1/p-JNK-2 and p-ERK1/p-ERK2 were positively correlated with the medium osmolarity. The inhibitors for JNK or ERK pathways, SB202190, PD98059 and doxycycline markedly suppressed the levels of phosphor-JNKs and/or ERKs, as well as these proinflammatory markers. Other investigators also showed that hyperosmolarity induced the pro-inflammatory cytokine and chemokines IL-6, IL-8 and monocyte chemotactic protein-1 in cultured human corneal epithelial cells [51]. The efficacy of doxycycline in treating ocular surface diseases may be due to its ability to suppress JNK and ERK signaling activation and inflammatory mediator production in the corneal epithelium.

Another hallmark of dry eye is cornea and conjunctiva metaplasia, where the normal epithelium undergoes terminal differentiation and becomes keratinized [52]. The cornea is a highly transparent tissue and this abnormal keratinization process can lead to corneal irregularity and blurred vision [53, 54]. In mice, we observed that desiccating stress induces expression of cornified envelope proteins, including involucrin and small proline-rich proteins 2a and 2b in both cornea and conjunctiva [21, 55]. We also observed that stress-associated pathway, such as JNK, ERK and p38 MAPK are activated in hours after desiccating stress starts [21, 43, 45].

We found increased levels of active phosphorylated JNK1 and JNK2 (JNK2 JNK1) in ocular surface epithelia treated with hypertonic saline in vivo and in cultured human corneal epithelial cells exposed to hyperosmolar media [45, 49, 56]. In vivo, we showed that the JNK2 protein but not JNK1, appears to have an essential role in desiccation-induced corneal epithelial disease by stimulating production of MMP-1, MMP-9, and cornified envelope precursors as JNK2KO mice were resistant to dry eye-induced changes [20].

4. Role of matrix metalloproteinases

The hallmark of dry eye disease is the increased permeability of corneal epithelium to fluorescent dyes, clinically observed as fluorescent punctate spots. Because epithelial corneal disease is responsible for the irritation and blurred vision symptoms reported by most dry eye patients, corneal epithelium health is very important. The epithelium is not bystander, but actively responds to desiccating stress by secreting inflammatory cytokines, chemokimes and matrix metalloproteinases (MMPs).

Matrix degrading enzymes including MMPs have been identified as important factors in the inflammatory and wound healing response of the ocular surface, particularly in dry eye and ocular burns. Their induction during wound healing is thought to play a role in extracellular matrix remodeling, cytokine activation, and regulation of angiogenesis [57]. The MMP family includes more than 25 members that can be divided into collagenases that degrade fibrillar collagen types I, II, and III (MMP-1, -8, -13); gelatinases that degrade collagen types IV, V, and VII and X as well as decorin, fibronectin, and laminin, that are found in basement membranes (MMP-2,-9); stromelysins (MMP-3, and -10); matrilysins that degrade proteoglycans, laminin, and glycoproteins (MMP-7 and -26); and the membrane-type MMPs that are bound to epithelial cell membranes, and can activate MMPs, according to their structure and substrate specificity (MMPs 14-17, and -24) [58-61]. Collectively they are able to degrade the entire extracellular matrix and basement membranes components. Barely detected in an unwounded cornea, MMPs are strongly induced during wound healing. Among these, MMP–9 plays a prominent role being produced by stressed cornea and conjunctival epithelial cells and has both matrix degrading and pro-inflammatory activities [62-64].

Several members of MMPs have been found to increase in the corneal epithelium after experimental dry eye and MMP-9 (Figure 2) [57]. MMP-9 has been found in tear fluid of dry eye patients [65]. Of special interest, we have shown that epithelium-secreted MMP-9 after experimental dry eye activates TGF-β [66], breaks-down the apical corneal epithelial tight junctions (Figure 3), facilitating corneal barrier dysfunction [21, 57, 67] and accelerating corneal desquamation [68].

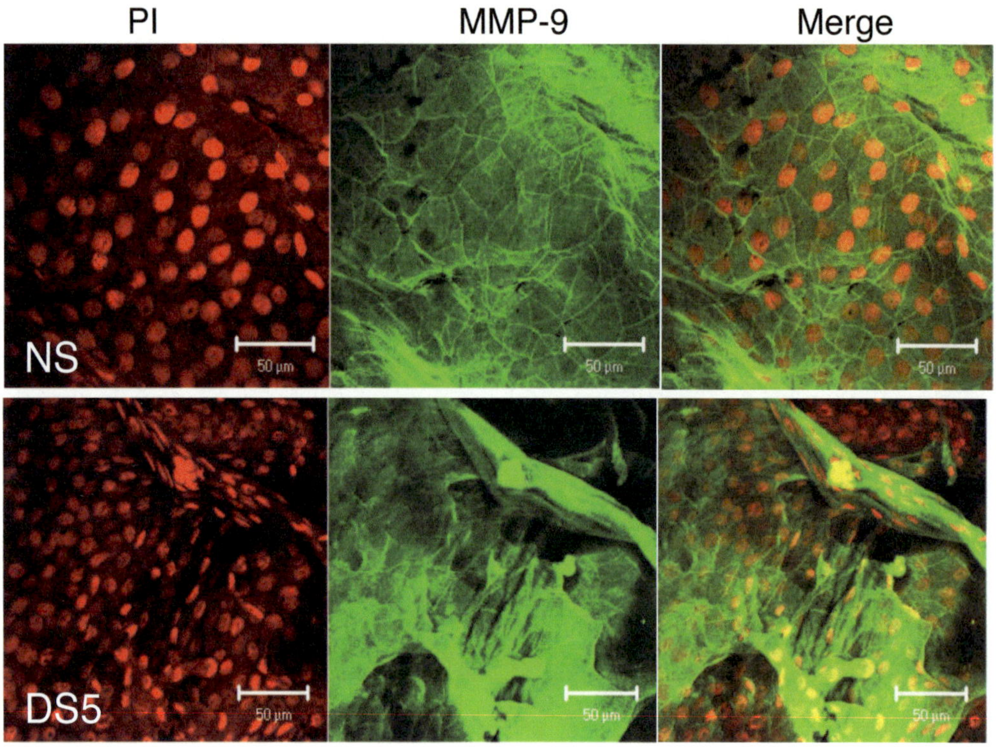

Figure 2. Laser scanning confocal microscopy of wholemount murine corneas stained for MMP-9 (in green) with propidium iodide nuclear counterstaining (PI, in red), organized into non-stressed (NS) and desiccating stress for 5 days (DS5).

MMP-9 knock-out mice are resistant to these changes, but exogenous topical administration of MMP-9 to MMP-9KO mice induced increased corneal permeability in similar range to wild-type control mice. Moreover, cultured human corneal epithelial cells treated with MMP-9 showed breakdown of tight junction proteins, notably occludin [67]. In human dry eye patients, increased MMP-9 mRNA transcripts in conjunctiva and increased MMP-9 activity in tears was noted compared to normal subjects; increased MMP-9 activity in tears positively correlated with symptom score, cornea and conjunctiva staining, low contrast visual acuity and inversely correlated with tear-break-up [54]. In a group of dry eye patients, we observed that tear MMP-9 activity levels increased as the severity of corneal disease progressed (Table 1) [54].

http://dx.doi.org/10.5772/57585

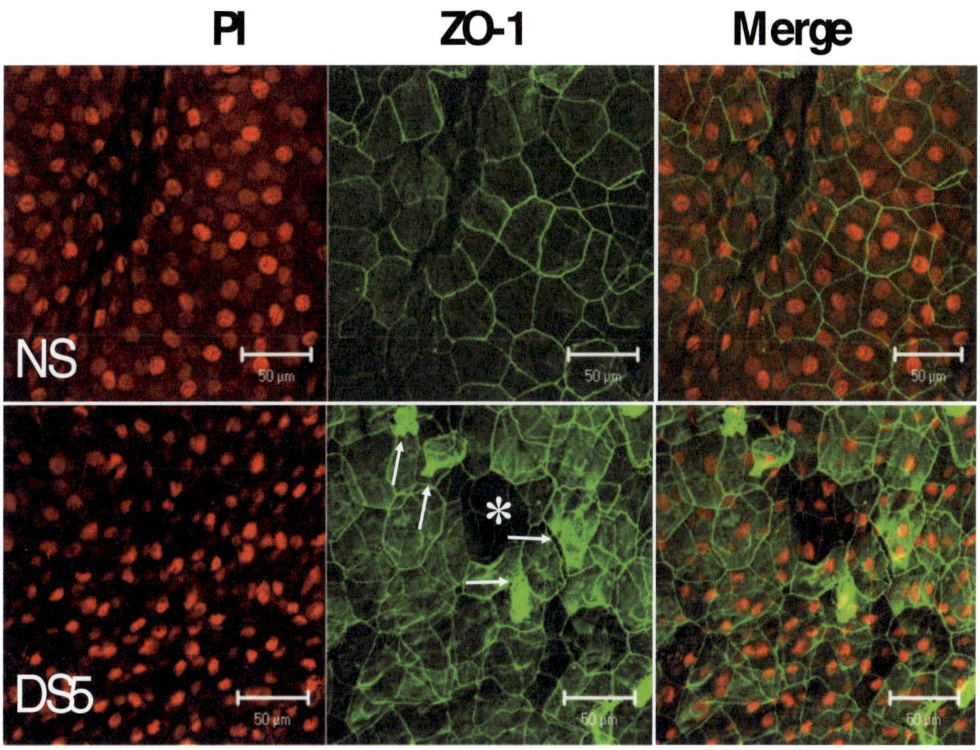

Figure 3. Laser scanning confocal microscopy of wholemount murine corneas stained for zona occludens 1 (ZO-1, in green) with propidium iodide nuclear counterstaining (PI, in red), organized into non-stressed (NS) and desiccating stress for 5 days (DS5). The NS controls show uniform cell with membrane staining while the DS5 corneas have increased apical cell loss (asterisk) and increase desquamation (arrows show either broken ZO-1 or cells that are rolling up).

Group	MMP-9 Activity (ng/mL)
Normal (n=18)	8.39 ± 4.70
Dysfunctional tear syndrome 1 (n=10)	62.40 ± 49.33**
Dysfunctional tear syndrome 2 (n=20)	58.84 ± 49.46**
Dysfunctional tear syndrome 3 (n=07)	116.99 ± 138.18**
Dysfunctional tear syndrome 4 (n=11)	360.25 ± 168.83**♦♦

Note: DTS=dysfunctional tear syndrome ** *P*<0.004 versus normal;♦♦*P* <0.007 versus normal and the other severity based DTS groups

Table 1. Tear MMP-9 activity levels among normal subjects and dry eye patients stratified by 4 levels of severity according to the Delphi Panel [69] [range from DTS1 (very mild) to DTS4 (severe dry eye)]

5. The conjunctiva acts as an exogenous lymphoid tissue

Similar to other mucosal tissues, the conjunctiva is covered with epithelium containing dendritic antigen presenting cells and a variety of intraepithelial lymphocyte (IEL) populations, lymphocytes that reside outside the lymphoid organs and in contact with epithelial cells in the gut, skin and lungs [70]. To date, several subsets of IELs have been identified in the mouse and human conjunctiva, including $CD4^+$, $CD8^+$, gammadelta $(\gamma\delta)^+$and NK^+ cells[71-74]. The CD103 integrin has been used as a marker for IEL in different mucosal sites because it mediates homing and retention of lymphocytes to the epithelium. Its ligand, E-cadherin is highly expressed on mucosal epithelial cells [75, 76].

An important breakthrough in recent studies is the discovery of a link between the ocular surface epithelium and immune cells. Soluble factors from immune cells have been found to be either pathogenic or homeostatic to cornea and conjunctiva epithelium. Early biopsies from Sjögren's Syndrome (SS) patients have shown lymphocytic infiltration in the lacrimal gland and activated T cells have been detected in the conjunctiva dry eye patients [77-82]. Animal studies using the adoptive transfer experiment showed that dry eye can be induced in T cell deficient nude mice that had never been exposed to desiccated stress by adoptively transferring $CD4^+$T cells from dry eye mouse model [83]. This landmark study showed that immunocompetent recipients will only develop disease when regulatory cells are depleted with antibody to CD25 [83]. Taken together, these experiments showed that: 1) dry eye is indeed an autoimmune disease, since goblet cell loss and $CD4^+$T infiltration was seen in naïve mice receiving cells but never subjected to DS; 2) confirmed the pathogenic role of $CD4^+$T cells as adoptive transfer of unfractionated or non-CD4+T cells had minimal effect; 3) showed that $CD4^+$T cells primed in vivo during DS will migrate back to ocular surface tissues and LG; 4) dry eye induces a systemic immune response, as adoptive transfer of splenic $CD4^+$T cells was sufficient to induce disease and 5) provided a mechanism to evaluate different components of the immune system.

T helper (Th) $CD4^+$T cells have been classically divided into Th-1, Th-2 and Th-17. Th-1 responses are important for controlling viral, fungal and intracellular bacterial infections. Th-1 cells are classically identified by the production of interferon-gamma (IFN-γ). Once committed, the Th-1 cells activate macrophages and induce IgG2a production by B cells. Th-2 responses are frequently found in allergic diseases, such as asthma, and are particularly important in the host response to parasites and helminthes in the gut. Th-2 cell differentiation is promoted by interleukin (IL)-4 and it is characterized by production of IL-4, IL-13 and IL-5. The Th-2 committed cells promote IgG1 and IgE class switching and eosinophil recruitment. Th-17 cells are important in responding to extracellular bacterial and fungal pathogens, by recruiting neutrophils and macrophages to infected tissues and have been implicated in autoimmunity [84-86].

Migration of CD4+T cells into the conjunctival and cornea in dry eye disease may be modulated by chemokine ligands produced by the surface epithelium that increase in dryness. Pathogenic CD4 cells that infiltrate the ocular surface tissues express receptors to these ligands [18, 87, 88].

http://dx.doi.org/10.5772/57585

5.1. Th-1 CD4+T cells in dry eye

Th-1 committed CD4+T cells secrete IFN-γ. CXCL9, CXCL10, CXCL11, IFN-γ inducible chemokines, are highly expressed after experimental desiccating stress in both cornea and conjunctiva [87-89] which will in turn attract more Th-1 cells, serving as an amplifying mechanism.

IFN-γ has been proposed as a biomarker for dry eye disease and SS because elevated IFN-γ, either protein or RNA levels, has been detected in tears [90-97], conjunctiva [96-100], saliva [101, 102], lacrimal [26, 103-108], submandibular glands [94, 103, 109-111], and blood [112, 113].

Increased IFN-γ concentration in tears of dry eye patients detected by ELISA was reported more than a decade ago. More sensitive immunoassays, such as Luminex and antibody microarrays used in subsequent studies have confirmed these early results [90, 92-96]. In addition to dry eye, increased tear IFN-γ concentration has also been found in patients with sicca symptoms after bone marrow transplantation [90] and in tears of SS patients [91, 93]. Among the various subsets of dysfunctional tear syndrome, those with meibomian gland disease (MGD) had significantly lower IFN-γ concentration than those without MGD [91, 92] and tear IFN-γ concentration was found to correlate with corneal fluorescein staining score [91]. It is possible that inflamed lacrimal glands in patients with SS are one source for their increased tear IFN-γ.

Similarly to tears [90], increased IFN-γ has been found in saliva of SS patients and its presence correlated with sicca symptoms [101]. Interestingly, increased Th1/Th2 ratios was observed in more severe SS cases [114-116], where increased Th-2 response correlated with milder SS [101, 102, 117, 118]. Virtually every mouse autoimmune model that mimics SS or even environmentally-induced mouse dry eye models have shown increased expression of IFN-γ in LG and submandibular gland [26, 103-109, 118]. Increased expression of IFN-γ mRNA has also been observed in the conjunctiva, both in dry eye patients and mice subjected to dry eye [18, 96-100]. We have shown that IFN-γ induces conjunctiva metaplasia and apoptosis and loss of conjunctival goblet cells [97, 119, 120]. IFN-γKO mice are resistant to dry eye induced changes but reconstitution of KO mice with exogenous IFN-γ induces goblet cell loss in similar magnitude as wild-type mice and this was accompanied by cornification and apoptosis of conjunctival epithelium [97, 120]. It has also been shown that IFN-γ significantly decreases epithelial mucin expression [121]. Adoptive transfer of CD4+T cells from donor mice exposed to desiccating stress that received anti-IFN-γ were less pathogenic to immunodeficient mice recipients, yielding less corneal apoptosis and greater number of PAS+filled goblet cells [119]. Mice that received subconjunctival injections of anti-IFN-γ antibody showed decreased corneal and conjunctival apoptosis [98, 119].

5.2. Th-17 and NK cells in dry eye

IL-17A is the signature cytokine of the new discovered Th subtype, Th-17. The differentiation of Th17 cells from naïve $CD4^{+}T$ cells is regulated by cytokines [122]. Transforming growth factor-β (TGF-β) and IL-6, broadly expressed by many cell types in the body, including dendritic and epithelial cells, are dominant in the initiation of Th17 cell differentiation [122-124]. IL-23, IL-1β and IL-21, which are products of activated dendritic cells, macrophages, activated T cell or inflamed epithelial cells, possibly expand and maintain the differentiated Th17 cells in the presence of IL-6 and TGF-β1 [122, 125, 126]. Furthermore, signal transducer and activator of transcription 3 (STAT3) has been found to mediate the initiation of Th17 cell differentiation by these inducing cytokines [127].

TGF-β is a critical factor in Th-17 differentiation. TGF-β is a pleiotropic cytokine that can have pro- or anti-inflammatory effects depending on the context. It regulates various biologic processes such as embryonic development, cell proliferation and differentiation, extracellular matrix synthesis, immune response, inflammation, and apoptosis [128]. TGF-β1 is produced by the human lacrimal gland (LG) and corneal and conjunctiva epithelia and has been detected in tears [129, 130]. Elevated levels of bioactive TGF-β1 in tears and elevated TGF-β1 mRNA transcripts in conjunctiva and minor salivary glands of human Sjögren's Syndrome (SS) patients has also been reported [18, 78, 131, 132].

We addressed the role of TGF-β in the Th-17 response in the conjunctiva by evaluating TGF-β dominant-negative TGF-β type II receptor (CD4-DNTGFβRII) mice. These mice have a truncated TGF-β receptor in $CD4^+$T cells, rendering them unresponsive to TGF-β. These mice exhibit an age-related dry eye phenotype at 14 weeks of age; however, when subjected to desiccating stress, we observed that DS improved their corneal barrier function and corneal surface irregularity, increased their number of PAS+GC, and lowered $CD4^+$T cell infiltration in conjunctiva. In contrast to WT, CD4-DNTGFβRII mice did not generate a Th-17 and Th-1 response, and they failed to upregulate MMP-9, IL-23, IL-17A, RORγT, IFN-γ and T-bet mRNA transcripts in conjunctiva. RAG1KO recipients of adoptively transferred CD4+T cells isolated from DS5 CD4-DNTGFβRII showed milder dry eye phenotype and less conjunctival inflammation than recipients of WT control [19].

Thrombospondin-1 (TSP-1) is an extracellular matrix protein that activates TGF-β1. When covalently bound to TGF-β1, the latency associated peptide (LAP) blocks its active site and renders the molecule inactive. This immature form of TGF-β1 naturally equilibrates with its active state via detachment from LAP. Thrombospondin-1 stabilizes the covalent binding sites on the disassociated LAP, thereby preventing its interaction and subsequent inhibition of TGF-β1 [133]. As a result, increased levels of TSP-1 in the presence of TGF-β1 are linked to greater levels of active TGF-β1 [133, 134]. Interestingly, similar to our findings in the CD4-DNTGFβRII mice, TSP-1KO mice had decreased corneal surface dye staining, increased number of conjunctival goblet cells and low levels of inflammatory cytokine mRNA transcripts in cornea tissue compared to WT mice. We also showed that adoptive transfer of WT bone-marrow DC into TSP-1KO reverted the TSP-1KO resistance to desiccating stress, showing that DC-derived TSP is critical for the immune dry eye phenotype [135].

The corneal epithelium responds quickly to different stressors. Cultured human corneal epithelial cells challenged by hyperosmotic media (450 mOsM), microbial components (polyI:C, flagellin, R837, and other TLR ligands) and TNF-alpha responded by significantly increasing expression of IL-6, TGF-β and IL-1β and IL-23 mRNA transcripts. Interestingly, when incubated with conditioned media of HCECs irritated by polyI:C or TNF-α, CD4^{+} T cells displayed increased mRNA levels of IL-17A, IL-17F, IL-22, CCL-20, and STAT3, increased IL-17 protein in the supernatant, and increased numbers of IL-17-producing T cells (Th17 cells). These findings demonstrate for the first time that Th17 differentiation can be promoted by cytokines produced by corneal epithelium that are exposed to hyperosmotic, microbial, and inflammatory stimuli [136].

Th17 cells can be identified by expression of CCR6 surface receptors [137-139]. CCR6 only ligand known, CCL20, is highly expressed after injuries to epithelium, including experimental desiccating stress [18]. Dry eye has been demonstrated to cause inflammation on the ocular surface, evidenced by increased levels of inflammatory cytokines (IL-1, IL-6, IL-17 and TNF-α) in the tear fluid and corneal and conjunctival epithelium, and an increased infiltration of DCs and T lymphocytes in the conjunctiva [18, 79, 83, 96, 136, 140-144]. Increased levels of IL-17, IL-23 and IL-6 were also found in saliva and salivary glands biopsies obtained from patients with the severe autoimmune dry eye condition, Sjögren's syndrome [145-147].

Evidence in mouse models of dry eye indicates that IL-17 stimulates production of MMP-3 and MMP-9 that contribute to disruption of corneal epithelial barrier function. Recent studies have shown that antibody neutralization of IL-17 ameliorated corneal barrier disruption in mice subjected to desiccating stress [18, 148] and decreased expression of MMP-3 and-9 mRNA transcripts in the corneal epithelium [18], providing a definitive link between epithelial and immune cells in this process.

5.3. Goblet Cells in dry eye

The conjunctival epithelium is part of the few tissues in the body where goblet cells are present, including the gut and the airway epithelia. Goblet cell loss is another clinical characteristic of ocular surface diseases, including dry eye, Stevens-Johnson and ocular graft-versus-host-diseases [149, 150]. Both NK and NKT cells are resident cells in conjunctiva [142]. NK cells are a subtype of lymphocytes that lack expression of the antigen receptors expressed by B and T cells; their name is derived from their ability to recognize and kill malignant cells. NKT cells are defined as NK cells that express conventional T cell receptor (TCR). Both cell types are important source of inflammatory cytokines, notably after encountering pathogens (viruses, bacteria and protozoans). NKT cells have been involved in mucosal immunity and in a variety of inflammatory/autoimmune diseases, such as experimental murine and human ulcerative colitis, asthma, multiple sclerosis and skin diseases (atopic dermatitis, psoriasis) [151-153].

Using isolation techniques, we identified that NKT-derived IL-13 is trophic factor for conjunctival goblet cells, as IL-13KO and STAT6KO strains had lower goblet cell density than their wild-type control mice [154]. In experimental murine dry eye, IL-13 significantly decreased in tears after 5 and 10 days in Th-1 prone C57BL/6 mice, while it increased in BALB/C mice that have been found to develop less severe corneal and conjunctival disease in response to desiccating stress [96].

NK cells participate in the initiation of the immune response by releasing IFN-γ [99] and IL-17A and by decreasing dendritic cell activation [142]. NK cells have been implicated in both the regulation and immunopathogenesis of dry eye disease since they are an early source of IFN-γ during the induction phase of experimental dry eye disease [99]. Systemic depletion of NK cells prior and during DS led to a decrease in the frequency of total and activated DCs, a decrease in T helper-17(+) cells in the cervical lymph nodes and generation of less pathogenic $CD4^+$T cells. B6.nude recipient mice of adoptively transferred $CD4^+$T cells isolated from NK-depleted DS5 donor mice showed significantly less corneal barrier disruption, lower levels of IL-17A, CCL20 and MMP-3 in the cornea epithelia compared to recipients of control $CD4^+$T cells [142].

5.4. Regulatory T Cells in dry eye

Resident $CD8^+$T cells have been found in the epithelium and stroma of normal human and mouse conjunctiva [97, 155], but their function remains unknown. In non-ocular tissues, $CD8^+$T cells have been found to have an immunoregulatory function. In the Lewis rat, peripheral tolerance to orally administered antigens was mediated by TGF-β secreting $CD8^+$T cells [156, 157]. In the iris, $CD8^+$T cells once activated in the presence of parenchymal cells, expressed and secreted enhanced amounts of TGF-β2 [158]. In certain conjunctival inflammatory conditions, including graft-versus-host disease, Sjögren's syndrome and human and experimental murine keratoconjunctivitis, a significant decrease in $CD8^+$T cells with concomitant increase in CD4/CD8 ratio in the conjunctiva has been observed [74, 97, 159].

We have identified that $CD8^+$ T cells can also function as regulatory cells. $CD8^+$ T cell depletion promoted generation of IL-17A producing $CD4^+$T cells via activation of dendritic cells in both the ocular surface and draining cervical lymph nodes in C57BL/6 mice subjected to DS. T cell-deficient nude recipient mice receiving adoptively transferred $CD4^+$T cells from $CD8^+$cell-depleted donors exposed to DS displayed increased $CD4^+$T cell infiltration and elevated IL-17A and CCL20 levels in the ocular surface, which was associated with greater corneal barrier disruption. Enhanced DS-specific corneal barrier disruption in CD8-depleted donor mice correlated with a Th17-mediated expression of MMP-3 and 9 in the recipient corneal epithelium. Co-transfer of $CD8^+CD103^+$Tregs did not affect the ability of DS-specific pathogenic $CD4^+$T cells to infiltrate and cause ocular surface disease in the nude recipients, showing that $CD8^+$cells regulate the afferent arm of DS-induced immune response. In summary, $CD8^+$regulatory cells suppress generation of a pathogenic Th17 response that plays a pivotal role in DS-induced disruption of corneal barrier function [160].

6. Therapeutic strategies: from bench side to clinic

Traditionally, dry eye was treated with palliative solutions and frequent instillation of artificial tears. With the change of paradigm and recognition of the role of inflammation in the disease, several other modalities of treatment entered the pipeline. Animal models have suggested potential agents/pathways.

Anti-protease therapy is very effective in treating dry eye associated corneal epithelial disease. Previously reported studies using our experimental dry eye model demonstrated that the

MMP inhibitor doxycycline and the steroid methylprednisolone was efficacious in decreasing gelatinolytic activity and levels of MMP-9 transcripts in corneal epithelium, as well as preventing the dry eye-induced increase in inflammatory cytokines IL-1 and TNF-α [161]. Doxycycline also improved corneal surface regularity and improved corneal barrier function [21]. At the cellular level, doxycycline preserved apical epithelial cell area and the tight-junction protein occludin, resulting in a decreased number of desquamating epithelial cells from the surface of the cornea [21, 68]. The inhibitory effect of doxycycline on MMP-9 was also confirmed on osmotically stressed cultured human corneal epithelial cells [67]. While there is no FDA approved anti-inflammatory agents, both steroid and doxycycline eyedrops have also been used with success in human dry eye patients [162, 163].

It has also been shown that manipulation of afferent (migration of DC into the regional lymph nodes) or efferent (migration of differentiated cells from the nodes and into the cornea and conjunctiva) can ameliorate development of dry eye disease [137, 164-167] indicating that therapeutic strategies that interfere with various points in this immune circle may have clinical significance.

Cyclosporine A 0.01 % emulsion (CsA), the only FDA-approved drug to treat dry-eye disease has been shown to modulate several arms of the immune response by decreasing HLA-DR expression in conjunctiva of dry eye patients [16, 168, 169] and decreasing expression of IL-17A and IFN-γ in conjunctiva of animals after desiccating stress [18]. One beneficial side effect from Cyclosporine emulsion is its significant effect increasing the amount of goblet cells in human patients. We observed similar findings in our animal model as well: CsA topical treatment prevented goblet cell loss, maintained the number of NK+cells in the conjunctiva increased IL-13 mRNA in NK+cells, and decreased IFN-γ and IL-17A mRNA transcripts in NK+and NK-populations, showing that CsA can act in both epithelial and immune compartments [154].

Novel therapeutic strategies based on the interruption of migration of $Th17^{+}CCR6^{+}$cells to the ocular surface or production of IL-17 have been shown to ameliorated dry eye disease in animal models of dry eye [18, 137, 142, 148, 165]. Exogenous administration of IL-13 to wild-type mice subjected to desiccating stress for 5 days prevented DS-induced goblet cell loss [154]. Recently, it has been made clear that strategies to neutralize IFN-γ may inhibit development of corneal and conjunctival disease in experimental dry eye. Neutralization of NK cells, early producers of IFN-γ (NK cells) following desiccating stress was found to decrease corneal fluorescein staining and inflammatory cytokine expression in the cornea and conjunctiva [99, 142] and also to decrease the Th-17 response.

7. Conclusions

This book chapter described the most recent advances in understanding the pathogenesis of dry eye disease. A significant amount of work has been performed using an environmentally-induced murine dry eye model. Inflammation is now recognized as important player in dry eye. While there is just one FDA-approved drug to treat dry eye, several other drugs are in the pipeline addressing different aspects of the disease and are potential new therapeutics.

Author details

Cintia S. de Paiva[1], Andrew J.W. Huang[2], De-Quan Li[1] and Stephen C. Pflugfelder[1*]

*Address all correspondence to: stevenp@bcm.edu

1 The Ocular Surface Center, Cullen Eye Institute, Department of Ophthalmology, Baylor College of Medicine, USA

2 Department of Ophthalmology and Visual Sciences, School of Medicine, Washington University, St. Louis, MO, USA

References

[1] Epidemiology Subcommittee: The definition and classification of dry eye disease: report of the Definition and Classification Subcommittee of the International Dry Eye WorkShop (2007). *Ocul Surf* 2007,5(2): 75-92.

[2] Moss SE, Klein R, Klein BE: Incidence of dry eye in an older population. *Arch Ophthalmol* 2004,122: 369-373.

[3] Schein OD, Munoz B, Tielsch JM, Bandeen-Roche K, West S: Prevalence of dry eye among the elderly. *Am J Ophthalmol* 1997,124: 723-728.

[4] Schaumberg DA, Sullivan DA, Buring JE, Dana MR: Prevalence of dry eye syndrome among US women. *Am J Ophthalmol* 2003,136: 318-326.

[5] Pflugfelder SC: Prevalence, burden, and pharmacoeconomics of dry eye disease. *Am J Manag Care* 2008,14: S102-S106.

[6] Yu J, Asche CV, Fairchild CJ: The economic burden of dry eye disease in the United States: a decision tree analysis. *Cornea* 2011,30: 379-387.

[7] Yamada M, Mizuno Y, Shigeyasu C: Impact of dry eye on work productivity. *Clinicoecon Outcomes Res* 2012,4: 307-312.

[8] Maeda N, Sato S, Watanabe H, Inoue Y, Fujikado T, Shimomura Y, Tano Y: Prediction of letter contrast sensitivity using videokeratographic indices. *Am J Ophthalmol* 2000,129: 759-763.

[9] Miljanovic B, Dana R, Sullivan DA, Schaumberg DA: Impact of dry eye syndrome on vision-related quality of life. *Am J Ophthalmol* 2007,143: 409-415.

[10] Ivers RQ, Cumming RG, Mitchell P, Attebo K: Visual impairment and falls in older adults: the Blue Mountains Eye Study. *J Am Geriatr Soc* 1998,46: 58-64.

[11] Sattin RW: Falls among older persons: a public health perspective. *Annu Rev Public Health* 1992,13: 489-508.

[12] Schiffman RM, Walt JG, Jacobsen G, Doyle JJ, Lebovics G, Sumner W: Utility assessment among patients with dry eye disease. *Ophthalmology* 2003,110: 1412-1419.

[13] Harris RA, Nease RF, Jr.: The importance of patient preferences for comorbidities in cost-effectiveness analyses. *J Health Econ* 1997,16: 113-119.

[14] Pflugfelder SC: Differential diagnosis of dry eye conditions. *Adv Dent Res* 1996,10: 9-12.

[15] Lemp MA: Evaluation and differential diagnosis of keratoconjunctivitis sicca. *J Rheumatol Suppl* 2000,61: 11-14.

[16] Brignole F, Pisella PJ, Goldschild M, De Saint JM, Goguel A, Baudouin C: Flow cytometric analysis of inflammatory markers in conjunctival epithelial cells of patients with dry eyes. *Invest Ophthalmol Vis Sci* 2000,41: 1356-1363.

[17] Kunert KS, Tisdale AS, Gipson IK: Goblet cell numbers and epithelial proliferation in the conjunctiva of patients with dry eye syndrome treated with cyclosporine. *Arch Ophthalmol* 2002,120: 330-337.

[18] de Paiva CS, Chotikavanich S, Pangelinan SB, Pitcher JI, Fang B, Zheng X, Ma P, Farley WJ, Siemasko KS, Niederkorn JY, Stern ME, Li D-Q, Pflugfelder SC: IL-17 disrupts corneal barrier following desiccating stress. *Mucosal Immunology* 2009, May; 2(3): 243-53

[19] de Paiva CS, Volpe EA, Gandhi NB, Zhang X, Zheng X, Pitcher JD, III, Farley WJ, Stern ME, Niederkorn JY, Li DQ, Flavell RA, Pflugfelder SC: Disruption of TGF-beta Signaling Improves Ocular Surface Epithelial Disease in Experimental Autoimmune Keratoconjunctivitis Sicca. *PLoS One* 2011,6: e29017. Epub 2011 Dec 14.

[20] de Paiva CS, Pangelinan SB, Chang E, Yoon KC, Farley WJ, Li DQ, Pflugfelder SC: Essential role for c-Jun N-terminal kinase 2 in corneal epithelial response to desiccating stress. *Arch Ophthalmol* 2009,127: 1625-1631.

[21] de Paiva CS, Corrales RM, Villarreal AL, Farley W, Li DQ, Stern ME, Pflugfelder SC: Apical corneal barrier disruption in experimental murine dry eye is abrogated by methylprednisolone and doxycycline. *Invest Ophthalmol Vis Sci* 2006,47: 2847-2856.

[22] Pitcher JI, de Paiva CS, Pelegrino FSA, McClellan AJ, Raince JK, Pangelinan SB, Rahimy E, Farley JW, Stern ME, Li D-Q, Pflugfelder SC: Pharmacological cholinergic blockade stimulates inflammatory cytokine production in the mouse lacrimal gland. *Invest Ophthalmol Vis Sci* 2011,16: 3221-7.

[23] Zoukhri D, Macari E, Kublin CL: A single injection of interleukin-1 induces reversible aqueous-tear deficiency, lacrimal gland inflammation, and acinar and ductal cell proliferation. *Exp Eye Res* 2007,84: 894-904.

[24] Mircheff AK, Wang Y, Thomas PB, Nakamura T, Samant D, Trousdale MD, Warren DW, Ding C, Schechter JE: Systematic variations in immune response-related gene transcript abundance suggest new questions about environmental influences on lacrimal gland immunoregulation. *Curr Eye Res* 2011,36: 285-294.

[25] Van Blokland SC, Versnel MA: Pathogenesis of Sjogren's syndrome: characteristics of different mouse models for autoimmune exocrinopathy. *Clin Immunol* 2002,103: 111-124.

[26] de Paiva CS, Hwang CS, Pitcher JD, III, Pangelinan SB, Rahimy E, Chen W, Yoon KC, Farley WJ, Niederkorn JY, Stern ME, Li DQ, Pflugfelder SC: Age-related T-cell cytokine profile parallels corneal disease severity in Sjogren's syndrome-like keratoconjunctivitis sicca in CD25KO mice. *Rheumatology (Oxford)* 2010,49: 246-258.

[27] Yang Z, Mu Z, Dabovic B, Jurukovski V, Yu D, Sung J, Xiong X, Munger JS: Absence of integrin-mediated TGFbeta1 activation in vivo recapitulates the phenotype of TGFbeta1-null mice. *J Cell Biol* 2007,176: 787-793.

[28] Cha S, Peck AB, Humphreys-Beher MG: Progress in understanding autoimmune exocrinopathy using the non-obese diabetic mouse: an update. *Crit Rev Oral Biol Med* 2002,13: 5-16.

[29] Sharma R, Bagavant H, Jarjour WN, Sung SS, Ju ST: The role of Fas in the immune system biology of IL-2R alpha knockout mice: interplay among regulatory T cells, inflammation, hemopoiesis, and apoptosis. *J Immunol* 2005,175: 1965-1973.

[30] McCartney-Francis NL, Mizel DE, Redman RS, Frazier-Jessen M, Panek RB, Kulkarni AB, Ward JM, McCarthy JB, Wahl SM: Autoimmune Sjogren's-like lesions in salivary glands of TGF-beta1-deficient mice are inhibited by adhesion-blocking peptides. *J Immunol* 1996,157: 1306-1312.

[31] McCartney-Francis NL, Mizel DE, Frazier-Jessen M, Kulkarni AB, McCarthy JB, Wahl SM: Lacrimal gland inflammation is responsible for ocular pathology in TGF-beta 1 null mice. *Am J Pathol* 1997,151: 1281-1288.

[32] Shull MM, Ormsby I, Kier AB, Pawlowski S, Diebold RJ, Yin M, Allen R, Sidman C, Proetzel G, Calvin D,.: Targeted disruption of the mouse transforming growth factor-beta 1 gene results in multifocal inflammatory disease. *Nature* 1992,359: 693-699.

[33] Von Bahr G: Konnte der flussigkeitsabgang durch die cornea von physiologischer bedeutung sein? *Acta Ophthalmol* 1941,19: 125-134.

[34] BALIK J: The lacrimal fluid in keratoconjunctivitis sicca; a quantitative and qualitative investigation. *Am J Ophthalmol* 1952,35: 1773-1782.

[35] Mishima S, Kubota Z, Farris RL. The tear flow dynamics in normal and in keratoconjunctivitis sicca cases. 1971:1801-1805.

[36] Gilbard JP, Farris RL, Santamaria J: Osmolarity of tear microvolumes in keratoconjunctivitis sicca. *Arch Ophthalmol* 1978,96: 677-681.

[37] Farris RL: Tear osmolarity-a new gold standard? *Adv Exp Med Biol* 1994,350: 495-503.

[38] Aragona P, Di Stefano G, Ferreri F, Spinella R, Stilo A: Sodium hyaluronate eye drops of different osmolarity for the treatment of dry eye in Sjogren's syndrome patients. *Br J Ophthalmol* 2002,86: 879-884.

[39] Gilbard JP, Rossi SR, Gray KL, Hanninen LA, Kenyon KR: Tear film osmolarity and ocular surface disease in two rabbit models for keratoconjunctivitis sicca. *Invest Ophthalmol Vis Sci* 1988,29: 374-378.

[40] Gilbard JP, Rossi SR, Gray KL, Hanninen LA: Natural history of disease in a rabbit model for keratoconjunctivitis sicca. *Acta Ophthalmol Suppl* 1989,192: 95-101.

[41] Gilbard JP, Carter JB, Sang DN, Refojo MF, Hanninen LA, Kenyon KR: Morphologic effect of hyperosmolarity on rabbit corneal epithelium. *Ophthalmology* 1984,91: 1205-1212.

[42] de Paiva CS, Corrales RM, Villarreal AL, Farley W, D.-Q L, Stern ME, Pflugfelder SC: Corticosteroid and doxycycline suppress MMP-9 and inflammatory cytokine expression, MAPK activation in the corneal epithelium in experimental dry eye. *Exp Eye Res* 2006,83: 526-535.

[43] Luo L, Li DQ, Corrales RM, Pflugfelder SC: Hyperosmolar saline is a proinflammatory stress on the mouse ocular surface. *Eye & Contact Lens* 2005,31(5): 186-93.

[44] Dursun D, Wang M, Monroy D, Li DQ, Lokeshwar BL, Stern M, Pflugfelder SC: Experimentally induced dry eye produces ocular surface inflammation and epithelial disease. *Adv Exp Med Biol* 2002,506: 647-655.

[45] Luo L, Li DQ, Doshi A, Farley W, Corrales RM, Pflugfelder SC: Experimental dry eye stimulates production of inflammatory cytokines and MMP-9 and activates MAPK signaling pathways on the ocular surface. *Invest Ophthalmol Vis Sci* 2004,45: 4293-4301.

[46] Kyriakis JM, Banerjee P, Nikolakaki E, Dai T, Rubie EA, Ahmad MF, Avruch J, Woodgett JR: The stress-activated protein kinase subfamily of c-Jun kinases. *Nature* 1994,369: 156-160.

[47] Galcheva-Gargova Z, Derijard B, Wu IH, Davis RJ: An osmosensing signal transduction pathway in mammalian cells. *Science* 1994,265: 806-808.

[48] Rosette C, Karin M: Ultraviolet light and osmotic stress: activation of the JNK cascade through multiple growth factor and cytokine receptors. *Science* 1996,274: 1194-1197.

[49] Li DQ, Chen Z, Song XJ, Luo L, Pflugfelder SC: Stimulation of matrix metalloproteinases by hyperosmolarity via a JNK pathway in human corneal epithelial cells. *Invest Ophthalmol Vis Sci* 2004,45: 4302-4311.

[50] Li DQ, Luo L, Chen Z, Kim HS, Song XJ, Pflugfelder SC: JNK and ERK MAP kinases mediate induction of IL-1beta, TNF-alpha and IL-8 following hyperosmolar stress in human limbal epithelial cells. *Exp Eye Res* 2006,82: 588-596.

[51] Cavet ME, Harrington KL, Ward KW, Zhang JZ: Mapracorat, a novel selective glucocorticoid receptor agonist, inhibits hyperosmolar-induced cytokine release and MAPK pathways in human corneal epithelial cells. *Mol Vis* 2010,16: 1791-1800.

[52] Pflugfelder SC, Huang AJW, Schuchovski PT, Pereira IC, Tseng SCG: Conjunctival cytological features of primary Sjogren syndrome. *Ophthalmology* 1990,97: 985-991.

[53] de Paiva CS, Lindsey JL, Pflugfelder SC: Assessing the severity of keratitis sicca with videokeratoscopic indices. *Ophthalmology* 2003,110: 1102-1109.

[54] Chotikavanich S, de Paiva CS, D.-Q L, Chen JJ, Bian F, Farley WJ, Pflugfelder SC: Production and Activity of Matrix Metalloproteinase-9 on the Ocular Surface Increase in Dysfunctional Tear Syndrome. *Invest Ophthalmol Vis Sci* 2009, 50(7):-3203.

[55] Corrales RM, de Paiva CS, Li DQ, Farley WJ, Henriksson JT, Bergmanson JP, Pflugfelder SC: Entrapment of conjunctival goblet cells by desiccation-induced cornification. *Invest Ophthalmol Vis Sci* 2011,52: 3492-3499.

[56] Luo L, Li DQ, Pflugfelder SC. Hyperosmolarity-induced apoptosis in human corneal epithelial cells is mediated by cytochrome c and MAPK pathways. *Cornea* 2007, 26:452-460.

[57] Corrales RM, Stern ME, de Paiva CS, Welch J, Li DQ, Pflugfelder SC: Desiccating stress stimulates expression of matrix metalloproteinases by the corneal epithelium. *Invest Ophthalmol Vis Sci* 2006,47: 3293-3302.

[58] Nagase H, Woessner JF, Jr.: Matrix metalloproteinases. *J Biol Chem* 1999,274: 21491-21494.

[59] Johnson LL, Dyer R, Hupe DJ: Matrix metalloproteinases. *Curr Opin Chem Biol* 1998,2: 466-471.

[60] Visse R, Nagase H: Matrix metalloproteinases and tissue inhibitors of metalloproteinases: structure, function, and biochemistry. *Circ Res* 2003,92: 827-839.

[61] Brejchova K, Liskova P, Hrdlickova E, Filipec M, Jirsova K: Matrix metalloproteinases in recurrent corneal melting associated with primary Sjorgen's syndrome. *Mol Vis* 2009,15: 2364-2372.

[62] Fini ME, Girard MT, Matsubara M: Collagenolytic/gelatinolytic enzymes in corneal wound healing. *Acta Ophthalmol Suppl* 1992: 26-33.

http://dx.doi.org/10.5772/57585

[63] Matsubara M, Girard MT, Kublin CL, Cintron C, Fini ME: Differential roles for two gelatinolytic enzymes of the matrix metalloproteinase family in the remodelling cornea. *Dev Biol* 1991,147: 425-439.

[64] Matsubara M, Zieske JD, Fini ME: Mechanism of basement membrane dissolution preceding corneal ulceration. *Invest Ophthalmol Vis Sci* 1991,32: 3221-3237.

[65] Afonso AA, Sobrin L, Monroy DC, Selzer M, Lokeshwar B, Pflugfelder SC: Tear fluid gelatinase B activity correlates with IL-1alpha concentration and fluorescein clearance in ocular rosacea. *Invest Ophthalmol Vis Sci* 1999,40: 2506-2512.

[66] Kim HS, Luo L, Pflugfelder SC, Li DQ: Doxycycline Inhibits TGF-{beta}1-Induced MMP-9 via Smad and MAPK Pathways in Human Corneal Epithelial Cells. *Invest Ophthalmol Vis Sci* 2005,46: 840-848.

[67] Pflugfelder SC, Farley W, Luo L, Chen LZ, de Paiva CS, Olmos LC, Li DQ, Fini ME: Matrix metalloproteinase-9 knockout confers resistance to corneal epithelial barrier disruption in experimental dry eye. *Am J Pathol* 2005,166: 61-71.

[68] Beardsely RM, de Paiva CS, Power DF, Pflugfelder SC: Desiccating stress decreases apical corneal epithelial cell size--modulation by the metalloproteinase inhibitor doxycycline. *Cornea* 2008,27: 935-940.

[69] Behrens A, Doyle JJ, Stern L, Chuck RS, McDonnell PJ, Azar DT, Dua HS, Hom M, Karpecki PM, Laibson PR, Lemp MA, Meisler DM, Del Castillo JM, O'Brien TP, Pflugfelder SC, Rolando M, Schein OD, Seitz B, Tseng SC, van SG, Wilson SE, Yiu SC: Dysfunctional tear syndrome: a Delphi approach to treatment recommendations. *Cornea* 2006,25: 900-907.

[70] Jameson JM, Sharp LL, Witherden DA, Havran WL: Regulation of skin cell homeostasis by gamma delta T cells. *Front Biosci* 2004,9: 2640-2651.

[71] Dua HS, Gomes JA, Jindal VK, Appa SN, Schwarting R, Eagle RC, Jr., Donoso LA, Laibson PR: Mucosa specific lymphocytes in the human conjunctiva, corneoscleral limbus and lacrimal gland. *Curr Eye Res* 1994,13: 87-93.

[72] Dua HS, Gomes JA, Donoso LA, Laibson PR: The ocular surface as part of the mucosal immune system: conjunctival mucosa-specific lymphocytes in ocular surface pathology. *Eye (Lond)* 1995,9 (Pt 3): 261-267.

[73] Hingorani M, Metz D, Lightman SL: Characterisation of the normal conjunctival leukocyte population. *Exp Eye Res* 1997,64: 905-912.

[74] Rojas B, Cuhna R, Zafirakis P, Ramirez JM, Lizan-garciia M, Zhao T, Foster CS: Cell populations and adhesion molecules expression in conjunctiva before and after bone marrow transplantation. *Exp Eye Res* 2005,81: 313-325.

[75] Cepek KL, Parker CM, Madara JL, Brenner MB: Integrin alpha E beta 7 mediates adhesion of T lymphocytes to epithelial cells. *J Immunol* 1993,150: 3459-3470.

[76] Cepek KL, Shaw SK, Parker CM, Russell GJ, Morrow JS, Rimm DL, Brenner MB: Adhesion between epithelial cells and T lymphocytes mediated by E-cadherin and the alpha E beta 7 integrin. *Nature* 1994,372: 190-193.

[77] Jones DT, Monroy D, Ji Z, Atherton SS, Pflugfelder SC: Sjogren's syndrome: cytokine and Epstein-Barr viral gene expression within the conjunctival epithelium. *Invest Ophthalmol Vis Sci* 1994,35: 3493-3504.

[78] Pflugfelder SC, Jones D, Ji Z, Afonso A, Monroy D: Altered cytokine balance in the tear fluid and conjunctiva of patients with Sjogren's syndrome keratoconjunctivitis sicca. *Curr Eye Res* 1999,19: 201-211.

[79] Solomon A, Dursun D, Liu Z, Xie Y, Macri A, Pflugfelder SC: Pro-and anti-inflammatory forms of interleukin-1 in the tear fluid and conjunctiva of patients with dry-eye disease. *Invest Ophthalmol Vis Sci* 2001,42: 2283-2292.

[80] Calonge M: The treatment of dry eye. *Surv Ophthalmol* 2001,45 Suppl 2: S227-S239.

[81] Stern ME, Gao J, Schwalb TA, Ngo M, Tieu DD, Chan CC, Reis BL, Whitcup SM, Thompson D, Smith JA: Conjunctival T-cell subpopulations in Sjogren's and non-Sjogren's patients with dry eye. *Invest Ophthalmol Vis Sci* 2002,43: 2609-2614.

[82] Kunert KS, Tisdale AS, Stern ME, Smith JA, Gipson IK: Analysis of topical cyclosporine treatment of patients with dry eye syndrome: effect on conjunctival lymphocytes. *Arch Ophthalmol* 2000,118: 1489-1496.

[83] Niederkorn JY, Stern ME, Pflugfelder SC, de Paiva CS, Corrales RM, Gao J, Siemasko K: Desiccating Stress Induces T Cell-Mediated Sjogren's Syndrome-Like Lacrimal Keratoconjunctivitis. *J Immunol* 2006,176: 3950-3957.

[84] Happel KI, Dubin PJ, Zheng M, Ghilardi N, Lockhart C, Quinton LJ, Odden AR, Shellito JE, Bagby GJ, Nelson S, Kolls JK: Divergent roles of IL-23 and IL-12 in host defense against Klebsiella pneumoniae. *J Exp Med* 2005,202: 761-769.

[85] Chung DR, Kasper DL, Panzo RJ, Chitnis T, Grusby MJ, Sayegh MH, Tzianabos AO: CD4+T cells mediate abscess formation in intra-abdominal sepsis by an IL-17-dependent mechanism. *J Immunol* 2003,170: 1958-1963.

[86] Huang W, Na L, Fidel PL, Schwarzenberger P: Requirement of interleukin-17A for systemic anti-Candida albicans host defense in mice. *J Infect Dis* 2004,190: 624-631.

[87] Yoon KC, Park CS, You IC, Choi HJ, Lee KH, Im SK, Park HY, Pflugfelder SC: Expression of CXCL9,-10,-11, and CXCR3 in the tear film and ocular surface of patients with dry eye syndrome. *Invest Ophthalmol Vis Sci* 2010,51: 643-650.

[88] Yoon KC, de Paiva CS, Qi H, Chen Z, Farley WJ, Li DQ, Pflugfelder SC: Expression of th-1 chemokines and chemokine receptors on the ocular surface of C57BL/6 mice: effects of desiccating stress. *Invest Ophthalmol Vis Sci* 2007,48: 2561-2569.

[89] Choi W, Li Z, Oh HJ, Im SK, Lee SH, Park SH, You IC, Yoon KC: Expression of CCR5 and its ligands CCL3,-4, and-5 in the tear film and ocular surface of patients with dry eye disease. *Curr Eye Res* 2012,37: 12-17.

[90] Riemens A, Stoyanova E, Rothova A, Kuiper J: Cytokines in tear fluid of patients with ocular graft-versus-host disease after allogeneic stem cell transplantation. *Mol Vis* 2012,18: 797-802.

[91] Lam H, Blieden L, de Paiva CS, Farley WJ, Stern ME, Pflugfelder SC: Tear Cytokine Profiles in Dysfunctional Tear Syndrome. *Am J Ophthalmol* 2009, 147: 198-205. Nov. 5 [Epub ahead of print].

[92] Enriquez-de-Salamanca A, Castellanos E, Stern ME, Fernandez I, Carreno E, Garcia-Vazquez C, Herreras JM, Calonge M: Tear cytokine and chemokine analysis and clinical correlations in evaporative-type dry eye disease. *Mol Vis* 2010,16: 862-873.

[93] Massingale ML, Li X, Vallabhajosyula M, Chen D, Wei Y, Asbell PA: Analysis of inflammatory cytokines in the tears of dry eye patients. *Cornea* 2009,28: 1023-1027.

[94] Mrugacz M, Kaczmarski M, Bakunowicz-Lazarczyk A, Zelazowska B, Wysocka J, Minarowska A: IL-8 and IFN-gamma in tear fluid of patients with cystic fibrosis. *J Interferon Cytokine Res* 2006,26: 71-75.

[95] Boehm N, Riechardt AI, Wiegand M, Pfeiffer N, Grus FH: Proinflammatory cytokine profiling of tears from dry eye patients by means of antibody microarrays. *Invest Ophthalmol Vis Sci* 2011,52: 7725-7730.

[96] Corrales RM, Villarreal A, Farley W, Stern ME, Li DQ, Pflugfelder SC: Strain-related cytokine profiles on the murine ocular surface in response to desiccating stress. *Cornea* 2007,26: 579-584.

[97] de Paiva CS, Villarreal AL, Corrales RM, Rahman HT, Chang VY, Farley WJ, Stern ME, Niederkorn JY, Li DQ, Pflugfelder SC: Dry Eye-Induced Conjunctival Epithelial Squamous Metaplasia Is Modulated by Interferon-{gamma}. *Invest Ophthalmol Vis Sci* 2007,48: 2553-2560.

[98] Zhang X, Chen W, de Paiva CS, Corrales RM, Volpe EA, McClellan AJ, Farley WJ, Li DQ, Pflugfelder SC: Interferon-{gamma} Exacerbates Dry Eye Induced Apoptosis in Conjunctiva via Dual Apoptotic Pathways. *Invest Ophthalmol Vis Sci* 2011.

[99] Chen Y, Chauhan SK, Saban DR, Sadrai Z, Okanobo A, Dana R: Interferon-{gamma}-secreting NK cells promote induction of dry eye disease. *J Leukoc Biol* 2011,89: 965-972.

[100] Chen Z, Mok H, Pflugfelder SC, Li DQ, Barry MA: Improved transduction of human corneal epithelial progenitor cells with cell-targeting adenoviral vectors. *Exp Eye Res* 2006,83: 798-806.

[101] Kang EH, Lee YJ, Hyon JY, Yun PY, Song YW: Salivary cytokine profiles in primary Sjogren's syndrome differ from those in non-Sjogren sicca in terms of TNF-alpha levels and Th-1/Th-2 ratios. *Clin Exp Rheumatol* 2011,29: 970-976.

[102] Pertovaara M, Antonen J, Hurme M: Th2 cytokine genotypes are associated with a milder form of primary Sjogren's syndrome. *Ann Rheum Dis* 2006,65: 666-670.

[103] Hayashi T, Shimoyama N, Mizuno T: Destruction of salivary and lacrimal glands by Th1-polarized reaction in a model of secondary Sjogren's syndrome in lupus-prone female NZB x NZWF(1) mice. *Inflammation* 2012,35: 638-646.

[104] Ogawa N, Ping L, Zhenjun L, Takada Y, Sugai S: Involvement of the interferon-gamma-induced T cell-attracting chemokines, interferon-gamma-inducible 10-kd protein (CXCL10) and monokine induced by interferon-gamma (CXCL9), in the salivary gland lesions of patients with Sjogren's syndrome. *Arthritis Rheum* 2002,46: 2730-2741.

[105] Viau S, Pasquis B, Maire MA, Fourgeux C, Gregoire S, Acar N, Bretillon L, Creuzot-Garcher CP, Joffre C: No consequences of dietary n-3 polyunsaturated fatty acid deficiency on the severity of scopolamine-induced dry eye. *Graefes Arch Clin Exp Ophthalmol* 2011,249: 547-557.

[106] Jie G, Jiang Q, Rui Z, Yifei Y: Expression of interleukin-17 in autoimmune dacryoadenitis in MRL/lpr mice. *Curr Eye Res* 2010,35: 865-871.

[107] Rahimy E, Pitcher JD, III, Pangelinan SB, Chen W, Farley WJ, Niederkorn JY, Stern ME, Li DQ, Pflugfelder SC, de Paiva CS: Spontaneous autoimmune dacryoadenitis in aged CD25KO mice. *Am J Pathol* 2010,177: 744-753.

[108] Pelegrino FS, Volpe EA, Gandhi NB, Li DQ, Pflugfelder SC, de Paiva CS: Deletion of interferon-gamma delays onset and severity of dacryoadenitis in CD25KO mice. *Arthritis Res Ther* 2012,14: R234.

[109] Kohashi M, Ishimaru N, Arakaki R, Hayashi Y: Effective treatment with oral administration of rebamipide in a mouse model of Sjogren's syndrome. *Arthritis Rheum* 2008,58: 389-400.

[110] Koarada S, Haruta Y, Mitamura M, Morito F, Tada Y, Ohta A, Nagasawa K: Ex vivo CD(+) T-cell cytokine expression from patients with Sjogren's syndrome following in vitro stimulation to induce proliferation. *Rheumatology (Oxford)* 2006,45: 392-399.

[111] Brookes SM, Price EJ, Venables PJ, Maini RN: Interferon-gamma and epithelial cell activation in Sjogren's syndrome. *Br J Rheumatol* 1995,34: 226-231.

[112] Szodoray P, Gal I, Barath S, Aleksza M, Horvath IF, Gergely P, Jr., Szegedi G, Nakken B, Zeher M: Immunological alterations in newly diagnosed primary Sjogren's syndrome characterized by skewed peripheral T-cell subsets and inflammatory cytokines. *Scand J Rheumatol* 2008,37: 205-212.

[113] Hagiwara E, Pando J, Ishigatsubo Y, Klinman DM: Altered frequency of type 1 cytokine secreting cells in the peripheral blood of patients with primary Sjogren's syndrome. *J Rheumatol* 1998,25: 89-93.

[114] Konttinen YT, Kemppinen P, Koski H, Li TF, Jumppanen M, Hietanen J, Santavirta S, Salo T, Larsson A, Hakala M, Sorsa T: T(H)1 cytokines are produced in labial salivary glands in Sjogren's syndrome, but also in healthy individuals. *Scand J Rheumatol* 1999,28: 106-112.

[115] Ajjan RA, McIntosh RS, Waterman EA, Watson PF, Franklin CD, Yeoman CM, Weetman AP: Analysis of the T-cell receptor Valpha repertoire and cytokine gene expression in Sjogren's syndrome. *Br J Rheumatol* 1998,37: 179-185.

[116] Giron-Gonzalez JA, Baturone R, Soto MJ, Marquez M, Macias I, Montes de OM, Medina F, Chozas N, Garcia-Perez S: Implications of immunomodulatory interleukins for the hyperimmunoglobulinemia of Sjogren's syndrome. *Cell Immunol* 2009,259: 56-60.

[117] van Woerkom JM, Kruize AA, Wenting-van Wijk MJ, Knol E, Bihari IC, Jacobs JW, Bijlsma JW, Lafeber FP, van Roon JA: Salivary gland and peripheral blood T helper 1 and 2 cell activity in Sjogren's syndrome compared with non-Sjogren's sicca syndrome. *Ann Rheum Dis* 2005,64: 1474-1479.

[118] Mitsias DI, Tzioufas AG, Veiopoulou C, Zintzaras E, Tassios IK, Kogopoulou O, Moutsopoulos HM, Thyphronitis G: The Th1/Th2 cytokine balance changes with the progress of the immunopathological lesion of Sjogren's syndrome. *Clin Exp Immunol* 2002,128: 562-568.

[119] Zhang X, Chen W, de Paiva CS, Volpe EA, Gandhi NB, Farley WJ, Li DQ, Niederkorn JY, Stern ME, Pflugfelder SC: Desiccating Stress Induces CD4(+) T-Cell-Mediated Sjogren's Syndrome-Like Corneal Epithelial Apoptosis via Activation of the Extrinsic Apoptotic Pathway by Interferon-gamma. *Am J Pathol* 2011,179: 1807-1814.

[120] Zhang X, Chen W, de Paiva CS, Corrales RM, Volpe EA, McClellan AJ, Farley WJ, Li DQ, Pflugfelder SC: Interferon-gamma exacerbates dry eye-induced apoptosis in conjunctiva through dual apoptotic pathways. *Invest Ophthalmol Vis Sci* 2011,52: 6279-6285.

[121] Albertsmeyer AC, Kakkassery V, Spurr-Michaud S, Beeks O, Gipson IK: Effect of pro-inflammatory mediators on membrane-associated mucins expressed by human ocular surface epithelial cells. *Exp Eye Res* 2010,90: 444-451.

[122] Veldhoen M, Hocking RJ, Atkins CJ, Locksley RM, Stockinger B: TGFbeta in the context of an inflammatory cytokine milieu supports de novo differentiation of IL-17-producing T cells. *Immunity* 2006,24: 179-189.

[123] Bettelli E, Carrier Y, Gao W, Korn T, Strom TB, Oukka M, Weiner HL, Kuchroo VK: Reciprocal developmental pathways for the generation of pathogenic effector TH17 and regulatory T cells. *Nature* 2006,441: 235-238.

[124] Mangan PR, Harrington LE, O'Quinn DB, Helms WS, Bullard DC, Elson CO, Hatton RD, Wahl SM, Schoeb TR, Weaver CT: Transforming growth factor-beta induces development of the T(H)17 lineage. *Nature* 2006,441: 231-234.

[125] Korn T, Mitsdoerffer M, Croxford AL, Awasthi A, Dardalhon VA, Galileos G, Vollmar P, Stritesky GL, Kaplan MH, Waisman A, Kuchroo VK, Oukka M: IL-6 controls Th17 immunity in vivo by inhibiting the conversion of conventional T cells into Foxp3+regulatory T cells. *Proc Natl Acad Sci U S A* 2008,105: 18460-18465.

[126] Nurieva RI, Chung Y, Hwang D, Yang XO, Kang HS, Ma L, Wang YH, Watowich SS, Jetten AM, Tian Q, Dong C: Generation of T follicular helper cells is mediated by interleukin-21 but independent of T helper 1, 2, or 17 cell lineages. *Immunity* 2008,29: 138-149.

[127] Yang XO, Panopoulos AD, Nurieva R, Chang SH, Wang D, Watowich SS, Dong C: STAT3 regulates cytokine-mediated generation of inflammatory helper T cells. *J Biol Chem* 2007,282: 9358-9363.

[128] Li MO, Wan YY, Sanjabi S, Robertson AK, Flavell RA: Transforming growth factor-beta regulation of immune responses. *Annu Rev Immunol* 2006,24: 99-146.

[129] Gupta A, Monroy D, Ji Z, Yoshino K, Huang AJW, Pflugfelder SC: Transforming growth factor beta-1 and beta-2 in human tear fluid. *Curr Eye Res* 1996,15: 605-614.

[130] Yoshino K, Garg R, Monroy D, Ji Z, Pflugfelder SC: Production and secretion of transforming growth factor beta (TGF-β) by the human lacrimal gland. *Curr Eye Res* 1996,15: 615-624.

[131] Zheng X, de Paiva CS, Rao K, Li DQ, Farley WJ, Stern M, Pflugfelder SC: Evaluation of the transforming growth factor-beta activity in normal and dry eye human tears by CCL-185 cell bioassay. *Cornea* 2010,29: 1048-1054.

[132] Sun D, Emmert-Buck MR, Fox PC: Differential cytokine mRNA expression in human labial minor salivary glands in primary Sjogren's syndrome. *Autoimmunity* 1998,28: 125-137.

[133] Murphy-Ullrich JE, Poczatek M: Activation of latent TGF-beta by thrombospondin-1: mechanisms and physiology. *Cytokine Growth Factor Rev* 2000,11: 59-69.

[134] Turpie B, Yoshimura T, Gulati A, Rios JD, Dartt DA, Masli S: Sjogren's syndrome-like ocular surface disease in thrombospondin-1 deficient mice. *Am J Pathol* 2009,175: 1136-1147.

[135] Gandhi NB, Su Z, Zhang X, Volpe EA, Pelegrino FS, Rahman SA, Li DQ, Pflugfelder SC, de Paiva CS: Dendritic cell-derived thrombospondin-1 is critical for the generation of the ocular surface Th17 response to desiccating stress. *J Leukoc Biol* 2013, 94:1293-301.

[136] Zheng X, Bian F, Ma P, de Paiva CS, Stern M, Pflugfelder SC, Li DQ: Induction of Th17 differentiation by corneal epithelial-derived cytokines. *J Cell Physiol* 2009,2009 Sep 10;222(1): 95-102.

[137] Coursey TG, Gandhi NB, Volpe EA, Pflugfelder SC, de Paiva CS. CCR6 KO Mice Are Resistant To Dry Eye Disease. *PLoS One* 2013, 8: e78508.

[138] Wang C, Kang SG, Lee J, Sun Z, Kim CH: The roles of CCR6 in migration of Th17 cells and regulation of effector T-cell balance in the gut. *Mucosal Immunol* 2009,2: 173-183.

[139] Hirota K, Yoshitomi H, Hashimoto M, Maeda S, Teradaira S, Sugimoto N, Yamaguchi T, Nomura T, Ito H, Nakamura T, Sakaguchi N, Sakaguchi S: Preferential recruitment of CCR6-expressing Th17 cells to inflamed joints via CCL20 in rheumatoid arthritis and its animal model. *J Exp Med* 2007,204: 2803-2812.

[140] Pflugfelder SC: Anti-inflammatory therapy of dry eye. *Am J Ophthalmol* 2004,137: 337-342.

[141] Turner K, Pflugfelder SC, Ji Z, Feuer WJ, Stern M, Reis BL: Interleukin-6 levels in the conjunctival epithelium of patients with dry eye disease treated with cyclosporine ophthalmic emulsion. *Cornea* 2000,19: 492-496.

[142] Zhang X, Volpe EA, Gandhi NB, Schaumburg CS, Siemasko KF, Pangelinan SB, Kelly SD, Hayday AC, Li DQ, Stern ME, Niederkorn JY, Pflugfelder SC, de Paiva CS: NK cells promote Th-17 mediated corneal barrier disruption in dry eye. *PLoS One* 2012,7: e36822.

[143] Zheng X, de Paiva CS, Li DQ, Farley WJ, Pflugfelder SC: Desiccating stress promotion of Th17 differentiation by ocular surface tissues through a dendritic cell-mediated pathway. *Invest Ophthalmol Vis Sci* 2010,51: 3083-3091.

[144] Solomon A, Rosenblatt M, Monroy D, Ji Z, Pflugfelder SC, Tseng SC: Suppression of interleukin 1alpha and interleukin 1beta in human limbal epithelial cells cultured on the amniotic membrane stromal matrix. *Br J Ophthalmol* 2001,85: 444-449.

[145] Katsifis GE, Rekka S, Moutsopoulos NM, Pillemer S, Wahl SM: Systemic and local interleukin-17 and linked cytokines associated with Sjogren's syndrome immunopathogenesis. *Am J Pathol* 2009,175: 1167-1177.

[146] Sakai A, Sugawara Y, Kuroishi T, Sasano T, Sugawara S: Identification of IL-18 and Th17 cells in salivary glands of patients with Sjogren's syndrome, and amplification of IL-17-mediated secretion of inflammatory cytokines from salivary gland cells by IL-18. *J Immunol* 2008,181: 2898-2906.

[147] Nguyen CQ, Hu MH, Li Y, Stewart C, Peck AB: Salivary gland tissue expression of interleukin-23 and interleukin-17 in Sjogren's syndrome: findings in humans and mice. *Arthritis Rheum* 2008,58: 734-743.

[148] Chauhan SK, El AJ, Ecoiffier T, Goyal S, Zhang Q, Saban DR, Dana R: Autoimmunity in dry eye is due to resistance of Th17 to Treg suppression. *J Immunol* 2009,182: 1247-1252.

[149] Nakamura T, Nishida K, Dota A, Matsuki M, Yamanishi K, Kinoshita S: Elevated expression of transglutaminase 1 and keratinization-related proteins in conjunctiva in severe ocular surface disease. *Invest Ophthalmol Vis Sci* 2001,42: 549-556.

[150] Pflugfelder SC, Tseng SCG, Yoshino K, Monroy D, Felix C, Reis BL: Correlation of goblet cell density and mucosal epithelial membrane mucin expression with rose bengal staining in patients with ocular irritation. *Ophthalmology* 1997,104: 223-235.

[151] Fuss IJ, Strober W: The role of IL-13 and NK T cells in experimental and human ulcerative colitis. *Mucosal Immunol* 2008,1 Suppl 1: S31-S33.

[152] Middendorp S, Nieuwenhuis EE: NKT cells in mucosal immunity. *Mucosal Immunol* 2009,2: 393-402.

[153] Matangkasombut P, Pichavant M, Dekruyff RH, Umetsu DT: Natural killer T cells and the regulation of asthma. *Mucosal Immunol* 2009,2: 383-392.

[154] de Paiva CS, Raince JK, McClellan AJ, Shanmugam KP, Pangelinan SB, Volpe EA, Corrales RM, Farley WJ, Corry DB, Li DQ, Pflugfelder SC: Homeostatic control of conjunctival mucosal goblet cells by NKT-derived IL-13. *Mucosal Immunol* 2011,4(4): 397-408. doi: 10.1038/mi.2010.82. Epub 2010 Dec 22.

[155] Sacks EH, Wieczorek R, Jakobiec FA, Knowles DM: Lymphocytic subpopulations in the normal human conjunctiva. A monoclonal antibody study. *Ophthalmology* 1986,93: 1276-1283.

[156] Lider O, Santos LM, Lee CS, Higgins PJ, Weiner HL: Suppression of experimental autoimmune encephalomyelitis by oral administration of myelin basic protein. II. Suppression of disease and in vitro immune responses is mediated by antigen-specific CD8+T lymphocytes. *J Immunol* 1989,142: 748-752.

[157] Miller A, Lider O, Weiner HL: Antigen-driven bystander suppression after oral administration of antigens. *J Exp Med* 1991,174: 791-798.

[158] Sugita S, Ng TF, Schwartzkopff J, Streilein JW: CTLA-4+CD8+T cells that encounter B7-2+iris pigment epithelial cells express their own B7-2 to achieve global suppression of T cell activation. *J Immunol* 2004,172: 4184-4194.

[159] Raphael M, Bellefqih S, Piette JC, Le HP, Debre P, Chomette G: Conjunctival biopsy in Sjogren's syndrome: correlations between histological and immunohistochemical features. *Histopathology* 1988,13: 191-202.

[160] Zhang X, Schaumburg CS, Coursey TG, Siemasko KF, Volpe EA, Gandhi NB, D.-Q L, Niederkorn JY, Stern ME, Pflugfelder SC, de Paiva CS. $CD8^+$Cells Regulate the T

helper-17 Response in an Experimental Murine Model of Sjögren Syndrome. Mucosal Immunol. 2014, 7:417-27.

[161] de Paiva CS, Corrales RM, Villarreal AL, Farley WJ, Li DQ, Stern ME, Pflugfelder SC: Corticosteroid and doxycycline suppress MMP-9 and inflammatory cytokine expression, MAPK activation in the corneal epithelium in experimental dry eye. *Exp Eye Res* 2006,83: 526-535.

[162] Pflugfelder SC, Maskin SL, Anderson B, Chodosh J, Holland EJ, de Paiva CS, Bartels SP, Micuda T, Proskin HM, Vogel R: A randomized, double-masked, placebo-controlled, multicenter comparison of loteprednol etabonate ophthalmic suspension, 0.5%, and placebo for treatment of keratoconjunctivitis sicca in patients with delayed tear clearance. *Am J Ophthalmol* 2004,138: 444-457.

[163] Dursun D, Kim MC, Solomon A, Pflugfelder SC: Treatment of recalcitrant recurrent corneal erosions with inhibitors of matrix metalloproteinase-9, doxycycline and corticosteroids. *Am J Ophthalmol* 2001,132: 8-13.

[164] Schaumburg CS, Siemasko KF, de Paiva CS, Pflugfelder ME, Stern ME: Ocular Surface Antigen Presenting Cells are Necessary for Activation of Autoreactive T cells and Development of Autoimmune Lacrimal Keratoconjunctivtis. *J Immunol* 2011,187(7): 3653-3662.

[165] Sadrai Z, Stevenson W, Okanobo A, Chen Y, Dohlman TH, Hua J, Amparo F, Chauhan SK, Dana R: PDE4 inhibition suppresses IL-17-associated immunity in dry eye disease. *Invest Ophthalmol Vis Sci* 2012,53: 3584-3591.

[166] Lee HS, Chauhan SK, Okanobo A, Nallasamy N, Dana R: Therapeutic Efficacy of Topical Epigallocatechin Gallate in Murine Dry Eye. *Cornea* 2011,30(12): 1465-1472.

[167] Goyal S, Chauhan SK, Zhang Q, Dana R: Amelioration of murine dry eye disease by topical antagonist to chemokine receptor 2. *Arch Ophthalmol* 2009,127: 882-887.

[168] Baudouin C, Brignole F, Pisella PJ, De Jean MS, Goguel A: Flow cytometric analysis of the inflammatory marker HLA DR in dry eye syndrome: results from 12 months of randomized treatment with topical cyclosporin A. Adv Exp Med Biol 2002,506: 761-769.

[169] Brignole F, Pisella PJ, De Saint JM, Goldschild M, Goguel A, Baudouin C: Flow cytometric analysis of inflammatory markers in KCS: 6-month treatment with topical cyclosporin A. Invest Ophthalmol Vis Sci 2001,42: 90-95.

Chapter 18

Advances in Pathogenesis of Behcet's Disease and Vogt-Koyanagi-Harada Syndrome

Peizeng Yang, Chaokui Wang, Shengping Hou,
Bo Lei, Aize Kijlstra and De-Quan Li

Additional information is available at the end of the chapter

http://dx.doi.org/10.5772/57586

1. Introduction

Uveitis is one of the leading causes of blindness in the world. It is estimated that uveitis accounts for 10%-15% of the blindness in the western world [1]. More importantly, the blindness caused by uveitis is mostly permanent and irreversible since the retina and optic nerve are damaged by inflammation.

Uveitis was previously defined as inflammation of the uveal tract, which is classically composed of the iris, ciliary body and choroid. Yet in common practice, uveitis refers to inflammation involving any intraocular structure and therefore carries the following names: iritis, iridocyclitis, parsplanitis, posterior uveitis, choroiditis, retinitis and retinal vasculitis. It is usually classified into infectious and noninfectious origins on the basis of predominant etiological characteristics. Behcet's disease (BD) is thought to be an autoinflammatory disease, while Vogt-Koyanagi-Harada (VKH) syndrome is an autoimmune disease. Therefore, we chose BD and VKH, which are two important representative entities among the noninfectious uveitis class, to discuss the recent advances in our knowledge on the pathogenesis of uveitis.

BD is a chronic systemic autoinflammatory disease, characterized by recurrent uveitis, skin lesions, oral and genital mucous ulcers, as well as some complications in central nervous system, gastrointestinal tract and thrombotic events [2]. A high prevalence of BD has been reported along the ancient Silk Road [3], from Asia to the Mediterranean basin countries, such as Turkey, Iraq, Iran, Korea and Japan. The clinical features of BD have been well documented in publications originating from the high incidence countries. Our research group has evaluated the clinical characteristics and associated ocular complications in a large group of consecutive Chinese BD patients and found that most patients presented a bilateral nongranulomatous anterior, posterior, or panuveitis with a chronic and relapsing course. Uveitis occurred mostly in male patients and in the age group from the second to fifth decade of life. Oral aphthae (100%), skin lesions (78%), and genital ulcers (57.9%) were the typical extraocular findings in patients with BD [4].

VKH syndrome is a well-established immune-mediated multi-organ disorder characterized by a bilateral granulomatous panuveitis frequently associated with extraocular findings including poliosis, vitiligo, alopecia, and central nervous system and auditory signs [5]. It is an autoimmune disease against melanocyte-associated antigens in genetically susceptible individuals. VKH mainly affects certain pigmented races, such as Asians and Native Americans [5-6]. Four clinical stages of uveitis could be developed in patients with VKH syndrome: prodromal, acute, convalescent, and chronic recurrent stages. A clinical analysis based on a large group (n=410) of uveitis patients with VKH syndrome performed by our group showed that the disease was diagnosed most often in young people without a gender predisposition. The intraocular manifestations typically began with choroiditis or chorioretinitis, serous retinal detachment, and optic disc edema, and then proceeded to anterior uveitis if appropriate treatment was not given during the first 2 weeks. Eventually, the eyes developed a recurrent generalized granulomatous uveitis. With regard to the extraocular manifestations, meningismus signs, tinnitus, and abnormal touch sensitivity of the hair frequently occurred before or concurrently with ocular involvement, whereas vitiligo and poliosis usually appear after the uveitis attack [7]. This is possibly due to the autoimmune attack against melanocytes at different sites of the body.

Although the etiology and pathogenesis of BD and VKH syndrome is not completely known, it is hypothesized that abnormalities in the regulation of the immune system and an immunogenetic predisposition are involved in the development of these diseases. Deregulation of Th1, Th17 and regulatory T cells and abnormalities in the associated molecules were found to be involved in the development of these diseases. Recently, two large genome-wide association studies (GWAS) from Japan and Turkey reported an association between single nucleotide polymorphism (SNP) of IL-10, IL-23R/IL-12RB2 gene and BD [8-9]. HLA-DR4 and HLA-DRw53 were reported to be highly associated with VKH syndrome [10], implicating that genetic factors contributed to the pathogenesis of BD and VKH syndrome. The aim of this chapter is to expound the pathogenesis of BD and VKH syndrome with emphasis on new insights in the area of immunoregulation and immunogenetics.

2. Th1 cells and cytokines in Behcet's disease and VKH syndrome

Th1 cells were the first subtype of T help cells that was reported to be involved in the pathogenesis of autoimmune diseases. IFN-γ is the hallmark cytokine of Th1 cells. A number of studies have determined the role of the Th1 cell and its specific cytokine repertoire in the pathogenesis of BD and VKH syndrome. The increased levels of IFN-γ and T-bet, which is considered as the critical transcriptional factor for Th1 cells, have been observed in the peripheral blood of the patients with active uveitis of BD and VKH syndrome [11-14]. Our study found that S-Ag specific T cells may be involved in the pathogenesis of BD via the production of Th1-dominant cytokines, but not Th17 cytokines [15]. The increased levels of Th1 cell specific cytokines and chemokines in the cerebrospinal fluid (CSF) of VKH patients and in the lesions of active BD patients were also reported [16-17]. El-Asrar et al found an increased levels of IFN-γ in the aqueous humor samples of uveitis from BD, VKH syndrome and HLA-B27-associated uveitis as compared with normal controls; and importantly, the levels of IFN-γ were higher in BD patients than in VKH and HLA-B27-associated uveitis [18], which suggests that IFN-γ may play more important role in the pathogenesis of BD.

In the murine uveitis models, previous reports suggested that Th1 played a pathogenic role during experimental autoimmune uveitis (EAU) development. It was shown that mice neutralized with monoclonal antibodies to IL-12, which drives Th1 differentiation, did not develop EAU [19]. In order to detect whether constitutive ocular expression of IFN-γ influences the course of EAU, Egwuagu et al generated transgenic rats with targeted expression of IFN-γ in the eye and found that IFN-γ markedly accelerated the onset and exacerbated the severity of rat EAU [20]. However, it has been reported that IFN-γ can also provide a protective role in this model. Genetic deletion or neutralization with antibodies against endogenous IFN-γ did not lead to a resistance of EAU induction and development, but rather aggravated the severity of uveitis [21-22]. Mice treated with IL-12 during the first week after immunization appeared to protect the animals from EAU through an IFN-γ-dependent mechanism. It has now been demonstrated that the role of IFN-γ in the development of uveitis is dependent on the stage of disease and the model of EAU that is being studied. IFN-γ confers protection when it is produced during the early stage of the disease. Th1 cells play an essential pathogenic role in the induction of the so called dendritic cell (DC) EAU model, which is induced by the infusion of uveitogenic interphotoreceptor retinoid-binding protein (IRBP) peptide-pulsed DCs. On the other hand, Th17 cells are essential to the induction of classical EAU, which is induced by the immunization with IRBP in the presence of strong adjuvants such as complete Freund's adjuvant and *B. pertusis* [23].

3. Th17 cells and cytokines in Behcet's disease and VKH syndrome

Th17 cells, characterized by their production of IL-17, have been reported be associated with the pathogenesis of many autoimmune diseases, including multiple sclerosis, rheumatoid arthritis and systemic lupus erythematosus (SLE). Th17 cells preferentially produce IL-17A, IL-17F, IL-21, and IL-22 [24]. IL-17A, also commonly called IL-17, plays a critical role in the development of allergy and autoimmune responses. IL-17F is mainly involved in mucosal host defense mechanisms, while not required for the induction of experimental autoimmune encephalomyelitis (EAE) and Collagen-induced arthritis (CIA) [25]. As yet no reports have appeared on the role of IL-17F in the pathogenesis of uveitis, thus, whether IL-17F is involved in human uveitis and EAU needs further investigation. This section aims to review studies regarding Th17 cells and related cytokines in the development of BD and VKH syndrome.

Various studies have shown that Th17 cells contribute to the pathogenesis of BD and VKH syndrome. The previous reports from ours and others have shown that the level of IL-17 by polyclonally stimulated peripheral blood mononuclear cells (PBMCs) and $CD4^{+}T$ cells, and the frequency of IL-17–producing $CD4^{+}T$ cells in PBMCs was higher in patients with active BD or VKH syndrome than the controls [11-12, 26]. Geri et al reported an increase of Th17 cells in peripheral blood and in CSF from active BD patients [27]. Animal studies showed that IL-17 may play a major role in the pathogenesis of EAU. The neutralization of IL-17 by monoclonal antibodies prevented or reversed the intraocular inflammation in the EAU model [28-30]. Adoptive transfer of Th17 cells could induce EAU in the absence of INF-γ [29]. These results indicate that IL-17 plays a proinflammatory and pathogenic role in autoimmune uveitis, and the blockade of IL-17 signaling may represent a therapeutic target in BD and VKH syndrome as well as in other Th17 cell-mediated autoimmune diseases.

IL-21, a member of the IL-2 family of cytokines, can drive Th17 differentiation in an autocrine manner [31-32]. We recently reported a higher level of serum IL-21 and IL-21 mRNA in PBMCs from patients having chronic or recurrent active VKH syndrome as compared with patients having inactive VKH syndrome or healthy controls. Moreover, in vitro experiments showed that IL-21 significantly increased IL-17 production, but had no influence on IFN-γ production by PBMCs or $CD4^{+}T$ cells obtained from either patients or healthy controls [33]. Geri et al observed higher levels of serum IL-21 and IL-21-producing $CD4^{+}T$ cells in BD patients. IL-21 was found to be able to drive Th1 and Th17 differentiation and suppressed the frequency of Treg cells. More importantly, they demonstrated the presence of IL-21-producing T cells in the CSF, choroid plexus, brain parenchyma inflammatory infiltrates and intracerebral blood vessels in active BD with CNS involvement [27]. These results suggest that IL-21 may be involved in the pathogenesis of BD and VKH syndrome and may represent a novel therapeutic target for these diseases. The pathogenic role of IL-21 in autoimmune uveitis is supported by animal models. IL-21R-deficient mice are resistant to EAU, and adoptive transfer of $IL\text{-}21R^{-/-}T$ cells reduced the EAU severity. Increased IL-21 in lymph nodes and spleens has been reported during the development of EAU [34-35]. All these findings provide evidence for a role of IL-21 in the pathogenesis of uveitis by promoting Th1 and Th17 cell responses and inhibiting Treg cell development.

IL-22, a member of the IL-10 cytokine family, has recently been reported to be involved in a number of human diseases, including mucosal-associated infections and inflammatory disorders of the intestine, skin and joints. In view of the biological function, controversial effects of IL-22 have been observed in different animal models and human disease. IL-22 seems to play a pathogenic role in experimental arthritis and dermatitis, whereas a protective effect was found in inflammatory bowel disease, experimental hepatitis and collagen-induced arthritis [36-37]. Sugita et al showed that the frequency of IL-22-producing T cell clones from aqueous humor of Behcet's uveitis was higher than that from normal controls. Furthermore, they demonstrated that CD4⁺T cells from PBMCs secrete increased amounts of IL-22 in BD patients with active uveitis. Higher IL-22 levels in the supernatants of stimulated PBMCs and CD4⁺T cells and an increased frequency of IL-22-producing CD4⁺T cells in BD patients with active uveitis were also reported by our group. In addition, increased IL-22 mRNA expression was found in erythema nodosum (EN) skin lesions, and positively correlated with the presence of EN [38]. The group of Nussenblatt reported an upregulated expression of IL-22 in PBMCs of clinical uveitis patients. IL-22 was shown to damage the physiological integrity of primary fetal retinal epithelium cells and induced their apoptosis [39]. These results suggest that an increased IL-22 may also be involved in the pathogenesis of BD. However, studies in a mouse model of uveitis showed that IL-22 can protect mice from the development of uveitis by inducing the generation of regulatory CD11b⁺antigen-presenting cells, which were able to convert pathogenic T cells into regulatory T cells [40]. As mentioned, the role of IL-22 in human clinical uveitis and animal models remains controversial and needs further investigation.

4. Molecules modulating Th1 or Th17 cells in Behcet's disease and VKH syndrome

The induction and maintenance of Th1 and Th17 cells requires a large set of molecules. The differentiation of Th17 cells from naïve CD4⁺T cells is regulated by cytokines [41]. Transforming growth factor-β (TGF-β) and IL-6, broadly expressed by many cell types in the body, including dendritic and epithelial cells, are dominant in the initiation of Th17 cell differentiation [42-45]; IL-23, IL-1β and IL-21, which are products of activated DCs, macrophages, activated T cell or inflamed epithelial cells, possibly expand and maintain the differentiated Th17 cells in the presence of IL-6 and TGF-β1 [31-32, 43, 46-47]. Furthermore, signal transducer and activator of transcription 3 (STAT3) has been found to mediate the initiation of Th17 cell differentiation by these inducing cytokines [48]. IL-12 is an important cytokine responsible for Th1 cell differentiation. IL-27 can induce Tr1 cell differentiation while inhibiting Th17 cell differentiation.

IL-6 has been shown to be a critical mediator of the autoimmune response and inflammation. Various studies have demonstrated that IL-6 was associated with disease activity in BD [49-50]. Studies by Norose et al showed that the level of IL-6 was significantly increased and correlated with the number of lymphocytes in aqueous humor from VKH patients [51]. The infiltrated T cells in the aqueous humor or PBMCs obtained from VKH patients showed an enhanced capability to secrete IL-6 as compared to normal controls [51-52]. Ozdamar et al found that serum levels of IL-6 were higher in BD patients with active uveitis than in those without uveitis [53]. A higher level of IL-6 was also reported in the CSF of patients with active BD with nervous system involvement [54-55]. A case report by Hirano et al showed that tocilizumab, a humanized anti-interleukin 6 receptor antibody, could suppress the clinical manifestations in a patient with refractory BD [56]. Consistent with observations in clinical uveitis, IL-6-deficient mice were not able to generate Th17 cells and were resistant to EAU. Systemic administration of anti-IL-6 receptor antibody ameliorated EAU by suppressing both systemic and regional Th17 responses [57-58]. Taken together, these findings suggest that IL-6 is involved in the pathogenesis of BD and VKH syndrome, and IL-6 blockade may provide a therapeutic efficacy in treating ocular inflammation in patients with BD or VKH syndrome.

IL-23, which is composed of a unique p19 subunit and a shared p40 subunit of IL-12, is essential in the survival and maintenance of pathogenic Th17 cells. Our earlier studies provided evidence for the involvement of IL-23 in the occurrence of uveitis in BD and VKH syndrome. Active uveitis in both diseases showed a higher level of IL-23 in the serum and supernatants of PBMCs as compared to inactive patients and normal controls [11-12]. IL-23p19 mRNA expression was increased in the EN-like skin lesions from BD patients [59]. Studies by Habibagahi et al showed that the IL-23 expression was strongly associated with the disease activity of uveitis with BD [60]. These results suggest that IL-23 may be a biomarker in the course of BD and VKH syndrome. Animal studies have shown that IL-23 is necessary for the induction of EAU due to its capacity to promote a Th17 effector response. It has been shown that IL-23KO mice are resistant to EAU and specific anti-IL-23 antibody prevented EAU induction [29]. These findings support the hypothesis that the IL-23/IL-17 pathway is involved in the pathogenesis of intraocular inflammation in BD and VKH syndrome.

IL-1β is a key proinflammatory cytokine that promotes Th17 cell differentiation. We recently observed a higher IL-1β production by peptidoglycan (PGN)/lipopolysaccharide (LPS)–induced monocyte-derived macrophages from active ocular BD patients [61]. Pay et al showed a significantly increased level of IL-1β in synovial fluid from BD patients as compared to that from osteoarthritis patients [62]. These results suggest that IL-1β may play a critical role in the pathogenesis of BD. The pathogenic role of IL-1β in uveitis was also proven directly by the observation that IL-1 receptor deficient mice were completely resistant to EAU [63].

IL-12, a heterodimeric cytokine composed of the subunits p40 andp35, is known to induce the differentiation of naïve $CD4^{+}$T cells into Th1 cells. Studies on the role of IL-12 in clinical uveitis have shown that IL-12 levels in plasma and PBMC culture supernatants were higher in BD with active uveitis [64-65]. Actual measurements of IL-12 in VKH syndrome have not yet been reported. Many studies have shown that Th1 cells are involved in VKH syndrome [13-14], which makes it likely that IL-12 is involved in the pathogenesis.

IL-27, a member of the IL-12 family of cytokines, has been shown to be able to inhibit Th17 cells and that it can induce regulatory Tr1 cells. IL-27 is composed of a unique p28 subunit and a shared EBI3 subunit with IL-35. Our studies on VKH found a decreased IL-27P28 mRNA expression by PBMCs and the lower IL-27 levels in the serum and supernatants of PBMCs in active VKH patients as compared to the inactive patients and normal controls, while the shared EBI3 mRNA expression was not different between the three groups. Furthermore, IL-27 was shown to inhibit the Th17 cell response in a direct manner on $CD4^{+}$T cells as well as by modulating DCs. Treatment with corticosteroids has been shown to upregulate IL-27 production in vivo and in vitro [66]. An increased levels of IL-27 have been reported in the serum of uveitis patients with BD [67]. Various animal models have been used to examine the role of IL-27 in autoimmune disease and found that the presence of IL-27 could protect mice from

EAE and CIA [68-69]. In the EAU model, an increased expression of IL-27 was observed at the peak of EAU, and further experiments showed that IL-27 could suppress the expansion of Th17 cells in the retina [70]. These observations suggest that an upregulated IL-27 response may contribute to the self-limited inflammation seen in the EAU model. Further clinical studies are needed in clinical uveitis and EAU to obtain further support whether IL-27 may be a potential therapeutic target for BD and VKH syndrome.

Tumor necrosis factor-alpha (TNF-α) is a proinflammatory cytokine that plays a significant role in the pathogenesis of many inflammatory and autoimmune diseases. It has been reported that the level of TNF-α was increased in the ocular fluids, serum and in the supernatants of stimulated $CD4^{+}$T cells from active uveitis patients with BD. Furthermore, TNF-α could induce the polarization of Th17 cells in BD patients [71-72]. A similar result was seen in the aqueous humor of VKH patients concerning the expression of TNF-α [18]. In the animal models of EAU it was shown that TNFR1-deficient mice were resistant to EAU through a TNFR1-dependent deficit in macrophage migration to the inflammatory site [73]. Treatment with systemic or local TNF-α inhibition with etanercept in the induction phase of EAU could effectively alleviate the severity of uveitis [74]. The pathogenic role of TNF-α in uveitis was also supported by experiments that showed that TNF-α could disrupt morphologic and functional barrier properties of polarized retinal pigment epithelium cells [75]. Thus, these results also indicate that TNF-α plays an important role in the pathogenesis of uveitis and has provided the basis as a major target for treating inflammatory and autoimmune eye diseases. In clinical trials, a number of reports have shown encouraging results in treating BD and VKH syndrome with anti-TNF-α antibody, such as infliximab [76-77].

A number of other immune-related molecules were also found to be associated with the pathogenesis of BD or VKH syndrome. Our most recent studies have revealed that other proinflammatory mediators, such as osteopontin (OPN), IL-7 and leptin, were also involved in the pathogenesis of BD and/or VKH syndrome. We observed the increased serum levels of OPN, IL-7 and leptin in patients with active BD and/or VKH syndrome, which may promote both Th1 and/or Th17 polarization [78-81]. Consistent with our findings, it has been shown that OPN aggravated the severity of EAU, and blockade of OPN with siRNA prevented the uveitis development [82-83]. IL-7 and leptin have been reported to be involved in the induction and progress of EAE, a model that shares many immunopathogenic mechanisms with EAU [84-85].

Other regulatory molecules may also play a critical role in controlling autoimmunity. 1,25-Dihydroxyvitamin D, miRNA155, IFN-α and IFN-β have all been shown to have an anti-inflammatory role in autoimmune disease. Levels of 1,25-Dihydroxyvitamin D3 and miRNA155 have been shown to be decreased in BD and VKH syndrome. Furthermore, 1,25-Dihydroxyvitamin D3 and miRNA155 were shown to inhibit Th17 cell responses [86-87], supporting its protective role in both BD and VKH syndrome. IFN-α has been effective in treating uveitis in patients with BD and our studies on the possible mechanisms showed that it could inhibit the Th17 cell response and was able to induce the expression of the regulatory cytokine IL-10 [88]. Studies in the animal model of uveitis showed that IFN-β exerted its inhibitory effect on EAU by inhibiting the Th1 and Th17 cell response [89], suggesting a protective role in uveitis.

5. Treg cells in Behcet's disease and VKH syndrome

Treg cells maintain the immune balance between effector and tolerogenic immune responses. It is well documented that a deficiency in Treg cells can result in the development of autoimmune disease and adoptive transfer of Treg cells effectively prevented and suppressed the severity of inflammation and/or autoimmune disease. Up to now, several subsets of Treg cells have been identified, such as the TGF-β-secreting Th3 regulatory cells [90], $CD8^+CD28^-$T cells [91] and NKT regulatory cells [92]. However, the best characterized subsets of $CD4^+$regulatory T cells are $CD4^+CD25^+FoxP3^+$Tregs and Tr1 cells that secrete IL-10 and lack FoxP3 expression. The important protective role played by these T-regulatory cells in the control of inflammatory and autoimmune disease has generated considerable interest in patients with noninfectious uveitis including BD and VKH syndrome.

$CD4^+CD25^+FoxP3^+$Tregs can be divided into two subpopulations: natural Treg cells (nTreg), which are develop as a distinct lineage of cells in the thymus, and the induced Treg cells (iTreg), which are generated in the periphery from naïve $CD4^+$T cells. They can also be induced in vitro. The difference and relative contributions in immune response of nTreg and iTreg cells are difficult to distinguish. A recent study found that a cell surface molecule neuropilin-1 was expressed on thymus-derived nTreg cells, but not on mucosa-generated $Foxp3^+$iTreg cells [93-94]. This marker can now be used to distinguish the subsets of $CD4^+CD25^+$Tregs. Our studies showed a decreased frequency of $CD4^+CD25^+$Treg cells and $CD4^+CD25^+Foxp3^+$Treg cells in the peripheral blood from active VKH patients. $CD4^+CD25^+$Treg cells from active VKH patients showed a diminished function in suppressing the proliferation of $CD4^+CD25^-$T cells and were less potent in inhibiting the production of IFN-γ and IL-13 by $CD4^+CD25^-$Tcells [95]. These results suggest that a decreased frequency and diminished function of $CD4^+CD25^+$Treg cells are associated with the active uveitis seen in VKH patients. However, Commodaro et al found no significant differences in the frequency of $CD4^+Foxp3^+$and $CD25^+Foxp3^+$T cells as well as no reduction in FOXP3 mRNA expression in mononuclear cells from VKH patients with active or inactive uveitis as compared with healthy controls [96]. The discrepancy may be due to the difference in Tregs subtypes investigated in the two studies (iTreg or nTreg). Patients with BD showed a significantly decreased frequency of Treg cells [27, 97], suggesting that the low level of Treg cells may contribute to the pathogenesis of ocular attacks in BD patients.

Tr1 cells are defined by their high expression of IL-10 and their ability to suppress antigen-specific effector T cell. Unlike $CD4^+CD25^+$Treg cells, which are present from birth, Tr1 cells are inducible cells and can be generated both in vitro and in vivo. It has been reported that IL-27 or CD46 activation in the presence of IL-2 can induce the differentiation of Tr1 cells [98-99]. A defect of CD46-mediated Tr1 cells has been reported in multiple sclerosis [98]. A study by our group revealed a decreased IL-10 production by naïve $CD4^+$T cells under Tr1 cell polarizing conditions in active VKH patients as compared with inactive VKH patients and healthy controls [66], suggesting that a defect of Tr1 cells might contribute to the pathogenesis of VKH syndrome.

Animal studies showed that Treg cells are involved in the remission of ocular inflammation. nTreg cells and iTreg cells induced by LPS-activated bone marrow dendritic cells inhibited the development of EAU. An increased frequency of $CD4^+CD25^+$Treg cells was associated with the EAU activity, and these Treg cells from EAU mice have a stronger ability to inhibit the proliferation of $CD4^+CD25^-$T cells and decreased IFN-γ production by $CD4^+CD25^-$T cells compared with those obtained from normal control mice. Moreover, transfer of $CD4^+CD25^+$Treg cells obtained from EAU mice on day 14 or 28 inhibited EAU induction [100]. These results suggest that the increased frequency and inhibitory effect of $CD4^+CD25^+$Treg cells in EAU mice may contribute to the monophasic nature and rapid resolution of EAU. Shao and his colleagues found that the suppressive function of Treg cells from animals with recurrent EAU was weaker than those from animals with the monophasic form, indicating that the dysregulation and malfunction of Treg cells in the eye contributed to disease recurrence [101]. Taken together, these results offer an explanation why the uveitis in the BD and VKH syndrome is recurrent while the uveitis in the EAU model is monophasic. The observations demonstrate the important role of $Foxp3^+$Treg cells in maintaining immune tolerance and preventing autoimmunity. Thus, it could be hypothesized that Treg cells in vitro expansion and adoptive transfer back to the patient might be a potential treatment for BD and VKH syndrome.

6. Genetic factors in Behcet's disease and VKH syndrome

The majority of BD is sporadic, but its familial aggregation has been reported [102-103]. BD can be found all over the world, however, its prevalence is particularly high in a peculiar region along the Silk Road extending from the Mediterranean basin to China [2, 104]. BD has been shown to be strongly associated with HLA-B51, which has been confirmed in different ethnic groups [105-106]. Previous studies showed that VKH syndrome is more prevalent in particular ethnic groups, particularly in pigmented groups [7] including Latin-American and Asian populations and displays a familial aggregation pattern [107]. Several HLA genes such as HLA-DR4 and HLA-DRw53, were strongly associated with VKH in a variety of ethnic groups [10, 108-109]. The aforementioned evidence as provided a strong genetic basis for BD and VKH confirmed by familial aggregation, geographical ethnic distribution, and strong association with especially Human leukocyte antigen (*HLA*) antigens. The genes associated with Behcet's disease and VKH syndrome are summarized in Tables 1 and 2, respectively.

6.1. Risk genes in Th1 cell pathway associated with Behcet's disease and VKH syndrome

STAT4, a transcription factor belonging to the Signal Transducer and Activator of Transcription protein family, is required for Th1 development of naive $CD4^+$T cells. Our study has identified an associated locus at STAT4 for BD in a Chinese Han population, and indicated that the risk SNP rs897200 in the STAT4 gene played a pathogenic role through an effect on

STAT4 transcription and IL-17 production [110]. The association of STAT4 with BD was confirmed in a Turkish population [111], suggesting that STAT4 is a common risk gene for BD in different ethnic cohorts.

C-C chemokine receptor type 1 (CCR1) and CCR3 play important roles in the accumulation and activation of inflammatory cells such as the Th1 cell. Recent studies showed that a locus at CCR1/CCR3 was associated with BD in Chinese Han and Turkish populations [111-112]. Functional studies showed a higher expression of CCR1 and migration of monocytes was found in individuals with the risk genotype [111], suggesting that impaired clearance of pathogens may contribute to the development of BD.

IL-18 is a proinflammatory cytokine that stimulates the production of IFN-γ in collaboration with IL-12 by Th1 cells. Studies from Turkish and Korean populations have shown the consistent association with BD in spite of inconsistent result in Korean cohorts [113].

TNF-α has been implicated in the pathogenesis of BD and anti-TNF-α represents an important treatment modality for BD patients [114]. A meta analysis showed an association of TNF-α gene polymorphisms with BD in various ethnic populations [115-117].

6.2. Risk genes in the Th17 cell pathway associated with Behcet's disease and VKH syndrome

Accumulative evidence supports the important role of the IL-23/Th17/IL-17 pathway in mediating chronic inflammatory or immune diseases such as BD and VKH syndrome [11, 95] and suggests the involvement of genes related to this pathway such as IL23R-IL12RB2, JAK1, STAT3, IL-1β, IL-6, IL17 and OPN in BD and VKH syndrome. We investigated the association of IL23R genes with BD in the Chinese Han population [118]. The results showed that two SNPs in IL23R were associated with the susceptibility to BD. Genome-wide association studies also confirmed the association of IL23R-IL12RB2 with BD in Japanese, Turkish and Iranian patients [8-9, 119]. Additionally, we identified the association of STAT3, JAK1, MCP-1 genes with BD in a Chinese Han population [120-122]. Other genes in the Th17 pathway such as IL-6 and IL-1β also showed an association with BD [123-124].

OPN, also known as bone sialoprotein I or early T-lymphocyte activation, may enhance T cell survival and proliferation, and promotes the responses of Th1 and Th17 cells during chronic inflammatory or immune mediated diseases. We examined the OPN serum level in VKH syndrome and the association of OPN polymorphisms and its receptors with this disease [80]. The results showed that the OPN level was significantly increased in the serum of active VKH patients and identified an association of this gene with VKH syndrome in a Chinese Han population. Furthermore, we found the association of JAK1, IL17F with VKH syndrome [125-126]. These studies suggest that genetic variants of cytokines associated to the Th17 pathway may play an important role in the development of BD and VKH syndrome.

6.3. Risk genes in the Treg cell pathway associated with Behcet's disease and VKH syndrome

Mir-146a, one of the miRNAs prevalently expressed in Treg cells, is known as a negative regulator of innate immunity in a variety of immune diseases [127]. We examined the associ-

http://dx.doi.org/10.5772/57586

ation of polymorphisms in mir-146a with BD and VKH syndrome in a Chinese Han population and found that a polymorphism in this gene was associated with BD but not with VKH syndrome [128].

7. Innate immunity in Behcet's disease and VKH syndrome

It has been reported that infection may be involved in the pathogenesis of BD and VKH syndrome. Most of the uveitis patients with BD or VKH syndrome have manifestations of a bacterial or viral infection before the prodromal stage [129-130], suggesting that infectious agents may be a triggering factor to the onset of these diseases. DCs serve as professional antigen-presenting cells and provide the first line of defense against pathologic infections. Toll-like receptors (TLRs) expressed on DCs play a critical role in innate immunity against these pathologic infections. Interaction of DCs with TLR ligands results in the secretion of a number of proinflammatory cytokines that can induce the differentiation of naïve $CD4^+$T cells into different $CD4^+$T cells, including Th1, Th17 and Treg cells. Kirino and his colleagues reported that an increased expression of TLR4 is associated with heme oxygenase-1 reduction in PBMCs from patients with BD, leading to augmented inflammatory responses [131]. The study by Do et al showed a higher level of TLR2 and TLR4 in monocytes from active BD patients [132]. Our recent study showed a higher expression of TLR2, TLR3, TLR4 and TLR8 by either PBMCs, $CD4^+$T cells or monocytes obtained from BD patients as compared with controls. Furthermore, significantly higher levels of IL-1β were produced by monocytes from active BD patients stimulated with known TLR ligands such as LPS and PGN [133]. These results suggest that a higher expression of TLR is associated with ocular Behcet's disease and may partly explain the mechanism by which infection was involved in the pathogenesis. It has been reported that DC deregulation was implicated in the pathogenesis of BD [134]. DCs play a critical role in determining the immune balance between self and non-self and this area is becoming a hotspot for researchers to develop tolerogenic DCs for treating autoimmune disease [135].

8. Summary

With the recent progress in immunology and genetics, environmental triggering factors such as viruses, bacteria or other molecular mimicry are thought to be participated in the outbreak of BD and VKH through interacting with TLRs. The imbalance of pathogenic Th1/Th17 and regulatory T cells and abnormalities in the associated immunoregulatory molecules with the abovementioned T cells are now supposed to be involved in the pathogenesis of these two diseases. The understanding of novel pathogenic mechanisms of both diseases may provide a foundation for developing new strategies to better treat the uveitis.

Genes	Odd Ratio	95% Confidence Interval	Ethnic	References
CCR1/CCR3	0.28	0.2–0.4	Chinese	[112]
CCR5	2.37	1.1- 5.1	Italian	[136]
CD40	1.98	1.38-2.83	Chinese	[137]
CPVL	2.26	1.47–3.45	Turkish	[138]
eNOS	1.88	1.27-2.49	Turkish	[139]
	3.2	1.4-7.3	Korean	[140]
	1.26	2.13-3.62	Tunisian	[141]
ERAP1	4.56	2.88-7.22	Turkish	[111]
FCRL3	0.7	0.5–0.9	Chinese	[142]
ICAM1	1.26	2.13-3.62	Tunisian	[143]
	4.2	1.9-9.3	Italian	[144]
IL1β	3.63	1.23–12.97	Turkish	[123]
IL4	3.40	1.72–7.12	Turkish	[145]
IL6	3.5	1.2-10.0	Korean	[124]
IL10	1.20	1.02-1.40	Iran	[119]
	1.45	1.34-1.58	Turkish, Arab, Greek, UK, Korean, Japanese	[9]
	1.45	1.32–1.60	Japanese, Turkish, Korean	[8]
IL12B	1.8	1.0–3.3	Japanese	[146]
IL18	1.48	1.10–1.97	Turkish	[147]
IL23R-IL12RB2	1.51	1.27–1.78	Iran	[119]
	1.28	1.18-1.39	Turkish	[9]
	1.35	0.95–1.91	Japanese,Turkish, Korean	[8]
	1.86	1.39 -2.49	Chinese	[118]
IRF-1	3.71	1.778-7.770	Korean	[148]
KIAA1529	2.04	1.45–2.88	Turkish	[138]
LOC100129342	1.84	1.32–2.58	Turkish	[138]
m.709G >A	1.40	1.0-1.97	Iranian	[149]
MCP1	1.51	1.05–2.17	Chinese	[122]

Genes	Odd Ratio	95% Confidence Interval	Ethnic	References
MDR1	3.03	1.41-6.54	Turkish	[150]
MIF	1.46	1.19–1.79	Chinese	[151]
miR-146a	1.33	1.17-1.52	Chinese	[128]
MMP2	0.6	0.44-0.87	Korean	[152]
MMP9	0.371	0.152-0.905	Korean	[153]
MTHFR	1.70	1.23–2.35	Turkish	[154]
NRAMP1	1.88	1.21-2.93	Turkish	[155]
PDGFRL	0.59	0.49–0.72	Chinese	[156]
Protein Z	6.8	2.6-17.9	Turkish	[157]
PTPN22	2.4	1.2 to 4.7	UK, Middle East	[158]
SLC11A1	0.60	0.37-0.95	Korean	[159]
STAT3	1.712	1.238–2.369	Chinese	[121]
STAT4	1.45	1.3-1.6	Chinese	[110, 160]
	1.27	1.17–1.37	Turkish	[111]
SUMO4	23.40	2.33-235.54	Korean	[161]
	1.41	1.01-1.97	Tunisian	[162]
	1.7	1.3–2.2	Chinese	[106]
TGFBR3	0.617	0.441-0.863	Chinese	[163]
TLR4	1.96	1.26-3.26	Korean	[164]
	1.67	1.08-2.60	Japanese	[165]
TNF-α	1.68	1.10-2.56	Moroccan	[116]
	3.08	1.73-5.47	Iranian Azeri Turk	[117]
TNFAIP3	2.03	1.65-2.49	Chinese	[166]
TREM-1	2.723	1.285-5.770	Korean	[167]
UBAC2	1.5	1.2-1.7	Chinese	[168]
UBASH3B	1.71	1.23–2.38	Turkish	[138]
VDR	1.89	1.32-2.71	Tunisians	[169]
VEGF	0.10	0.011-0.875	Korean	[170]

Table 1. Summary of the associated genes with Behcet's disease

Author details

Peizeng Yang[1*], Chaokui Wang[1], Shengping Hou[1], Bo Lei[1], Aize Kijlstra[2] and De-Quan Li[3*]

*Address all correspondence to: peizengycmu@126.com; dequanl@bcm.tmc.edu

1 The First Affiliated Hospital of Chongqing Medical University, Chongqing Key Lab of Ophthalmology, Chongqing Eye Institute, Chongqing, P. R. China

2 University Eye Clinic Maastricht, Maastricht, Netherlands

3 Ocular Surface Center, Cullen Eye Institute, Department of Ophthalmology, Baylor College of Medicine, Houston, Texas, USA

References

[1] Wakefield D.,J.H. Chang. Epidemiology of uveitis. Int Ophthalmol Clin 2005; 45(2): 1-13.

[2] Sakane T., M. Takeno, N. Suzuki,G. Inaba. Behcet's disease. N Engl J Med 1999; 341(17):1284-91.

[3] Evereklioglu C. Current concepts in the etiology and treatment of Behcet disease. Surv Ophthalmol 2005; 50(4):297-350.

[4] Yang P., W. Fang, Q. Meng, Y. Ren, L. Xing,A. Kijlstra. Clinical features of chinese patients with Behcet's disease. Ophthalmology 2008; 115(2):312-318 e4.

[5] Moorthy R.S., H. Inomata,N.A. Rao. Vogt-Koyanagi-Harada syndrome. Surv Ophthalmol 1995; 39(4):265-92.

[6] Murakami S., Y. Inaba, M. Mochizuki, A. Nakajima,A. Urayama. [A nation-wide survey on the occurrence of Vogt-Koyanagi-Harada disease in Japan]. Nihon Ganka Gakkai Zasshi 1994; 98(4):389-92.

[7] Yang P., Y. Ren, B. Li, W. Fang, Q. Meng,A. Kijlstra. Clinical characteristics of Vogt-Koyanagi-Harada syndrome in Chinese patients. Ophthalmology 2007; 114(3):606-14.

[8] Mizuki N., A. Meguro, M. Ota, S. Ohno, T. Shiota, T. Kawagoe, N. Ito, J. Kera, E. Okada, K. Yatsu, Y.W. Song, E.B. Lee, N. Kitaichi, K. Namba, Y. Horie, M. Takeno, S. Sugita, M. Mochizuki, S. Bahram, Y. Ishigatsubo,H. Inoko. Genome-wide association studies identify IL23R-IL12RB2 and IL10 as Behcet's disease susceptibility loci. Nat Genet 2010; 42(8):703-6.

[9] Remmers E.F., F. Cosan, Y. Kirino, M.J. Ombrello, N. Abaci, C. Satorius, J.M. Le, B. Yang, B.D. Korman, A. Cakiris, O. Aglar, Z. Emrence, H. Azakli, D. Ustek, I. Tugal-Tutkun, G. Akman-Demir, W. Chen, C.I. Amos, M.B. Dizon, A.A. Kose, G. Azizlerli,

B. Erer, O.J. Brand, V.G. Kaklamani, P. Kaklamanis, E. Ben-Chetrit, M. Stanford, F. Fortune, M. Ghabra, W.E. Ollier, Y.H. Cho, D. Bang, J. O'Shea, G.R. Wallace, M. Gadina, D.L. Kastner,A. Gul. Genome-wide association study identifies variants in the MHC class I, IL10, and IL23R-IL12RB2 regions associated with Behcet's disease. Nat Genet 2010; 42(8):698-702.

[10] Islam S.M., J. Numaga, Y. Fujino, R. Hirata, K. Matsuki, H. Maeda,K. Masuda. HLA class II genes in Vogt-Koyanagi-Harada disease. Invest Ophthalmol Vis Sci 1994; 35(11):3890-6.

[11] Chi W., P. Yang, B. Li, C. Wu, H. Jin, X. Zhu, L. Chen, H. Zhou, X. Huang,A. Kijlstra. IL-23 promotes CD4+T cells to produce IL-17 in Vogt-Koyanagi-Harada disease. J Allergy Clin Immunol 2007; 119(5):1218-24.

[12] Chi W., X. Zhu, P. Yang, X. Liu, X. Lin, H. Zhou, X. Huang,A. Kijlstra. Upregulated IL-23 and IL-17 in Behcet patients with active uveitis. Invest Ophthalmol Vis Sci 2008; 49(7):3058-64.

[13] Li B., P. Yang, H. Zhou, X. Huang, H. Jin, L. Chu, Y. Gao, L. Zhu,A. Kijlstra. Upregulation of T-bet expression in peripheral blood mononuclear cells during Vogt-Koyanagi-Harada disease. Br J Ophthalmol 2005; 89(11):1410-2.

[14] Liu X., P. Yang, X. Lin, X. Ren, H. Zhou, X. Huang, W. Chi, A. Kijlstra,L. Chen. Inhibitory effect of Cyclosporin A and corticosteroids on the production of IFN-gamma and IL-17 by T cells in Vogt-Koyanagi-Harada syndrome. Clin Immunol 2009; 131(2): 333-42.

[15] Zhao C., P. Yang, H. He, X. Lin, L. Du, H. Zhou,A. Kijlstra. Retinal S-antigen Th1 cell epitope mapping in patients with Behcet's disease. Graefes Arch Clin Exp Ophthalmol 2009; 247(4):555-60.

[16] Ben Ahmed M., H. Houman, M. Miled, K. Dellagi,H. Louzir. Involvement of chemokines and Th1 cytokines in the pathogenesis of mucocutaneous lesions of Behcet's disease. Arthritis Rheum 2004; 50(7):2291-5.

[17] Miyazawa I., T. Abe, K. Narikawa, J. Feng, T. Misu, I. Nakashima, J. Fujimori, M. Tamai, K. Fujihara,Y. Itoyama. Chemokine profile in the cerebrospinal fluid and serum of Vogt-Koyanagi-Harada disease. J Neuroimmunol 2005; 158(1-2):240-4.

[18] El-Asrar A.M., S. Struyf, D. Kangave, S.S. Al-Obeidan, G. Opdenakker, K. Geboes,J. Van Damme. Cytokine profiles in aqueous humor of patients with different clinical entities of endogenous uveitis. Clin Immunol 2011; 139(2):177-84.

[19] Yokoi H., K. Kato, T. Kezuka, J. Sakai, M. Usui, H. Yagita,K. Okumura. Prevention of experimental autoimmune uveoretinitis by monoclonal antibody to interleukin-12. Eur J Immunol 1997; 27(3):641-6.

[20] Egwuagu C.E., J. Sztein, R.M. Mahdi, W. Li, C. Chao-Chan, J.A. Smith, P. Charukamnoetkanok,A.B. Chepelinsky. IFN-gamma increases the severity and accelerates the

onset of experimental autoimmune uveitis in transgenic rats. J Immunol 1999; 162(1): 510-7.

[21] Caspi R.R., C.C. Chan, B.G. Grubbs, P.B. Silver, B. Wiggert, C.F. Parsa, S. Bahmanyar, A. Billiau,H. Heremans. Endogenous systemic IFN-gamma has a protective role against ocular autoimmunity in mice. J Immunol 1994; 152(2):890-9.

[22] Fukushima A., T. Yamaguchi, W. Ishida, K. Fukata, K. Udaka,H. Ueno. Mice lacking the IFN-gamma receptor or fyn develop severe experimental autoimmune uveoretinitis characterized by different immune responses. Immunogenetics 2005; 57(5): 337-43.

[23] Damsker J.M., A.M. Hansen,R.R. Caspi. Th1 and Th17 cells: adversaries and collaborators. Ann N Y Acad Sci 2010; 1183:211-21.

[24] Korn T., E. Bettelli, M. Oukka,V.K. Kuchroo. IL-17 and Th17 Cells. Annu Rev Immunol 2009; 27:485-517.

[25] Iwakura Y., H. Ishigame, S. Saijo,S. Nakae. Functional specialization of interleukin-17 family members. Immunity 2011; 34(2):149-62.

[26] Hamzaoui K., E. Bouali, I. Ghorbel, M. Khanfir, H. Houman,A. Hamzaoui. Expression of Th-17 and RORgammat mRNA in Behcet's Disease. Med Sci Monit 2011; 17(4):CR227-34.

[27] Geri G., B. Terrier, M. Rosenzwajg, B. Wechsler, M. Touzot, D. Seilhean, T.A. Tran, B. Bodaghi, L. Musset, V. Soumelis, D. Klatzmann, P. Cacoub,D. Saadoun. Critical role of IL-21 in modulating TH17 and regulatory T cells in Behcet disease. J Allergy Clin Immunol 2011; 128(3):655-64.

[28] Peng Y., G. Han, H. Shao, Y. Wang, H.J. Kaplan,D. Sun. Characterization of IL-17+interphotoreceptor retinoid-binding protein-specific T cells in experimental autoimmune uveitis. Invest Ophthalmol Vis Sci 2007; 48(9):4153-61.

[29] Luger D., P.B. Silver, J. Tang, D. Cua, Z. Chen, Y. Iwakura, E.P. Bowman, N.M. Sgambellone, C.C. Chan,R.R. Caspi. Either a Th17 or a Th1 effector response can drive autoimmunity: conditions of disease induction affect dominant effector category. J Exp Med 2008; 205(4):799-810.

[30] Zhang R., J. Qian, J. Guo, Y.F. Yuan,K. Xue. Suppression of experimental autoimmune uveoretinitis by Anti-IL-17 antibody. Curr Eye Res 2009; 34(4):297-303.

[31] Nurieva R., X.O. Yang, G. Martinez, Y. Zhang, A.D. Panopoulos, L. Ma, K. Schluns, Q. Tian, S.S. Watowich, A.M. Jetten,C. Dong. Essential autocrine regulation by IL-21 in the generation of inflammatory T cells. Nature 2007; 448(7152):480-3.

[32] Korn T., E. Bettelli, W. Gao, A. Awasthi, A. Jager, T.B. Strom, M. Oukka,V.K. Kuchroo. IL-21 initiates an alternative pathway to induce proinflammatory T(H)17 cells. Nature 2007; 448(7152):484-7.

[33] Li F., P. Yang, X. Liu, C. Wang, S. Hou,A. Kijlstra. Upregulation of interleukin 21 and promotion of interleukin 17 production in chronic or recurrent Vogt-Koyanagi-Harada disease. Arch Ophthalmol 2010; 128(11):1449-54.

[34] Wang L., C.R. Yu, H.P. Kim, W. Liao, W.G. Telford, C.E. Egwuagu,W.J. Leonard. Key role for IL-21 in experimental autoimmune uveitis. Proc Natl Acad Sci U S A 2011; 108(23):9542-7.

[35] Liu L., Y. Xu, J. Wang,H. Li. Upregulated IL-21 and IL-21 receptor expression is involved in experimental autoimmune uveitis (EAU). Mol Vis 2009; 15:2938-44.

[36] Sarkar S., X. Zhou, S. Justa,S.R. Bommireddy. Interleukin-22 reduces the severity of collagen-induced arthritis in association with increased levels of interleukin-10. Arthritis Rheum 2013; 65(4):960-71.

[37] Sanjabi S., L.A. Zenewicz, M. Kamanaka,R.A. Flavell. Anti-inflammatory and pro-inflammatory roles of TGF-beta, IL-10, and IL-22 in immunity and autoimmunity. Curr Opin Pharmacol 2009; 9(4):447-53.

[38] Cai T., Q. Wang, Q. Zhou, C. Wang, S. Hou, J. Qi, A. Kijlstra,P. Yang. Increased expression of IL-22 is associated with disease activity in Behcet's disease. PLoS One 2013; 8(3):e59009.

[39] Li Z., B. Liu, A. Maminishkis, S.P. Mahesh, S. Yeh, J. Lew, W.K. Lim, H.N. Sen, G. Clarke, R. Buggage, S.S. Miller,R.B. Nussenblatt. Gene expression profiling in autoimmune noninfectious uveitis disease. J Immunol 2008; 181(7):5147-57.

[40] Ke Y., D. Sun, G. Jiang, H.J. Kaplan,H. Shao. IL-22-induced regulatory CD11b+APCs suppress experimental autoimmune uveitis. J Immunol 2011; 187(5):2130-9.

[41] Zheng X., F. Bian, P. Ma, C.S. De Paiva, M. Stern, S.C. Pflugfelder,D.Q. Li. Induction of Th17 differentiation by corneal epithelial-derived cytokines. J Cell Physiol 2010; 222(1):95-102.

[42] Zhou L., Ivanov, II, R. Spolski, R. Min, K. Shenderov, T. Egawa, D.E. Levy, W.J. Leonard,D.R. Littman. IL-6 programs T(H)-17 cell differentiation by promoting sequential engagement of the IL-21 and IL-23 pathways. Nat Immunol 2007; 8(9):967-74.

[43] Veldhoen M., R.J. Hocking, C.J. Atkins, R.M. Locksley,B. Stockinger. TGFbeta in the context of an inflammatory cytokine milieu supports de novo differentiation of IL-17-producing T cells. Immunity 2006; 24(2):179-89.

[44] Mangan P.R., L.E. Harrington, D.B. O'Quinn, W.S. Helms, D.C. Bullard, C.O. Elson, R.D. Hatton, S.M. Wahl, T.R. Schoeb,C.T. Weaver. Transforming growth factor-beta induces development of the T(H)17 lineage. Nature 2006; 441(7090):231-4.

[45] Bettelli E., Y. Carrier, W. Gao, T. Korn, T.B. Strom, M. Oukka, H.L. Weiner,V.K. Kuchroo. Reciprocal developmental pathways for the generation of pathogenic effector TH17 and regulatory T cells. Nature 2006; 441(7090):235-8.

[46] Manel N., D. Unutmaz,D.R. Littman. The differentiation of human T(H)-17 cells requires transforming growth factor-beta and induction of the nuclear receptor ROR-gammat. Nat Immunol 2008; 9(6):641-9.

[47] Hunter C.A. New IL-12-family members: IL-23 and IL-27, cytokines with divergent functions. Nat Rev Immunol 2005; 5(7):521-31.

[48] Yang X.O., A.D. Panopoulos, R. Nurieva, S.H. Chang, D. Wang, S.S. Watowich,C. Dong. STAT3 regulates cytokine-mediated generation of inflammatory helper T cells. J Biol Chem 2007; 282(13):9358-63.

[49] Adam B.,E. Calikoglu. Serum interleukin-6, procalcitonin and C-reactive protein levels in subjects with active Behcet's disease. J Eur Acad Dermatol Venereol 2004; 18(3): 318-20.

[50] Nalbant S., B. Sahan, M. Durna, D. Ersanli, M. Kaplan, O. Karabudak,M. Unal. Cytokine profile in Behcet uveitis. Bratisl Lek Listy 2008; 109(12):551-4.

[51] Norose K., A. Yano, X.C. Wang, T. Tokushima, J. Umihira, A. Seki, M. Nohara,K. Segawa. Dominance of activated T cells and interleukin-6 in aqueous humor in Vogt-Koyanagi-Harada disease. Invest Ophthalmol Vis Sci 1994; 35(1):33-9.

[52] Norose K.,A. Yano. Melanoma specific Th1 cytotoxic T lymphocyte lines in Vogt-Koyanagi-Harada disease. Br J Ophthalmol 1996; 80(11):1002-8.

[53] Ozdamar Y., N. Berker, G. Bahar, E. Soykan, T. Bicer, S.S. Ozkan,J. Karakaya. Inflammatory mediators and posterior segment involvement in ocular Behcet disease. Eur J Ophthalmol 2009; 19(6):998-1003.

[54] Akman-Demir G., E. Tuzun, S. Icoz, N. Yesilot, S.P. Yentur, M. Kurtuncu, M. Mutlu,G. Saruhan-Direskeneli. Interleukin-6 in neuro-Behcet's disease: association with disease subsets and long-term outcome. Cytokine 2008; 44(3):373-6.

[55] Wang C.R., C.Y. Chuang,C.Y. Chen. Anticardiolipin antibodies and interleukin-6 in cerebrospinal fluid and blood of Chinese patients with neuro-Behcet's syndrome. Clin Exp Rheumatol 1992; 10(6):599-602.

[56] Hirano T., N. Ohguro, S. Hohki, K. Hagihara, Y. Shima, M. Narazaki, A. Ogata, K. Yoshizaki, A. Kumanogoh, T. Kishimoto,T. Tanaka. A case of Behcet's disease treated with a humanized anti-interleukin-6 receptor antibody, tocilizumab. Mod Rheumatol 2012; 22(2):298-302.

[57] Hohki S., N. Ohguro, H. Haruta, K. Nakai, F. Terabe, S. Serada, M. Fujimoto, S. Nomura, H. Kawahata, T. Kishimoto,T. Naka. Blockade of interleukin-6 signaling suppresses experimental autoimmune uveoretinitis by the inhibition of inflammatory Th17 responses. Exp Eye Res 2010; 91(2):162-70.

[58] Yoshimura T., K.H. Sonoda, N. Ohguro, Y. Ohsugi, T. Ishibashi, D.J. Cua, T. Kobayashi, H. Yoshida,A. Yoshimura. Involvement of Th17 cells and the effect of anti-IL-6 therapy in autoimmune uveitis. Rheumatology (Oxford) 2009; 48(4):347-54.

[59] Lew W., J.Y. Chang, J.Y. Jung,D. Bang. Increased expression of interleukin-23 p19 mRNA in erythema nodosum-like lesions of Behcet's disease. Br J Dermatol 2008; 158(3):505-11.

[60] Habibagahi Z., M. Habibagahi,M. Heidari. Raised concentration of soluble form of vascular endothelial cadherin and IL-23 in sera of patients with Behcet's disease. Mod Rheumatol 2010; 20(2):154-9.

[61] Liang L., X. Tan, Q. Zhou, Y. Zhu, Y. Tian, H. Yu, A. Kijlstra,P. Yang. IL-1beta triggered by peptidoglycan and lipopolysaccharide through TLR2/4 and ROS-NLRP3 inflammasome-dependent pathways is involved in ocular Behcet's disease. Invest Ophthalmol Vis Sci 2013; 54(1):402-14.

[62] Pay S., H. Erdem, A. Pekel, I. Simsek, U. Musabak, A. Sengul,A. Dinc. Synovial proinflammatory cytokines and their correlation with matrix metalloproteinase-3 expression in Behcet's disease. Does interleukin-1beta play a major role in Behcet's synovitis? Rheumatol Int 2006; 26(7):608-13.

[63] Su S.B., P.B. Silver, R.S. Grajewski, R.K. Agarwal, J. Tang, C.C. Chan,R.R. Caspi. Essential role of the MyD88 pathway, but nonessential roles of TLRs 2, 4, and 9, in the adjuvant effect promoting Th1-mediated autoimmunity. J Immunol 2005; 175(10): 6303-10.

[64] Guenane H., D. Hartani, L. Chachoua, O.S. Lahlou-Boukoffa, F. Mazari,C. Touil-Boukoffa. [Production of Th1/Th2 cytokines and nitric oxide in Behcet's uveitis and idiopathic uveitis]. J Fr Ophtalmol 2006; 29(2):146-52.

[65] Belguendouz H., D. Messaoudene, D. Hartani, L. Chachoua, M.L. Ahmedi, K. Lahmar-Belguendouz, O. Lahlou-Boukoffa,C. Touil-Boukoffa. [Effect of corticotherapy on interleukin-8 and-12 and nitric oxide production during Behcet and idiopathic uveitis]. J Fr Ophtalmol 2008; 31(4):387-95.

[66] Wang C., Y. Tian, B. Lei, X. Xiao, Z. Ye, F. Li, A. Kijlstra,P. Yang. Decreased IL-27 expression in association with an increased Th17 response in Vogt-Koyanagi-Harada disease. Invest Ophthalmol Vis Sci 2012; 53(8):4668-75.

[67] Shen H., L.P. Xia,J. Lu. Elevated levels of interleukin-27 and effect on production of interferon-gamma and interleukin-17 in patients with Behcet's disease. Scand J Rheumatol 2013; 42(1):48-51.

[68] Fitzgerald D.C., B. Ciric, T. Touil, H. Harle, J. Grammatikopolou, J. Das Sarma, B. Gran, G.X. Zhang,A. Rostami. Suppressive effect of IL-27 on encephalitogenic Th17 cells and the effector phase of experimental autoimmune encephalomyelitis. J Immunol 2007; 179(5):3268-75.

[69] Pickens S.R., N.D. Chamberlain, M.V. Volin, A.M. Mandelin, 2nd, H. Agrawal, M. Matsui, T. Yoshimoto,S. Shahrara. Local expression of interleukin-27 ameliorates collagen-induced arthritis. Arthritis Rheum 2011; 63(8):2289-98.

[70] Amadi-Obi A., C.R. Yu, X. Liu, R.M. Mahdi, G.L. Clarke, R.B. Nussenblatt, I. Gery, Y.S. Lee,C.E. Egwuagu. TH17 cells contribute to uveitis and scleritis and are expanded by IL-2 and inhibited by IL-27/STAT1. Nat Med 2007; 13(6):711-8.

[71] Sugita S., Y. Kawazoe, A. Imai, Y. Yamada, S. Horie,M. Mochizuki. Inhibition of Th17 differentiation by anti-TNF-alpha therapy in uveitis patients with Behcet's disease. Arthritis Res Ther 2012; 14(3):R99.

[72] Evereklioglu C., H. Er, Y. Turkoz,M. Cekmen. Serum levels of TNF-alpha, sIL-2R, IL-6, and IL-8 are increased and associated with elevated lipid peroxidation in patients with Behcet's disease. Mediators Inflamm 2002; 11(2):87-93.

[73] Raveney B.J., D.A. Copland, A.D. Dick,L.B. Nicholson. TNFR1-dependent regulation of myeloid cell function in experimental autoimmune uveoretinitis. J Immunol 2009; 183(4):2321-9.

[74] Busch M., D. Bauer, M. Hennig, S. Wasmuth, S. Thanos,A. Heiligenhaus. Effects of systemic and intravitreal TNF-alpha inhibition in experimental autoimmune uveoretinitis. Invest Ophthalmol Vis Sci 2013; 54(1):39-46.

[75] Shirasawa M., S. Sonoda, H. Terasaki, N. Arimura, H. Otsuka, T. Yamashita, E. Uchino, T. Hisatomi, T. Ishibashi,T. Sakamoto. TNF-alpha disrupts morphologic and functional barrier properties of polarized retinal pigment epithelium. Exp Eye Res 2013; 110:59-69.

[76] Khalifa Y.M., M.R. Bailony,N.R. Acharya. Treatment of pediatric vogt-koyanagi-harada syndrome with infliximab. Ocul Immunol Inflamm 2010; 18(3):218-22.

[77] Cantini F., L. Niccoli, C. Nannini, O. Kaloudi, E. Cassara, M. Susini,I. Lenzetti. Efficacy of infliximab in refractory Behcet's disease-associated and idiopathic posterior segment uveitis: a prospective, follow-up study of 50 patients. Biologics 2012; 6:5-12.

[78] Liu L., P. Yang, H. He, X. Lin, L. Jiang, W. Chi, C. Zhao,H. Zhou. Leptin increases in Vogt-Koyanagi-Harada (VKH) disease and promotes cell proliferation and inflammatory cytokine secretion. Br J Ophthalmol 2008; 92(4):557-61.

[79] Chu M., P. Yang, S. Hou, F. Li, Y. Chen,A. Kijlstra. Behcet's disease exhibits an increased osteopontin serum level in active stage but no association with osteopontin and its receptor gene polymorphisms. Hum Immunol 2011; 72(6):525-9.

[80] Chu M., P. Yang, R. Hu, S. Hou, F. Li, Y. Chen,A. Kijlstra. Elevated serum osteopontin levels and genetic polymorphisms of osteopontin are associated with Vogt-Koyanagi-Harada disease. Invest Ophthalmol Vis Sci 2011; 52(10):7084-9.

[81] Yang Y., X. Xiao, F. Li, L. Du, A. Kijlstra,P. Yang. Increased IL-7 expression in Vogt-Koyanagi-Harada disease. Invest Ophthalmol Vis Sci 2012; 53(2):1012-7.

[82] Iwata D., M. Kitamura, N. Kitaichi, Y. Saito, S. Kon, K. Namba, J. Morimoto, A. Ebihara, H. Kitamei, K. Yoshida, S. Ishida, S. Ohno, T. Uede, K. Onoe,K. Iwabuchi. Prevention of experimental autoimmune uveoretinitis by blockade of osteopontin with small interfering RNA. Exp Eye Res 2010; 90(1):41-8.

[83] Kitamura M., K. Iwabuchi, N. Kitaichi, S. Kon, H. Kitamei, K. Namba, K. Yoshida, D.T. Denhardt, S.R. Rittling, S. Ohno, T. Uede,K. Onoe. Osteopontin aggravates experimental autoimmune uveoretinitis in mice. J Immunol 2007; 178(10):6567-72.

[84] Liu X., S. Leung, C. Wang, Z. Tan, J. Wang, T.B. Guo, L. Fang, Y. Zhao, B. Wan, X. Qin, L. Lu, R. Li, H. Pan, M. Song, A. Liu, J. Hong, H. Lu,J.Z. Zhang. Crucial role of interleukin-7 in T helper type 17 survival and expansion in autoimmune disease. Nat Med 2010; 16(2):191-7.

[85] Matarese G., A. Di Giacomo, V. Sanna, G.M. Lord, J.K. Howard, A. Di Tuoro, S.R. Bloom, R.I. Lechler, S. Zappacosta,S. Fontana. Requirement for leptin in the induction and progression of autoimmune encephalomyelitis. J Immunol 2001; 166(10): 5909-16.

[86] Tian Y., C. Wang, Z. Ye, X. Xiao, A. Kijlstra,P. Yang. Effect of 1,25-dihydroxyvitamin D3 on Th17 and Th1 response in patients with Behcet's disease. Invest Ophthalmol Vis Sci 2012; 53(10):6434-41.

[87] Zhou Q., X. Xiao, C. Wang, X. Zhang, F. Li, Y. Zhou, A. Kijlstra,P. Yang. Decreased microRNA-155 expression in ocular Behcet's disease but not in Vogt Koyanagi Harada syndrome. Invest Ophthalmol Vis Sci 2012; 53(9):5665-74.

[88] Liu X., P. Yang, C. Wang, F. Li,A. Kijlstra. IFN-alpha blocks IL-17 production by peripheral blood mononuclear cells in Behcet's disease. Rheumatology (Oxford) 2011; 50(2):293-8.

[89] Sun M., Y. Yang, P. Yang, B. Lei, L. Du,A. Kijlstra. Regulatory effects of IFN-beta on the development of experimental autoimmune uveoretinitis in B10RIII mice. PLoS One 2011; 6(5):e19870.

[90] Weiner H.L. Induction and mechanism of action of transforming growth factor-beta-secreting Th3 regulatory cells. Immunol Rev 2001; 182:207-14.

[91] Najafian N., T. Chitnis, A.D. Salama, B. Zhu, C. Benou, X. Yuan, M.R. Clarkson, M.H. Sayegh,S.J. Khoury. Regulatory functions of CD8+CD28-T cells in an autoimmune disease model. J Clin Invest 2003; 112(7):1037-48.

[92] Taniguchi M., M. Harada, S. Kojo, T. Nakayama,H. Wakao. The regulatory role of Valpha14 NKT cells in innate and acquired immune response. Annu Rev Immunol 2003; 21:483-513.

[93] Weiss J.M., A.M. Bilate, M. Gobert, Y. Ding, M.A. Curotto de Lafaille, C.N. Parkhurst, H. Xiong, J. Dolpady, A.B. Frey, M.G. Ruocco, Y. Yang, S. Floess, J. Huehn, S. Oh, M.O. Li, R.E. Niec, A.Y. Rudensky, M.L. Dustin, D.R. Littman,J.J. Lafaille. Neuropilin 1 is expressed on thymus-derived natural regulatory T cells, but not mucosa-generated induced Foxp3+T reg cells. J Exp Med 2012; 209(10):1723-42, S1.

[94] Yadav M., C. Louvet, D. Davini, J.M. Gardner, M. Martinez-Llordella, S. Bailey-Bucktrout, B.A. Anthony, F.M. Sverdrup, R. Head, D.J. Kuster, P. Ruminski, D. Weiss, D. Von Schack,J.A. Bluestone. Neuropilin-1 distinguishes natural and inducible regulatory T cells among regulatory T cell subsets in vivo. J Exp Med 2012; 209(10):1713-22, S1-19.

[95] Chen L., P. Yang, H. Zhou, H. He, X. Ren, W. Chi, L. Wang,A. Kijlstra. Diminished frequency and function of CD4+CD25high regulatory T cells associated with active uveitis in Vogt-Koyanagi-Harada syndrome. Invest Ophthalmol Vis Sci 2008; 49(8): 3475-82.

[96] Commodaro A.G., J.P. Peron, J. Genre, C. Arslanian, L. Sanches, C. Muccioli, L.V. Rizzo,R. Belfort, Jr. IL-10 and TGF-beta immunoregulatory cytokines rather than natural regulatory T cells are associated with the resolution phase of Vogt-Koyanagi-Harada (VKH) syndrome. Scand J Immunol 2010; 72(1):31-7.

[97] Nanke Y., S. Kotake, M. Goto, H. Ujihara, M. Matsubara,N. Kamatani. Decreased percentages of regulatory T cells in peripheral blood of patients with Behcet's disease before ocular attack: a possible predictive marker of ocular attack. Mod Rheumatol 2008; 18(4):354-8.

[98] Astier A.L., G. Meiffren, S. Freeman,D.A. Hafler. Alterations in CD46-mediated Tr1 regulatory T cells in patients with multiple sclerosis. J Clin Invest 2006; 116(12): 3252-7.

[99] Murugaiyan G., A. Mittal, R. Lopez-Diego, L.M. Maier, D.E. Anderson,H.L. Weiner. IL-27 is a key regulator of IL-10 and IL-17 production by human CD4+T cells. J Immunol 2009; 183(4):2435-43.

[100] Sun M., P. Yang, L. Du, H. Zhou, X. Ren,A. Kijlstra. Contribution of CD4+CD25+T cells to the regression phase of experimental autoimmune uveoretinitis. Invest Ophthalmol Vis Sci 2010; 51(1):383-9.

[101] Ke Y., G. Jiang, D. Sun, H.J. Kaplan,H. Shao. Ocular regulatory T cells distinguish monophasic from recurrent autoimmune uveitis. Invest Ophthalmol Vis Sci 2008; 49(9):3999-4007.

[102] Berman L., B. Trappler,T. Jenkins. Behcet's syndrome: a family study and the elucidation of a genetic role. Ann Rheum Dis 1979; 38(2):118-21.

[103] Gul A., M. Inanc, L. Ocal, O. Aral,M. Konice. Familial aggregation of Behcet's disease in Turkey. Ann Rheum Dis 2000; 59(8):622-5.

[104] Verity D.H., J.E. Marr, S. Ohno, G.R. Wallace,M.R. Stanford. Behcet's disease, the Silk Road and HLA-B51: historical and geographical perspectives. Tissue Antigens 1999; 54(3):213-20.

[105] de Menthon M., M.P. Lavalley, C. Maldini, L. Guillevin,A. Mahr. HLA-B51/B5 and the risk of Behcet's disease: a systematic review and meta-analysis of case-control genetic association studies. Arthritis Rheum 2009; 61(10):1287-96.

[106] Hou S., P. Yang, L. Du, H. Zhou, X. Lin, X. Liu,A. Kijlstra. SUMO4 gene polymorphisms in Chinese Han patients with Behcet's disease. Clin Immunol 2008; 129(1): 170-5.

[107] Rutzen A.R., G. Ortega-Larrocea, I.R. Schwab,N.A. Rao. Simultaneous onset of Vogt-Koyanagi-Harada syndrome in monozygotic twins. Am J Ophthalmol 1995; 119(2): 239-40.

[108] Zhao M., Y. Jiang,I.W. Abrahams. Association of HLA antigens with Vogt-Koyanagi-Harada syndrome in a Han Chinese population. Arch Ophthalmol 1991; 109(3): 368-70.

[109] Zhang X.Y., X.M. Wang,T.S. Hu. Profiling human leukocyte antigens in Vogt-Koyanagi-Harada syndrome. Am J Ophthalmol 1992; 113(5):567-72.

[110] Hou S., Z. Yang, L. Du, Z. Jiang, Q. Shu, Y. Chen, F. Li, Q. Zhou, S. Ohno, R. Chen, A. Kijlstra, J.T. Rosenbaum,P. Yang. Identification of a susceptibility locus in STAT4 for Behcet's disease in Han Chinese in a genome-wide association study. Arthritis Rheum 2012; 64(12):4104-13.

[111] Kirino Y., G. Bertsias, Y. Ishigatsubo, N. Mizuki, I. Tugal-Tutkun, E. Seyahi, Y. Ozyazgan, F.S. Sacli, B. Erer, H. Inoko, Z. Emrence, A. Cakar, N. Abaci, D. Ustek, C. Satorius, A. Ueda, M. Takeno, Y. Kim, G.M. Wood, M.J. Ombrello, A. Meguro, A. Gul, E.F. Remmers,D.L. Kastner. Genome-wide association analysis identifies new susceptibility loci for Behcet's disease and epistasis between HLA-B*51 and ERAP1. Nat Genet 2013; 45(2):202-7.

[112] Hou S., X. Xiao, F. Li, Z. Jiang, A. Kijlstra,P. Yang. Two-stage association study in Chinese Han identifies two independent associations in CCR1/CCR3 locus as candidate for Behcet's disease susceptibility. Hum Genet 2012; 131(12):1841-50.

[113] Jang W.C., S.B. Park, Y.H. Nam, S.S. Lee, J.W. Kim, I.S. Chang, K.T. Kim,H.K. Chang. Interleukin-18 gene polymorphisms in Korean patients with Behcet's disease. Clin Exp Rheumatol 2005; 23(4 Suppl 38):S59-63.

[114] Arida A., K. Fragiadaki, E. Giavri,P.P. Sfikakis. Anti-TNF agents for Behcet's disease: analysis of published data on 369 patients. Semin Arthritis Rheum 2011; 41(1):61-70.

[115] Touma Z., C. Farra, A. Hamdan, W. Shamseddeen, I. Uthman, H. Hourani,T. Arayssi. TNF polymorphisms in patients with Behcet disease: a meta-analysis. Arch Med Res 2010; 41(2):142-6.

[116] Radouane A., M. Oudghiri, A. Chakib, S. Bennani, I. Touitou,M. Barat-Houari. SNPs in the TNF-alpha gene promoter associated with Behcet's disease in Moroccan patients. Rheumatology (Oxford) 2012; 51(9):1595-9.

[117] Bonyadi M., Z. Jahanafrooz, M. Esmaeili, S. Kolahi, A. Khabazi, A.A. Ebrahimi, M. Hajialilo,S. Dastgiri. TNF-alpha gene polymorphisms in Iranian Azeri Turkish patients with Behcet's Disease. Rheumatol Int 2009; 30(2):285-9.

[118] Jiang Z., P. Yang, S. Hou, L. Du, L. Xie, H. Zhou,A. Kijlstra. IL-23R gene confers susceptibility to Behcet's disease in a Chinese Han population. Ann Rheum Dis 2010; 69(7):1325-8.

[119] Xavier J.M., F. Shahram, F. Davatchi, A. Rosa, J. Crespo, B.S. Abdollahi, A. Nadji, G. Jesus, F. Barcelos, J.V. Patto, N.M. Shafiee, F. Ghaderibarim,S.A. Oliveira. Association study of IL10 and IL23R-IL12RB2 in Iranian patients with Behcet's disease. Arthritis Rheum 2012; 64(8):2761-72.

[120] Hou S., J. Qi, Q. Zhang, D. Liao, Q. Li, K. Hu, Y. Zhou, A. Kijlstra,P. Yang. Genetic variants in the JAK1 gene confer higher risk of Behcet's disease with ocular involvement in Han Chinese. Hum Genet 2013.

[121] Hu K., S. Hou, Z. Jiang, A. Kijlstra,P. Yang. JAK2 and STAT3 polymorphisms in a Han Chinese population with Behcet's disease. Invest Ophthalmol Vis Sci 2012; 53(1): 538-41.

[122] Hou S., P. Yang, L. Du, Z. Jiang, L. Mao, Q. Shu, H. Zhou,A. Kijlstra. Monocyte chemoattractant protein-1-2518 A/G single nucleotide polymorphism in Chinese Han patients with ocular Behcet's disease. Hum Immunol 2010; 71(1):79-82.

[123] Ozcimen A.A., K. Dilek, U. Bingol, H. Saricaoglu, A. Sarandol, O. Taskapilioglu, M. Yurtkuran, M.A. Yurtkuran,H.B. Oral. IL-1 cluster gene polymorphisms in Turkish patients with Behcet's disease. Int J Immunogenet 2011; 38(4):295-301.

[124] Chang H.K., W.C. Jang, S.B. Park, S.M. Han, Y.H. Nam, S.S. Lee, J.U. Kim,H.S. Lee. Association between interleukin 6 gene polymorphisms and Behcet's disease in Korean people. Ann Rheum Dis 2005; 64(2):339-40.

[125] .Hu K., S. Hou, F. Li, Q. Xiang, A. Kijlstra,P. Yang. JAK1, but not JAK2 and STAT3, confers susceptibility to Vogt-Koyanagi-Harada (VKH) syndrome in a Han Chinese population. Invest Ophthalmol Vis Sci 2013; 54(5):3360-5.

[126] Shu Q., P. Yang, S. Hou, F. Li, Y. Chen, L. Du,Z. Jiang. Interleukin-17 gene polymorphism is associated with Vogt-Koyanagi-Harada syndrome but not with Behcet's disease in a Chinese Han population. Hum Immunol 2010; 71(10):988-91.

[127] Tang Y., X. Luo, H. Cui, X. Ni, M. Yuan, Y. Guo, X. Huang, H. Zhou, N. de Vries, P.P. Tak, S. Chen,N. Shen. MicroRNA-146A contributes to abnormal activation of the type I interferon pathway in human lupus by targeting the key signaling proteins. Arthritis Rheum 2009; 60(4):1065-75.

http://dx.doi.org/10.5772/57586

[128] Zhou Q., S. Hou, L. Liang, X. Li, X. Tan, L. Wei, B. Lei, A. Kijlstra,P. Yang. MicroRNA-146a and Ets-1 gene polymorphisms in ocular Behcet's disease and Vogt-Koyanagi-Harada syndrome. Ann Rheum Dis 2012.

[129] Sugita S., H. Takase, T. Kawaguchi, C. Taguchi,M. Mochizuki. Cross-reaction between tyrosinase peptides and cytomegalovirus antigen by T cells from patients with Vogt-Koyanagi-Harada disease. Int Ophthalmol 2007; 27(2-3):87-95.

[130] Narikawa S., Y. Suzuki, M. Takahashi, A. Furukawa, T. Sakane,Y. Mizushima. Streptococcus oralis previously identified as uncommon 'Streptococcus sanguis' in Behcet's disease. Arch Oral Biol 1995; 40(8):685-90.

[131] Kirino Y., M. Takeno, R. Watanabe, S. Murakami, M. Kobayashi, H. Ideguchi, A. Ihata, S. Ohno, A. Ueda, N. Mizuki,Y. Ishigatsubo. Association of reduced heme oxygenase-1 with excessive Toll-like receptor 4 expression in peripheral blood mononuclear cells in Behcet's disease. Arthritis Res Ther 2008; 10(1):R16.

[132] Do J.E., S.Y. Kwon, S. Park,E.S. Lee. Effects of vitamin D on expression of Toll-like receptors of monocytes from patients with Behcet's disease. Rheumatology (Oxford) 2008; 47(6):840-8.

[133] Liu X., C. Wang, Z. Ye, A. Kijlstra,P. Yang. Higher expression of Toll-like receptors 2, 3, 4 and 8 in ocular Behcet's disease. Invest Ophthalmol Vis Sci 2013.

[134] Pay S., I. Simsek, H. Erdem,A. Dinc. Immunopathogenesis of Behcet's disease with special emphasize on the possible role of antigen presenting cells. Rheumatol Int 2007; 27(5):417-24.

[135] Harry R.A., A.E. Anderson, J.D. Isaacs,C.M. Hilkens. Generation and characterisation of therapeutic tolerogenic dendritic cells for rheumatoid arthritis. Ann Rheum Dis 2010; 69(11):2042-50.

[136] Atzeni F., L. Boiardi, B. Casali, E. Farnetti, D. Nicoli, P. Sarzi-Puttini, N. Pipitone, I. Olivieri, F. Cantini, F. Salvi, R. La Corte, G. Triolo, D. Filippini, G. Paolazzi,C. Salvarani. CC chemokine receptor 5 polymorphism in Italian patients with Behcet's disease. Rheumatology (Oxford) 2012; 51(12):2141-5.

[137] Chen F., S. Hou, Z. Jiang, Y. Chen, A. Kijlstra, J.T. Rosenbaum,P. Yang. CD40 gene polymorphisms confer risk of Behcet's disease but not of Vogt-Koyanagi-Harada syndrome in a Han Chinese population. Rheumatology (Oxford) 2012; 51(1):47-51.

[138] Fei Y., R. Webb, B.L. Cobb, H. Direskeneli, G. Saruhan-Direskeneli,A.H. Sawalha. Identification of novel genetic susceptibility loci for Behcet's disease using a genome-wide association study. Arthritis Res Ther 2009; 11(3):R66.

[139] Oksel F., G. Keser, M. Ozmen, K. Aksu, G. Kitapcioglu, A. Berdeli,E. Doganavsargil. Endothelial nitric oxide synthase gene Glu298Asp polymorphism is associated with Behcet's disease. Clin Exp Rheumatol 2006; 24(5 Suppl 42):S79-82.

[140] Kim J.U., H.K. Chang, S.S. Lee, J.W. Kim, K.T. Kim, S.W. Lee,W.T. Chung. Endothelial nitric oxide synthase gene polymorphisms in Behcet's disease and rheumatic diseases with vasculitis. Ann Rheum Dis 2003; 62(11):1083-7.

[141] Ben Dhifallah I., H. Houman, M. Khanfir,K. Hamzaoui. Endothelial nitric oxide synthase gene polymorphism is associated with Behcet's disease in Tunisian population. Hum Immunol 2008; 69(10):661-5.

[142] Li K., M. Zhao, S. Hou, L. Du, A. Kijlstra,P. Yang. Association between polymorphisms of FCRL3, a non-HLA gene, and Behcet's disease in a Chinese population with ophthalmic manifestations. Mol Vis 2008; 14:2136-42.

[143] Ben Dhifallah I., E.F. Karray, F. Sassi,K. Hamzaoui. Intercellular adhesion molecule 1 K469E gene polymorphism is associated with presence of skin lesions in Tunisian Behcet's disease patients. Tissue Antigens 2010; 75(1):74-8.

[144] Boiardi L., C. Salvarani, B. Casali, I. Olivieri, G. Ciancio, F. Cantini, F. Salvi, R. Malatesta, M. Govoni, F. Trotta, D. Filippini, G. Paolazzi, D. Nicoli, E. Farnetti,L. Macchioni. Intercellular adhesion molecule-1 gene polymorphisms in Behcet's Disease. J Rheumatol 2001; 28(6):1283-7.

[145] Oral H.B., K. Dilek, A.A. Ozcimen, O. Taskapilioglu, U. Bingol, A. Sarandol, H. Saricaoglu, M. Yurtkuran,M.A. Yurtkuran. Interleukin-4 gene polymorphisms confer Behcet's disease in Turkish population. Scand J Immunol 2011; 73(6):594-601.

[146] Yanagihori H., N. Oyama, K. Nakamura, N. Mizuki, K. Oguma,F. Kaneko. Role of IL-12B promoter polymorphism in Adamantiades-Behcet's disease susceptibility: An involvement of Th1 immunoreactivity against Streptococcus Sanguinis antigen. J Invest Dermatol 2006; 126(7):1534-40.

[147] Htoon J., A. Nadig, T. Hughes, S. Yavuz, H. Direskeneli, G. Saruhan-Direskeneli,A.H. Sawalha. IL18 polymorphism is associated with Behcet's disease but not lupus in patients from Turkey. J Rheumatol 2011; 38(5):962-3.

[148] Lee Y.J., S.W. Kang, J.K. Song, H.J. Baek, H.J. Choi, Y.D. Bae, H.J. Ryu, E.Y. Lee, E.B. Lee,Y.W. Song. Associations between interferon regulatory factor-1 polymorphisms and Behcet's disease. Hum Immunol 2007; 68(9):770-8.

[149] Xavier J.M., N.M. Shafiee, F. Ghaderi, A. Rosa, B.S. Abdollahi, A. Nadji, F. Shahram, F. Davatchi,S.A. Oliveira. Association of mitochondrial polymorphism m.709G>A with Behcet's disease. Ann Rheum Dis 2010; 70(8):1514-6.

[150] Rustemoglu A., U. Gul, G. Gumus-Akay, M. Gonul, S. Yigit, N. Bozkurt, A. Karadag, E. Piskin, A. Sunguroglu,A. Kadikiran. MDR1 gene polymorphisms may be associated with Behcet's disease and its colchicum treatment response. Gene 2012; 505(2):333-9.

[151] Zheng X., D. Wang, S. Hou, C. Zhang, B. Lei, X. Xiao, A. Kijlstra,P. Yang. Association of macrophage migration inhibitory factor gene polymorphisms with Behcet's disease in a Han Chinese population. Ophthalmology 2012; 119(12):2514-8.

[152] Park K.S., Y. Min, S.R. Park, E.H. Kim, D.J. Lee, D. Bang,E.S. Lee. Matrix metalloproteinase-2,-9,-12, and tissue inhibitor of metalloproteinase 2 gene polymorphisms and cutaneous expressions in patients with Behcet's disease. Tissue Antigens 2012; 79(5): 333-9.

[153] Lee Y.J., S.W. Kang, H.J. Baek, H.J. Choi, Y.D. Bae, E.H. Kang, E.Y. Lee, E.B. Lee,Y.W. Song. Association between matrix metalloproteinase 9 promoter polymorphisms and Behcet's disease. Hum Immunol 2010; 71(7):717-22.

[154] Karakus N., S. Yigit, G. Kalkan, A. Rustemoglu, A. Inanir, U. Gul, G.S. Pancar, S. Akkanet,O. Ates. Association between the methylene tetrahydrofolate reductase gene C677T mutation and colchicine unresponsiveness in Behcet's disease. Mol Vis 2012; 18:1696-700.

[155] Ates O., L. Dalyan, G. Hatemi, V. Hamuryudan,A. Topal-Sarikaya. Genetic susceptibility to Behcet's syndrome is associated with NRAMP1 (SLC11A1) polymorphism in Turkish patients. Rheumatol Int 2009; 29(7):787-91.

[156] Hou S., X. Xiao, Y. Zhou, X. Zhu, F. Li, A. Kijlstra,P. Yang. Genetic variant on PDGFRL associated with Behcet disease in Chinese Han populations. Hum Mutat 2013; 34(1):74-8.

[157] Demir H.D., F.N. Yalcindag, A. Ozturk,N. Akar. Intron F G79A polymorphism of the protein Z gene in Turkish Behcet patients. Curr Eye Res 2012; 37(7):630-2.

[158] Baranathan V., M.R. Stanford, R.W. Vaughan, E. Kondeatis, E. Graham, F. Fortune, W. Madanat, C. Kanawati, M. Ghabra, P.I. Murray,G.R. Wallace. The association of the PTPN22 620W polymorphism with Behcet's disease. Ann Rheum Dis 2007; 66(11): 1531-3.

[159] Kim S.K., W.C. Jang, S.B. Park, D.Y. Park, K.T. Bang, S.S. Lee, J.B. Jun, D.H. Yoo,H.K. Chang. SLC11A1 gene polymorphisms in Korean patients with Behcet's disease. Scand J Rheumatol 2006; 35(5):398-401.

[160] Hou S., A. Kijlstra,P. Yang. The genetics of Behcet's disease in a Chinese population. Front Med 2012; 6(4):354-9.

[161] Park G., H.S. Kim, J.Y. Choe,S.K. Kim. SUMO4 C438T polymorphism is associated with papulopustular skin lesion in Korean patients with Behcet's disease. Rheumatol Int 2012; 32(10):3031-7.

[162] Kamoun M., I. Ben Dhifallah, E. Karray, L. Zakraoui,K. Hamzaoui. Association of small ubiquitin-like modifier 4 (SUMO4) polymorphisms in a Tunisian population with Behcet's disease. Clin Exp Rheumatol 2010; 28(4 Suppl 60):S45-9.

[163] Chen Y., P. Yang, F. Li, S. Hou, Z. Jiang, Q. Shu,A. Kijlstra. Association analysis of TGFBR3 gene with Vogt-Koyanagi-Harada disease and Behcet's disease in the Chinese Han population. Curr Eye Res 2012; 37(4):312-7.

[164] Horie Y., A. Meguro, M. Ota, N. Kitaichi, Y. Katsuyama, Y. Takemoto, K. Namba, K. Yoshida, Y.W. Song, K.S. Park, E.B. Lee, H. Inoko, N. Mizuki,S. Ohno. Association of TLR4 polymorphisms with Behcet's disease in a Korean population. Rheumatology (Oxford) 2009; 48(6):638-42.

[165] Meguro A., M. Ota, Y. Katsuyama, A. Oka, S. Ohno, H. Inoko,N. Mizuki. Association of the toll-like receptor 4 gene polymorphisms with Behcet's disease. Ann Rheum Dis 2008; 67(5):725-7.

[166] Li H., Q. Liu, S. Hou, L. Du, Q. Zhou, Y. Zhou, A. Kijlstra, Z. Li,P. Yang. TNFAIP3 gene polymorphisms confer risk for Behcet's disease in a Chinese Han population. Hum Genet 2013; 132(3):293-300.

[167] Jung E.S., S.W. Kim, C.M. Moon, D.J. Shin, N.H. Son, E.S. Kim, H.J. Lee, S.P. Hong, T.I. Kim, W.H. Kim,J.H. Cheon. Relationships between genetic polymorphisms of triggering receptor expressed on myeloid cells-1 and inflammatory bowel diseases in the Korean population. Life Sci 2011; 89(9-10):289-94.

[168] Hou S., Q. Shu, Z. Jiang, Y. Chen, F. Li, F. Chen, A. Kijlstra,P. Yang. Replication study confirms the association between UBAC2 and Behcet's disease in two independent Chinese sets of patients and controls. Arthritis Res Ther 2012; 14(2):R70.

[169] Karray E.F., I. Ben Dhifallah, K. Ben Abdelghani, I. Ben Ghorbel, M. Khanfir, H. Houman, K. Hamzaoui,L. Zakraoui. Associations of vitamin D receptor gene polymorphisms FokI and BsmI with susceptibility to rheumatoid arthritis and Behcet's disease in Tunisians. Joint Bone Spine 2012; 79(2):144-8.

[170] Nam E.J., S.W. Han, S.U. Kim, J.H. Cho, K.H. Sa, W.K. Lee, J.Y. Park,Y.M. Kang. Association of vascular endothelial growth factor gene polymorphisms with behcet disease in a Korean population. Hum Immunol 2005; 66(10):1068-73.

[171] Du L., P. Yang, S. Hou, X. Lin, H. Zhou, X. Huang, L. Wang,A. Kijlstra. Association of the CTLA-4 gene with Vogt-Koyanagi-Harada syndrome. Clin Immunol 2008; 127(1):43-8.

[172] Hu K., P. Yang, Z. Jiang, S. Hou, L. Du,F. Li. STAT4 polymorphism in a Chinese Han population with Vogt-Koyanagi-Harada syndrome and Behcet's disease. Hum Immunol 2010; 71(7):723-6.

[173] Li H., Q. Liu, S. Hou, L. Du, Q. Zhou, Y. Zhou, A. Kijlstra,P. Yang. TNFAIP3 gene polymorphisms in a Chinese Han population with Vogt-Koyanagi-Harada syndrome. PLoS One 2013; 8(3):e59515.

Chapter 19

Ibopamine – A New Alpha-Adrenergic and D1-Dopaminergic Drug

Italo Giuffré

Additional information is available at the end of the chapter

http://dx.doi.org/10.5772/58380

1. Introduction

Ibopamine (3,4 di-isobutyrrylester of N-methyldopamine) at 2% concentration, when instilled in the conjunctival sac, stimulates ocular D1-dopaminergic and α-adrenergic receptors [1,2]. It is a pro-drug of epinine (N-methyldopamine) (Figure 1). It has positive inotropic effects: it improves cardiac function and it is effective in the treatment of congestive heart failure. The pharmacological ocular characteristics of ibopamine are as follows:

- It increases aqueous humor production following D1-dopaminergic stimulation;
- It is a provocative test for evaluating the function of aqueous humor outflow structures;
- It can be used to treat ocular hypotension;
- It induces a noncycloplegic mydriasis (α-adrenergic action);
- It is very useful, apart from genetic testing, to detect a predisposition to ocular hypertension and even glaucoma in relatives of glaucoma patients.

In the conjunctival sac, ibopamine is fastly hydrolysed to epinine by the esterases of the aqueous humor and ocular tissues. This hydrolysis suggests that epinine is the active component of the molecule. The half-life of ibopamine in the aqueous humor is short (about 2 minutes) and epinine formation precedes the mydriatic effect [3,4] (Figure 1). It has been proved that after the instillation of ibopamine, only epinine can be found in the aqueous humor [3].

When hydrolysed to epinine, ibopamine stimulates the α-adrenergic and D1 dopaminergic receptors. The mydriatic effect of ibopamine is due to the stimulation of the α-adrenergic receptors of the dilating muscle of the pupil. Since ibopamine has no effect on the ciliary muscle, the mydriasis is not accompanied by cycloplegia. Mydriasis can be antagonized and

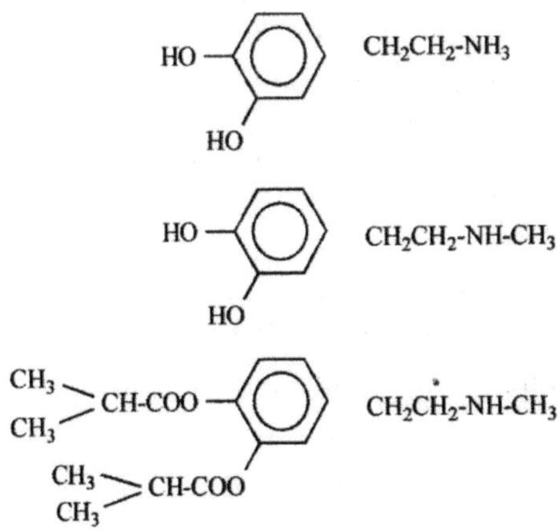

Figure 1. Dopamine → Epinine → Ibopamine (3,4 dyisobutyrrilester of N-methyldopamine).

reversed by pre-treatment by α-blocking agents (such as thymoxamine and dapiprazole). Some Randomized Clinical Trials (RCTs) show that the D1 dopaminergic activity of the drug increases aqueous humor production and intraocular pressure (IOP) in open-angle glaucoma (POAG) patients [5].

Ibopamine has low toxicity both at systemic and local levels. LD_{50} is 2056 mg/Kg, 4930 mg/Kg and 1786 mg/Kg in mice, rats and guinea pigs respectively. Ibopamine is well tolerated without any significant change to the haematological and behavioural parameters. 2% ibopamine eye drops show that ibopamine is well tolerated at local level, without systemic side-effects and tachyphylaxis phenomena. One drop of 2% ibopamine contains 1 mg of the compound, while the oral dosage is higher than 400 mg/day. Electrophysiological assessment showed that ibopamine is not retinotoxic at all [6].

2. Clinical use

2.1. Non-cycloplegic mydriatic activity

In binocular indirect examination of fundus oculi with scleral indentation, fluorescein and indocyanine angiography, and in the laser treatment of retinal lesions, ibopamine can induce a fast, short-lasting (2-3 hours) maximal mydriasis without cycloplegic effects or local a/or systemic side-effects [7]. The mydriatic effect of ibopamine can be prolonged if repeatedly administered (every 30 minutes). Ibopamine-induced mydriasis can be reversed by local application of α-blockers such as thymoxamine and dapiprazole. Ibopamine can substitute phenylephrine in association with tropicamide a/or cyclopentolate to avoid the typical discomfort of cycloplegia mostly in adults [7]. Ibopamine eye drops is effective in inducing pre-operative mydriasis, without effects on the cardiovascular system [7]. In the post-operative period ibopamine can induce a fast and short-lasting mydriasis to induce pupil dilatation.

http://dx.doi.org/10.5772/58380

2.2. Pathophysiology of IOP

2% ibopamine eye drops increases IOP only in patients suffering from POAG. Ibopamine is useful in different ways:

- Physiological studies on IOP;
- Evaluation of trabecular outflow pathways (pressure-dependent outflow);
- Treatment of ocular hypotony.

The instillation of ibopamine increases the IOP only in about 96% of eyes with POAG [8,9,10] (Figures 2, 3). In normal eyes, 2% ibopamine does not significantly affect IOP, with a possible mild hypotensive effect (1-2 mmHg) (Figure 4). The IOP, in POAG patients, increases by a maximum value of 10-11 mmHg within 45 minutes from the instillation and lasts about 180 minutes [7,8,9,10,11,12,13,14]. To observe this effect, 2 drops of 2% ibopamine have been instilled 5 minutes apart, and IOP was measured 45 minutes after the first instillation. The ibopamine provocative test shows a significant correlation with the highest intraocular pressure in the diurnal tension curve in glaucoma patients [15]. Indeed, in glaucoma patients with early visual field defect, the ibopamine provocative test has shown better sensitivity/specificity than the water drinking test [16]. Ibopamine test does not modify the results of visual field tests in normal individuals [17].

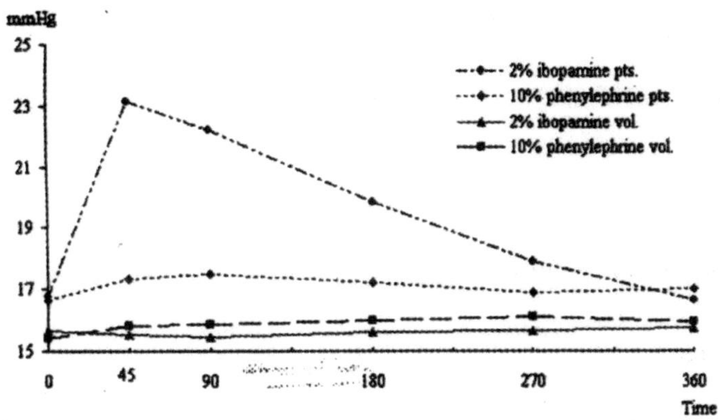

	Maximum increase	Area under the curve
Ibo pts. vs. Ibo vol.	p = 0.0001	p = 0.0001
Ibo pts. vs. Phn pts.	p = 0.0001	p = 0.0001
Ibo vol. vs. Phn vol.	p = n.s.	p = 0.01
Phn pts. vs. Phn vol.	p = n.s.	p = n.s.

Figure 2. Effect on the intraocular pressure of 2% ibopamine and 10% phenylephrine in glaucomatous patients and in normal volunteers.

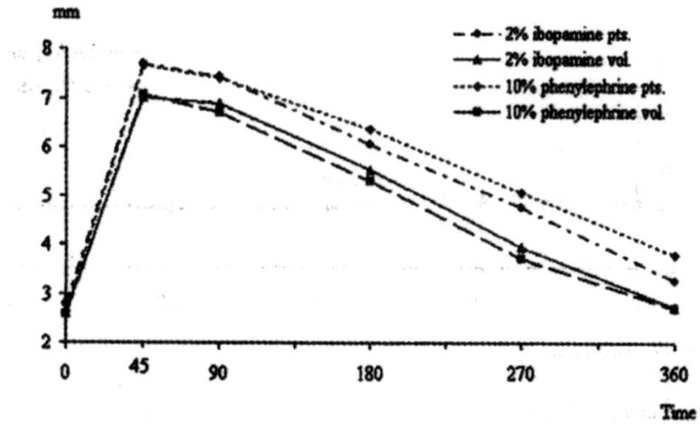

	Maximum increase	Area Under the Curve
Ibo pts. vs. Ibo vol.	p = n.s.	p = n.s.
Ibo pts. vs. Phn pts.	p = n.s.	$p < 0.05$
Ibo vol. vs. Phn vol.	p = n.s.	p = n.s.
Phn pts. vs. Phn vol.	p = n.s.	p = 0.0002

Figure 3. Effect on the pupillary diameter of 2% ibopamine and 10% phenylephrine in glaucomatous patients and in normal volunteers.

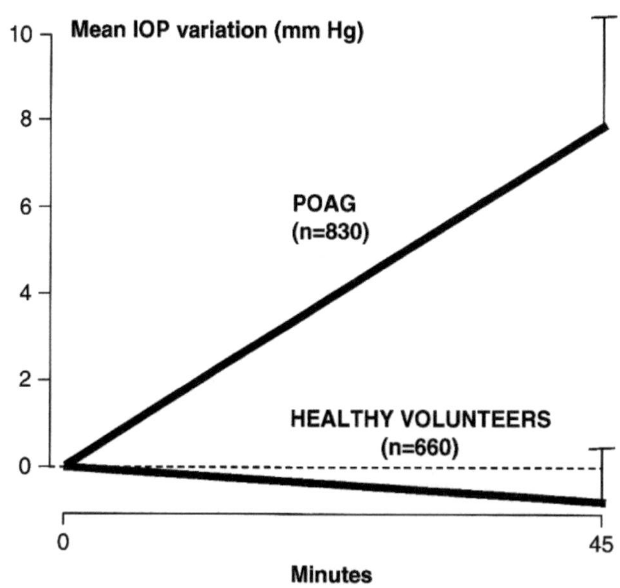

Figure 4. ibopamine induces a transient ocular hypertensive effect (mean, 8.31±2.14 mmHg) in 96% of eyes of patients affected by POAG, whereas in healthy eyes there is a reduction of intraocular pressure (IOP) by 1 to 2 mmHg.

Several studies have been performed to assess the following issues:

- Identification of the responsible receptor (agonist and antagonist);
- Evaluation of the change of the aqueous humor dynamics;
- Evaluation of ibopamine effects when the outflow system was experimentally impaired.

Only the D1 agonist substances, such as fenoldopam, have the same effect as ibopamine on IOP in POAG patients. D1 agonist drugs increase the IOP only in POAG, but never in healthy eyes, stressing the involvement of D1 dopaminergic receptors on the mechanism stimulating the aqueous humor production.

The hypertensive effect of ibopamine in POAG is completely counteracted by the pre-treatment with a selective antagonist of the D1 receptors such as SCH23390. A clear receptorial antagonism for IOP has been identified. Ocular anti-hypertensive drug, such as β-blockers and α-agonists do not antagonize the hypertensive effects of ibopamine in POAG [14]. The partial antagonism performed by glycerol is due to an osmotic reduction of the vitreous mass.

When there is a marked increase of aqueous humor production, due to the D1 dopaminergic effect of ibopamine, the healthy eye increases its outflow mantaining the homeostasis. Instead, in glaucomatous eyes, the impaired trabecular outflow fails to maintain the hydrodynamic equilibrium and IOP increases. Fluorophotometry proves that the D1 dopaminergic stimulation, induced by 2% ibopamine, undoubtedly increases the aqueous humor production.

Ibopamine, when instilled, prior to the Laminaria, into the healthy rabbit eyes does not significantly affect the IOP, while in the eyes treated with Laminaria digitata induces ocular hypertension.

3. Provocative test in glaucoma

Ibopamine 2% eye drops have a positive pressure effect in 50% of suspected normal-tension glaucoma eyes and may differentiate between eyes with normal trabecular outflow capacity and eyes with increased resistance in the trabecular meshwork that are ready to have pressure peaks and deterioration to glaucoma [18].

A long-term treatment with corticosteroids can induce ocular hypertension. They increase the IOP by interfering with the aqueous humor outflow system. By administering dexamethasone at two different concentrations (0.1 and 1%) in eyes suffering from allergic conjunctivitis, the ibopamine test was positive, in a dose-dependent manner, from 33 to 50%.

Ibopamine test is useful in detecting an impairment of the outflow system also in patients affected by psudoexfoliative syndrome (PEX) [19]. This test is also positive when PEX syndrome is unilateral. It exerts a significant additive effect on mydriasis of PEX eyes induced with 10% phenylephrine-0.5% tropicamide with only minimal increase in IOP [20].

The ibopamine test is positive in 44.33% of offspring of one glaucoma parent without glaucomatous damage. It signifies an impaired function of the outflow structures and, therefore, a predisposition to intraocular hypertension and possible glaucoma in some years [21,22].

Ocular hypotony is a pathological condition of the IOP when it decreases to values below 6-7 mmHg. IOP values below 4 mmHg usually cause progressive damage to the eye [23]. Ocular hypotony can be caused by a damage to ciliary body from trauma or inflammation. In the treatment of ocular hypotony, ibopamine can be administerd every 3 hours or 3-4 times daily, associated to corticosteroid therapy [24,25].

4. Conclusion

In conclusion, 2% ibopamine eye drops test is a useful pharmacological tool allowing us to study the pathophysiology of hydrodynamic disorders and in evaluating the outflow impairment. It is useful as a therapeutic drug in ocular hypotony secondary to filtering surgery, vitreo-retinal surgery or long-lasting uveitis. That's why its use is adviced in all the Ophthalmological Department in EU and USA.

Author details

Italo Giuffré*

Address all correspondence to: italogiuffre@libero.it

Department of Ophthalmology – Medical School – Catholic University of Roma, Italy

References

[1] Virno M., Taverniti L., Motolese E. et al. Ibopamina: nuovo midriatico non cicloplegico (nota preliminare). Boll. Ocul. 1986; 65: 11-2.

[2] Virno M., Taverniti L., De Gregorio F et al. Increase in aqueous humor production following D1 receptors activation by means of ibopamine. Int. Ophthalmol. 1997; 20: 141-6.

[3] Soldati L., Gianesello V., Galbiati I. et al. Ocular pharmacokinetics and pharmacodynamics in rabbits of ibopamine, a new mydriatic agent. Exp. Eye Res. 1993; 56: 247-54.

[4] Ugahary L.C., Ganteris E., Veckeneer M. et al. Topical ibopamine in the treatment of chronic ocular hypotony attributable to vitreoretinal surgery, uveitis, or penetrating trauma. Am. J. Ophthalmol. 2006; 141: 571-3.

[5] De Gregorio F., Pecori-Giraldi J, Pannarale L. et al. Ibopamine in glaucoma diagnostics: a new pharmacological provocative test. Int. Ophthalmol. 1997; 20: 151-5.

[6] Giuffre' I., Falsini B., Gari M.A., Balestrazzi E. Pattern-electroretinogram assessment during ibopamine test in ocular hypertension. Eur. J. Ophthalmol. 2013 Jun 24; 23 (6): 819-22.

[7] Giuffre' I., Taverniti L., Di Staso S. The effects of 2% ibopamine eye drops on the intraocular pressure and pupil motility of patients with open-angle glaucoma. Eur. J. Ophthalmol. 2004; 14; 6:508-13.

[8] Giuffre' I. Ibopamine stimulates α-adrenergic receptors and D1 dopaminergic receptors in the eye. Curr. Drug Therapy 2007, 2: 1-7.

[9] Magacho L., Costa M.L., Dessimoni A., de Avila M.P. Comparison between the 1% and 2% ibopamine provocative test in primary open-angle glaucoma patients: sensitivity, specificity and tolerability. Arq. Bras Oftalmol. 2006 Sep-Oct; 69 (5): 695-9.

[10] Ullrich K., Craig J.E., Landers J. The ibopamine challenge test can be used to differentiate glaucoma suspects from glaucoma patients. Clin. Experiment. Ophthalmol. 2013 Sep. 3.

[11] Marchini G., Babighian S., Tosi R. et al. Comparative study of the effects of 2% ibopamine, 10% phenylephrine, and 1% tropicamide on the anterior segment. Invest. Ophthalmol. Vis. Sci. 2003; 44: 281-9.

[12] Boles Carenini B., Brogliatti B., Boles Carenini A. et al. Ibopamine: a new drug and its use as provocative test for the diagnosis of glaucoma. New Trends Ophthalmol. 1992; 7: 3.

[13] Nuti A., Ciappetta R., Diadori A., Frezzotti R. Ibopamine provocative test in the diagnosis of hydrodynamic disorders. Exp. Eye Res. 1992; 55 (suppl.): S185.

[14] Virno M., Pecori-Giraldi J., Taverniti L. et al. Indagini sul meccanismo d'azione dell'aumento tensionale di ibopamina nell'iperteso oculare. Boll. Ocul. 1989; 68 (suppl. 2): 379-84.

[15] Pecori-Giraldi J., De Gregorio F., Carbone F. et al. Curva tonometrica e positivita' al test della ibopamina nella prima diagnosi di glaucoma. Boll. Ocul. 1994; 73 (suppl. 2): 319-23.

[16] Magacho L., Reis R., Pigini M.A., Avila M.P. 2% ibopamine vs. water-drinking test as a provocative test for glaucoma. Arq. Bras. Oftalmol. 2008 Jul-Aug; 71 (4): 499-503.

[17] Pigini M.A., Avila M.P., Magacho L. Effects of 2% ibopamine eye drops on the results of computerized visual field. Arq. Bras. Oftalmol. 2009 May-Jun; 72 (3): 365-9.

[18] Kniestedt C., Romppainen T., Gloor B.P., Sturmer J. Positive ibopamine provocative test in normal-tension glaucoma suspects. Klin. Monbl. Augenheilkd 2007 Apr; 224 (4): 255-9.

[19] Di Staso S., D'Andrea D., Giuffre' I. et al. Test dell'ibopamina nella sindrome da pseudoesfoliazione. Boll. Ocul. 1994; 73 (suppl. 2): 325-30.

[20] Scuderi G.L., Regine F., Perdicchi A. et al. Efficacy of 2% ibopamine on the dilation of patients with pseudoexfoliation syndrome. Eur. J. Ophthalmol. 2010 Jan-Feb; 20 (1): 120-3.

[21] Pecori-Giraldi J., Damiano A., Gabrielli A. et al. Ocular hypertension induced by ibopamine early discloses glaucoma suspects among relatives of glaucomatous patients. Boll. Ocul. 2002; 81: 91.

[22] Virno M., Sanpaolesi R., Pecori-Giraldi J. et al. Ibopamine: D1-dopaminergic agonist in the diagnosis of glaucoma. J. Glaucoma 2013; 22: 5-9.

[23] Pivetti Pezzi P., Da Dalt S., La Cava M. et al. Ibopamine treatment in chronic hypotony secondary to long-lasting uveitis. A case report. Eur. J. Ophthalmol. 2000; 10: 332-4.

[24] Ganteris-Gerritsen E., Ugahary L.C., Jansen J. et al. Six months treatment with ibopamine in patients with hypotony after vitreoretinal surgery for retinal detachment, uveitis or penetrating trauma. Retina 2012 Apr; 32 (4): 742-7.

[25] Virno M., De Gregorio F., Pannarale L., Arrico L. Topical ibopamine and corticosteroids in the treatment of post-surgery ocular hypotony. Int. Ophthalmol. 1997; 20:147-50.

Chapter 20

Clinical Research Progress of Glaucomatocyclitic Crisis

He-Zheng Zhou, Wen-Shan Jiang, Han-Guang Jie,
Chang Feng, Wen-Qiang Zhang, Qian Ye,
Jian-Guo Wu, Yan-Ping Song and Qin Ding

Additional information is available at the end of the chapter

http://dx.doi.org/10.5772/58348

1. Introduction

1.1.Definition

Glaucomatocyclitic crisis was initially described in detail by Posner and Schlossman in 1948, so it was also called Posner – Schlossman syndrome (PSS). PSS is a special form of anterior uveitis with glaucoma, mainly seen in young adults, characterized by non-granulomatousiri-docyclitis with significant elevation of intraocular pressure. In most cases, the disease takes an acute form of recurrent and monocular onset.

1.2. Morbidity

This disease is often seen in people aged from 20 to 50, and rarely in people above 60 years old. Five percent or less of PSS cases were reported in people above 60 years old [3]. The disease is rare in Western countries, it was reported that 19 in one million people have suffered from PSS in Finland [4]. As PSS is a kind of disease attacks intermittently, it is difficult to diagnose PSS in intermittent period for the lack of diagnostic signs and investigate the morbidity with epidemiology methods. We used the full text VIP Chinese literature retrieval system and Medeline retrieval system to find PSS reports from 1975 to 2011 in both English and Chinese literature and divided into review, case, experimental study and clinical report four categories, then analyzed the regional distribution of the authors and cases (Chinese reports were divided into the Yangtze river and the other, English reports were divided into Asia and the other).

The report which contained the most number of cases was chosen if there were more than two from a same author statistical results shows that 1262 cases were reported by 33 Chinese clinical reports in which 991 cases were reported by 20 reports from the area near the Yangtze river, and 271 cases were reported by 13 reports from the other area. The other 211 cases were reported by 16 English clinical reports in which 144 cases were reported by 7 reports from the Asia area and 67 cases reported by 9 reports from the other area. The results above suggest that there are much more literature and cases related to PSS in the area near the Yangtze river and infer that the prevalence of PSS in that area may be higher.

Literature types	Region	Review	Case	Experimental research	Clinical report	Aggregate
Chinese	Near the Yangtze river basin	0	11	1	20	32
	Other areas	2	11	0	13	26
English	Asia	2	0	2	7	11
	Other areas	3	12	0	9	24
Aggregate		7	34	3	49	93(total)

Table 1. The regional distribution of the authors

1.3. Possible etiology

1. Many factors were considered to be related to the onset of PSS, such as allergy, fatigue, mental fatigue, mental stress, decreased body resistance, infection, hypothalamic disorders, autonomic dysfunction, abnormal reactions of ciliary vascular and nervous system and abnormal development in angle of anterior chamber.[1]

2. Recent research had confirmed that concentration of prostaglandins (PGs) in the anterior chamber aqueous increased obviously in the PSS cases, especially that of PGE. [5]

3. Infection by herpes virus.

The conclusion that PSS was caused by herpes simplex virus (HKS) was reported by Yainamotos in 1995, and was confirmed by many following researches. A recent report showed that antiviral treatment reduced the frequency of the outbreak of the disease. [6-7]

It was reported that aqueous humor of a binocular PSS case was collected after suffering from herpes viral keratitis for five months with anterior chamber paracentesis, then DNA of cytomegalovirus (CMV) and HKS were measured by means of quantitative polymerase chain reaction(PCR), the results showed CMV was positive but HKS was negative. It was speculated that CMV which belongs to herpes virus genera would also lead to PSS. It was considered that PSS is not a separate disease, but a kind of anterior uveitis relating to infections of herpes virus.

A study from Singapore showed that the CMV DNA of aqueous humor was positive for 24 of 104 anterior uveitis cases with monocular high IOP, in which 18 cases were PSS, 5 cases were Fuchs heterochromic iridocyclitis (FHI). [8]Another study showed CMV DNA was positive in 35 of 67 PSS cases (52.2%) and in 15 of 35 FHI cases (41.7%). Although the keratic precipitates (KP) in CMV DNA positive anterior uveitis cases was consider to be accompanied with an endothelial halo, clinical difference was not so significant between CMV DNA positive and negative cases as less aqueous humor in sample and weak sensitivity of detection method. In 2008, aqueous analysis for CMV by PCR was performed in 103 eyes of 102 patients with presumed PSS or FHI at the Singapore National Eye Centre. Their records were reviewed for clinical features and human immunodeficiency virus (HIV) status of the CMV-positive patients. The main parameters were age, gender, maximum intraocular pressure, endothelial cell count, endothelial changes, PCR results, and presence of uveitic cataract and/or glaucoma. It was found that there was no clinically detectable differences between CMV-positive and negative presumed PSS eyes. CMV-positive presumed FHI patients are more likely to be male, older at diagnosis or have nodular endothelial lesions. [9]

4. Helicobacter pylori infection.

It was reported in South Korean that there was a significant difference of the positive rate of helicobacter pylori serum antibody between cases with PSS (80%) and cases without PSS (56.2%). In another prospective study, 40 cases with PSS and 73 cases without PSS received serologic analysis for the presence of H. pylori infection by an enzyme-linked immunosorbent assay. The positive rate of serum anti-H. pylori IgG was compared between the two groups. It was proved that H. pylori infection occurred significantly more often in PSS patients. This study suggests that exposure to H. pylori infection is associated with PSS in Korea. [10]

1.4. Clinical features of typical cases [1, 2, 3, 11, 12, 13]

1. In most cases, the disease always attacks the identical eye repeatedly, binocularly affected cases is not common; PSS results in paroxysmal increase of IOP repeatedly, which reaches as high as 40 to 60 mmHg, and lasts for 1 to 14 days generally, 1 month occasionally, 2 months rarely; interval of onset is from months to 2 years;

2. Symptoms are not obvious, just mild discomfort for most cases;

3. Eyesight is normal generally, blurred vision when suffers from corneal edema at onset;

4. Pupil becomes slightly bigger with normal reaction to light, and never adheres to lens;

5. The KP of PSS appeared in a few days after or before the elevation of IOP with number of 1 to 25, took a form of hoar and suet-shaped and disappeared days to 1 month after the IOP returned normal, distributed mainly in the inferior part of the cornea or concealed in the trabecular meshwork. There were no or at most a few planktonic cells in aqueous while the flare was negative.There is no inflammatory cell in vitreous body (See Figure 1);

6. The anterior chamber angle is open, no matter IOP is normal or elevated; visual field and fundus of most cases are normal generally, but a reversible expanding of vascular shadow may occur during an acute onset.

7. Coefficient of outflow facility (C value) descends in episodes and recovers in intermission; various stimulation tests for glaucoma are negative in intermission;

8. The forms of onset of PSS could be divided into three kinds: KP, high IOP and intermediate type, according to relationship between KP and IOP.

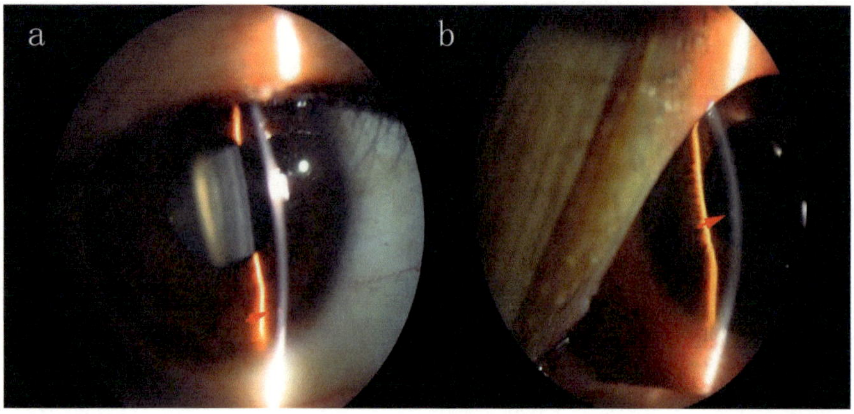

Figure 1. Anterior segment of a case with PSS in episodes. Arrows indicate the typital hoar and suet-shaped KP.

Typical case

A patient complained of her blurred vision two months ago, examination in other hospital showed: conjunctiva of her left eye wasn't congestive and the cornea was edematous mildly, IOP: 34/ 18(R/L) mmHg; there were some round lipid-like KP in the left cornea, aqueous flare(-). She came to our hospital on June 7, 2012, ophthalmologic examination: vision was 0.5/ 1.5(R/L), best corrected vision of left eye was 1.2(-1.25DS), IOP: 18/ 13 (R/L) mmHg. Her right eye was normal, conjunctiva of her left eye wasn't congestive and there were five rounds lipid-like KP in the left cornea, binocular C/D was 0.4. Her KP faded away after the treatment of chloromethyl and pranopulin (three times a day) for three weeks. Examination of FFA, ICGA and Virus screening were normal on July 10.The measurement of her 24 hours IOP performed two weeks after she ceased the drugs was 20-14mmHg(R), 15-12 mmHg (L). The result of her visual field and the OCT for glaucoma was normal. She was diagnosed as PSS in left eye and suggested to be observed and treated timely.

1.5. Treatment of typical cases in episodes

1. Anti-inflammation: Corticosteroid drugs is needed in most cases, but it should not be used too long at a time, so as not to cause the corticosteroid glaucoma.

2. It is a better select in some cases to apply non-steroidal anti-inflammatory drugs (NSAIDs) such as eye drops of pranoprofen, indomethacin and flufenamic acid.

3. Reducing IOP: Eye drops of epinephrine, timolol, or clonidine was needed singly or jointly for common patient, carbonic anhydrase inhibitor orally when the IOP is higher than 30mmHg and mannitol of intravenous drip when the IOP is higher than 40mmHg.

4. The antiviral treatment systemically or implanting long-acting agents may be helpful to reduce the frequency of attack, but it has worrying and serious side effects and costs too much. [12]

1.6. The outstanding clinical questions and the main points of the chapter

It was considered in the early years that PSS have a favorable prognosis without glaucomatous damage of optic disk and visual field, however, a number of authors have confirmed that part of the PSS cases suffered from glaucomatous damage similar to that in primary glaucoma patients in recent years. A lot of questions remained vague such as monocular or binocular explode, age of onset, the detailed features of its IOP and KP, the incidence and degree and relating factors of glaucomatous damage, especially the clinical approaches via which the damage occurred and disease complicated with PSS. These brought about to two undesirable consequences: on the one hand, PSS patients were misdiagnosed as primary glaucoma and received incorrect treatment even led to serious adverse consequences due to the lack of knowledge on the clinical characteristics of PSS; on the other hand, most cases of PSS combined with primary glaucoma especially those with primary angle-closed glaucoma were failed to be diagnosed correctly without delay, thus the best opportunity of treatment was lost ; severe damage occurred.

In recent decades, although there were some clinical observations reported by a number of authors on these clinical problems mentioned above, no report of continuous and systematic study was found. A mountain of work in this field had been done in our hospital and some research results were obtained. A brief introduction of our results will be shown in this chapter in combination with the research achievements of other authors.

2. The main results of our clinical research

The main results of our clinical research included 4 fields as follows: the clinical characteristics of PSS; the glaucomatous optic nerve damage in PSS patients; the clinical approach of optic nerve damage in PSS patients; other diseases concomitant with PSS.

2.1. Study on the clinical characteristics of the PSS

The research about clinical characteristics of the PSS included four aspects: clinical observation and analysis of monocular primary open-angle glaucoma(POAG) and binocular PSS; clinical features of elderly PSS patients; characteristics and clinical value of the intraocular pressure and the C-value in PSS patients ; the characteristic of postural intraocular pressure change in PSS patients.

2.1.1. Clinical observation and analysis of monocular primary open-angle glaucoma and binocular PSS

Background: As we knew, most of POAG patients are binocularly involved, while monocular attack is one of typical features of PSS. However, clinically suspected monocular POAG patients are not rare and binocular PSS cases are often reported. So following questions should be put forward based on the facts as follows [3, 11, 14]: Does monocular POAG really exist? What are the differences between monocular and binocularly involved PSS cases? Is there any relationship between the monocular POAG and binocular PSS?

Objects and methods: A long-term, systematic clinical observation and analysis were completed on 121 cases with tentative diagnosis of POAG (22 cases of monocular) and 126 cases of PSS (17 cases of which was binocular). (See figure2)

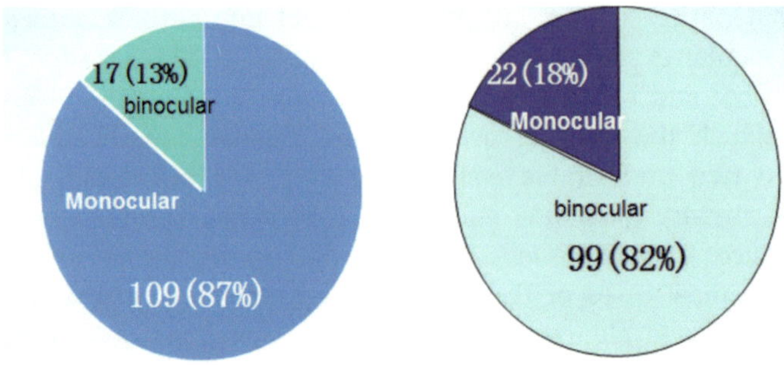

Figure 2. Distribution of monocular and binocular cases in PSS and POAG

Results

1. Glaucomatous visual field damage of monocular/ binocular PSS and binocular POAG

analysis of the clinical data of patients without doubt with the chi-square test showed: (1) The incidence of glaucomatous visual field damage in binocular PSS (15/16) was much higher than that in monocular cases(30/85), (X^2=27.43, P<0.01). (2) The damage in 26 of 30 monocular cases were in early stage, while that in 9 of 15 binocular cases were in middle/ last stage, the difference was significant(X^2=3.53, P<0.01). (3) There is no significant difference in incidence and degree of glaucomatous visual field damage between binocular PSS and binocular POAG.(See Table 2)

2. Visual field damage in binocular PSS

15 of 17 binocular PSS cases were confirmed with glaucomatous visual field damage, that was much more serious than in monocular cases; however, no remarkable difference was found between the course of disease in monocular and binocular cases. (See Figure3)

The result suggests that the course of disease cannot explain the severity of visual field damage in binocular PSS. We speculate that binocular PSS may be more relevant to POAG essentially through the following two ways. First, the insufficiency in adjusting IOP results in combination with POAG in some cases; secondly, the weak resistance of optic nerve to high IOP make it easy for a cumulative effect of high intraocular pressure during attacks of pure PSS to bring about visual field damage.

2. Results of clinical follow-up to monocular POAG

The results of clinical follow-up observation on the 22 cases with clinically suspected monocular POAG are as follows: 15 of the 22 cases were confirmed not to be POAG, 9 of them had been proved to be PSS. Although no definite diagnoses were made in the other 7 cases, but

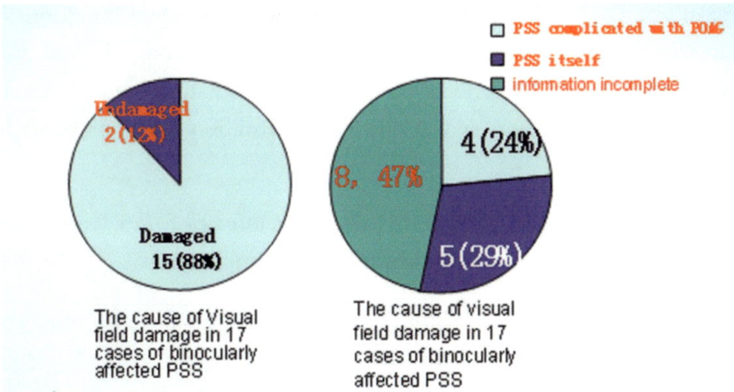

Figure 3. Results of visual field examination and defect in binocular PSS.

clinical manifestations contradictory with POAG were found in most cases, 3 of them were suspected of PSS.(See Figure4)

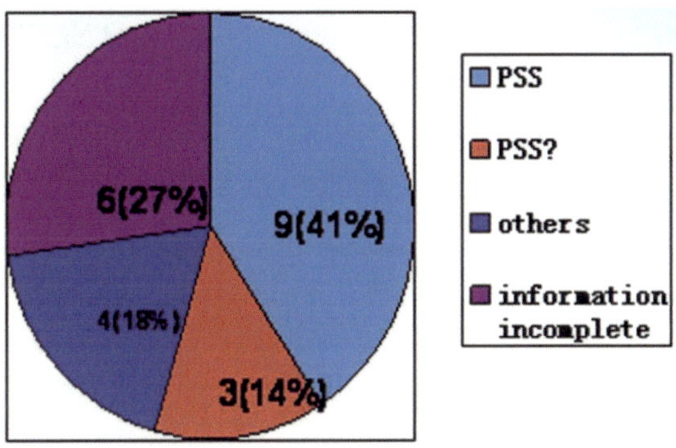

Figure 4. Results of clinical follow-up to monocular POAG.

The result suggests that the diagnosis of monocular POAG should be very careful, in addition to angle closure glaucoma and other secondary glaucoma, PSS which appears late or last transitorily should not be ignored. Close attention to slit lamp examination for KP and its relationship with IOP should be paid for such cases.

All in all, it cannot be stated too strongly: we should be very deliberative when making a diagnosis of monocular POAG or binocular PSS, as half part of suspicious monocular POAG cases were confirmed with PSS after clinical follow-up, and there was a closer connection between binocular PSS and POAG. [15]

2.1.2. Clinical observation of aged PSS cases

Background: Among the cases of PSS, the 50s are rare; the 60s are seldom. What is the feature of the aged PSS cases?

Objects and methods: The clinical data of 14 cases aged above 50 with a definite diagnosis of PSS collected in the past 4 years were summarized and analyzed. Clinical data met all the requirements were obtained in 11cases. The cases aged from 50 to 73 years old, with an average of 61.4 years. One case had a course of the disease beyond 30 years, 4 beyond 10 years and 6 beyond 5 years.

Results: Visual acuity of more than half of the cases was inferior to 0.5, 9 of 11 cases had visual field damage that was of moderate or advanced stage in most cases.

Conclusion: The aged PSS cases had a longer course of the disease and much more frequent and serious visual function damage. [16, 17, 18]

2.1.3. The characteristics and clinical value of the intraocular pressure and the C-value in PSS cases

Background: It is generally acknowledged that IOP of the attacked eye increased and C-value of attack eye decreased in episodes, and both were normal in intermission. Individual author reported that the IOP of the affected eye was lower than that of the fellow one in part of cases, and C-value was higher. It was not confirmed that whether this phenomenon could be considered as the unique characteristic of PSS and what clinical significance should it mean. [3, 19, 20]

Objective and methods: Binocular IOP measurement and tonography were done in 90 cases of PSS; According to the symptom, sign and results of examination for IOP, fundus, visual field, our cases were divided into 3 groups. Group A (typical type): with a normal optic disc, visual field and the diagnostic tests for glaucoma in intermission. Group B (development type): with a damaged optic disc and visual field; except for high intraocular pressure in episodes, binocular IOP and C values were normal. Group C (mixed type): with a damaged optic disc, visual field and abnormal results of binocular IOP, IOP diurnal variation and C value in both episodes and intermission. Another group case of primary glaucoma with a great fluctuation and difference in IOP level between his or her right and left eye was taken as the control group.

Results: IOP of PSS cases in group A and B increased in episodes, and were obviously higher than that of the fellow eye; C-value of them decreased and was lower. In intermission, binocular IOP and C-value turned normal, moreover, IOP of attacked eye was lower than that of the fellow one, and its C-value was higher. It means that binocular IOP and C-value in episodes and intermission were crossed-over.

Crossed-over phenomenon of binocular IOP and C-value had not appeared in the control group (primary glaucoma) as well as Group C (PSS combined with POAG).

Conclusion: Such an inference could be deduced based on our results that Crossed-over phenomenon of IOP and C-value was one characteristic for pure PSS cases, it is conducive to distinguish pure PSS from primary glaucoma and PSS combined with POAG to observe this phenomenon.

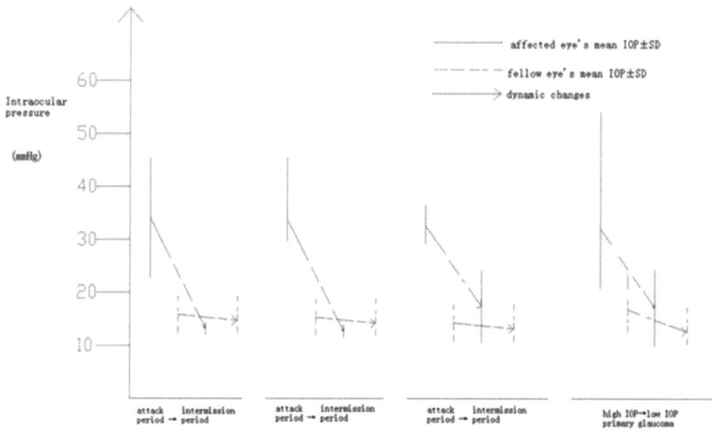

Figure 5. The difference of C-value and its dynamic changes between 3 PSS groups (A, B, C) and primary glaucoma

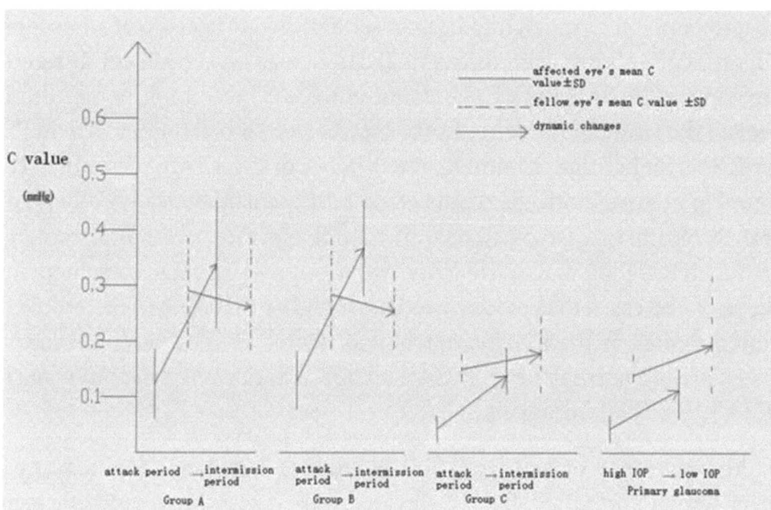

Figure 6. The difference of IOP and its dynamic changes between 3 PSS groups (A, B, C) and primary glaucoma

2.1.4. The characteristics of postural IOP change in PSS cases

Background: It is well known that the recumbent IOP is higher than sedentary one in most of people; however, such an IOP change in PSS cases was not reported so far.

Objective: The cases of PSS with regular IOP change, 42 cases of POAG and 61 cases of PACG with a great wave in IOP level. [21]

Methods: IOP measurement was performed with a handheld applanation tonometer before and after lying for five and thirty minutes, and a tonography was finished 1~3 days before or after postural IOP measurement. (See Figure7)

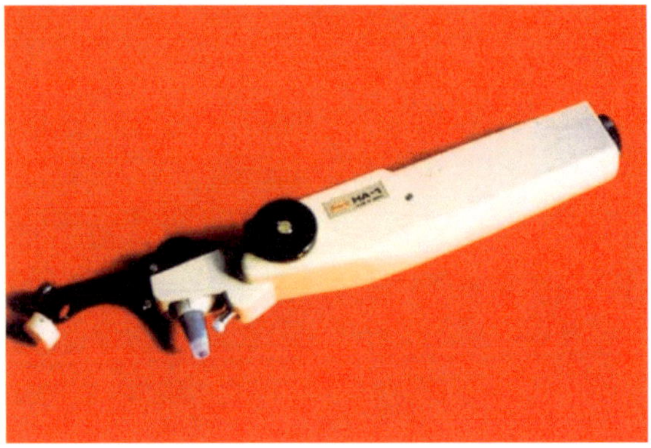

Figure 7. Handheld applanation tonometer.

Results: 1) Recumbent IOP is much higher than sedentary one in cases of all groups, however, their rising degrees after lying were different.2) There was no significant difference in rising degrees after lying in three kinds of glaucoma when IOP was high; when the IOP turned normal, however, the rising degrees in POAG, PACG were much higher than in PSS. 3) When the sedentary IOP is higher than 24mmHg, the number of cases with recumbent IOP elevated more than 5mmHg in three kinds glaucoma wasn't different statistically; When the sedentary IOP is lower than 24mmHg, cases with recumbent IOP elevated more than 5mmHg were rare in PSS group, much less than that in the other two groups. 4) The IOP increment after lying in the attacked eye of PSS cases in episodes was much higher than that of the fellow eye and the both eye in intermission. 5) The IOP increment was related to C value significantly for POAG when IOP was high and normal, for PACG when IOP was normal only; but wasn't related for PSS no matter IOP was high or normal.

Conclusion: Measurement of postural IOP change is beneficial to diagnose suspicious glaucoma cases with a normal or slightly elevated IOP, it may be as valuable as tonography clinically but more convenient, comfort and safer than tonography, complications such as corneal scratches were rarely seen in the measurement of postural IOP change

Discussion: Different pathogenesis of the three kinds of glaucoma brought about the different pattern in correlation between the IOP increment and C value in different conditions. PACG is caused by the closed anterior chamber angle, when the IOP is high, the increased IOP is related to C value significantly as the closed anterior chamber angle loses the ability to reduce IOP, however, the adjustability recovery as the anterior chamber angle open partly when the IOP is low. Degeneration of trabecular meshwork which result in more and more futile eduction function of aqueous humour was the primary mechanism for the increased IOP in POAG, so the IOP increment in POAG cases is related to C value significantly whenever the

IOP is high or low as the adjustability for IOP had been declining eventually. PSS is a secondary glaucoma for which the intermittent increased release of PGs maybe the primary mechanism. Increases PGs may expand the blood vessels and recedes eduction function of trabecular meshwork. On the contrary, the diluent PGs in remission promotes eduction function of aqueous humour and inturn IOP and C value to normal or even better. Therefore, there is no significant correlation between the IOP increment and C value no matter IOP was high or normal. [20, 22, 23]

2.2. The visual field damage in PSS cases

Although reports about that glaucomatous optical neural damage occurred in some cases of PSS were constantly released for past twenty years, we saw little of the systematic research aimed at the incidence, severity and probable relating facts of the damage. [3, 9]

2.2.1. Incidence and severity of the damage

Objective: To study the incidence and severity of the visual field damage in PSS cases.

Methods: Visual field examinations at regular intervals with perimeter of Goldmann or Humphrey 750 type were completed in 145 cases of PSS followed up for 5 to 15 years and 166 cases of POAG observed meanwhile (as the control). [17]

Results: The prevalence of visual field damage in PSS and POAG was 35.43% and 93.42% (P<0.001), 72.11% of the field damage in PSS cases was of early or suspected stage, 78.92% of that in POAG cases was of middle or late stage(P<0.001), 10% of PSS cases suffered a field damage of middle or late stage, 2 became absolute blind and one case had developed into bullous keratitis at last.(See Figure8)

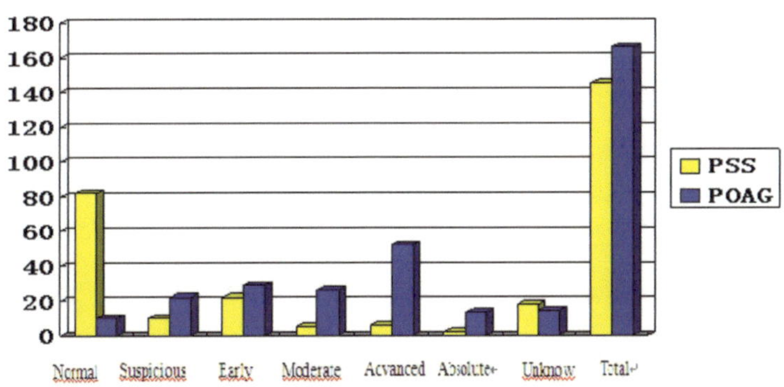

Figure 8. The stage distribution of visual field damage in PSS and POAG.

Conclusions: Even though the visual field damage in cases of PSS was less and slighter than that in cases of POAG, it is necessary to treat PSS efficiently and timely, as recurrent attacks of PSS for long period would result in a sad outcome like POAG.

2.2.2. The characteristic of the visual field damage in PSS

Objective: To study the characteristic of the visual field damage in PSS.

Methods: Compare the visual field damage in glaucoma cases with higher and lower IOP (PSS belongs to that with higher IOP). [24]

Results: 1) The visual field damage in cases with lower IOP is less and slighter than that in cases with higher IOP. 2) Paracentral, arcuate and ring scotoma was more seen in cases with normal IOP, while constriction of visual field and nasal field were more common in cases with higher IOP. 3) Most of the visual field damages in cases with higher IOP come from the periphery. (See Figure 9)

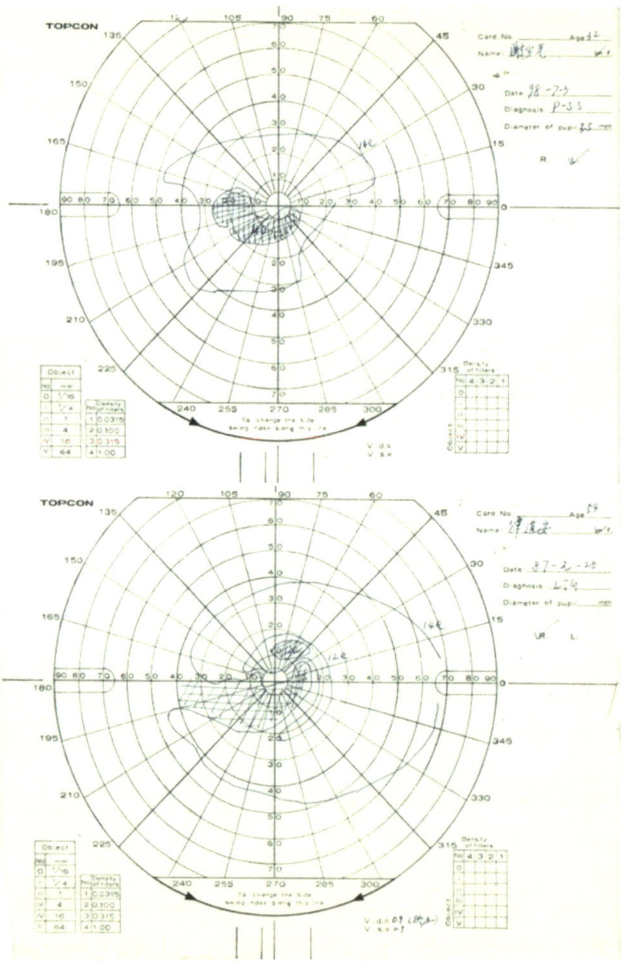

Figure 9. Visual field of a PSS case and a LTG case. The visual field damages in PSS case exist in the periphery area(A), on the contrary, those in glaucoma case with normal IOP exist in the centre area(B).

Conclusions: There are difference in visual field defects between higher IOP patients and lower IOP patients.

2.2.3. Relating factors of the visual field damage in PSS

Objective: To study the relating factors of the visual field damage in PSS.

Methods: Analysis the clinical data of 145 PSS cases and 166 POAG cases for recent 15 years.Results about the incidence and severity of visual field damage in the two kinds of glaucoma had been showed above.

Results: 1) Compared with the undamaged group of PSS, the damaged cases were older and with longer course of the disease while there was no remarkable difference in the averaged IOP value during crisis. 2) There was a much higher risk for the visual field damage in binocular cases of PSS. Most of the cases of PSS reported were monocular affected, but later, there were reports about some binocularly affected cases. In our study, 15 of the 35 cases with definite damage were binocularly affected while only one of the 82 cases without damage was affected binocularly. It needs further study to determine whether there is different pathological mechanism for the monocular and binocularly involved cases of PSS. 3) IOP manifestation: although no great difference in the average IOP value during crisis was found between the two groups of PSS, the damage group showed a higher average IOP between crises and included much more cases with an abnormal diurnal and nocturnal variance of IOP or without the IOP crossed-over phenomenon than the undamaged group. These data indicated that the adjustment of IOP between crises was insufficient in those PSS patients with visual field damage. Loss of IOP crossed-over phenomenon meant that other than PSS there were some factors affecting the IOP. [25]

Conclusions: These data indicated that the harmful effect of the raised IOP during crises of PSS on the optic disc could be accumulated.

2.3. The clinical approach of optic nerve damage in Posner Schlossman syndrome

In recent years a number of authors have confirmed that glaucomatous optic nerve damage similar to that in primary glaucoma cases occurred in part of the PSS cases, but the clinical approach of the occurrence was not reported. Clinical data of cases with PSS during a period of 25 years in our hospital was collected and analyzed, and four clinical approaches via which the damage occurred in PSS cases were deduced.

Propose

To investigate the clinical approaches of optic nerve damage in PSS patients.

Methods

208 cases with PSS during the recent 25 years collected in our hospital(male 124 cases, female84 cases), from 9 to 71 years old, with an average of 39.56±12.80. Diagnosis standard for PSS was basically accorded to clinical features described by Posner and Schlossman, except for the cases who suffered binocularly or had damage were contained in. [23, 26]

Research project of first diagnosis at the first attendance in our hospital

History, eyesight, intraocular pressure of episode and intermission, depth of anterior chamber, gonioscope or UBM, intraocular pressure during 24 hours in intermission without eyedrops more than five days, panretinal scope or OCT, FFA in episode of part cases, and so on.

Analytical methods

1. Analysis for damage

Standard: repeatable glaucomatous visual field damage and corresponding fundus performance

2. Stage division standard of glaucomatous visual field damage(see Table2)

Without defect	static visual field: no more than 2 clusters of spots with sensitivity reduces more than 5dB, no spot with sensitivity reduces more than 5dB; dynamic visual field: no nasal step and temporal quadrantanopsia more than 10 degrees, no significantly constriction of visual field (except for refractive interstitial lesions and retinopathy)
Early stage	paracentral scotoma, nasal step, temporal quadrantanopsia, arcuate scotoma not linked with physiological blind spot
Moderate stage	arcuate scotoma linked with physiological blind spot, nasal hemianopsia,ring scotoma, constriction of visual field more than 30 degrees,
Advanced stage	tubular visual field
Absolute stage	no light perception

Table 2. Staging standard of glaucomatous visual field defect

3. Classification method

According to the results of comprehensive and dynamical analysis of the clinical data of each cases and classification method as shown in table 3, each case was discriminated for the clinical approach of optic nerve damage. [20,21,22,24,27,28]

	A		B		C		D	
	Early stage	Later stage	Early stage	later stage	Early stage	later stage	Early stage	later stage
Age of onset	middle-aged and aged people		middle-aged and aged people		most middle-aged and aged people		middle-aged and aged people	
Family history of glaucoma	usually not		usually not		sometimes have		most have	
Monocular/ binoculus	monocular		monocular		monocular KP, binocular high IOP or eyes alternate		monocular KP,binocular high IOP	
Typical PSS course	positive	positive	positive	negative	Intermittent attack with binocular high IOP		positive	negative

			A		B		C		D	
			Early stage	Later stage	Early stage	later stage	Early stage	later stage	Early stage	later stage
IOP	Episodes	Sick eye	rise	rise	rise	rise	higher	higher	rise	rise
		another eye	normal	normal	normal	normal	high	high	high*/normal	high*/normal
	Intermission	Sick eye	normal	normal	normal	rise	high	high	high*/normal	high*/normal
		another eye	normal	normal	normal	normal	high	high	high*/normal	high*/normal
	Cross phenomenon of IOP		positive		positive	negative	negative	negative	positive */ negative	positive */ negative
	IOP of 24 hours in period of intermittent		normal	normal	normal	abnormal	abnormal	abnormal	abnormal */ normal	abnormal */ normal
Anterior chamber depth			normal	normal	normal	normal	normal	normal	A little shallow	Very shallow
Anterior chamber angle			medium width	medium width	medium width	medium width	medium width	medium width	narrow II-III	narrow III-IV

Table 3. Classification method of the clinical approach for optic nerve damage in PSS

Results

1. Incidence and stage distribution of glaucomatous optic nerve damage

190 cases of 208 patients with PSS had a set of complete material. There were 71 cases (34.1%) with optic nerve damage, in which 12 cases (16.9%) regarded as suspicious damage, 59 cases(83.1%) regarded as definite damage.

Stage distribution of glaucomatous optic nerve damage was shown in Table 4:

Early stage	Moderate stage	Advanced stage	Absolute stage	total
35	11	11	2	59
59.32%	18.64%	18.64%	3.39%	100%

Table 4. Stage of glaucomatous optic nerve damage in 59 cases regarded as clear damage

2. The clinical approach of optic nerve damage

Four clinical approaches via which the damage occurred in PSS were deduced, they were represented as Type A, B, C and D.

Type A Cumulative effect of repeated episode of high intraocular pressure of pure PSS leads to visual field damage: 27 cases

Type B Recurrent attacks of PSS which results in secondary trabecular meshwork damage causes secondary open-angle glaucoma: 6 cases

Type C PSS combined with primary open-angle glaucoma: 19 cases

Type D PSS combined with primary closed-angle glaucoma: 7 cases

Composition of the clinical approach in 59 cases regarded as definite glaucomatous optic nerve damage was showed in Figure10

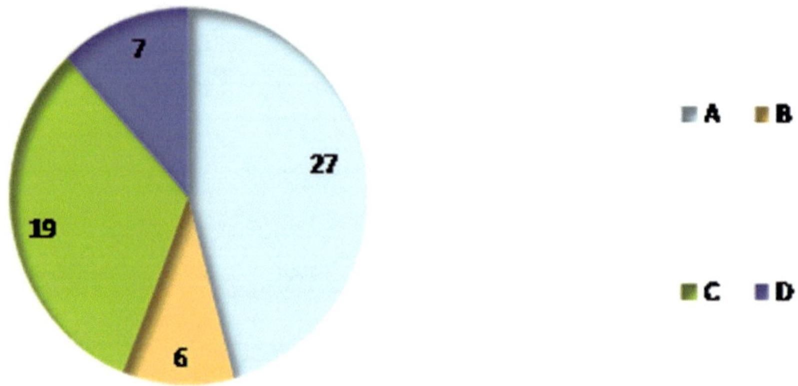

Figure 10. The distribution of clinical approach of optic nerve damage in PSS.

Distribution of stage of visual field damage in different optic nerve damage approacheswas showed in Table 5.

	Early stage	moderate stage	advanced stage	absolute stage	total
Type A	17	7	1	2	27
Type B	2	2	2	0	6
Type C	5	7	7	0	19
Type D	2	3	2	0	7

Table 5. Visual field damage in different type of PSS patients

There is no significant difference in the stage distribution of visual field damage in different type of PSS patients. (X^2=6.904, P>0.05).Make the early and moderate stage as one group, advanced and absolute stage as another group, Statistical result shows that there is significant difference in the stage distribution of visual field damage in different type of PSS patients. The incidence of early stage of glaucomatous visual field damage in Type A (63%) was higher. While 7 of 19 Type C cases were in advanced stage.

Conclusion: Most cases in type A suffered an early stage damage, and most in other types suffered a moderate or advanced stage damage, but there were 2 cases in type A who had gone to absolute stage.

http://dx.doi.org/10.5772/58348

Discussion

1. The clinical approach of optic nerve damage in Posner-Schlossman syndrome.

In the past PSS was considered to be a self-limited disease and has a favorable prognosis, however, in recent years a number of authors have confirmed that part of the PSS cases suffered glaucomatous optic nerve damage similar to those in primary glaucoma cases, but the incidence, degree, related factors and clinical approach of the occurrence is unknown. This part focused on the clinical approach of optic nerve damage in Posner-Schlossman syndrome after aforementioned researches. Reports about optic nerve damage caused by PSS combined with primary open-angle glaucoma were common; the other types were seldom reported. Systematic research aiming at this question has never been seen so far at home and abroad. We determined the damage approach by analyzing each patient's clinical data dynamically and comprehensively according to the discrimination method established on the basis of relating literatures and the results of our long-term systematic study, and got the conclusion that there were four clinical approaches via which the damage occurred. Beyond all question, further research, supplement and correct is necessary in this field, but the method and result of our study may be a wind vane for the further researches.

2. Clinical features and treatment principle for cases with damage from different clinical approach

(1) Type A Cumulative effect of repeated episodes of high intraocular pressure of pure PSS leads to damage

Clinical features

Except for visual field damage, type A cases complied with the basic characteristics of typical PSS: monocular attacked; intermittently onset of high intraocular pressure with hoar and suet-shaped KP ; normal intraocular pressure(including 24 hours intraocular pressure) of the fellow eye in episode and the both eyes in intermission ; Crossed-over phenomenon and postural changes of IOP; normal anterior chamber depth; wide anterior chamber angle; visual field change of vascular shadow usually appears in episode and recover in intermission at the initial in most cases, and true visual field damage is of mild and early stage usually, but loss of light perception can be seen in a few cases; the attack lasts a long time frequently in middle-aged and aged people for long course, also with higher IOP; heterochromia iridis occurred in later stage in some cases. (See Figure11) [20, 22, 29]

Treatment principle

Enough attention should be paid to treatment for each attack, in which the most important is controlling intraocular pressure timely and effectively. Surgery is necessary for the cases with excessive frequent attacks, heavy damage or obvious progress of his damage.

The surgery method and the time: glaucoma valve or EX-press glaucoma filtration device implantation may be suit for cases with excessive frequent attack, high IOP but light inflammation (intermission or episodes); trabeculectomy could be selected for cases with low attack frequency, high IOP as well as severe inflammation (intermission only).

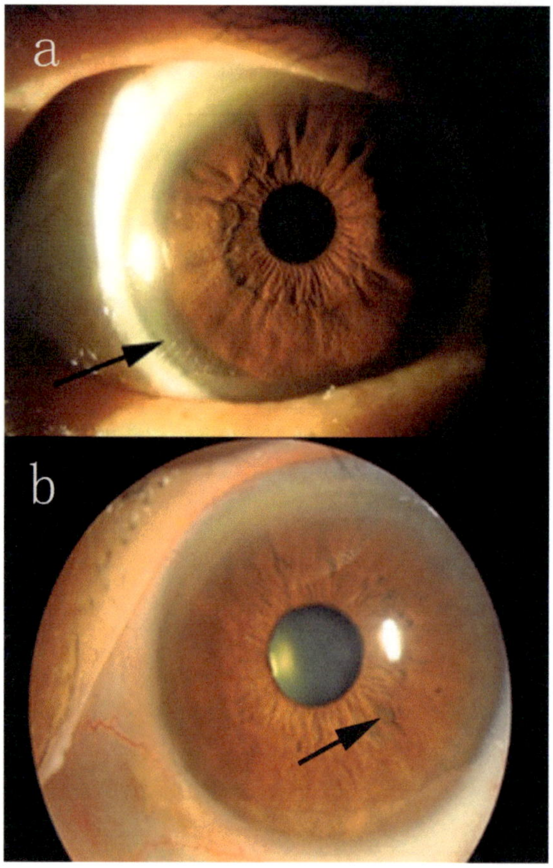

Figure 11. The iridis of a PSS patient.(A)is that of the normal eye,(B) is that of the affected eye.

Typical cases 1) A patient visited our hospital and was diagnosed as glaucomatocyclitis crisis of left eye in other hospital six years ago. In the initial stage, she attacked once or twice per year with duration of 3~7 days for each attack and ceased spontaneously, then the frequency of attack increased and the duration extended. This attack happened one month before this visits to our hospital and stop one week ago without use of any drug. Examination at first visit: Vision 1.0(OU), IOP19.7mmHg(R), 12mmHg (L), anterior chambers of both eyes were not shallow, iris color was symmetrical, KP (-).Fundus examination: C/D0.3(R) 0.6(L), there wasn't other abnormalities. She was diagnosed as secondary glaucoma of left eye. On September 13 (10 days after withdrawal), the 24 hours IOP of both eyes were measured: right eye: 14-18mmHg, left eye 12-14mmHg, Corneal thickness: right eye: 584μm, left eye: 575μm. She was diagnosed as "glaucomatocyclitis crisis in left eye." Another onset lasted for more than 10 days, IOP of the left eye was 43mmHg, there was 2hoar and suet--like KP and faded iris pigment in left eye. There were total seven attacks in one year, with the duration from 1 week to 20 days, during one of which the KP appeared 9day after the occurrence. 24 hours IOP during this episode: right

Eye: 14-19mmHg, left Eye: 23-29mmHg; iris depigmentation of her left eye exacerbated, no abnormal was found with fundus angiography. The recent onset occurred in September this year, the medication of hormone and pranopulin continued for 3 months, with another minor attack during thatthis period.

She made another visit to our hospital one year later. It was found that the iris of her left eye appeared a typical "rain dozen sand samples", meanwhile, there were two off-white round medium-sized lipid-like KP and she was diagnosed as "left eye glaucomatocyclitic crisis with heterochromatic iris." Since then, the attack occurred more frequently, with frequency of 1 to 2 times per month, the visual field damage exacerbated. She was hospitalized in our department, and the surgery of glaucoma valve implantation was performed. Postoperative intraocular pressure: 19mmHg for her right eye and 6mmHg for her left eye:, visual acuity1.0 left eye (with pin hole) for her both eye, and the syndrome did not attack postoperation. (Clinical data please see Figure 12)

Typical Case 2)

A patient was hospitalized in our hospital for the reason of "intermittent pain of left eye for 25years, decrease of vision for 20 years, blind for 1 year". The patient had a history of intermittent episodes of pain and blurred vision with his left eye for 25 years, which occurred 1 to 2 times per month with the duration of 3 to 5 days, and than self-cured. In many hospitals he was diagnosed as "glaucomatocyclitic crisis" and treated with medication irregularly The occurrence becomes more frequently in the recent 10 years, and the duration longer, and the vision recessions gradually. In the intermittent period, he was hospitalized for systematic examination. The visual acuity was 1.0 for his right eye and no light perception for his left eye. All the results of IOP, tonography, 24 hours IOP measurement and other tests during the intermittent period were normal for his both eyes. The result of the medical examination at this hospitalization showed as following: his right eye had a corrected visual acuity of 1.0, IOP 14mmHg, C/D 0.4, wide anterior chamber angle; his left eye had no light perception, intraocular pressure 56mmHg, C / D1.0, width of N1 ~ N3 for the anterior chamber angle with some small limited adhesions; corneal edema, a dozen of round lipid-like KP.

Without any treatment, the IOP of his fell to 14mmHg within one week. All results of examinations including 24 hours IOP measurement, drinking water experiment, dark room prone test for his right eye were normal. Laboratory results of systemic body check were normal.

His left eye still had attacks of PSS after he left hospital and each attack was self-limited. The IOP and 24-hour IOP during the intermittent period were measured to be normal, and his left eye had an IOP lower than that of his right eye, a typical IOP cross phenomenon appeared every time. Three years later, the fundus and visual field of his right eye kept normal. (Clinical data see Figure 13)

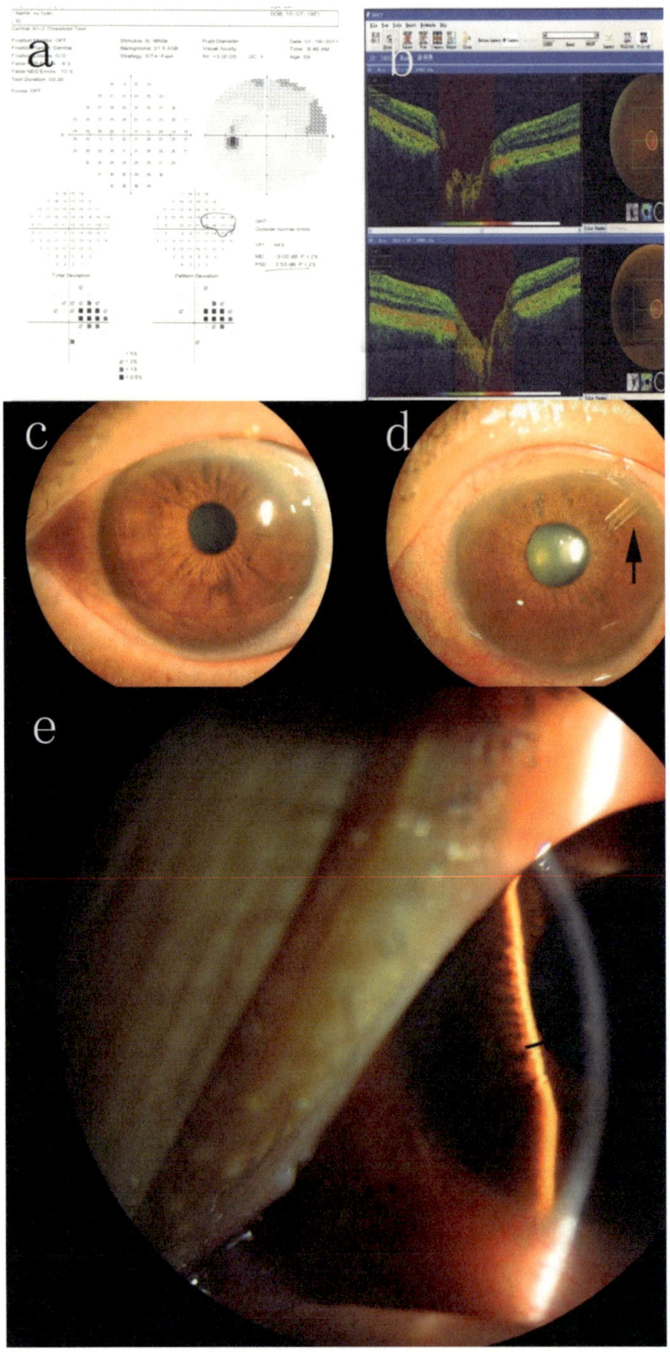

Figure 12. Clinical data of a cases suffered from PSS with glaucomatous optic nerve damage combined with heterochromia iris (Clinical number 488368).Visual field (A) and Optical Coherence Tomography (B) indicate glaucoma damages;Anterio segment of normal right eye(C) and left eye(D),arrow shows heterochmia iris and KP in the attacked eye(E).

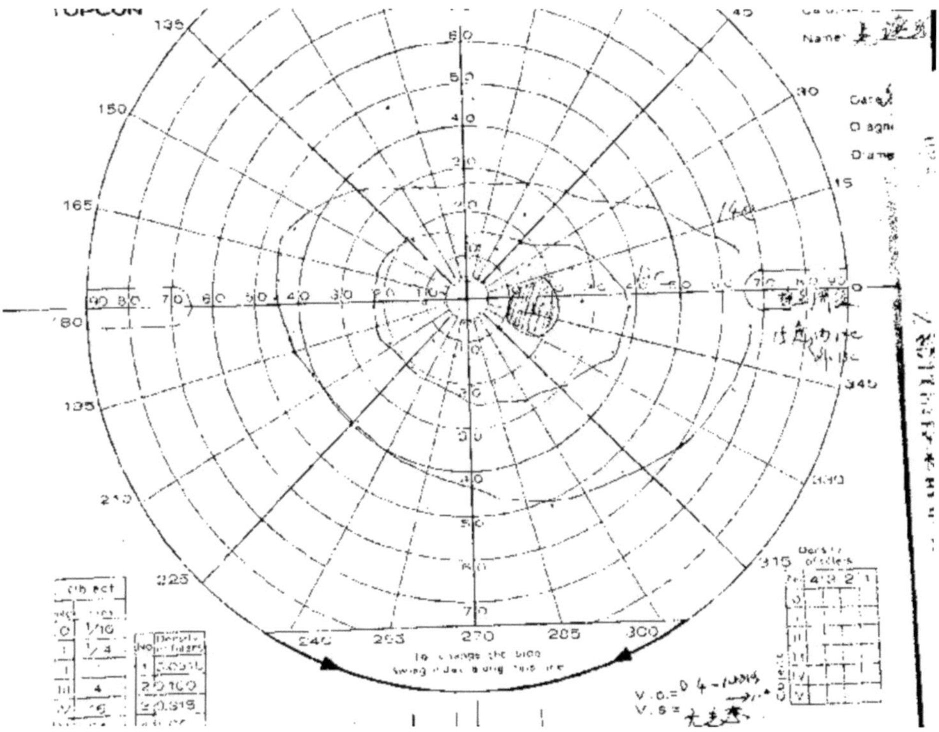

Figure 13. Visual field of the right eye of patient (Clinical number 241163).PSS results in blind of his left eye, but the visual field of his right eye without PSS is normal.

(2) Type B secondary open-angle glaucoma from secondary damage to trabecular meshwork by recurrent attacks of PSS

Clinical features

Type B cases complied with the basic characteristics (above mentioned) of typical PSS in early stage. These characteristics lost eventually as the damage to trabecular meshwork gradually accelerated, the attack takes place more frequently and lasts a longer and longer time with a higher and higher IOP, and serious visual field damage developed at last.[30, 31] However, the fundus, visual field, IOP in intermittent and episode of the fellow eye maintained normal. Patients of this type usually had a long course of the disease with an older age.

Treatment principle

It is necessary to reduce IOP with drugs according to extent and characteristics of elevated IOP and diminish inflammation with hormone of weak effect on elevating IOP for short time, for example, lotemax. PGA is useful and myotic is prohibitive. Surgery or other treatment (SLT, trabeculectomy, glaucoma valve or EX-press implantation) should be taken into account according to the IOP level controlled by drugs in intermittent and the situation of visual field damage.

Typical case

A patient was diagnosed as "left eye PSS" with the complain of vision decline associated with distending pain of his left eye in other hospitals five years ago. The medical records of other hospitals showed: IOP and other relating examinations of the right eye in episode and these in intermittent period of his both eyes was normal at the initial stage. The visual acuity decreased gradually, IOP fluctuated from 32 to 48 mmHg in recent years. He was hospitalized in our hospital three times, the results of clinical observation showed: IOP including 24 hours IOP in intermittent period, the fundus and visual field of his right eye appeared normal; while IOP of his left eye was high frequently and higher when PSS attacked, 24 hours IOP in intermittent period appeared abnormal including the highest IOP and IOP variation. The left eye was diagnosed as secondary open-angle glaucoma from secondary damage to trabecular meshwork by recurrent attacks of PSS, and then a trabecuectomy was performed on his left eye. Postoperative IOP of his left eye was from 12 to 10mmHg in intermittent period, 20 to 31 mmHg in episodes, while his right eye kept normal in all ways. (Clinical data see Figure 14)

(3) Type C PSS combined with primary open-angle glaucoma

Clinical features

Monocular/ binocular paroxysmal increased IOP with mild cyclitis; wide anterior chamber angle; binocular abnormal IOP and visual field damage; high average IOP; great fluctuation of IOP level; absence of IOP cross phenomenon; PSS attacks at the same eye in most cases; at the two eyes alternately or at the same time in a few cases; visual field damage was serious, and more serious in the eye often attacked by PSS.[27, 32]

Treatment principle

Enough attention should be given to the treatment for cases of this type, whose incidence reached up to 31% as reported. Drug treatment is similar to that of POAG, but in episode of PSS, corticosteroid is useful transitorily, while PGA and myotic is prohibitive. Indication of surgery is similar to that of POAG, but classical trabeculectomy should be performed in intermission, and the effect and safety of non-penetrating trabeculectomy, implantation of Ahmed glaucoma valve or EX-PRESS Glaucoma Filtration Device has not been confirmed. Laser trabeculoplasty(ALT), Selective laser trabeculoplasty (SLT) or Pneumatic trabeculoplasty (PNT) should be adopted in intermission, however, there has no related report. [11, 33, 34, 35]

Typical cases

A patient reported of discomfort and blurred vision of her left eye for more than 1 year, the patient was diagnosed as POAG in other hospital 10 days ago. Clinical date of that time showed: KP (-), IOP16.3/42.7(R/L), and she was treated with Travoprost Eye Drops to her left eye and brimonidine and brinzolamide to the both eye. 1 week after treatment, her IOP turned to 36/17(R/L), the treatment had been changed to travoprost, brimonidine and brinzolamide for the both eye. The results of examination in our hospital showed as follows: visual acuity R1.0 (-1.25DS),L0.05(-3.75DS), IOP17(OU); absence of conjunctiva hyperemia; cup/disc ratios 0.8 OD and0.9OS,and inferior RNFLD(by OCT:) in the both eye; severe glaucomatous visual

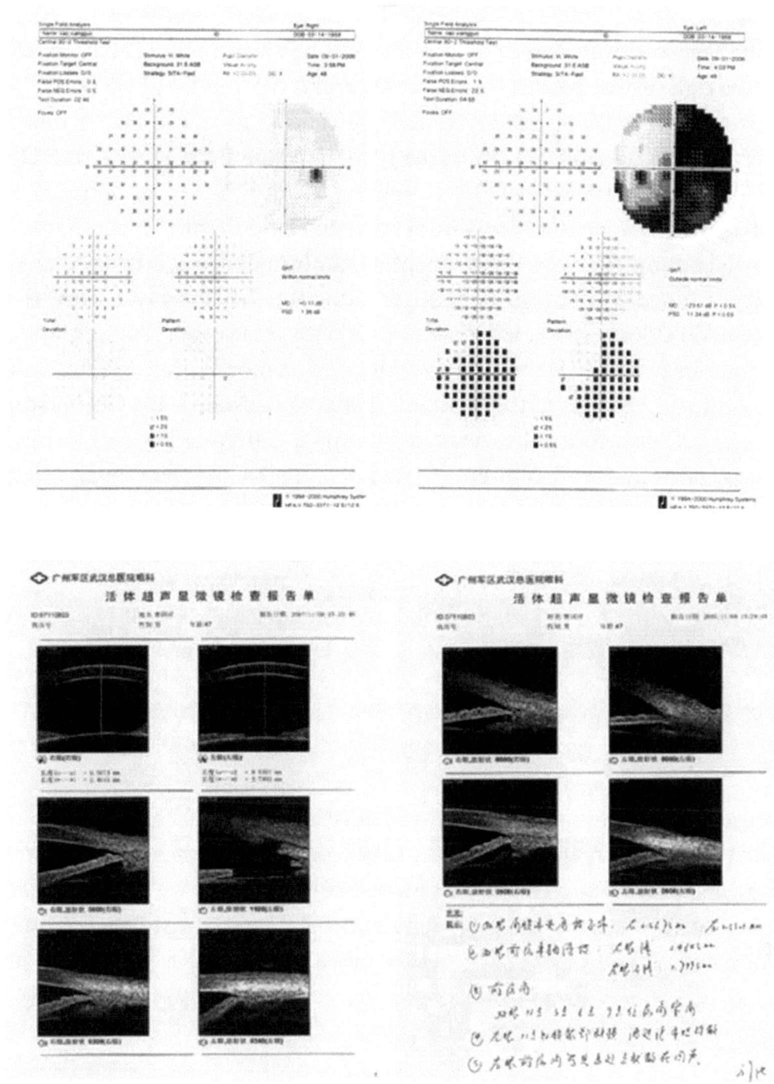

Figure 14. Clinical data of a patient suffered from PSS with glaucomatous optic nerve damange due to secondary open angle glaucoma (Clinical number 813064).Normal visual field in right eye(A) and advanced visual field defect in left eye (B);UBM shows the normol right eye and the affected left eye post-operation(C).

field damage in both eye, extended latent time and descended amplitude on VEP; CCT:540/520 (R/L),corneal endothelium cells 1730/2747(R/L); center anterior chamber depth ≥3.0mm and open anterior chamber angle in every direction for the both eye by UBM. She was diagnosed as binocular POAG, and treated successively with travatan, alphagan and brinzolamide to binoculus, but her IOP was not controlled well. Thus, a trabeculectomy was performed the left eye. Two weeksafter the operation, the filtration bubble turned fibrosed, and IOP increased. By 3 times of pin-delamination with 5-fluorouracil and eyeball massage, IOP was controlled on 12 to 14 mmHg. Her right eye was treated with travatan, carteolol hydrochloride and brimonidine, IOP wascontrolled from 12 to 14 mmHg. She was discharged from hospital. Four months later, the right eye appeared 5 small rounds and mutton-fat like KP, IOP increased to 19mmHg. A week later, KP played down, IOP descended to 12 mmHg. A month later; KP appeared again, IOP increased to 37, after treatment in hospital for a week, the IOP decreased to 12 mmHg. She was diagnosed as POAG combined with PSS. Two months later PSS of her right attacked again, IOP increased to 44 mmHg; visual field damage has progressed remarkably. FFA showed optic atrophy without any other abnormal. She was hospitalized again, and a implantation of Ahmed valve to her right eye was done on the next day. During the operation, the valve appeared out of control; we dealt it well with removable restraint line processing; the IOP and anterior chamber stability was controlled. 2 month after the operation, the IOP increased to 22 mmHg because of the draining disc was packaged. By pin-delamination and eyeball massage, IOP was controlled near to 20mmHg. Carteolol hydrochloride was added and the IOP was controlled well in intermittent, but PSS attacked frequently and the IOP was out of control during episode. She was hospitalized once more and the right eye was treated with no-penetrating glaucoma surgery. One month after surgery, the IOP was controlled well, binocular IOP was 10mmHg. 2 month after surgery, PSS attackwas seen in her right eye again, IOP increased to 20 mmHg. This attack faded a week later and IOP of her both maintained 14mmHg below until now. (Clinical data please see Figure 15)

(4) Type D PSS combined with primary closed-angle glaucoma

Research status

Except for our data, there had been only two individual reports about PSS combined with PCAG in China and none in abroad. Cases of PSS combined with PCAG at home are much more than those in abroad due to the higher incidence of PCAG as well as PSS at home. In 2004 we reported 6 cases and completed a systematic clinical analysis. It was often reminded by many ophthalmologists that cases of PSS had be mistaken as PACG, but enough attention has not been paid to this type of PSS. [18, 28, 36, 37, 38]

Clinical features

There is a typical history of PSS attack with binocular shallow anterior chamber and narrow or closed anterior chamber angle. PSS hardly attacked synchronously with PACG, the anterior chamber angle is open in episodes of PSS. Type D cases complied with the basic characteristics of typical PSS in early stage: binocular IOP is normal in intermission; with cross phenomenon of IOP; however, when PACG became more advanced, although the IOP of the PSS attacked eye was much higher than that of the unattacked eye in the episode of PSS, binocular IOP turned higher than normal even in intermission of PSS without obvious cross phenomenon. Most cases were diagnosed as PACG previously, PSS appeared after the treatment for PACG had been completed and the anterior chamber angle been opened, a few cases were typical PSS with narrow anterior chamber angle when they were young; PACG appeared as anterior chamber angle became narrower and narrower with age. Most of the cases of this type were elder with a longer course of PSS and a more advanced visual field damage.

http://dx.doi.org/10.5772/58348

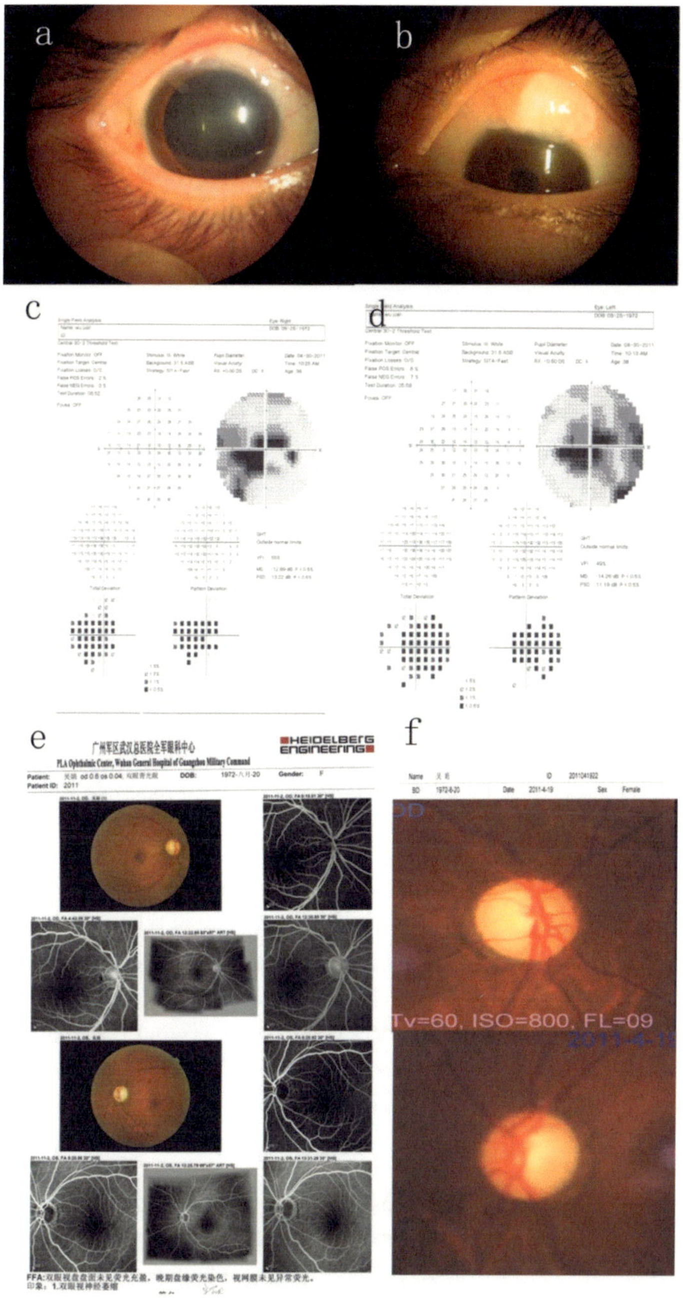

Figure 15. Clinical data of patient suffered from PSS(right eye) with glaucomatous optic nerve damange combined with POAG(both eye),the right eye is treated with Ahmed value implantation surgery(A),the left eye is treated with normal trabeculectomy(B), visual field of right eye(C) and left eye(D)show typical glaucoma damages,the fundus angiography indicates no vasular disorder except of optic atrophy(E) and the optic cups of right eye and lefr eye are non-symmetrical.

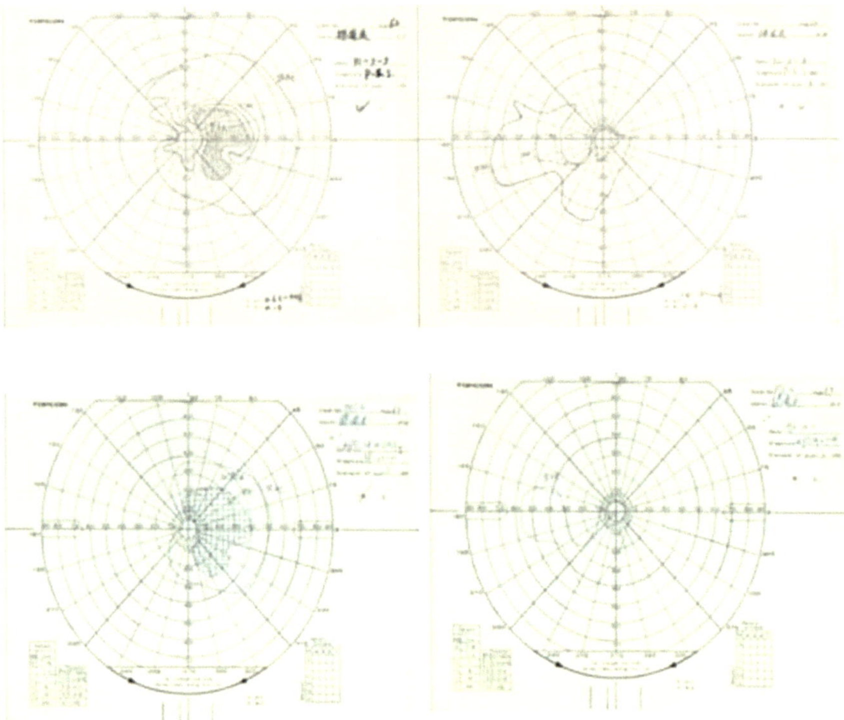

Figure 16. Visual field of patient (Clinical number 232036)with binocular PSS combined with POAG. After drug treatment,the damage of binocular visual field between 1991(A) and 1998(B) has no significant advance.

Diagnosis standard

The first is that the anterior chamber angle is open when PSS is diagnosed at episode, either in the intermission of PACG or after PACG was treated with Laser/surgery/drug; the second is that the cases complied with the basic characteristics of typical PSS described by Posner-Schlossman. In our study, 2 cases was diagnosed as PSS at a younger age with binocular narrow anterior chamber angle (first was narrow II, narrow III-IV four years later), 5 cases was diagnosed as PSS after treatment of PACG (similar to the two cases reported at home).[28, 39]

Diagnostic summary

To find out PACG complicated with PSS as soon as possible, it is necessary to carry out a set of comprehensive and careful examinations relating to PACG in the intermission of PSS for PSS patients with factors as follows: the old-aged, with a serious visual field damage, longer course of the disease, with a shallow anterior chamber or an narrow anterior chamber angle, and binocularly attacked.

When IOP appeared as repeated, intermittent and sudden elevation in a patient with PACG whose anterior chamber angle had been opened and the IOP been controlled well for a period after treatment by means of laser and/or surgery and/or drugs, it is very important to pay sufficient attention to the depth of the binocular anterior chamber and anterior chamber angle when the IOP is higher, and to make clinical follow-up observations for KP and its relationship with IOP, so as to ascertain whether PSS is the cause of elevating IOP, so that unnecessary surgery can be avoided.

Treatment principles

According to condition of PACG, laser and/or surgery and/or drugs may become options.

Laser treatment:

1. Indications of that for cases of PSS combined with PACG is similar to that PACG patients, except for that examination and treatment should be done in the intermission of PSS;
2. Curative effect on cases with typical cross phenomenon of IOP should be better;
3. The iris surrounding excision mouth by laser must be thoroughly penetrated and the hole should be big enough;
4. Corticosteroids and drugs for reducing IOP should be sufficient after laser operation;
5. It is import to pay attention to the treatment for PSS which continue to attack after laser therapy, and to the monitor of IOP and its dynamic change. Additional drug treatment even trabeculectomy should be adopted timely when necessary;[27]

It is necessary to prevent the attack of PACG in either episodes or intermission of PSS for these untreated PACG cases with the appropriate use of miosis drug.

Typical cases 1)

A patient was diagnosed as "PSS" in our hospital because of pain and discomfort of his right eye, then he was diagnosed as "acute angle-closure glaucoma " in other hospital because of severe sore of his both eyes and switched to our hospital after remission seven years later.

Examination revealed mutton-fat like KP in the right eye. His right eye was diagnosed as PSS combined with PACG with analysis by synthesis combining history and test results of IOP, fundus, visual field and anterior chamber angle. The right eye was treated with "glaucoma drainage surgery" and the left eye with "YAG laser iridectomy ".

IOP of his both appeared stable for six months after operation, then the right eye was attacked by PSS once again. This attack of PSS appeared as typical KP, open angle and slightly increased IOP. (Clinical data please see Figure 17)

Typical cases 2)

A patient came to our clinic because of "repeated intermittent attacks of eye pain and impaired vision for her left eye and right eye as well for more than 14 years". She was treated with YAG laser iridotomy in other hospital for PACG binocularly twice each. Her left eye had been still attacked intermittently ever since. Clinical date from her medical record showed that KP and IOP rising appeared nearly simultaneously on each episode and the IOP turned persistently higher than normal even if in intermission since 2 years ago and the drugs could not control the IOP well. Examination at this time showed: Vision R 1.0, L 0.4; IOP R 14 mmHg and L 46

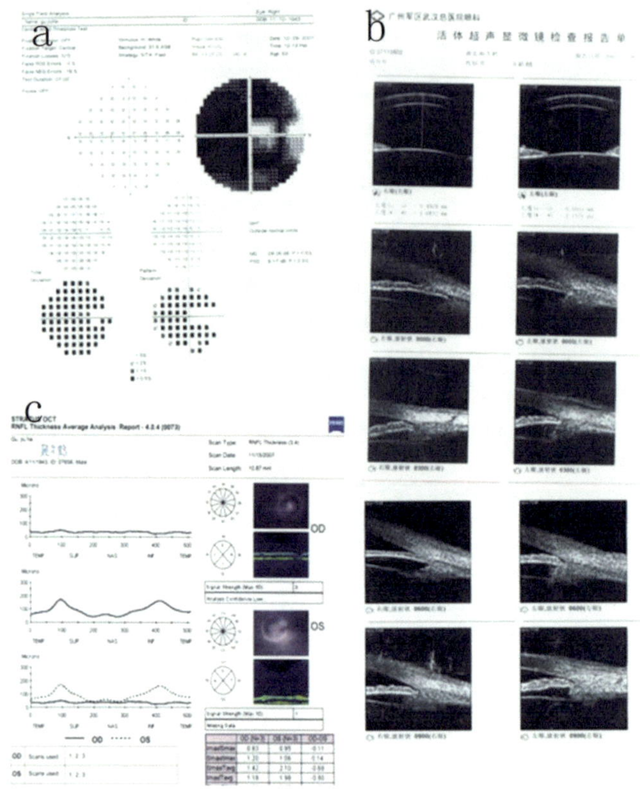

Figure 17. Typical clinical data of patient (Clinical number :406013)with diagnosis of right PSS combined with binocular PACG and treatment with classical trabeculectomy.The visual field show advanced glaucoma damange (A),OCT(C) also shows retinal nerve fiber layer defect.UBM indicate binocular closed angle(B).

mmHg; two mutton-fat like KP in the left eye ; shallow anterior chamber and angle multiple adhesions in both eyes; several trace of laser therapy on iris of her both eye, the only peetrated hole on the right eye be covered with fibrous membrane, and that on the left eye be too small; cup/disc ratios R 0.4and L 0.8.A diagnosis of "binocular PACG complicated with PSS in left eye" was established. A complementary laser therapy was given to her right eye just at that moment; after this laser therapy, her right had been kept well until now with only the help of 2% Carteolol Hydrochloride eye drops twice a day. Three weeks later, when this attack of PSS faded away, she was hospitalized in our hospital, and a trabeculectomy was performed on her left eye, and she was discharged 10 days after a IOP of 14mmHg. Six weeks after the surgery, an attack of PSS occurred with a IOP of 32mmHg and lasted a week; such attack occurred once or twice a year after that with a maximal IOP of 25mmHg. The IOP in intermission had maintained near 15mmHg during the first 4 years, but the result of 24h IOP measurement showed 13~20mmHg in the right eye and 15~24mmHg in the left eye. Iris heterochromia appeared in the left eye. Such a therapeutic schedule was established and kept 3 years since then: 2% Carteolol Hydrochloride Eye Drops twice a day to the both eye in intermission of PSS; 2% Carteolol twice a day plus brimonidine 3 times a day with shortly use of Lotemax for the left eye during episode of PSS. IOP of the both eye maintained15mmHg or below, and the visual field maintained stable in the 3 years. Several attacks of PSS had been recorded with a IOP up to 40mmHg, and her visual field turned worsen, and "rain dozen sand-like" appearance in the iris of her left eye got more pronounced in the last 2 years. She was hospitalized once more, and another trabeculectomy was performedon the left eye near the first one, at the end of which the two filtering blebs (an original and a just manufactured) were merged into one. She was discharged with an IOP of 12mmHg; the left eye was no longer attacked after this trabeculectomy, and the IOP kept stable.(Clinical data see Figure 18)

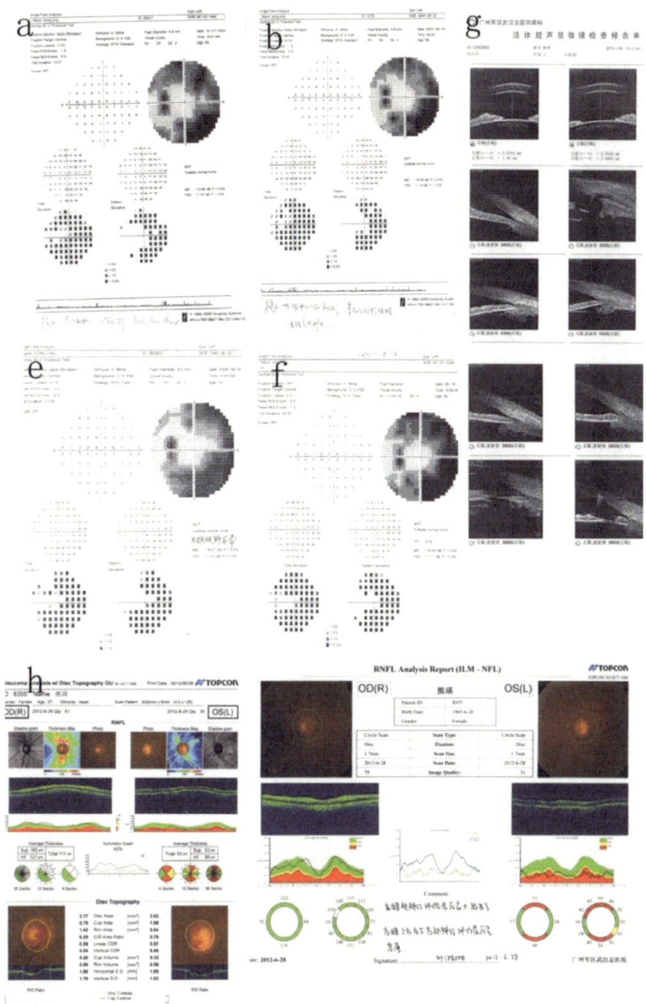

Figure 18. Typical clinical data of patient (Clinical number :341555)with diagnosis of left PSS combined with binocular closed-angle glaucoma. The visual fields of right eye(A) and left eye(B) become worse 4years later(C) and (D),UBM indicate binocular aqueous humour outflow after the 1 st trabeculectomy(E) and the OCT results show serious retinal nerve fiber layer defect in left eye(F).

3. Differential diagnosis and main points in diagnosis and treatment of complications of PSS

On the one hand, PSS is often misdiagnosed as other diseases, other diseases are often misdiagnosed as PSS; on the other hand, PSS can also be merged with or cause other diseases. Although the differential diagnosis of these conditions is complex, but we should be able to complete the work well through a careful clinical observation and analyzation rely on the basic characteristics of PSS described by Posner and Schlossman and new discoveries introduced above.,,.

3.1. The differential diagnosis of PSS and other diseases.

3.1.1. Analysis the situation of misdiagnosis

There were a total of 37 articles about misdiagnosis of PSS among the domestic documents about PSS since 1990. Here are the results of our analysis of these documents.

1. Other diseases misdiagnosed as PSS

There were 5 cases in which Fuchs syndrome was misdiagnosed as PSS, in 5 cases viral keratitis misdiagnosed as PSS and in 4 cases acute retinal necrosis misdiagnosed as PSS.

2. PSS misdiagnosed as other diseases

There were 76 cases of PSS misdiagnosed as acute angle-closure glaucoma, 42 misdiagnosed as iridocyclitis, 42 cases misdiagnosed as primary open-angle glaucoma, 22 cases misdiagnosed as uveitis, 4 cases misdiagnosed as conjunctivitis, 4 cases misdiagnosed as Fuch's syndrome, 1 case misdiagnosed as high intraocular pressure and1 case misdiagnosed as keratitis.

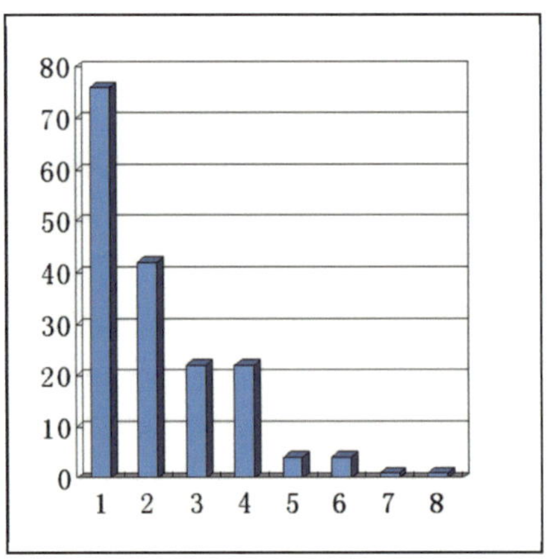

1. misdiagnosed as acute angle-closure glaucoma
2. misdiagnosed as iridocyclitis
3. misdiagnosed as POAG
4. misdiagnosed as uveitis
5. misdiagnosed as conjunctivitis
6. misdiagnosed as Fuch 's syndrome
7. misdiagnosed as high intraocular pressure
8. misdiagnosed as keratitis

Figure 19. Number of cases of PSS misdiagnosed as other diseases

3. About the harms of misdiagnosis for the patients.PSS patients were misdiagnosed as primary glaucoma and inappropriate treated, even the surgery that should not be done had been performed. Primary glaucoma merged with PSS were missed diagnosis, result in the lost the optimal timing of treatment. Such diseases as Fuch's syndrome, acute retinal necrosis and viral keratitis were misdiagnosed as PSS, lead to the delay of treatment.

	PSS	POAG	PCAG
age at first onset	usually under the age of 50 years	middle-aged or older	
KP	Yes, accompany with elevated IOP	No	pigmented KP sometimes after a outburst
Anterior chamber angle			or closed
Affected eye	most	most binocular	binocular, usually
Visual field damage	Little and light, more began in the peripheral, usually	usually binocular and centrally located	more binocular, often irregular
IOP	In episodes the is normal, in intermission both eyes are normal	invariably	Invariably or paroxysmal
IOP cross	Yes	No	No in chronic cases, Yes in acute cases sometimes after an outburst
postrualar IOP change	Not related to C value no matter IOP is high or low	Related to C value no matter IOP is high or low	Related to C value only when IOP is high

Table 6. The key points about differential diagnosis between PSS and POAG or PACG

3.1.2. The differential diagnosis of several kinds of common diseases

1. The differential diagnosis of PSS and other glaucomaThe differential diagnosis between PSS and POAG or PACG can be carried out in reference to table 7. [23 24, 27, 28, 40]

2. The differential diagnosis of PSS and other uveitis

The characteristics of common uveitis

Iridocyclitis: Ciliary hyperemia, eyesight drops significantly, smaller KP, aqueous humor of turbidity, fast and heavy adhesion of iris, higher or lower IOP.

Choroiditis: significantly dropped vision, with or without KP, vitreous of turbidity, no iris adhesion usually, lower IOP, corresponding pathological changes in retinal and choroiditis.

All uveitis: ciliary hyperemia, significantly dropped vision, KP in most cases, muddy aqueous humor, vitreous of turbidity, fast and heavy adhesion of iris, higher or lower IOP, corresponding pathological changes in retinal and choroiditis.

Intermediate uveitis: a kind of uveitis limited in the pars plana of ciliary body, peripheral retina and vitreous base, without any clinical symptoms in some cases or with muscae volitantes, blurred vision and temporary myopia in most cases, normal or mild declined vision in most cases but significant vision loss in case with cystoid macular edema and other complications or sudden severe vision loss in case with acute vitreous hemorrhage, retinal detachment,, mild to moderate anterior segment inflammation in most cases but severe ciliary hyperemia, a large number of KP, obvious aqueous flare and a lot of inflammatory cells in the anterior chamber in a few cases at first onset with severe anterior segment reaction occasionally, change in the vitreous and the pars plana of ciliary body (the most common and important performance of the disease) such as vitreous inflammatory cells, snow ball turbidity due to cell agglutination, snowbank like lesion stretches from the pars plana and vitreous base into vitreous cavity, vitreous degeneration, hemorrhage and hyperplastic vitreous retinopathy at late stage, a variety of retinopathy, such as macular edema, diffuse retinal edema, retinal vasculitis and perivascular inflammation, exudation, hemorrhage, retinal neovascularization, hyperplastic retinopathy, retinal detachment, usually normal IOP in early time but a persistent high IOP once elevated, sporadic KP with no association with IOP.

3. The differential diagnosis of PSS and keratitis

Keratitis

Sign Obvious hyperaemia, matrix and endothelial change, KP with different forms mainly distributed in lesion site of the cornealand seldom inhealthy area.

Characteristics The eye with angle-closure glaucoma induced by keratitis have the basic characteristics of angle-closure glaucoma; A monocular open-angle glaucoma would occurred in the affected eye if keratitis spread to the trabecular meshwork with an intraocular pressure changes over the cornea edema.

Course of disease:They are not self-limited and repeated outbreaks tend to occur.

3.2. Main points in diagnosis and treatment of complications of PSS

Other kinds of glaucoma which PSS concurred with or lead to were not introduced before. PSS can also concur with or cause iris heterochromia, ischemic optic neuropathy, complicated cataract and other diseases, such as retinal detachment. Main points in diagnosis and treatment of these complications were briefly introduced as follows:

3.2.1. PSS combined with iris heterochromia

Typical cases

Case 1) A patient consulted at our hospital because his left eye suffered from intermittent recurrent pain and blurred vision for more than one year. Intraday examinations showed: best corrected visual acuity is 1.0/ 0.6(R/L), IOP: 16.7/ 13.7(R/L) mmHg, FFA in both eyes are normal, optic cup in his left eye is expand. He was suspected of glaucoma. Intermittent recurrent pain and blurred vision kept to attack his left eye for more than half a year after then. These attacks usually ceased a few days late, with or without the help of 0.5% timolol eye drop and other drugs. During this period, the highest IOP record of his left eye was 35mmHg with a normal record of his right eye. The patient returned to our hospital one year later after stopping use of any drugs for two weeks. Ophthalmologic examination at this time showed: visual acuity1.2

http://dx.doi.org/10.5772/58348

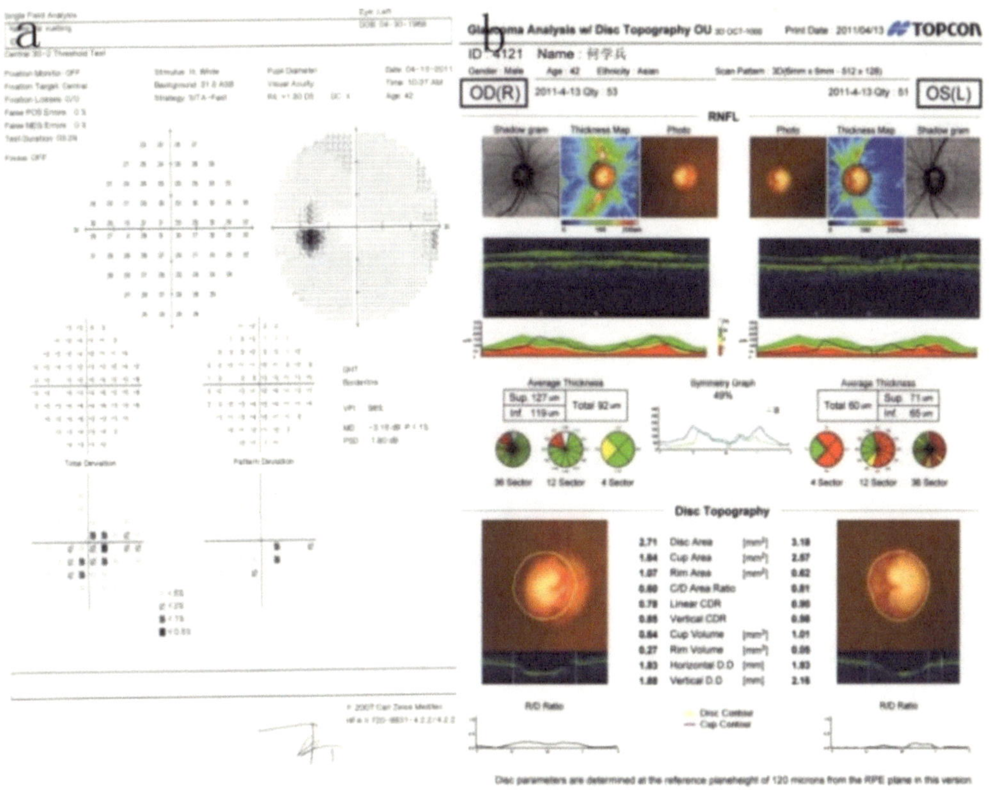

Figure 20. Typical clinical data of patient (ID :11041302)with diagnosis of left PSS combined with iris heterochromia. The visual fields of left eye show nasal defect (A) ,binocular OCTresults indicate ocular cups expand (B)and (C) obvious retinal nerve fiber layer defect (C).

both eyes, IOP 17/15(R/L)mmHg, a lot of small lipid-like KP in the inferior of the left cornea, "rain dozen sand-like" appearance in the iris of his left eye, C/D rate 0.6/0.7(R/L),CCT 553/560(R/L). Results of his visual field and OCT showed in Figure below. UBM showed wide-angle in the both eyes. Fundus fluorescein angiography and contrast sensitivity revealed no special finds. 24 hours IOP measurements (2 weeks after KP disappeared): 13~16/ 12~15(R/L)mmHg. Diagnosis of "PSS complicated with iris heterochromia" for his left eye was confirmed than. He was asked to treat every onset of the disease in time with drugs dropping IOP as well as anti-inflammatory medicine. (Clinical data see Figure 20)

Case 2) A patient was admitted to our hospital because her right eye suffered from repeated episodes of pain with blurred vision for more than nine years, and her vision decreased 3 months, with a primary diagnosis of "secondary glaucoma" for her right eye. A lot of intermittent recurrent pain and blurred vision had attacked her right eye from nine years ago, 2 or 3 times a year. Each attack lasted about one week, than resolved spontaneously. Three months ago her sense of vision went to recession. She felt that her right eye was attacked again recent days, so she can to our hospital. Ophthalmologic examination in this time showed: visual

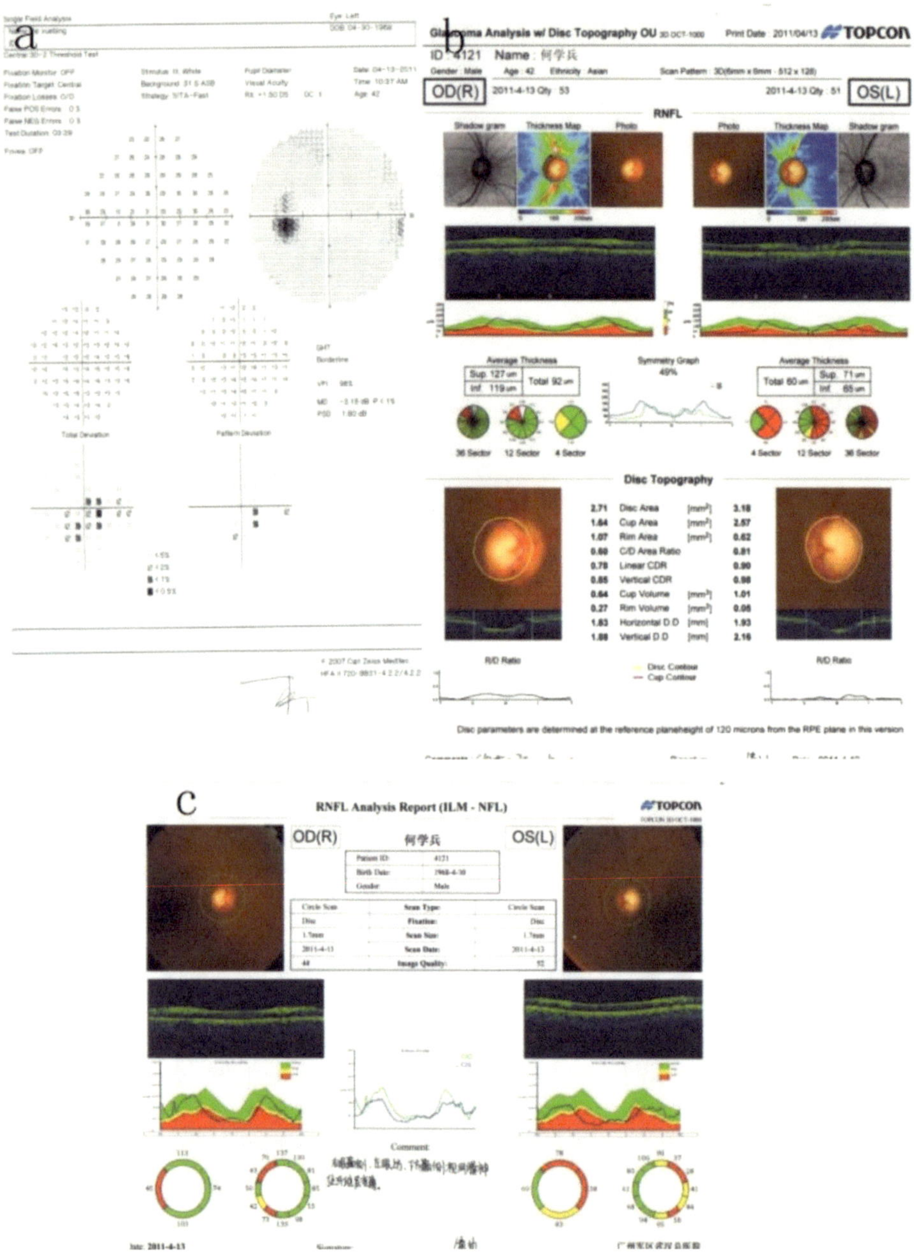

Figure 21. Typical clinical data of patient (ID :11041302)with diagnosis of left PSS combined with iris heterochromia. The visual fields of left eye show nasal defect(A),binocular OCT results indicate ocular cups expand(B) and (C) obvious retinal nerve fiber layer defect (C).

acuity: 0.15/ 1.0(R/L), IOP: 43/12(R/L) mmHg, mist edema in her cornea of her right eye with a lot of fat-like KP, pale and "rain scatting beach-like" appearance in her left iris with a round pupil about 3mm in diameter, her optic disk appeared pale in color with a C/D 0.9, her anterior chamber was not shallow, ultrasound biomicroscopy (UBM) showed a wide angle in both eye. Her left eye showed no KP with a C/D less 0.3. Her systemic examination and routine inspection and examination showed no special finds. Treatment with drugs dropping IOP such as carteolol and brimonidine and mannitol as well as steroids loteprednol kept about a week, KP significantly reduced but the intraocular pressure is still high. Operation of Ahmed valve implantation was performed on her right eye two weeks later. She was discharged a week postoperative with an IOP of 9mmHg in the operated eye. Her IOP was controlled well with fewer attacks of PSS and a stable visual field in the recent 3 years after the surgery. (Clinical data see Figure 21)

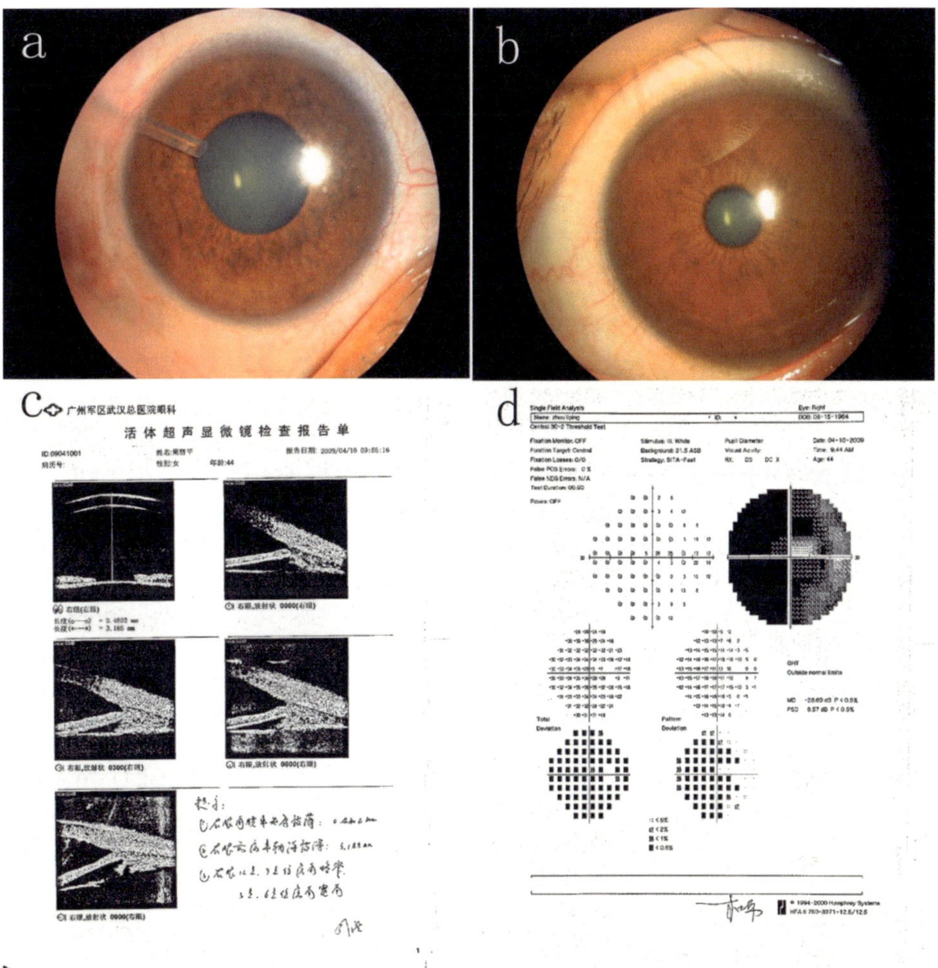

Figure 22. Typical clinical data of patient (Clinical number :437614)with diagnosis of right PSS combined with iris disorder. The right eye is after Ahmed implantation and arrow indicate iris heterochromia(A),the left eye is normal(B).UBM indicate a wild angle in right eye (C),but the visual field show serious damanges in right eye(D).

Discussion

1. Clinical performance of PSS complicated with iris heterochromia

Four cases of PSS complicated with iris heterochromia were reported [40]. They were two males and two females aged 35 to 45 years. In addition to typical PSS performance, the iris showed "rain scatting sand-like" appearance in all of the 4 patients. All of them are monocular repeatedly attacked at the same eye. Each attack kept 3 to 7 days with a significantly increased IOP up to30.00 ~ 60.00mnHg and a few of fat-like KP, than relieve itself or extinct with the help of medication. Intraocular pressure (including 24 hours intraocular pressure) in intermittent period appeared normal after discontinuation of all medication with a typical crossed-over phenomenon.

2. Key-points in the differential diagnosis between PSS complicated with iris heterochromatic and FHI (Fuchs heterochromic iridicyclitis).The two diseases are different clinically in the following five aspects: the attacked eye and sex of patients, manifestation of intraocular pressure, character of KP, appearance of the Lens and glaucomatous damage of optic nerve and visual field.

(1) The attacked eye and sex of patients

Most of PSS cases had monocular presentation, a few of cases were binocular, but usually one eye was affected at a time, in extremely rare cases was binocularly attacked simultaneously. Male patients were more common than female in PSS. FH is generally believed that no gender more predisposed than the other more than 90% of the cases were monocularly affected.

(2) Manifestation of intraocular pressure

The IOP in patients of PSS with iris heterochromatic appeared as an intermittent and abruptly rising when the attack comes with the appearance of typical KP in pure PSS patients. IOP elevation in patients of PSS with iris heterochromatic usually lasted 3 ~ 10days, and then turned to subside spontaneously with the disappearance of the KP after this period, it is also sensitive to drugs dropping IOP and anti-inflammatory medicine. On the contrary, IOP of patient with FH appeared normal in the initial stage for a long time, after that, elevated in part of the cases gradually; however, once the intraocular pressure elevated, it often appeared persistently higher, although there maybe some fluctuations. The elevated IOP and KP in patient with FH had no characteristic of intermittent, were difficult to be controlled and poorly responded to corticosteroids therapy. The IOP in patients with PSS complicated with iris heterochromia kept the characteristic of crossed-over, that is, the IOP of the attacked eye was higher than that of contra lateral eye during the episode but lower(3 ~ 5mmHg) than the other eye between attacks. IOP in patients with Fuchs syndrome had no such characteristic, once elevated; it is always higher if untreated.

(3) Keratic Precipitates

The KP in patient with PSS complicated with iris heterochromia appeared only in a short period during the attack in most cases. This KP is of following characteristics: small round suet-like, medium sized, isolated, with no pigment in initial stage, mainly located in the lower part of the cornea, usually disappeared naturally within a few days after or before IOP reduction. On the contrary, KP in patients with Fuchs syndrome has different characteristics as following: persistence for very long time even always in most cases, white transparent small dot or star-like coexisting with pigmented KP, diffuse distribution in the cornea, sometimes connected each other with fibrous filaments, poor response to corticosteroids therapy. (Clinical data see Figure 22)

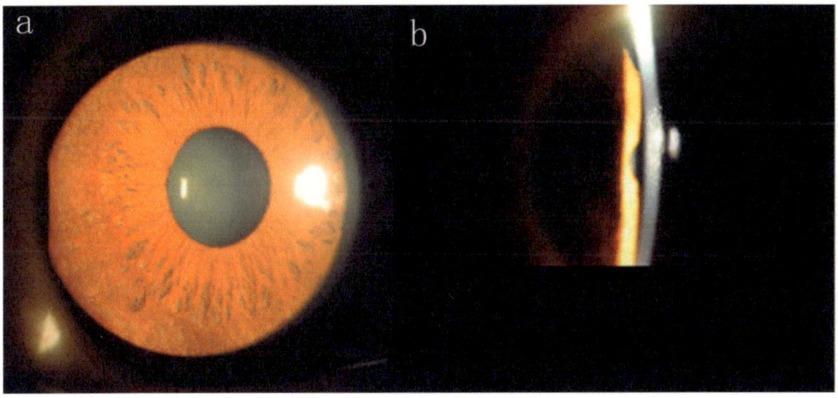

Figure 23. Heterochromatic iris and KP in FHI. There is a typical iris such as "rain dozen sand-like"(A) arrow shows a lot of star-like KPs(B).

(4) Lens situation

Fuchs syndrome complicated with cataract is common at later stage; however the complicated cataract is uncommon in the PSS cases with iris heterochromia.

(5) Glaucomatous retinal and visual damage

Glaucomatous damage in PSS cases appeared later and to a lesser extent, however that of FH cases occur earlier and quicker.

3.2.2. PSS combined with ischemic optic neuropathy

Typical cases

A patient came to our hospital because her vision of the left eye sudden dropped 2 months ago. She was examined 2 months ago: visual acuity: 1.0/ 0.5(R/L) IOP: 17.3/ 15(R/L) mmHg. The optic disc of her left eye was pale, visual field showed an inferior fan like defect. Fundus fluorescein angiography(FFA) of her left eye showed ischemic optic neuropathy. The anterior segment, fundus, vision, and FFA of her right eye were normal. She was diagnosed as "left eye ischemic optic neuropathy". She was admitted to our hospital, and examinations showed: visual acuity: 1.0/ 0.15(R/L). IOP: 17.3/ 50.62(R/L), anterior chamber of both eyes were not shallow, Right eye showed no abnormality. Left cornea had mild edema and there was a medium size fat-like KP below the pupil. The boundary of optic papillae in left eye was clear, the color was off white, and the C / D was about 0.3,the angle of left eye was N1 ~ N2. Systemic examination such as X-ray, electrocardiogram and routine laboratory tests were normal. Visual field of right eye was normal and that of the left eye showed a centripetal narrow with an inferior fan like defect. She was diagnosed as "Left eye PSS, complicated with ischemic optic neuropathy", and treated with drugs for reducing IOP and nutrition curing to optic nerve for about a weak. She was discharged with IOP 12mmHg disappeared KP, vision 0.2 of her left eye. (Clinical data see Figure 23)

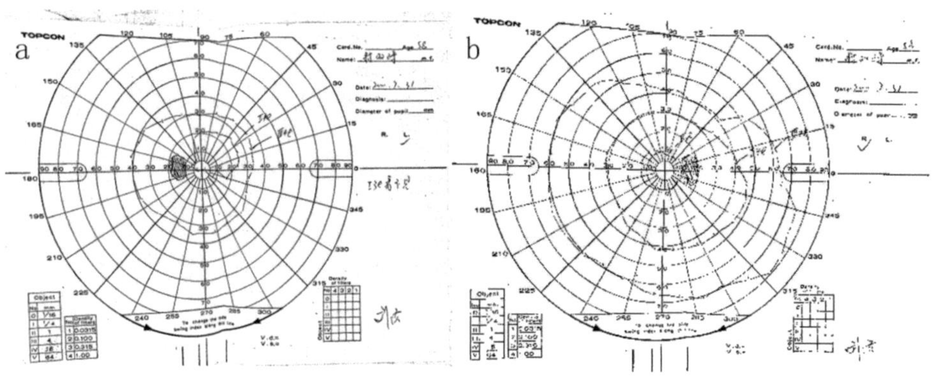

Figure 24. visual field of patient (Clinical number :294450) The case suffered from left eye PSS combined with ischemic optic neuropathy. inferior visual field defect and serious contraction of left(A),and that of the normal right eye(B).

Discussion

In 2003 1 case of PSS complicated with non-arteritic anterior ischemic optic neuropathy (AION) was reported. The vision of the case improved significantly after the attack of PSS had been controlled, but the vision and optic neuropathy damaged continually. The authors emphasized that the IOP of PSS patients complicated with AION should be promptly controlled as it is one of the risk factors [41]. It is useful to use drugs with dual role of reducing IOP and improving retinal blood supply in intermittent period. Our case appeared a sudden vision loss and significant discomfort two months ago. The result of examinations in other hospital such as visual field defect of arcuate below and FFA supported the diagnosis of left eye ischemic optic neuropathy. Results of examinations, reaction to treatment and course of the disease during her hospitalization in our hospital In July 2000 conformed with diagnostic criteria of PSS. The structure of the optic nerve, damage of blood vessels and blood state are related to ischemic optic neuropathy, the severely sudden rising of IOP during attack of PSS maybe the inducing factors. So it is necessary to reduce the IOP during each attack of PSS as soon and effective as possible for the cases of PSS combined with ischemic optic neuropathy or with the risk factors for that.

3.2.3. PSS combined with rhegmatogenous retinal detachment

Typical cases

A patient was hospitalized in our hospital for the reason that there was shadow before his right eye with a diagnose of rhegmatogenous retinal detachment. The IOP of his right eye elevated to 29 mmHg 3 days after hospitalization and a fat-like KP appeared in his right eye, than he was diagnosed as rhegmatogenous retinal detachment combined with PSS. Retinal detachment surgery (Condensation+cerclage+scleral pressure technique) were done after reducing IOP with the treatment of drugs. Postoperative recovery was good. PSS recurred 4 months later and recovered 5 days late.

Discussion

The pathogenesis of PSS combined with rhegmatogenous retinal detachment is unknown. Increased concentration of PG (especially PGE) resulted from retinal S-antigen entered into the vitreous cavity after blood-eye barrier breakdown during the formation of retinal breaks may leads to the inflammation of the uvea, and the higher concentration of PGs and inflammatory products results in the IOP elevation.

3.2.4. PSS combined with cataract

Typical cases

A patient complained of recurrent pain and decreased vision of her right eye for four years. Results of examinations intraday showed: visual acuity:0.08/ 0.4(R/L); corrected visual acuityR: 0.3(-0.75DS/1.50DC*111),L: 0.9(-1.25DS/-0.50DC*83) ;IOP: 12/ 14(R/L) mmHg; a few of time worn pigmented KP on the central and lower part of her clear corneal; round pupil about3mm in diameter; normal iris, opacification of posterior capsule of lens; C/D of optic papillaeo.4.Her left eye appeared normal. She was hospitalized with the diagnosis of PSS and was treated with carteolol, brimonidine, mannitol for reducing IOP, tobradex for anti-inflammation and methycobal to maintain optic nerve. She was discharged once the attack of PSS faded away every time. The PSS attacked her1 to 2 month a time, her vision of right eye declined gradually without other discomfort. (Clinical data see Figure 24)

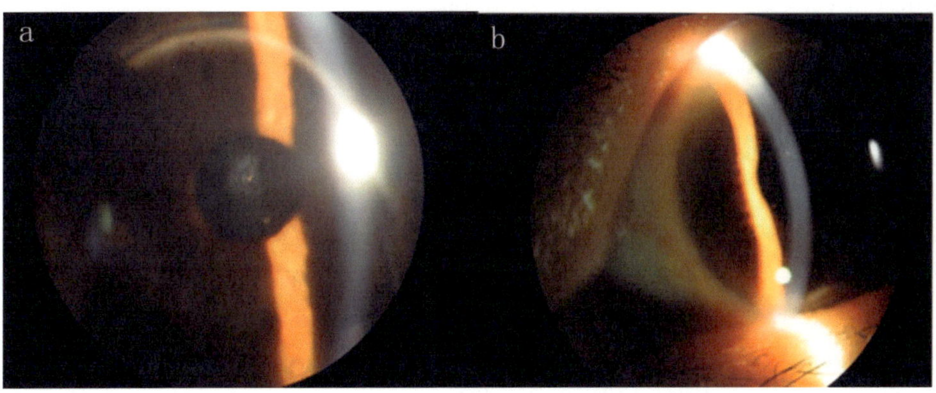

Figure 25. Anterior segment slit-lamp photography of patient (Clinical number 394998) with the diagnosis of PSS combined with cataract.Arrows show an opacities area at posterior capsule (A) and few typical fat-shaped KPs(B).

Discussion

The possible pathogenesis: repeated onset of IOP elevation and anterior segment inflammation cause disorders of nutrition and metabolism of the lens.

Surgical opportunity: Cataract surgery should be done after the inflammation has been subsidized for more than 3 months. The rest of the indication is the same to the conventional cataract. Considering the PSS is an inflammation of the nature of the disease and the literature PSS patients of corneal endothelial cell density is low, PSS patients combined cataract surgery methods should also do more thinking. Femtosecond laser cataract surgery with accurate positioning, and the advantage of less influence on corneal endothelial, compared with the phaco, whether merger of cataract in patients with PSS has advantages, is worth our discussion.[42]

Prospect

With the deepening of the research on PSS, the pathogenic factors, pathogenesis, clinical characteristics, especially the clinical pathway via which the glaucoma optic nerve damage occurred in PSS cases will become clearer. For example, if hormone treatment was used excessively in PSS cases, would glueoeortieoid-induced glaucoma take place? If a poor blood supply to the optic disc of a patient with PSS or a weak structure of the papilla of optic nerve or a lower intracranial pressure, in such cases, would a normal-tension glaucoma appear? All these problems need to be continuously explored through our joint efforts.

Author details

He-Zheng Zhou*, Wen-Shan Jiang, Han-Guang Jie, Chang Feng, Wen-Qiang Zhang, Qian Ye, Jian-Guo Wu, Yan-Ping Song and Qin Ding

*Address all correspondence to: zhoueye@qq.com

Department of Ophthalmology, Wuhan General Hospital of Guangzhou Command, China

References

[1] Posener A, Schlossman A. Syndrome of unilateral attacks of glaucoma with cyclic-symptoms. Arch opthalmol.1948,39:5-28

[2] Theodore FH. Observation on glaucomatocycliticcrisis(Posner Schloddman Syndrome).Br J Ophthalmol.1952,36:207-213

[3] Dao-Ping Lu, Ran-Ran Xi. [Clinical analyzation of 177 cases with Posner SchloddmanSyndrome]. Chin J Ophthalmology. 1982,18:34-37

[4] Paivonsalo HT, Tuminen J, Vaahtoranta LH, et al. Incidence and prevalence of differ-entuneitis,entilies in Filand. Acta Ophthalmology Scand.1997, 75:76~81.

[5] Kanjiro M. The relationship between elevation of intraocular pressure and prosta-glandin in cases with glaucomatocyclitic crisis. clinical ophthalmology. 1975,29:689-692

[6] Yamamoto S, Pavan-Langston D, Tada R, et al. Possible role of herpes simplex viru-sin the origin of Posner-Schlossman syndrome. Am J Ophthalmol.1995, 119: 796-798

[7] Yang SY, Chen MJ, Chen KH, et al. Cytomegalovirus and herpes simplex virus as-causes of bilateral anterior uveitis in an immunocompetent patient. J Chin Med As-soc. 2011,74:48-50

[8] Blich-Michel E, Dussaix E, Cerqueti P, et al. Possible role of cytomegalovirus infec-tion in the etiology of the Posner-Schlossman syndrome. IntOphthalmol. 1987,11:95-96

[9] Chee SP, Jap A. Presumed Fuchs heterochromiciridocyclitis and Posner-Schlossman-syndrome: comparison of cytomegalovirus-positive and negative eyes. Am2008,146:883-889

[10] CY Choi, MS Kim, JM Kim, SH Park, KH Park, C Hong. Association between Helico-bacter pylori infection and Posner–Schlossman syndrome. Eye. 2010, [11] Zhi-Hui Li, Xun-ChuanJi, Shu-Chu Chen, et al. [The Long-term follow-up of PosnerSchloddman Syndrome]. Chin J Ophthalmology. 1982,18:306-308

[11] Nan-Xiang Peng. [Clinical analyzation of 52 cases with Posner Schloddman Syn-drome].Contemporary Medicine.2008, 5:141-141

[12] Wen-Xue Hu. [Clinical observation of early stage of Posner-Schlossman syn-drome].Int J Ophthalmology. 2011; 11: 1980-1982

[13] Puri P, Verma D. Bilateral glaucomatocyclitic crisis in a patient with Holmes Adie-syndrome. J Postgrad Med.1998,44:76-77

[14] Yu-Hong Wang, Xing-Huai Sun. [Clinical analysization of the the operative effect in-patients with glaucomatocyclitic crisis]. Chinese Journal of Practical Ophthalmology. 2005, 10:23-30

[15] Wen-Bing Zhou, Shou-Xiong Peng. [glaucomatocyclitic crisis and Primary Open-an-gle Glaucoma]. Chinese Ophthalmic Res.1994,12:34-36

[16] He-Zheng Zhou, Yuan-Hong Du. [The related factors about Posner-Schlossman syn-drome damage of visual field].Chinese Journal of Practical Ophthalmology. 2002,10:768~769

[17] Hua-Xin Chen, He-Zheng Zhou, Bai-Chuan Wang et al.[The Clinical Observation of14 cases elderly Posner-Schlossmansyndrome]. Military medical journal of South-China. 2007; 21: 43-45

[18] Raitta C, Vannas A. Glaucomatocyclitic crisis. Arch Ophthalmology. 1977, 95:608-612

[19] He-Zheng Zhou, Yi-Jia Yang. [Characteristics and clinical value of the intraocular-pressure and the C-value in Posner Schloddman Syndrome]. Chinese Journal ofPractical Ophthalmology.1992, 10:143-145

[20] Ying-Bo Shui, Hou-Ren Wei. [Influence of Postural Change on Intraocular Pressureof Normal Eyes]. Chinese Ophthalmic Res. 1987; 3 : 182-185

[21] He-Zheng Zhou. [Tonography and postural change of intraocular pressure in patients with glaucoma]. Chinese Journal of Practical Ophthalmology.1991,9:598-602

[22] He-Zheng Zhou, Wen-Shan Jiang. [Differential diagnosis of Posner-Schlossman syndrome]. Military medical journal of South China.2012,2:32-35

[23] He-Zheng Zhou, Yuan-Hong Du, Yan-Ping Song, Guang-Jie Wang, Jian-Guo Wu. [Visual field damage of glaucomatocyclitic crisis and its relating factors]. Fourth MilMed Univ.2001,22:1674-1677

[24] Yi-Lin Tang. [Clinical analysis of damage of visual field with Posner Schlossmanps-syndrome]. International Journal of Ophthalmology. 2010,10:1204-1205

[25] Jap A, Sivakumar M, Chee SP. Is Posner-Schlossman syndrome benign? Ophthalmology.2001,108:913-991

[26] He-Zheng Zhou, Bai-Chuan Wang, Xiong Zhou. [Unilateral Primary Open-Angle-Glaucomaand BilateralPosner-Schlossman syndrome]. Chin J Misdiagn. 2001,1:334-336

[27] He-Zheng Zhou, Wen-Qiang Zhang, Bai-ChuanWang. [Glaucomatocyclitic crisiswith primary close-Angle glaucoma]. International Journal of Ophthalmology,2004,4(5): 844-847

[28] Darchuk V, Sampaolesi J, Mato L, Nicoli C, SampaolesiR.Optic nerve head behavior-in Posner-Schlossman syndrome. IntOphthalmol,2001;23:373-379

[29] Rong-Xin Wu. [Operative effect in 1 Case with Posner-Schlossman syndrome].Ocular-trauma professional eye disease magazine. 2002,24:328

[30] Lei Sheng, Yu-Pu Li, Gui-LanLan. [1 Case of Posner-Schlossmansyndrome].Chinese-Journal of Practical Ophthalmology.2008,26:572

[31] Bo Zhao, Da-Yong Bai, Hui Zhao.et al. [Posner-Schlossman syndrome and primaryopen-angle glaucoma]. Chin J Pract Ophthalmology. 2004,22:142-143

[32] Xiu-Feng Ke, Dan-Ning Z, Li Yuan. [Observation the clinical operation curative effectof Posner-Schlossman syndrome]. Chinese Journal of Practical Ophthalmology. 2007,6:642-643

[33] Dinakaran S, Kayarkar V. Trabeculectomy in the management of Posner-Schlossman-syndrome. Ophthalmic SurgLasers.2002,33:321-322

[34] Stavrou P, Murray PI. Does trabeculectomy influence the course of uveitis? OculImmunolInflamm. 1999,7:103-108

[35] Xiao-Ping Zhang, Ji-Zhong Chen, Ru-Yong Song,[Analyze the Diagnostic of Posner-Schlossman syndrome]. Journal of clinical ophthalmology.2002,10:137-139

[36] Jin-Fu Ying, Ling-Ling Wu, [Posner-Schlossman syndrome complicated with Primary Closed-Angle Glaucoma]. Chinese Journal of Practical Ophthalmology. 1993.11:491-492

[37] Chang-lin Zhao, Han-Ping Xie. [A case report of primary angle closure glaucoma accompanied by glaucomatocyclitic crisis]. Acta Academiae Medicinae Militaris Tertiae. 2004.10.25; 26: 1798

[38] Li-Hong Guan. [2 cases of Posner-Schlossman syndrome complicated with Primary Closed-Angle Glaucoma]. Modern Medicine & Health. 2008, 24: 152

[39] Wen-Shan Jiang, He-ZhengZhou,Yun-Hui Chen, Ling Hong [Differential diagnosisof the Posner-Schlossman syndrome with heterochromic iris and the Fuchs syndrome—clinial report about three cases]. International Journal of Ophthalmology, 2009; 9 (9): 1762-1763

[40] Irak I, Katz BJ, Zabriskie NA, Zimmerman PL.Posner-Schlossman syndrome andnonarteritic anterior ischemic optic neuropathy. J Neuroophthalmol. 2003,23: 264-267

[41] Schultz T, Conrad – Hengerer I, Hengerer FH, et al. Intraocular pressure variation during femtosecond laser – assisted cataract surgery using a fluid–filled interface. J Cataract Refract Surg 2013; 39 (1): 22–27

Chapter 21

Excitotoxicity and Glaucoma

Makoto Ishikawa, Takeshi Yoshitomi and
Yukitoshi Izumi

Additional information is available at the end of the chapter

http://dx.doi.org/10.5772/57605

1. Introduction

Glutamate is a major excitatory neurotransmitter in the visual perception pathway. In the retina, rod and cone photoreceptor cells continuously release glutamate and partially depolarized in darkness, and light decreases the glutamate release in a graded manner. The photoreceptor signals are transmitted to bipolar cells and horizontal cells. The two-types of bipolar cells, ON-and OFF-bipolar cells, continuously release glutamate in lightness and in darkness, respectively [1,2]. Bipolar cells respond to light with sustained and graded potential as photoreceptor cells do. Bipolar cell signals are then transmitted to ganglion cells, which produce action potentials as a signal transduction to the brain via the axon of the ganglion cell.

Glutamate released from the presynaptic terminals diffuse to bind to the glutamate receptors on the postsynaptic membrane via the synaptic cleft. Retinal glutamate receptors are mainly located in the outer plexiform layer where glutamatergic synapses connect photoreceptors to bipolar and horizontal cells; and also in the inner plexiform layer which contains the bulk of glutamatergic synapses from bipolar cells to ganglion cells and amacrine cells [3-6].

Multiple glutamate receptor types have been identified. Though glutamate will bind onto all glutamate receptors, each receptor is characterized by its sensitivity to specific glutamate analogues and by the features of the glutamate-elicited current. Glutamate receptors are divided into three groups, N-methyl-D-aspartate (NMDA) receptors, AMPA (α-amino-3-hydroxyl-5-methyl-4-isoxazole-propionate)/kainic acid receptors (non-NMDA receptors), and metabotropic receptors. NMDA and non-NMDA receptors are called ionotropic glutamate receptors, and form ion channel pores for ion influx and efflux, when glutamate binds to the receptor [7-9].

When glutamate is in excess, glutamate binds to cell surface ionotropic glutamate receptors, triggering massive Ca^{2+}influx and activation of pro-apoptotic signaling cascades. It can become toxic to the retinal neurons [10-13]. Olney (1969)coined the term excitotoxicity to describe the process of neuronal death caused by excessive or prolonged activation of receptors for excitatory amino acid neurotransmitters [14]. Like excitotoxicity has been considered as an important contributor to the retinal ganglion cell death in ischemic retinal diseases such as vascular occlusions [15] or diabetic retinopathy [16-18] excitotoxicity may be involved in ganglion cell death in glaucoma [19].

Although massive glutamate release is characteristic for the ischemic retinal diseases [20-22], this is not necessarily required for pathogenesis of glaucoma. In fact, several studies were unable to detect the elevation of extracellular concentration of glutamate in vitreous humor samples from experimental animals with ocular hypertension, and in human glaucoma [23-27]. Correspondingly, it has been revealed that retinal glial cells play critical roles in the prevention of excitotoxocity. For example, Müller cells are responsible for the uptake of excess glutamate via GLAST (Glutamate Aspartate Transporter) [28.29], which is essential to maintain physiological concentrations of glutamate. Glutamate at physiological levels can be neurotoxic, if glutamate metabolism is impaired. Therefore, it is considered that impaired metabolism of glutamate more likely contributes to the excitotoxic injury even if glutamate is not in excess.

This review summarizes the present knowledge regarding the glutamate metabolism in glaucoma and the possible neuroprotective therapy of glaucoma.

2. Glutamate uptake and glaucoma

Glutamate released from the presynaptic terminals reaches the receptor molecules of the postsynaptic plasma membrane; but majority of glutamate are taken up by Müller glia or by retinal neurons via glutamate transporters. Glutamate transported into Müller glia is amidated to glutamine by a glutamate degrading enzyme, glutamine synthetase [30-33] (Figure 1).

2.1. Physiology of glutamate transporters

Glutamate uptake is mediated by five distinct glutamate transporters (EAAT1-5): GLAST (EAAT1) [34], GLT-1 (EAAT2) [35], EAAC1 (EAAT3) [36], EAAT4 [37] and EAAT5 [38]. In five EAATs, GLAST (EAAT1) and GLT-1 (EAAT2) are the major glutamate transporters in the retina. GLAST is mainly expressed in the Müller cells, whereas GLT1 and EAAC1 are in retinal neurons. We describe the physiological roles of GLAST and GLT-1, respectively.

a. GLAST

GLAST is the prominent glutamate transporter in the retina, and mainly expressed in the Müller cells [10, 31-33, 39, 40]. Müller cells remove the majority of glutamate from extracellular sites [41-47]. When Müller glial uptake is pharmacologically blocked, extracellular glutamate concentration increase [48], and severe excitotoxicity is induced [48, 49]. In GLAST KO mice, the Vmax for Müller glial glutamate transport is suppressed by 50%, suggesting that approximately 50% of glutamate is taken up via GLAST, another 40% through electroneutral, sodium-dependent (presently undefined) glutamate transporters, and 10% via sodium-independent

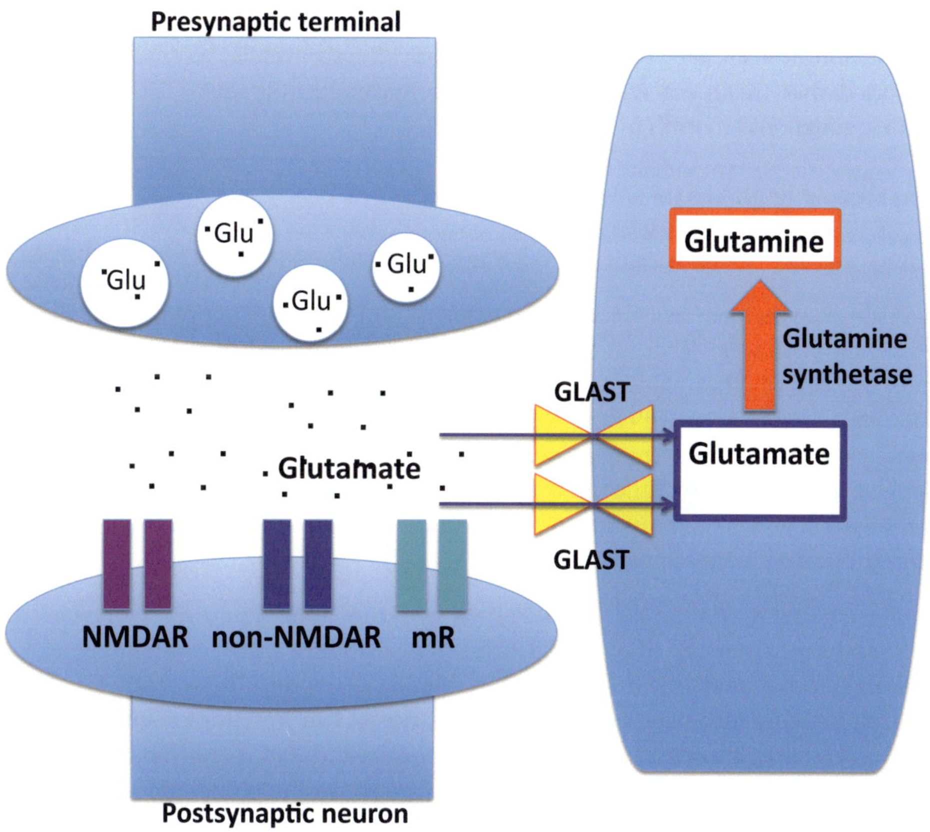

Figure 1. After release from the presynaptic terminal, glutamate binds to the post-synaptic glutamate receptors.Then, excess of glutamate is transported into the Mulller glia via glial glutamate transporter, GLAST, and catalyzed by glutamine synthetase to the nontoxic amino acid glutamine. Glutamate is also transported into retinal neurons via neuronal glutamate transporter, GLT-1.

transporters or exchangers [50]. Although antisense GLAST fails to induce apparent excitotoxicity [51], antisense suppresses the b-wave and oscillatory potentials of electrocardiogram [46, 51], and doubles total glutamate levels in the retina [50]. These results indicate that GLAST is essential to maintain the homeostasis of glutamate metabolism and physiological neural functions. In support of this, it has been shown that retinas from mice with targeted deletions of GLAST are extremely sensitive to ischemic insults [46].

b. GLT-1

GLT-1 (EAAT2) is the neuronal glutamate transporter, and exists in several distinct forms, including the originally described form (GLT-1, also referred as GLT-1a), along with GLT-1b (also called GLT1v) and GLT1c [48]. GLT-1a appears to be associated mainly with a population of amacrine cells and bipolor cells, whereas GLT-1b is associated with cone photoreceptors and subpopulations of bipolar cells [52,53]. GLT-1c is normally only expressed by the photoreceptors in the mammalian retina [54]. GLT1 knockout mice appear to exhibit minimal compromise of retinal function, suggesting that GLAST is essential for the maintenance of normal synaptic transmission [46, 49]. However, it is still controversial because other researchers reported that treatment with antisense oligonucleotides against GLT-1 induced the excitotoxic ganglion cell death in the rat retina [42].

2.2. Impairment of glutamate removal in glaucoma

a. GLAST

Some studies have shown that GLAST expression diminishes [55-57] or remains stable [58] in experimental glaucoma, whereas others have reported increased expression [59]. Thus, it remains unclear whether elevated intraocular pressure (IOP) alters glutamate uptake by modulating GLAST. After experimental IOP elevation in rats, Holcombe et al. (2008) [47] immunohistochemically determined the glutamate transport activity as aspartate uptake into Müller glia, and found that Müller glial uptake is normal even IOP is as high as 70 mmHg but compromised at 80 mmHg or higher. These results suggest that GLAST is functional as long as retinal perfusion is maintained.

We [60] used a rat *ex vivo* model incubating rat eye cups under hydrostatic pressure at the bottom of a deep cylinder. Such acute high pressures can induce retinal ischemia clinically and in *in vivo* glaucoma models [61-63] but not in this *ex vivo* model. The advantages of *ex vivo* hydrostatic pressure model include better preservation of eyecup samples without ischemia, making it possible to investigate direct effects of pressure-induced retinal injury on glutamate metabolism. In this acute *ex vivo* model, axonal damage of the retinal ganglion cells were prominent, and Western blot and real-time RT-PCR analyses revealed that 75 mm Hg pressure depressed GLAST expression [64]. Administration of glutamate receptor blockers prevented axonal damages, indicating that IOP elevation induces excitotoxicity via depression of GLAST. It should be also noticed that IOP elevation can depress GLAST activity even if retinal perfusion is preserved.

Harada et al. (2007) [65] show that GLAST-deficient mice demonstrate spontaneous RGC loss and optic nerve degeneration in spite of normal IOP. In GLAST-deficient mice, administration of glutamate receptor blockers prevented RGC loss.

These findings suggest that glutamate transporters are necessary to prevent glaucomatous excitotoxic retinal damages.

b. GLT-1

GLT-1, the main neuronal glutamate transporter in the retinal neurons, is reported to be down-regulated in glaucomatous eyes in rats [58, 66] and mice [57]. By contrast, Park et al. [58] reported that the expression of GLT-1 was expressed in cone photoreceptors and the level of expression in some cone bipolar cells was significantly increased in *in vivo* glaucoma model. They also demonstrated that GLAST expression in Müller cells remained stable during the experimental period. These results suggest that integrity of GLT-1 may be a prerequisite for the maintenance of glutamate homeostasis in the retina undergoing glaucoma [67].

Sullivan et al. (2006) [68] reported the expressional changes of the splice variant of GLT-1 (GLT-1c) in the glaucoma eyes. In normal eyes of humans and rats, GLT-1c is expressed only in photoreceptors. In glaucoma, additional robust expression of GLT-1c is detected in retinal ganglion cells, including occasional displaced ganglion cells [106]. The new induction of GLT-1c expression by retinal ganglion cells may imply abnormalities in glutamate homeostasis in glaucomatous RGCs. The same authors said that GLT-1c may be a useful indicator of the extent of stress of the RGCs and thus a tool for examining outcomes of potential therapeutic and experimental interventions.

2.3. Neuroprotection by upregulation of glutamate transporters

Several studies [56, 64] revealed that the expression of the major glutamate transporter, GLAST, decreases after pressure loading. Therefore, agents that effectively enhance glutamate transporter function may serve as potential therapeutics against the pressure-induced injury. Enhancement of glutamate transport is developing into a new strategy for reducing excitotoxicity also in brain injury and neurodegenerative disease [69-71]. Lee et al. (2009) [72] reported that tamoxifen, estrogen modulator, possessed neuroprotective properties against excitotoxicity by the up-regulation of GLAST at protein and mRNA levels in the mannganese-induced excitotoxicity. Estradiol and its derivative also reported to increase GLAST expression, though these drugs have not been applied to glaucoma patients.

Recently, the daily treatment with 17β-estradiol (E2) eye drops resulted in significant E2 concentration in the retina with concomitant profound neuroprotective therapeutic benefits, even in the presence of continually elevated IOP [73]. However, E2 eye drop induces the adverse effect to other organs induced by stimulation of estrogen receptors. It seems safe to apply E2 eye drops to postmenopausal women. Taking all above into consideration, there is a long way to go before topical estrogen drops becomes a new therapeutics of glaucoma.

3. Enzymatic degradation of glutamate and glaucoma

In the Müller cells, glutamate is rapidly converted into glutamine by the glia-specific enzyme, glutamine synthetase [33]. Glutamine synthetase is specifically localized in the cytosol of Müller cells [74].Glutamine synthetase catalyzes the following reaction,

$$\text{Glutamate} + NH^{4+} + ATP \rightarrow \text{glutamine} + ADP + P_i + H^+,$$

in the presence of Mn^{2+}or Mg^{2+}.

The activity of the glutamine synthetase influences the rate of the glutamate uptake by the Müller cells [41]. The rapid metabolization of glutamate to glutamine causes a stronger driving force for the glutamate uptake in the Müller cells than in neurons, which have intracellular free glutamate concentrations two orders of magnitude higher than the Müller cells [75]. A prerequisite for an effective glutamate-glutamine cycle in Müller cells would be the regulated coordination between glutamate uptake and glutamate degradation [39].

The activity of glutamine synthetase is stimulated by glucocorticoids [76,77]. In chick embryo retinas the stimulated glutamine synthetase by glucocorticoids is correlated with amounts of released glutamine from Müller glia, suggesting that the activity of glutamine synthetase influences glutamate uptake [78]. Conversely, it is also reported that basic fibrogrowth factor (bFGF) suppresses the activity of glutamine synthetase presumably through inhibition of glucocorticoid actions [79].

Glutamine, synthesized from glutamate in Müller glia, is the major source of glutamate found in retinal neurons. MSO, an inhibitor of glutamine synthetase, rapidly abolish free glutamate from bipolar cells and retinal ganglion cells [80]. Therefore, glutamine synthetase is a key enzyme in glutamate-glutamine cycle.

3.1. Impairment of glutamate metabolism and glaucoma

Several studies have shown increases in the expression of glutamine synthetase [78] after pressure elevation [81,82], whereas others have reported decreases. Thus, it remains controversial whether elevated IOP alters glial cell glutamate metabolism as a potential mechanism of retinal excitotoxicity [83].

In primary glaucoma in dogs [84], decreases in immunoreactivity of glutamine synthetase were associated with glutamate redistribution. These decreases in glutamine synthetase occurred even in mildly damaged regions of retina before retinal thinning. Reactive Müller cells were seen primarily in chronic primary glaucoma in severely damaged regions. Decreases in glutamine synthetase may potentiate ischemia-induced early glutamate redistribution and neuronal damage in canine primary glaucoma.

We (2010) [60] reported that pressure elevation induced reduction of glutamine synthetase activity compared with control pressure in an acute*ex vivo* model. The result suggests that the neural degeneration observed during pressure elevation is caused by impaired glial glutamate metabolism.

Although GLAST and the activities of glutamine synthetase are intimately intertwined [85], both are simultaneously suppressed by high pressure-loading. Thus, it is also possible that suppression of GLAST and the activities of glutamine synthetase occur separately during pressure-loading [86]. However, a series of observations using acute *ex vivo* model suggest that during pressure-loading, the impairment of GLAST expression precedes the depression of glutamine synthetase activity. Pharmacologic inhibition of glutamine synthetase activity with MSO fails to modulate GLAST expression, whereas inhibition of GLAST with TFB-TBOA substantially suppresses glutamine synthetase activity. Based on these findings, it is hypothesize that during pressure-loading, impairment of GLAST takes place first and results in downregulation of activities of glutamine synthetase as a secondary effect [62], though it is also possible that changes in the activities of glutamine synthetase influence GLAST activities [78].

http://dx.doi.org/10.5772/57605

3.2. Neuroprotection by upregulation of glutamine synthetase

Hydrocortisone, which is shown to increase the expression of glutamine synthetase in the Müller cells, is considered as neuroprotectve against excitotoxicity [87-89]. Upregulation of glutamine synthetase by hydrocortisone may be related to the fact that the upstream region of the glutamine synthetase gene contains a glucocorticoid response element that can bind the glucocorticoid receptor protein [53]. Glutamine synthtase was also reported upregulated by taurine supplementation in the diabetic retina [90]. These agents that effectively enhance glutamine synthetase function and expression may serve as potential therapeutics against the pressure-induced injury.

4. Glutamate receptors

The excitotoxicity is predominantly mediated by the overstimulation of NMDA receptors due to their extreme permeability to calcium ions [94]. Many researchers have concluded, therefore, that excitotoxicity occurs, in part, via NMDA receptors activation [99,100]. There is still remained a possibility that glutamate acts via non-NMDA receptors to initiate neurotoxicity [101-105]. However, the role of non-NMDA receptorsin pathogenesis of glaucoma has not been elucidated.

We describe the present knowledge concerning the molecular function of NMDA receptors and its relation to excitotoxicity.

a. NMDA receptors

Retinal ganglion cells express abundant NMDA receptors [106-109]. A number of studies demonstrated that ganglion cells are extremely vulnerable to exogenously applied NMDA, which inducesganglion cell degeneration.It has been also shown that NMDA receptor antagonists are neuroprotective in experimental glaucoma models [110-117]. NMDA receptors permit the influx of sodium ions (Na^+) and calcium ions (Ca^{2+}) and the efflux of potassium ions (K^+).

Although all NMDA receptors express the NR1 subunit [122,123,124], NR2 subunits are major determinants of the functional properties of NMDA receptor [125]. Recently, Bai et al. (2013) [126] reported the roles of the four different NR2 subtypes (NR2a, NR2b, NR2c, NR2d) in NMDA-induced retinal cell death using mice lacking specific NR2 subunits. They also evaluated the neuroprotective effect of 7-hydroxy-6-methoxy-2-methyl-1-(2-(4-(trifluoromethyl)phenyl)ethyl)-1,2,3,4-tetra-hydro-isoquinoline hydrochloride (HON0001) [127], an specific NR2b antagonist, on ganglion cell degeneration due to glutamate excitotoxicity in GLAST-deficient mice. As the results, NR2b-and NR2d-deficiency protected ganglion cells from NMDA-induced excitotoxicity. Pharmacological inhibition of the NR2b subunit by HON0001 attenuated ganglion cell loss in GLAST deficient mice. These findings suggest that NR2b-and NR2d-containing NMDA receptors play a critical role in NMDA receptor-mediated excitotoxicity in the retina. Based on these findings,inhibition of NR2b and NR2d activity is a potential therapeutic strategy for the treatment of retinal neurodegeneration induced by excitotoxicity.

The same authors demonstrate that NR2d deficiency attenuates ganglion cell loss in GLAST-deficient mice [126]. Furthermore, Dock3, a guanine nucleotide exchange factor, binds to the NR2d C-terminal domain and reduces the expression of NR2d, thereby protects ganglion cells from excitotoxicity. These results suggest that NR2d is involved in the excitotoxic ganglion cell death, and that the interaction between NR2d and Dock3 may have a neuroprotective effect. These findings indicate the possibility that NR2d and Dock3 might be therapeutic targets for glaucoma.

b. Neuroprotection by NMDA receptor antagonists

Classical pharmacological approaches for reducing excitotoxicity have focused on antagonism of glutamate receptors. Memantine is an uncompetitive NMDA antagonist, binding near the Mg^{2+}site within the ion channel [128]. The degree of blockade of the NMDA receptors is changed according to the concentration of memantine [128]. Memantine is a neuroprotective agent that has completed phase III clinical trial in patients with glaucoma [129, 130]. The trial showed that memantine was ineffective by the primary end point, with the variable mechanisms of retinal ganglion apoptosis being offered as an explanation [131].

A recent study demonstrated that NR2c-and NR2d-containing NMDA receptors are the primary targets of memantine [132]. It has been reported that memantine prevents the loss of retinal ganglion cells in GLAST knockout mice, a model of normal tension glaucoma (NTG), suggesting that NR2d-containing receptors may be involved in ganglion cell loss in glaucoma [125, 126]. It was also demonstrated that Mg^{2+}regulates the sensitivity of NMDA receptors to memantine [133]. In a physiological concentration (1 mM) of extracellular Mg^{2+}, memantine exerts a more potent blocking effect at NR2c and NR2d subunits than at NR2a and NR2b subunits. These findings suggest that NR2c-and NR2d-containing NMDA receptors are likely to be the main targets of memantine.

5. Concluding comments

Glutamate accumulation in extracellular spaces can be potentially neurotoxic if glutamate is not removed in an appropriate manner. It should be noticed that excitotoxicity does not always due to excess of glutamate. Extracellular glutamate level duringretinal ischemia may not be sufficient to induceneuronal damage under normal conditions. This suggeststhat clearance of glutamate is essential in preventingretinal excitotoxicity. In glaucomatous models, glutamate metabolism can be impaired by inhibition of glutamate transporter and glutamine synthetase, resulting in excitotoxic glaucomatous damages of retinal ganglion cells. A series of observations using ex vivo glaucomatous model suggest that during pressure-loading, the impairment of glutamate transporter expression precedes the depression of glutamine synthetase activity. Therefore, it is also possible that changes in the activities of glutamine synthetase influence GLAST activities.Agents that effectively enhance glutamate transporter function may serve as

http://dx.doi.org/10.5772/57605

potential therapeutics against the pressure-induced injury. Enhancement of glutamine synthetase may be a therapeutic strategy for reducing excitotoxicity.

Acknowledgements

I thank Yoko Hayami, and Sanae Takaseki (Department of Ophthalmology Akita Graduate University School of Medicine) for instructions and suggestions. This work was supported by JSPS KAKENHI Grant Numbers 24592666 to M.I.

Author details

Makoto Ishikawa[1*], Takeshi Yoshitomi[1] and Yukitoshi Izumi[2]

*Address all correspondence to: mako@med.akita-u.ac.jp

1 Department of Ophthalmology, Akita Graduate University Faculty of Medicine, Akita, Japan

2 Department of Psychiatry, Washington University School of Medicine, St. Louis, M.O., USA

References

[1] Crevetto, L, & Piccolino, M. Synaptic trans-mission between photoreceptors and horizontal cells in the turtle retina. Science (1974)., 183, 417-419.

[2] Dowling, J. E, & Ripps, H. Effect of magnesium on horizontal cell activity in the skate retina. Nature London(1973)., 242, 101-103.

[3] Gruender, T, Kohler, K, Kaletta, A, & Guenther, E. The distribution and developmental regulation of NMDA receptor subunit proteins in the outer and inner retina of the rat. J. Neurobiol (2000)., 44, 333-342.

[4] Lagrèze, W. A, Darstein, M, Feuerstein, T. J, Otto, T, & Landwehrmeyer, G.B. NMDA receptor subunit mRNA expression in human retinal ganglion cells.Graefe's Archives of Clinical & Experimental Ophthalmology (2000)., 238, 486-490.

[5] Lukasiewicz, P. Synaptic mechanisms that shape visual signaling at the inner retina. Progress in Brain Research (2005).. 147, 205-218.

[6] Peng, Y. W, Blackstone, C. D, Huganir, R. L, &Yau, K. W, Distribution of glutamate receptor subtypes in the vertebrate retina. Neuroscience (1995)., 66, 483-497.

[7] Thoreson, W. B, & Witkovsky, P. Glutamate receptors and circuits in the vertebrate retina. Progress in Retinal and Eye Research(1999)., 18, 765-810.

[8] Massey, S. C, & Miller, R. F. Excitatory amino acid receptors of rod-and cone-driven horizontal cells in the rabbit retina. Journal of Neurophysiology (1987)., 57, 645-59.

[9] Massey, S. C, & Miller, R. F. N-methyl-D-aspartate receptors of ganglion cells in rabbit retina. Journal of Neurophysiology (1990)., 63, 16-30.

[10] Lucas, D. R, & Newhouse, J. P. The toxic effect of sodium l-glutamate on the inner layers of the retina. Archives of Ophthalmology (1957)., 58, 193–201.

[11] Sisk, D. R, & Kuwabara, T. Histologic changes in the inner retina of albino rats following intravitreal injection of monosodium l-glutamate. Graefe's Archives of Clinical&Experimental Ophthalmology (1985)., 223, 250–258.

[12] Olney, J. W. The toxic effects of glutamate and related compounds in the retina and the brain, Retina(1982)., 2, 341–359.

[13] Vorwerk, C. K, Lipton, S. A, Zurakowski, D, Hyman, B. T, Sabel, B. A, &Dreyer, E. B. Chronic low-dose glutamate is toxic to retinal ganglion cells. Toxicity blocked by memantine. Invest igative Ophthalmology & Visual Science (1996)., 37, 1618–1624.

[14] Olney J. W. Glutaate-induced retinal degeneration in neonatal mice. Electron microscopy of the acutely evolving lesion. Journal of Neuropatholgy & Experimental Neurology(1969)., 28(3):455-74.

[15] Ju, W. K, &Kim, K. Y. Measuring glutamate receptor activation-induced apoptotic cell death in ischemic rat retina using the TUNEL assay. Methods in Molecular Biology(2011)., 740:149-56.

[16] Casson, R. J. Possible role of excitotoxicity in the pathogenesis of glaucoma. Clinical & Experimental Ophthalmology (2006)., 34, 54-63.

[17] Kaur, C, Foulds, W. S, & Ling, E. A. Hypoxia-ischemia and retinal ganglion cell damage.
Clinical Ophthalmology(2008)., 2, 879-889.

[18] Hernández, C, & Simó, R. Neuroprotection in diabetic retinopathy.
Current Diabtes Report (2012).,12, 329-337.

[19] Vorwerk C. K, Gorla M. S, &Dreyer, E. B. An experimental basis for implicating excitotoxicity in glaucomatous optic neuropathy. Survey of Ophthalmology(1999)., 43 Suppl 1, S142-150.

[20] Choi, D. W, &Rothman, S. M. The role of glutamate neurotoxicity in hypoxicischemic neuronal death. Annual Review of Neuroscience (1990)., 13, 171-182.

[21] Bertram, K. M, Bula, D. V, Pulido, J. S, Shippy, S. A, Gautam, S, Lu, M. J, Hatfield, R. M, Kim, J. H, Quirk, M. T, &Arroyo, J. G. Amino-acid levels in subretinal and vitreous fluid of patients with retinal detachment. Eye(2008).,22, 582-589.

[22] Diederen, R.M. H, La Heij, E. C, Deutz, N.E. P, Kijlstra, A, Kessels, A.G. H, van Eijk, H.M. H, Liem, A.T. A, Dieudonné, S, & Hendrikse, F. Increased glutamatelevels in the vitreous of patients with retinal detachment. Experimantal Eye Research (2006)., 83, 45-50.

[23] Carter-Dawson, L, Crawford, M.L. J, Harwerth, R. S, Smith, E. L, Feldman, R, Shen, F. F, Mitchell, C. K, & Whitetree, A. Vitreal glutamate concentration in monkeys with experimental glaucoma. Investigative Ophthalmology & Visual Science(2002)., 43, 2633e2637.

[24] Honkanen, R. A, Baruah, S, Zimmerman, M. B, Khanna, C. L, Weaver, Y. K, Narkiewicz, J, Waziri, R, Gehrs, K. M, Weingeist, T. A, Boldt, H. C, Folk, J.C., Russell, S. R, &Kwon, Y. H. Vitreous amino acid concentrations in patients with glaucoma undergoing vitrectomy. Archives of Ophthalmology (2003)., 121, 183-188.

[25] Kwon, Y. H, Rickman, D. W, Baruah, S, Zimmerman, M. B, Kim, C.S., Boldt, H. C, Russell, S. R, &Hayreh, S. S. Vitreous and retinal amino acid concentrations in experimental central retinal artery occlusion in the primate. Eye (2004)., 19, 455-463.

[26] Levkovitch-Verbin, H, Martin, K. R, Quigley, H. A, Baumrind, L. A, Pease, M. E, & Valenta, D. Measurement of amino acid levels in the vitreous humor of rats after chronic intraocular pressure elevation or optic nerve transection. Journal of Glaucoma (2002)., 11, 396-405.

[27] Wamsley, S, Gabelt, B. T. Dahl, D. B, Case, G. L, Sherwood, R. W. May, C.A., Hernandez, M. R,& Kaufman, P.L. Vitreous glutamate concentration and axon loss in monkeys with experimental glaucoma. Archives of Ophthalmology(2005)., 123, 64-70.

[28] Barnett, N. L Pow, D. V, &Bull, N. D. Differential perturbation of neuronal and glial glutamate transport systems in retinal ischemia. Neurochemistry International(2001)., 39(4), 291-299.

[29] Otori, Y, Shimada, S, Tanaka, K, Ishimoto, I. Tano, Y, & Tohyama, M. Marked increase in glutamate-aspartate transporter (GLAST/GluT-1) mRNA following transient retinal ischemia. Molecular Brain Research (1994)., 27, 310–314.

[30] Derouiche, A, & Rauen, T. Coincidence of L-glutamate/L-aspartate transporter (GLAST) and glutamine synthetase (GS) immunoreactions in retinal glia: evidence for coupling of GLAST and GS in transmitter clearance. Journal of Neuroscience Research (1995)., 42, 131-143.

[31] Higgs, M. H, & Lukasiewicz, P. D. Glutamate uptake limits synaptic excitation of retinal ganglion cells. Journal of Neuroscience (2002)., 19, 3691–3700.

[32] Matsui, K, Hosoi, N, & Tachibana, M. Active role of glutamate uptake in the synaptic transmission from retinal nonspiking neurons. Journal of Neuroscience (1999)., 19, 6755–6766.

[33] Bringmann, A, Pannicke, T, Biedermann, B, Francke, M, Iandiev, I, Grosche, J, Wiedemann, P, Albrecht, J, & Reichenbach, A. Role of retinal glial cells in neurotransmitter uptake and metabolism. Neurochemistry International (2009)., 54, 143-160.

[34] Storck, T, Schulte, S, Hofmann, K, &Stoffel, W. Structure, expression, and functional analysis of a Na(+)-dependent glutamate/aspartate transporter from rat brain. Proceedings ofthe National Acaddemy of Sciences of the United States of America(1992)., 89:10955–10959.

[35] Pines, G, Zhang, Y, & Kanner, B. I. Glutamate 404 is involved in the substrate discrimination of GLT-1, a (Na++K+)-coupled glutamate transporter from rat brain. Journal of Biological Chemistry (1995)., 270,17093-17097.

[36] Kanai, Y, & Hediger, M. A. Primary structure and functional characterization of a high-affinity glutamate transporter. Nature(1992)., 360, 467-471.

[37] Fairman, W. A, Vandenberg, R. J, Arriza, J. L, Kavanaugh, M. P, & Amara, S. G. An excitatory amino-acid transporter with properties of a ligand-gated chloride channel. Nature(1995)., 375, 599-603.

[38] Arriza, I. L, Eliasof, S, Kavanaugh, M. P, & Amara, S. G. Excitatory amino acid transporter 5, a retinal glutamate transporter coupled to a chloride conductance. Proceedings ofthe National Acaddemy of Sciences of the United States of America(1997)., 94, 4155-4160.

[39] Rauen, T, & Wiessner, M. Fine tuning of glutamate uptake and degradation in glial cells: common transcriptional regulation of GLAST1 and GS. Neurochemistry International (2000)., 37, 179–189.

[40] Kanai, Y, & Hediger, M. A. The glutamate/neutral amino acid transporter family SLC1: molecular, physiological and pharmacological aspects. Pflugers Archiv(2004)., 447, 469–479.

[41] Rauen, T, Taylor, W. R, Kuhlbrodt, K, & Wiessner, M. High-affinity glutamate transporters in the rat retina: a major role of the glial glutamate transporter GLAST-1 in transmitter clearance. Cell &Tissue Research (1998)., 291, 19–31.

[42] Rauen, T. Diversity of glutamate transporter expression and function in the mammalian retina. Amino Acids(2000)., 19, 53–62.

[43] Pow, D. V, Barnett, N. L, & Penfold, P. Are neuronal transporters relevant in retinal glutamate homeostasis? Neurochemistry International (2000)., 37, 191–198.

[44] White, R. D, & Neal, M. J. The uptake of L-glutamate by the retina. Brain Research (1976)., 111, 79–93.

http://dx.doi.org/10.5772/57605

[45] Ladanyi, M, & Beaudet, A. In-vivo labeling of (3H)D-aspartate uptake sites in monkey retina. Cell & Tissue Research (1986)., 243, 59–63.

[46] Harada, T, Harada, C, Watanabe, M, Inoue, Y, Sakagawa, T, Nakayama, N, Sasaki, S, Okuyama, S, Watase, K, Wada, K, & Tanaka, K. Functions of the two glutamate transporters GLAST and GLT-1 in the retina. Proceedings ofthe National Acaddemy of Sciences of the United States of America(1998).,95, 4663–4666.

[47] Holcombe, D. J, Lengefeld, N, Gole, G. A, &Barnett, N. L. (The effects of acute intraocular pressure elevation on rat retinal glutamate transport. Acta Ophthalmologica Scandinavia, (2008)., 86, 408–414.

[48] Sarthy, V. P, Pignataro, L, Pannicke, T. Weick, M, Reichenbach, A, Harada, T, Tanaka, K, &Marc, R. Glutamate transport by retinal Mülle cells in glutamate/aspartate transporter-knockout mice. Glia(2005)., 49, 184–196.

[49] Barnett, N. L, & Pow, D. V. Antisense knockdown of GLAST, a glial glutamate transporter, compromises retinal function. Investigative Ophthalmology & Visual Science (2000)., 41, 585–591.

[50] Izumi, Y, Shimamoto, K, Benz, A. M, Hammerman, S. B, Olney, J. W, &Zorumski, C. F. Glutamate transporters and retinal excitotoxicity. Glia (2002). 39, 58–68.

[51] Reye, P, Sullivan, R, Fletcher, E. L, & Pow, D. W. Distribution of two splice variants of the glutamate transporter GLT1 in the retinas of humans, monkeys, rabbits, rats, cats, and chickens. Journal of Comparative Neurology (2002)., 445, 1–12.

[52] Reye, P, Sullivan, R, &Pow, D. V. Distribution of two splice variants of the glutamate transporter GLT-1 in the developing rat retina. Journal of Comparative Neurology (2002)., 447, 323–330.

[53] Rauen, T, Wiessner, M, Sullivan, R, Lee, A, & Pow, D. V. A new GLT1 splice variant: cloning and immunolocalization of GLT1c in the mammalian retina and brain,. Neurochemistry International (2004)., 45, 1095–1106.

[54] Naskar, R, Vorwerk, C. K, &Dreyer, E. B. Concurrent downregulation of a glutamate transporter and receptor in glaucoma. Investigative Ophthalmology & Visual Science (2000)., 41, 1940–1944.

[55] Martin, K. R, Levkovitch-Verbin, H, Valenta, D., L, Baumrind, L, Pease, M. E, &Quigley, H. A. Retinal glutamate transporter changes in experimental glaucoma and after optic nerve transection in the rat. Investigative Ophthalmology & Visual Science (2002)., 43, 2236–2243.

[56] Schuettauf, F, Thaler, S. Bolz, S, Kalbacher, S. H, Mankowska, A, Zurakowski, D, Zrenner, E, & Rejdak, R. Alterations of amino acids and glutamate transport in the DBA/2J mouse retina; possible clues to degeneration. Graefe's Archives of Clinical&Experimental Ophthalmology (2007)., 245, 1157–1168.

[57] Park, C. K, Cha, J, Park, S. C, Lee, P. Y, Kim, J. H, Kim, H. S, Kim, S. A, Kim, I. B, & Chun, M. H. "Differential expression of two glutamate transporters, GLAST and GLT-1, in an experimental rat model of glaucoma. Experimental Brain Research (2009).. 197, 101–109.

[58] Ishikawa, M, Yoshitomi, T, Zorumski, C. F, & Izumi, Y. Effects of acutely elevated hydrostatic pressure in a rat ex vivo retinal preparation, Investigative Ophthalmology & Visual Science (2010)., 51,6414-6423.

[59] Park, S. W., Kim, K. Y, Lindsey, J. D, Dai, Y, Heo, H. Nguyen, D. H, Ellisman, M. H, Weinreb, R. N, & Ju, W. K. A selective inhibitor of drp1, mdivi-1, increases retinal ganglion cell survival in acute ischemic mouse retina. Investigative Ophthalmology & Visual Science (2011)., 52, 2837-2843.

[60] Yoneda, S, Tanaka, E, Goto, W, Ota, T, & Hara, H. Topiramate reduces excitotoxic and ischemic injury in the rat retina. Brain Research (2003)., 967, 257-266.

[61] Whitlock, N. A, Agarwal, N. Ma, J. X, & Crosson, C. E. Hsp27 upregulation by HIF-1 signaling offers protection against retinal ischemia in rats. Investigative Ophthalmology & Visual Science (2005)., 46, 1092-1098.

[62] shikawa, M, Yoshitomi, T, Zorumski, C. F., & Izumi, Y. Downregulation of glutamine synthetase via GLAST suppression induces retinal axonal swelling in a rat ex vivo hydrostatic pressure model. Investigative Ophthalmology & Visual Science (2011).. 52, 6604-6616.

[63] Harada T, Harada, C, Nakamura, K, Quah, H. M, Okumura, A, Namekata, Saeki, K, Aihara, M, Yoshida, H, Mitani, A, &Tanaka, K. The potential role of glutamate transporters in the pathogenesis of normal tension glaucoma. Journal of Clinical Investigation (2007)., 117, 1763–1770.

[64] Russo, R, Cavaliere, F, Varanom G. P, Milanese, M, Adornetto, A, Nucci, C, Bonanno, G, Morrone, L. A, Corasaniti, M. T, & Bagetta, G. Impairment of Neuronal Glutamate Uptake and Modulation of the Glutamate Transporter GLT-1 Induced by Retinal Ischemia. PLoS One(2013)., 8, e69250.

[65] Persson, M, & Rönnbäck, L. Microglial self-defence mediated through GLT-1 and glutathione. Amino Acids(2012)., 42, 207-219.

[66] Sullivan, R. K, Woldemussie, E, Macnab, L, Ruiz, G, Pow, DV. Evoked expression of the glutamate transporter GLT-1c in retinal ganglion cells in human glaucoma and in a rat model. Investigative Ophthalmology & Visual Science(2006)., 47(9):3853-3859.

[67] Shi, J, Zhang, Y. Q, & Simpkins, J. W. Effects of 17beta-estradiol on glucose transporter 1 expression and endothelial cell survival following focal ischemia in the rats. Experimantal Brain Research (1997)., 117, 200–206.

[68] Namekata, K, Harada, C, Guo, X, Kikushima, K, Kimura, A, Fuse, N, Mitamura, Y, Kohyama, K, Matsumoto, Y, Tanaka, K, & Harada, T. Interleukin-1 attenuates normal

tension glaucoma-like retinal degeneration in EAAC1-deficient mice. Neuroscience Letter (2009)., 465, 160-164.

[69] Dhandapani, K. M, & Brann, D. W. Protective effects of estrogen and selective estrogen receptor modulators in the brain. Biology of Reproduction (2002)., 67, 1379–1385.

[70] Lee, E. S, Sidoryk, M, Jiang, H, Yin, Z, & Aschner, M. Estrogen and tamoxifen reverse manganese-induced glutamate transporter impairment in astrocytes. Journal of Neurochemistry (2009)., 110, 530-544.

[71] Prokai-Tatrai, K, Xin, H, Nguyen, V, Szarka, S, Blazics, B, Prokai, L, & Koulen, P. 17β-estradiol eye drops protect the retinal ganglion cell layer and preserve visual function in an in vivo model of glaucoma. Molecular Pharmacology (2013)., 10, 3253-3261.

[72] Riepe, R. E, &Norenburg, M. D. Müller cell localisation of glutamine synthetase in rat retina. Nature(1977)., 268(5621):654-655.

[73] Marc, R. E, Murry, R. F, & Basinger, S. F. Pattern recognition of amino acid signatures in retinal neurons. Journal of Neuroscience (1995)., 15, 5106–5129.

[74] Gorovits, R, Yakir, A, Fox, L. E, & Vardimon, L. Hormonal and non-hormonal regulation of glutamine synthetase in the developing neural retina. Brain Research & Molecular Brain Research (1996)., 43, 321–329,

[75] Vardimon L. Neuroprotection by glutamine synthetase. Israel Medical Association Journal(2000)., Suppl:46-51

[76] Shaked, I, Ben-Dror, I, &Vardimon, L. Glutamine synthetase enhances the clearance of extracellular glutamate by the neural retina. Journal of Neurochemistry(2002)., 83(3):574-580.

[77] Kruchkova, Y, Ben-Dror, I, Herschkovitz, A, David, M, Yayon, A, &Vardimon, L. Basic fibroblast growth factor: a potential inhibitor of glutamine synthetase expression in injured neural tissue. Journal of Neurochemistry (2001).,77(6), 1641-1649.

[78] Pow, D. V, &Robinson, S. R. Glutamate in some retinal neurons is derived solely from glia. Neuroscience. (1994).,60(2), 355-366

[79] Izumi, Y., Hammerman, S. B., Kirby, C. O., Benz, A. M, Olney, J. W, & Zorumski, C. F. Involvement of glutamate in ischemic neurodegeneration in isolated retina. Visual Neuroscience (2003)., 20, 97-107.

[80] Shen, F, Chen, B, J., Danias, J, Lee, K. C, Lee, K. H, Su, Y, Podos, S. M, &Mittag, T. W. Glutamate-induced glutamine synthetase expression in retinal Müller cells after short-term ocular hypertension in the rat. Investigative Ophthalmology & Visual Science (2004)., 45, 3107–3111.

[81] Zeevalk, G. D, &Nicklas, W. J. Evidence that the loss of the voltage-dependent Mg2+block at the N-methyl-D-aspartate receptor underlies receptor activation dur-

ing inhibition of neuronal metabolism. Journal of Neurochemistry (1992).. 59, 1211–1220.

[82] Chen, C-H, Alyahya, K, Gionfriddo, J. R, Dubielzig, R. R, &Madl, J. E. Loss of glutamate synthetase immunoreactivity from the retina in canine primary glaucoma, Veterinary Ophthalmology (2008)., 11, 150–157.

[83] Derouiche, A, & Rauen, T. Coincidence of L-glutamate/L-aspartate transporter (GLAST) and glutamine synthetase (GS) immunoreactions in retinal glia: evidence for coupling of GLAST and GS in transmitter clearance. Journal of Neuroscience Research (1995)., 42:131–143.

[84] Jablonski, M. M, Freeman, N. E, Orr, W. E, Templeton, J. P, Lu, L, Williams, R. W, & Geisert, E. E. Genetic pathways regulating glutamate levels in retinal Mülle cells. Neurochemical Research (2011)., 36, 594–603.

[85] Carter-Dawson, L, Crawford, M. L, Harwerth, R. S, Smith, E. L, Feldman, R, Shen, F. F, Mitchell, C. K, & Whitetree, A. Vitreal glutamate concentration in monkeys with experimental glaucoma.
Investigative Ophthalmology & Visual Science (2002).., 43:2633-2637.

[86] Louzada-Junior, P, Dias, J. J, Santos, W. F, Lachat, J. J, Bradford, H. F, & J. Coutinho-Netto. Glutamate release in experimental ischaemia of the retina: an approach using microdialysis. Journal of Neurochemistry (1992).,59, 358–363.

[87] Neal, M. J, Cunningham, J. R, Hutson, P. H, & Hogg,, J. Effects of ischemia on neurotransmitter release from the isolated retina. Journal of Neurochemistry(1994)., 62, 1025–1033.

[88] Zeng, K, Xu, H, Mi, M, Zhang, Q, Zhang, Y, Chen, K, Chen, F, Zhu, J, Yu, X. Dietary taurine supplementation prevents glial alterations in retina of diabetic rats. Neurochemical Research(2009)., 34(2), 244-54.

[89] Zuo, ZF, Zhang, Q, Liu, XZ. Protective effects of curcumin on retinal Müller cell in early diabetic rats. International Journal of Ophthalmology(2013)., 6(4):422-424.

[90] El-Remessy, A. B, Khalifa, Y, Ola, S, Ibrahim, A. S, &Liou, GI. Cannabidiol protects retinal neurons by preserving glutamine synthetase activity in diabetes. Molecular Vision(2010)., 16:1487-95

[91] Shen, X, Xie, B, Cheng, Y, Jiao, Q, &Zhong Y. Effect of pigment epithelium derived factor on the expression of glutamine synthetase in early phase of experimental diabetic retinopathy. Ocular Immunology & Inflammation(2011).,19(4), 246-254.

[92] Ferreira, I. L, Duarte, C. B, &Carvalho, A. P. Ca2+influx through glutamate receptor-associated channels in retina cells correlates with neuronal cell death.Europian Journal of Pharmacology(1996)., 302:153-162.

[93] Osborne, N.N, DeSantis, L, Bae, J. H, Ugarte, M, Wood, J.P. M. Nash, M. S, & Chidlow, G. Topically applied betaxolol attenuates NMDA-induced toxicity to ganglion

cells and the effects of ischaemia to the retina. Experimental Eye Research(1999)., 69, 331–342.

[94] Osborne, N.N, Safa, R, &Nash, M.S. Photoreceptors are preferentially affected in the rat retina following permanent occlusion of the carotid arteries. Vision Research (1999).. 39, 3995–4002.

[95] Osborne, N. N, Ugarte, M, Chao, M, Chidlow, G, Bae, J. H, Wood, J.P.M., &Nash, M. S. Neuroprotection in relation to retinal ischemia and relevance to glaucoma. Survey of Ophthalmology (1999).. 43 (Suppl. 1), 102–128.

[96] Osborne, N. N, Wood, J.P. M, Chidlow, G, Bae, J. H, Melena, J, &Nash, M. S., Ganglion cell death in glaucoma: what do we really know? British Journal of Ophthalmology(1999).83, 980–986.

[97] Olney, J. W, Price, M. T, Salles, K. S, Labruyere, J, Ryerson, R, Mahan, K, Frierdich, G, & Samson, L. L-homocysteic acid: an endogenous excitotoxic ligand of the NMDA receptor. Brain Research Bulletin (1987)., 19, 597–602.

[98] el-Asrar A. M, Morse P. H, Maimone, D, Torczynski, E, &Reder, A. T. MK-801 protects retinal neurons from hypoxia and the toxicity of glutamate and aspartate. Investigative Ophthalmology &Visual Science(1992)., 33(12):3463-3468.

[99] Izumi, Y, Hammerman, S. B, Kirby, C. O, Benz, A. M, Olney, J. W, &Zorumski, C. F. Involvement of glutamate in ischemic neurodegeneration in isolated retina. Visual Neuroscience (2003)., 20, 97-107.

[100] Romano, C, Price, M. T, Almli, T, Olney, J. W. Excitotoxic neurodegeneration induced by deprivation of oxygen and glucose in isolated retina. Investigative Ophthalmology & Visual Science(1998)., 39(2), 416-23.

[101] Lees, G. J, & Leong, W. Differential effects of NBQX on the distal and local toxicity of glutamate agonists administered intrahippocampally. Brain Research (1993).. 628, 1–7.

[102] Osborne, N. N,&Herrera, A. J. The effect of experimental ischaemia and excitatory amino acid agonists on the GABA and serotonin immunoreactivities in the rabbit retina. Neuroscience (1994).59,1071–1081.

[103] Weber, M, Bonaventure, N, &Sahel, J. A. Protective role of excitatory amino acid antagonists in experimental retinal ischemia. Graefes Archives of Clinical & Experimental Ophthalmology (1995)., 233, 360–365.

[104] Massey, S. C. Cell types using glutamate as a neurotransmitter in the vertebrate retina. In: Osborne, N.N., Chader, G.J. (Eds.), Progress in Retinal Research. Pergamon Press, Oxford, (1990)., pp. 399–425.

[105] Dixon D. B, &Copenhagen, D. R. Two types of glutamate receptors differentially excite amacrine cells in the tiger salamander retina. Journal of Physiology(1992)., 449, 589-606

[106] Diamond, J. S, &Copenhagen, D. R. The contribution of NMDA and non-NMDA receptors to the light-evoked input-output characteristics of retinal ganglion cells. Neuron(1993).,11(4), 725-38.

[107] Cohen, E. D, &Miller, R. F. The role of NMDA and non-NMDA excitatory amino acid receptors in the functional organization of primate retinal ganglion cells.Visual Neuroscience(1994).,11(2), 317-32.

[108] Dong, C-J, Guo, Y, Agey, P, Wheeler, L, & Hare, W.A, Alpha-2 adrenergic modulation of NMDA receptor function as a major mechanism of RGC protection in experimental glaucoma and retinal excitotoxicity. Investigative Ophthalmology & Visual Science(2008)., 49, 4515-4522.

[109] Hare, W. A, WoldeMussie, E, Lai, R. K, Ton, H, Ruiz, G, Chun, T, & Wheeler, L. Efficacy and safety of memantine treatment for reduction of changes associatedwith experimental glaucoma in monkey, I: functional Measures. Investigative Ophthalmology & Visual Science (2004)., 45, 2625-2639.

[110] Lam, T. T, Abler, A.S., Kwong, J.M. K, Tso, M.O. M. N-methyl-D-aspartate (NMDA)-induced apoptosis in rat retina. Investigative Ophthalmology & Visual Science(1999)., 40, 2391-2397.

[111] Manabe, S, &Lipton, S. Divergent NMDA signals leading to proapoptotic and antiapoptotic pathways in the rat retina. Investigative Ophthalmology & Visual Science (2003).. 44, 385-392.

[112] Reichstein, D, Ren, L, Filippopoulos, T, Mittag, T, & Danias, J., Apoptotic retinal ganglion cell death in the DBA/2 mouse model of glaucoma. Experimental Eye Research (2007)., 84, 13-21.

[113] Russo, R, Cavaliere, F, Berliocchi, L, Nucci, C, Gliozzi, M, Mazzei, C., Tassorelli, C, Corasaniti, M. T, Rotiroti, D, Bagetta, G, &Morrone, L. A. Modulation of prosurvival and death-associated pathways under retinal ischemia/reperfusion: effects of NMDA receptor blockade. J.ournal of Neurochemistry (2008)., 107, 1347-1357.

[114] Schuettauf, F, Stein, T, Choragiewicz, T, Rejdak, R, Bolz, S, Zurakowski, D. Varde, M, Laties, A, & Thaler, S. Caspase inhibitors protect against NMDAmediated retinal ganglion cell death. Clinical & Experimental Ophthalmology (2010)., 39, 545-554.

[115] Shimazawa, M, Yamashima, T, Agarwal, N, & Hara, H. Neuroprotective effects of minocycline against in vitro and in vivo retinal ganglion cell damage. BrainResearch (2005)., 1053, 185-194

[116] Kutsuwada, T, Kashiwabuchi, N, Mori, H, Sakimura, K, Kushiya, E, Araki, K, Meguro, H, Masaki, H, Kumanishi, T, Arakawa, M, &Mishina, M. Molecular diversity of the NMDA receptor channel. Nature (1992)., 358, 36–41.

[117] Moriyoshi, K, Masu, M, Ishii, T, Shigemoto, R, Mizuno, N, &Nakanishi, S. Molecular cloning and characterization of the rat NMDA receptor. Nature(1991).,354(6348), 31-37.

[118] Ikeda, K, Nagasawa, M, Mori, H, Araki, K, Sakimura, K, Watanabe, M, Inoue, Y, &Mishina, M. Cloning and expression of the epsilon 4 subunit of the NMDA receptor channel. FEBS Letter (1992)., 313(1), 34-38.

[119] Meguro, H, Mori, H, Araki, K, Kushiya, E, Kutsuwada, T, Yamazaki, M, Kumanishi, T, Arakawa, M, Sakimura, K, &Mishina, M. Functional characterization of a heteromeric NMDA receptor channel expressed from cloned cDNAs. Nature(1992) 357 (6373), 70-4.

[120] Ishii, T, Moriyoshi, K, Sugihara, H, Sakurada, K, Kadotani, H, Yokoi, M, Akazawa, C, Shigemoto, R, Mizuno, N, Masu, M, &Shigetada N. Molecular characterization of the family of the N-methyl-D-aspartate receptor subunits. Journal of Biological Chemistry(1993).,268(4), 2836-43

[121] Monyer, H, Sprengel, R, Schoepfe,r R, Herb, A, Higuchi, M, Lomeli, H, Burnashev, N, Sakmann, B, &Seeburg, P. H. Heteromeric NMDA receptors: molecular and functional distinction of subtypes. Science (1992).,256(5060), 1217-21

[122] Nakanishi, S. Molecular diversity of glutamate receptors and implications for brain function. Science(1992).,258(5082), 597-603.

[123] Bai, N, Aida, T, Yanagisawa, M, Katou, S, Sakimura, K, Mishina, M, & Tanaka, K. NMDA receptor subunits have different roles in NMDA-induced neurotoxicity in the retina. Molecular Brain(2013)., 6:34e

[124] Bai, N, Hayashi, H, Aida, T, Namekata, K, Harada, T, Mishina, M, &Tanaka, K. Dock3 interaction with a glutamate-receptor NR2D subunit protects neurons from excitotoxicity. Molecular Brain (2013)., 6:22e.

[125] Suetake-Koga, S, Shimazaki, T, Takamori, K, Chaki, S, Kanuma, K, Sekiguchi, Y, Suzuki, T., Kikuchi, T, Matsui, Y, & Honda, T. In vitro and antinociceptive profile of HON0001, an orally active NMDA receptor NR2B subunit antagonist. Pharmacology Biochemistry and Behavior (2006)., 84:134-141.

[126] Lipton, S. A. Possible role for memantine in protecting retinal ganglion cells from glaucomatous damage. Survey of Ophthalmology(2003)., (Suppl 1), S38-S46.

[127] Reisberg, B, Doody, R, Stoffler, A, Schmitt, F, Ferris, S, & Mobius, H. J. Memantine in moderate-to-severe Alzheimer's disease. New England Journal of Medicine (2003)., 348, 1333–1341.

[128] Baltmr, A, Duggan, J, Nizari, S, Salt, T. E & Cordeiro, M. F. Neuroprotection in glaucoma-Is there a future role? Experimental Eye Research (2010)., 91, 554-566.

[129] Osborne, N. N. Pathogenesis of ganglion "cell death" in glaucoma and neuroprotection: focus on ganglion cell axonal mitochondria. Progress in Brain Research(2008)., 173, 339–352

[130] Roberts, P. D, Spiros, A, &Geerts, H. Simulations of symptomatic treatments for Alzheimer's disease: computational analysis of pathology and mechanisms of drug action. Alzheimer's Research & Therapy(2012).,4(6), 50.

[131] Wrighton, D. C, Baker, E. J, Chen, P. E, &Wyllie, D. J. Mg2+and memantine block of rat recombinant NMDA receptors containing chimeric NR2A/2D subunits expressed in Xenopus laevis oocytes. Journal of Physiology(2008).,586(1), 211-225.

Chapter 22

Regional Immune, Hormonal and Mediatory Mechanisms Responsible for Function of "Immune Privilege of an Eye" at Senile and Complicated Cataracts

Artashes A. Zilfyan and Arto V. Zilfyan

Additional information is available at the end of the chapter

http://dx.doi.org/10.5772/58229

1. Introduction

Nowadays, in current biology and medicine the subject of wide discussion present paracrine and autocrine immune, endocrine and mediatory mechanisms functioning of which in all the integrative systems of the organism are realized due to principles of interregulation and interdependence. It is not excluded that similar mechanisms are also engaged in eye tunics, moreover that the hematoophthalmic barrier is characterized by a more stable selective permeability (as compared to other histohematic barriers) towards a wide range of endogenous active biological compounds of immune, hormonal and mediatory origin.

In this concern, to our mind, studies aimed at elucidation of autonomous mechanisms engaged in sustaining the immune and endocrine homeostasis in the eye tunics are rather promising.

Hence, during the last 40 years the subject of special investigation became scientific research works relevant to the aspects of pathogenesis "active immunological tolerance" originating in eye tunics as a response to baring of antigenic determinants in eye tunics and tissues at a wide range of ophthalmological diseases. The entire symptom complex of *in situ* occurring immunological reactions is defined in modern ophthalmology as "anterior chamber associated immune deviation" (ACAID).

At the same time, regional mechanisms responsible for ACAID function are studied rather insufficiently.

In the mentioned aspect, cells identified in certain eye tunics should become the subject of specific discussion; besides their "main functions' these cells are provided with the immune, hormonal and mediatory activity as well. The matter is *in situ* synthesis of transforming growth factor-$_{\beta\text{-}2}$, cortisol, fibronectin, availability of receptors to prolactin and prostaglandins E_2.

This chapter will bring to the attention of readers the analysis of scientific evidence and our own research findings obtained during the last 10 years in respect of possible regional immune, hormonal and mediatory mechanisms engaged in formation and abolition of ACAID function.

To avoid artificially expanded volume of this chapter, we considered to be expedient to supplement the narrative description of own research results with Tables and Schemes, excluding all the methodic approaches to selection of patient cohorts, methods of investigation, which were comprehensively presented within our previous studies (Zilfyan A., 2009; 2012; 2013).

We should only mention those groups of patients under study in the aqueous humor of which we determined the spectrum of the above-mentioned endogenously active substances of the immune, hormonal and mediatory nature.

The first (control) group included patients with senile non-complicated cataract, the second group involved patients with cataracts occurring on the background of primary open-angle glaucoma and the third group embraced patients with cataracts on the background of glaucoma and pseudoexfoliative syndrome, the fourth group made patients with cataracts on the background of "arterial hypertension", the fifth group – cataracts on the background of diabetes mellitus and the sixth group was composed of patients with cataract on the background of previous eye injury.

To our mind, it was rather reasonable that we did not include in the current chapter issues dealing with the role of intracorporeal resident gram-negative and gram-positive microorganisms, as well as viruses, *Chlamidiae*, *Toxoplasmas*, etc. Despite the bulk of evidence-frequently of contradictory character – mechanisms of "bacterial translocation" of the above-mentioned microorganisms in the aspect of their passage through the hematoophthalmic barrier and/or penetration of their secretion and decomposition products into the eye tunics are almost none-investigated.

Similar approach was used by us regarding the role of pro-and anti-inflammatory immunocytokines, because of a known controversy of available scientific data on their role in mechanisms responsible for formation of reactions responsible for ACAID function. The controversial character of scientific publications to a known extent is connected with dose-dependent and pleiotropic potencies of immunocytokines even towards the same "immunocompetent" cells localized in the eye tunics.

2. Immune shifts in mechanisms of formation and abolition of the active immunological tolerance responsible for ACAID function

The term "immune privilege of an eye" implies the entire complex of regional immune cell-mediated and humoral reactions aimed at prevention of inflammatory and dystrophic

http://dx.doi.org/10.5772/58229

processes development in tunics and fluid sections (slices) of an eye under conditions of a wide range of ophthalmologic maladies.

At the same time, this term first of all reflects the state of "local immune homeostasis" under conditions of normal functioning of an eye. The complete cascade of local protective/adaptive mechanisms is aimed to form immunological processes, which in total are defined as anterior chamber associated immune deviation (ACAID). To our mind based on available scientific publications, the general scheme of immunopathological process can be presented as the following chronologically occurring stages:

1. As a result of interaction of different pathogenetic factors there occurs "baring" (uncovering) of antigenic determinants (Orge Y., Gungor S., 1984; D'Orazio T., Niederkorn J., 1998; Sonoda A. et al., 2000; Camelo S. et al., 2005).

2. As a response to acquiring of antigenic properties by tissues of an eye in the region of damage (injury) there occurs no activation of the antibody formation process, as reactions of active immunological tolerance there prevail to dominate (Murray P. et al., 1990; Lightman S., Towler H., 1992; Fu T. et al., 2004; Kitaichi N. et al., 2005).

3. No formation of immune complexes occurs as under conditions of pathology there is engaged the regional mechanism preventing activation of the compliment (Streilein J., Stein-Streilein J., 2000).

4. Mechanisms of immune suppression (inhibition of antibody formation) are conditioned by targeted (directed) activation of T-suppressory and killer (killing) subpopulation (Wilbanks C., Streilein J., 1990; Muhaya M. et al., 1999).

5. Directed activation of T-killer lymphocytes occurs due to production of TGF_{β} (Streilein J. et al., 1992; Abrahamian A. et al., 1995; Fleenor D. et al., 2006).

6. The high level of CD_8 is mainly conditioned by the fact that in the region of eye tissues damage there occurs activation of the main histocompatibility class I complex, which functions as the initial factor ensuring triggering of receptor mechanisms underlying activation and proliferation of T-killer lymphocyte populations (Nishi O. et al., 1982; Martin W. et al., 1995; Bakunowicz L. et al., 1997; Muhaya M. et al., 1999).

It should be emphasized that certain pathogenetic mechanisms/links underlying induction and course of ACAID in case of non-complicated and complicated cataracts are currently the subject of a wide discussion (Orge Y., Gungor S., 1984; Uenoyama K. et al., 1989; Streilein J. et al., 1992; Zhou Z. et al., 1996; Cinatl et al., 2000; Robinson M. et al., 2000; Kawakami M. et al., 2005).

As a rule, the main reason of ACAID induction is 1-or 2-stage surgical intervention, as a result of which there occurs "baring" (uncovering) of antigenic determinants of lens tissues. As a result, in the "immunocompetent" tunics of an eye there occurs the synthesis of specific autoantibodies targeted to tissues of lens; by this latter are caused local processes of autoimmune aggression are caused being conditioned by the damaging action of both autoantibodies and locally formed immune complexes.

The activation of reactions of local humoral immunity is accompanied by significant increase of IgG levels in aqueous humor (in anterior and posterior chambers of eyes), due to which the aqueous humor is a rather informative media for studies on mechanisms of both formation and abolition of ACAID. At the same time, all the above-mentioned links underlying abolition of ACAID in case of cataracts are studied rather insufficiently.

It should be emphasized that regional immune mechanisms responsible for *in situ* formation of the active immunological tolerance, which ensures the ACAID function, is most comprehensively studied at senile non-complicated cataracts. At the same time, only single, sometimes even contradictory evidence is available on the course of the regional immune reactions engaged at complicated cataracts.

In our previous investigation (Zilfyan A., 2009) we studied the shifts of CD_4, CD_8 and IgG in the aqueous humor of patients with complicated cataracts: at cataracts on the background of primary open-angle glaucoma, pseudoexpfoliative glaucoma, diabetes mellitus, arterial hypertension, prior eye trauma.

The results of enzyme immunoassays for CD_4 and CD_8 in aqueous humor of patients are presented as Table 1.

Study groups (n=40)	Indices studied					
	CD_4			CD_8		
	M	*m*	*p*	*M*	*m*	*p*
I	10.7	± 2.1		53.9	±5.3	
II	28.4	±3.6	<0.0005	22.05	±5.4	<0.0005
III	30.2	±2.9	<0.0005	18.15	±2.3	<0.0005
IV	14.2	±2.4	*<0.25*	48.8	±4.2	<0.25
V	11.0	±2.5	"/>0.4	50.21	±2.54	<0.4
VI	17.5	±2.0	<0.025	33.7	±4.99	<0.005

Notes: *M* – mean; *m* – standard error of mean; *p* – confidence interval (indices of complicated cataracts as related to senile cataracts).

Table 1. The content of CD_4 (*unit/ml*) and CD_8 (*unit/ml*) in aqueous humor of patients with senile and complicated cataracts.

As obvious from the Table, at complicated cataracts (study groups II and III) already in presurgery period in the aqueous humor there was a marked decrease of CD_8 on the background of CD_4 increase in the aqueous humor of the same cohort of patients.

It is rather remarkable that upon the 2-factor statistical analysis strong reverse correlation dependence was revealed between the studied indices (correlation index made-0.893 and-0.940, appropriately). Apparently, at complicated cataracts in study groups II and III the antigenic determinants in post-barrier eye tunics were bared already in pre-surgery period;

relatively high levels of IgG revealed in the aqueous humor of the specified cohort of patients signified to this latter (Table 2).

Study groups (n=40)	IgG content		
	M	*m*	*p*
I	9.025	±0.73	
II	16.82	±2.20	<0.005
III	25.05	±2.25	<0.0005
IV	8.75	±1.71	"/>0.40
V	10.1	±0.74	<0.25
VI	14.57	±2.05	<0.025

Notes: *M* – mean; *m* – standard error of mean; *p* – confidence interval (indices of complicated cataracts as related to senile cataracts).

Table 2. IgG content (*IU/ml*) in the aqueous humor of patients with senile and complicated cataracts.

It appears, that in this precise case the intercellular mechanisms, which are conditioned by the cooperative activity of B-helper subpopulations and B-lymphocytic populations in the immune competent eye tunics and, first of all, of the ciliary body, are engaged in eye tunics; these latter eventually bring to the synthesis of anti-tissue autoantibodies. The performed 2-factor correlation analysis also signifies in favour of this circumstance: strong direct correlation dependence was revealed between CD_4 and IgG high levels in the aqueous humor of patients of the II and III study groups (correlation index made-0.891 and-0.935, appropriately). It should be mentioned that similar picture of immunological shifts was also observed in study group VI, i.e. at cataracts occurring on the background of trauma. Therefore, it is not excluded that prior trauma can be considered as a provoking factor bringing forth impairment of the immune homeostasis. In the aqueous humor of patients from all other study groups of complicated cataracts (groups IV and V) we registered CD_8, CD_4 and IgG indices similar to those registered in the aqueous humor of patients with senile cataracts.

The results of performed immunological analysis for IgG determination in aqueous humor of patients with senile and complicated cataracts are conformed by available data of scientific publications. In particular, N. Stambuk et al. (1994) established that IgG level in aqueous humor of patients with complicated cataracts was significantly higher than in patients with senile cataracts.

Thus performed, the comparative analysis in all study groups, though with due circumspection, signifies that at senile cataracts and, in all probability, at cataracts occurring on the background of diabetes mellitus and arterial hypertension during the pre-surgery period the regional immune homeostasis is not disturbed, i.e. only those mechanisms are engaged, which ensure the function of ACAID at norm.

At the same time, based on the studies performed by the above-mentioned authors (Lightman S., Towler H., 1992; Sonoda A. et al., 2000; Fu T. et al., 2004; Camelo S. et al., 2005; Kitaichi N. et al., 2005) it is difficult to consider if there is adequacy of inflammatory process, which occurs in eye post-barrier tunics as a response to surgery-related trauma, to what extent the local protective mechanisms work characterizing the immune deviation as related to "bared" autoantigens of the specified tunics. To our mind, it is possible to judge about the character and intensity of the inflammatory process in eye post-barrier tissues only under conditions of the lens transplantation into heterogenous sites of the organism. This problem was successfully solved by Japanese researchers already in 1989 (Uenoyama K. et al., 1989). The authors performed experiments aimed to study tissue specific shifts upon lens transplantation into the eye and intraperitoneally. Due to the complex approach with the use of cytological, immune-histochemical and electron microscopy methods the authors revealed that the degree of inflammatory reaction, the intensity of lymphomacrophagial infiltration were considerably more expressed at the site of lens transplantation, i.e.-in the peritoneum.

At the same time, even in patient with senile non-complicated cataract the surgery-related trauma might provoke disturbance of ACAID function, because as a response to baring of eye tunics antigenic determinants there occurrs the regional autoimmune process. The post-surgery period in those patients and the performed corrective therapy in the prevailing majority of cases proceed without complications; this latter allows us considering that the traumatic injury occurring in the course of surgery intervention is fraught with development of *in situ* immunopathological disorders, which are of exceptionally temporary, transient character.

3. Cortisol-and prolactin-dependent mechanisms responsible for formation and abolition of the ACAID function

In current scientific publications there is only scarce evidence according to which in certain eye tunics the cells of epithelial genesis and fibroblastic line – apart from their main function – also possess the hormone-producing property to synthesize cortisol (Chong A., Aw S., 1986). Due to experimental studies (Southern A. et al., 1979), the presence of receptors to glucocorticoids in cells of ciliary body and the cornea was established, whereas translocation of glucocorticoids from the surface towards the cell nuclei occurred during a rather short period of time. It is reasonable to mention another circumstance of no less importance. The authors failed to reveal similar mechanism of reception and translocation, which is characteristic for glucocorticoids, as related to a wide range of hormones: testosterone, estradiol, progesterone, T_3 and T_4. It was established that biological effects of cortisol are realized within the sclera, cornea, ciliary body and, mostly important, in the lens capsule (Kasavina B. et al., 1977). According to S. Rauz and associates (2001; 2003), cortisol is secreted in the ciliary body of both actually healthy contingent and in patients with the primary open-angle glaucoma.

Currently, the opinion dominates that the fundamental function of cortisol in eye tunics is sustaining the optimal level of intraocular pressure. Furthermore, this function has a dual

http://dx.doi.org/10.5772/58229

realization: through regulation of the regional immune homeostasis and potentiating the adrenergic effect towards the system of vascularization in specific eye tunics (Jacob E. et al., 1996; Rauz S. et al., 2001).

Nowadays, the role of prolactin appears more disputable. At cataracts and uveitides the presence of prolactin was revealed in the anterior chamber of the eye (Pleyer U. et al., 1991). Efforts were done to interpret biological effects of prolactin within the specific eye structures functioning. In particular, S. Duenas and co-workers (2004) allow for the possibility of intraocular synthesis of prolactin within the blood vessels of retina. At retinopathies, the mentioned authors revealed a high level of prolactin in the anterior chamber of the eye. It is important to emphasize that authors did not reveal any correlation dependence between prolactin levels in the anterior chamber of the eye and in blood serum. Despite the fact that of prolactin revealment in tunics and liquid media of the eye, the role of this hormone in the integrative activity of the eye remains unstudied.

To our mind, the role of in situ produced hormones, cortisol and prolactin, in eye tissues is more versatile and is far beyond the functions ensuring processes of ion exchange and intraocular pressure regulation.

We propose a hypothesis according to which cortisol and prolactin play an important role in establishment of ACAID function through modulation of immunological processes in the aspects of both activation and/or inhibition of specific T-and B-populations and also targeted synthesis of cytokines with adaptogenic spectrum of action.

The mentioned supposition is confirmed by literary data, according to which in the mammalian organism cortisol and prolactin possess immunomodulatory functions. In particular, it is established that prolactin and cortisol at physiological concentrations maintain the stability of the immune homeostasis. However, at high concentrations cortisol acts as a factor that selectively inhibits the activity of T-killer and T-helper cytotoxic lymphocytes (Pazirandeh A. et al., 2002; Lindeman D., Racke K., 2003; Visser J. et al., 2003), while prolactin activates a number of cytokines (IL-I, VI, TNF, as well as γ-IFN in central and periphery organs of immunogenesis (Matera L., 1986; Yarilin A., Belyakov I., 1996). Furthermore, prolactin – in a dose dependent mode – activates B-lympocytic population (Berczi I. et al., 1981; McMurrey R. et al., 1991; Lahat N. et al., 1993).

As shown by the results of our earlier performed immune enzyme assays (Zilfyan A., 2009; 2012; 2013) (Table 3) in the aqueous humor of patients with complicated cataracts (cataract occurring on the background of primary open-angle and pseudoexfoliative glaucoma and cataract occurring on the background of preceding trauma) the level of cortisol significantly increased as compared to control.

The highest indices were recorded by us in aqueous humor of the III group patients: at cataracts occurring on the background of pseudoexfoliative glaucoma.

Until present it was considered to be established that the main function of cortisol in the eye tunics was to regulate the intraocular pressure (Jacob E. et al., 1996; Rauz S. et al., 2001). At the same time, due to results obtained, a supposition might be done: the revealed high concen-

Study groups (n=40)	Cortisol content					
	aqueous humor			blood serum		
	M	*m*	*p*	*M*	*m*	*p*
I	12.90	± 0.64		56.90	±4.15	
II	23.38	±1.46	<0.0005	64.84	±7.28	<0.25
III	30.4	±1.56	<0.0005	50.70	±6.91	<0.25
IV	14.10	±0.61	*<0.1*	115.60	±16.88	<0.005
V	9.70	±2.69	<0.25	70.50	±10.41	<0.25
VI	14.05	±0.69	<0.25	68.60	±8.13	<0.25

Notes: *M* – mean; *m* – standard error of mean; *p* – confidence interval (indices of complicated cataracts as related to senile cataracts).

Table 3. The content of cortisol (*pg/ml*) in blood serum and aqueous humor of patients with senile and *complicated cataracts.*

trations of cortisol in the aqueous humor of patients from study groups II, VI and, especially, from group III might produce alterative (damaging) action towards immunocompetent cells of the anterior chamber of the eye, because the cytotoxic effect of cortisol immunocompetent cells of organs of immunogenesis and blood is considered to be established long ago (Bell P., Munck A., 1973; Carr D., Blalock J. et al., 1989). Moreover, we considered it reasonable to the interpret data obtained on shifts of cortisol content in aqueous humor of patients with cataracts taking into account rather informative evidence on dose-dependent impact of cortisol towards the functional state of lymphocytic populations (Pazirandeh A. et al., 2002). The authors studied the direct hormonal influence of endogenous levels of glucocorticoids to thymocytes and peripheral T-lymphocytic subpopulations in transgenic mice with the altered sensitivity to glucocorticoids. According to mentioned researchers, 2-fold increase of sensitivity to glucocorticoids in the organism of transgenic mice was accompanied with the profound alterative changes in thymocytes followed by a marked increase in number of all T-lymphocytic subpopulations in the cortical layer of thymus.

To our mind, it is not ruled out that in mechanisms of ACAID formation and functioning precisely similar cortisol-dependent mechanism of reactions balanced functioning – simultaneously ensuring processes of proliferation and apoptosis of T-lymphocytic subpopulations in tunics and anterior chamber of an eye – is engaged.

At the same time, we cannot exclude that cortisol high concentrations recorded by us in the aqueous humor of patients from study groups II, III and VI might be the provoking factor in the aspect of an abrupt enhancement of apoptosis processes in the immunocompetent cells of eye tunics and the cells of inflammatory reaction in the anterior chamber of the eye.

http://dx.doi.org/10.5772/58229

As seen in studies performed by our group a conclusion might be drawn that in organisms of mammals cortisol plays an important role in processes promoting ACAID functioning (Zilfyan A., 2009; Zilfyan A.A., Zilfyan A.V., 2013).

Moreover, at complicated cataracts (groups II, III and IV), especially at cataracts occurring on the background of the open-angle and pseudoexfoliative glaucoma, we should assign to cortisol an important role in mechanisms infringing the normal course of immunological reactions in tunics and the anterior chamber of an eye ensuring ACAID – in the aspect of abolishing the processes promoting *in situ* active and immunological tolerance.

Significant shifts were also observed on the part of prolactin determined in the aqueous humor of patients with complicated cataracts. In particular, in the aqueous humor of patients with complicated cataracts (study groups II, III and VI) relatively high level of prolactin was recorded. In the remaining patients with complicated cataracts (study groups IV, V) indices of prolactin were similar to those determined in aqueous humor of patients with senile cataracts (Table 4).

Study groups (n=40)	Prolactin content					
	aqueous humor			blood serum		
	M	*m*	*p*	*M*	*m*	*p*
I	0.34	±0.045		7.0	±3.6	
II	1.10	±0.08	<0.0005	9.5	±1.6	<0.10
III	2.23	±0.22	<0.0005	9.1	±2.2	<0.25
IV	0.300	±0.046	*<0.40*	7.50	±0.57	<0.25
V	0.49	±0.09	<0.10	6.40	±1.45	<0.40
VI	14.05	±0.07	*p*<0.0005	10.90	±3.66	<0.25

Notes: *M* – mean; *m* – standard error of mean; *p* – confidence interval (indices of complicated cataracts as related to senile cataracts).

Table 4. The content of prolactin (*ng/ml*) in aqueous humor and blood serum of patients with senile and complicated cataracts.

In the available literature the evidence on the role of prolactin in mechanisms of ACAID formation is lacking.

At the same time it is known that the organism of mammals prolactin possesses a profound stimulant action towards the specific subpopulations of lymphocytes and the cells of monocyte and lymphocyte line – in the aspect of synthesizing a number of immunocytokines: tumor necrosis factor alpha,-beta ($TNF_{\alpha,\beta}$), interleukins-IL-I, IL-II, IL-VI and γ-interferon. It is known that at senile and complicated cataracts relatively high levels of some pro-and anti-inflammatory cytokines (TNF, IL-I, IL-II, IL-IV, IL-VI, IL-X) are determined in the aqueous humor (Stambuk N. et al., 1994; Slepova O.S. et al., 1998; Patel J. et al., 2006; Sawada H., et al., 2010).

In consideration of the existing immune endocrine interrelations of prolactin and proinflammatory cytokines we can suppose that relatively high prolactin concentrations revealed by us in the aqueous humor of study groups II and III patients might be the cause of the enhanced synthesis of proinflammatory cytokines by immonocompetent cells of some eye tunics and cells of lymphocyte-monocyte line localized in the aqueous humor. This is one of the probable prolactin-dependent mechanisms underlying infringement of ACAID function at complicated cataracts.

Under conditions of pathology, i.e. at complicated cataracts, in the anterior chamber of the eye there might be also engaged another prolactin-dependent mechanism bringing to ACAID abolition. It is not excluded that prolactin acts as a co-factor participating in activation of *in situ* reaction of humoral immunity through the selective effect to B-cellular populations of eye tunics and the inflammatory exudates of the anterior chamber of the eye. Apparently, under conditions of increased prolactin content in the aqueous humor with precedent baring of antigenic determinants of eye tunics, prolactin in its turn stimulates the antigen-dependent function of B-lymphocyte populations. In favour of the proposed supposition also signify rather informative literary data depicting a direct dose-dependent stimulant effect of prolactin to the B-lymphocyte populations (Berczi I. et al., 1981; McMurray R. et al., 1991; Lahat N. et al., 1993).

On the base of our own findings and comparing them with the available scientific data on the role of prolactin in the immunological processes and its revealment in the anterior chamber of the eyes the following conclusion might be drawn. Prolactin-dependent mechanisms, which, on the one hand, stimulate the local synthesis of proinflammatory cytokines and, on the other hand, activate processes of *in situ* B-lymphocyte populations proliferation and thus worsen the course of an earlier developed autoimmune process in post-barrier tunics and the anterior chamber of the eye, are also engaged in mechanisms of ACAID abolition at complicated cataracts.

4. Fibronectin and prostaglandins E_2-dependent mechanisms responsible for abolition of reactions promoting the ACAID function

In our previous studies (Zilfyan A., 2009; 2012) data were presented on the important role of fibronectin and PgE_2 produced in the eye tunics regarding the mechanisms of disorders in the drainage function of the trabecular meshwork and the increase of intraocular pressure at complicated cataracts: cataracts occurring on the background of primary open-angle and pseudoexfoliative glaucoma.

At the same time, till present, the role of fibronectin and prostaglandins E_2 (PgE_2) at senile non-complicated cataract and complicated cataracts never became the subject of a special investigation.

Only scarce evidence is available that fibronectin is produced by keratocytes of the cornea, ciliary body and cells of the trabecular meshwork of the eye (Tripathi B., et al., 2004; Hindman

http://dx.doi.org/10.5772/58229

H. et al., 2010; Wordinger R.J. et al., 2007). The enhanced synthesis of fibronectin in the mentioned eye tunics might bring to activation of fibroplastic processes finally terminating in fibrosis of the eye tunics, including the lens. However, the role of fibronectin in processes of ACAID function formation and abolition is not studied. At the same time it is considered to be established that fibronectin might enhance phagocytosis; on the surface of macrophages there are receptors to fibronectin (Kuznik B. et al., 1989). Therefore, it is not excluded that fibronectin at a number of eye diseases might play a leading role in activation of macrophages of the eye tunics and the anterior chamber of the eye: both in the aspect of phagocytosis and synthesis of pro-inflammatory cytokines: interleukin-I (IL-I) and tumor necrosis factors alpha and beta ($TNF\text{-}_{\alpha,\beta}$) (Slepova O. et al., 1998; Sawada H. et al., 2010).

As demonstrated by our results of the performed immune enzyme assays, in patients of the study group II, i.e. at cataracts occurring on the background of primary open-angle and pseudoexfoliative glaucoma, relatively high indices of fibronectin were revealed in the aqueous humor (Table 5).

Study groups (n=40)	**Fibronectin content**		
	M	*m*	*p*
I	11.26	± 0.099	
II	20.71	±2.37	<0.005
III	33.83	±5.97	<0.005
IV	13.43	±2.57	*<0.25*
V	12.76	±1.14	*<0.25*
VI	12.04	±1.12	<0.40

Notes: *M* – mean; *m* – standard error of mean; *p* – confidence interval (indices of complicated cataracts as related to senile cataracts).

Table 5. The content of fibronectin (*ng/ml*) in the aqueous humor of patients with senile and complicated cataracts.

The highest indices of the cytokine were recorded by us in the aqueous humor of patients with cataract occurring on the background of pseudoexfoliative glaucoma (as compared to indices of the control group).

In all other study groups of patients with complicated cataracts low indices of fibronectin were determined in the aqueous humor; these indices were similar to those recorded in the aqueous humor of patients with senile cataracts.

Let us consider the role of fibronectin in processes of ACAID function formation and abolition. It is considered to be established that macrophages of eye tunics and aqueous humor play a role of in processes of pro-and anti-inflammatory cytokines synthesis; the balanced synthesis of mentioned cytokines ensures the normal course of reactions supporting ACAID.

Study groups (n=40)	Prostaglandins E_2 content		
	M	*m*	*p*
I	43.05	± 4.13	
II	66.11	±7.40	<0.01
III	76.64	±7.78	<0.005
IV	48.03	±3.02	*<0.25*
V	49.60	±6.37	*<0.25*
VI	58.96	±2.81	<0.25

Notes: *M* – mean; *m* – standard error of mean; *p* – confidence interval (indices of complicated cataracts as related to senile cataracts).

Table 6. Shifts in content of PgE_2 *(pg/ml)* in the aqueous humor of patients with senile and complicated cataracts.

As already mentioned by us earlier, at a number of diseases, including the complicated cataracts, this balance is broken and macrophages begin to produce immunocytokines – primarily of the proinflammatory – character: TNF_2 and IL I. Therefore, a role of no less importance should be assigned to macrophages in processes of abolishing reactions responsible for ACAID function.

At the same time, it is considered to be established that fibronectin has an ability to activate the cytokine function of macrophages. Hence, it is not excluded that at complicated cataracts fibronectin-dependent mechanisms are engaged in mechanisms of ACAID functions infringement; specified mechanisms are realized at the level of the regional monocyte-macrophageal system.

In our further research the shifts in PgE_2content in the aqueous humor of patients with senile and complicated cataracts were studied. There is only rather scarce literature on synthesis of prostaglandins in eye tunics. The local synthesis of prostaglandins was revealed only in epithelial cells of the lens capsule and was proved by experiments of O. Nishi and co-workers (1982), who performed model *in vitro* tests; in case of cataract surgery the isolated lens was placed in the incubation medium. Alongside with incubation time increase the content of prostaglandins in the incubation medium markedly increased. At the same time, in some eye tunics – the ciliary body, retina, sclera and trabecular meshwork of the anterior chamber angle receptors to PgE_2 were identified (Toris C. et al., 2008). The role of PgE_2 in maintaining the drainage function is widely discussed (Podos S. et al., 1972).

However, the role of PgE_2 in mechanisms of ACAID formation and infringement is almost not investigated. As shown by results of our own studies, the level of PgE_2 in aqueous humor of patients from study groups II, III and VI markedly increased as compared to the level of PgE_2 in the aqueous humor of the control group patients (Table 6).

The highest values were observed in aqueous humor of patients with cataract on the background of pseudoexfoliative glaucoma. In all other groups of complicated cataracts low indices

http://dx.doi.org/10.5772/58229

were recorded in the aqueous humor; these indices were similar to those determined in aqueous humor of the control group patients. The high level of PgE_2 at complicated cataracts (study groups II, III, VI) might be considered as a factor bringing to disorder of the eye trabecular meshwork drainage function; moreover that on its cells receptors to PgE_2 were revealed. Despite the presence of receptors to PgE_2 in different eye tunics, epithelial cells of the lens capsule are the only possible source of PgE_2 local synthesis. Therefore, it is not ruled out that in complicated cataracts the lens cells are engaged in an enhanced synthesis of E_2 group prostaglandins, which might influence the course and duration of reactions promoting abolition of the ACAID function.

Our supposition is also grounded by data of scientific publications dealing with the functional activity of PgE_2 towards the numerous integrative systems of the organism, including the immune system. In particular, it is considered to be established long ago, that PgE_2 inhibit the synthesis of cytotoxic lymphocytes: T-suppressor and T-killer lymphocyte subpopulations. Hence, it is not excluded, that the high level of PgE_2 in the aqueous humor of patients with complicated cataracts (study groups II, III and VI) might be considered as a factor producing immunosuppressive action to cytotoxic lymphocytes localized in eye tunics and the aqueous humor; the latter is fraught with abolishing the reactions responsible for *in situ* abolition of ACAID function.

This is the precise reason for formation of "favourable" conditions for *in situ* intensification of autoimmune reactions in the post-surgery period under conditions of infringed integrity of the lens capsule and baring of its antigenic determinants; moreover, at complicated cataracts the immune stimulant mechanisms aimed at activation of T-cytotoxic lymphocytes is infringed already at the pre-surgery stage.

The investigation of E.L. Nelson (1976) also signified to the important role of prostaglandins in induction of local inflammatory processes. According to author, different traumatic injuries of the eye are followed with the enhanced synthesis of E_2 and $F_{2\alpha}$ in the iris and other eye tissues, as a result of which the content of mentioned prostaglandins in the aqueous humor is significantly increased. The enhancement of mentioned processes is accompanied with vasodilatation, increased permeability of micro-vessels, and increased protein content in the aqueous humor.

Apart from this, the mentioned author proposed a supposition, according to which at traumatic injuries of the eye leucocytes of inflammatory exudates in the aqueous humor might serve as a source of prostaglandins synthesis.

Furthermore, as considered by the authors, the cascade of molecular and cellular processes at induction of inflammatory process in eye tunics is eventually terminated by the reaction that, to a considerable degree, is conditioned by prostaglandins. On the other hand, the high level of PgE_2 in the aqueous humor, to a known extent, reflects *in situ* formation of protective-adaptive mechanisms – in the aspect of correlation of synthesis processes of specific pro-inflammatory cytokines produced in the post-barrier tunics of the eye as well.

It is a common knowledge that prostaglandins of E and F group inhibit the synthesis of IL I in macrophages and leucocytes. Apparently, the similar mechanism is engaged in post-barrier eye tunics both at norm and in case of some eye diseases. The following fact signifies in favour of the latter circumstance: at endotoxin-induced experimental uveitis in rabbit despite the expressed inflammatory reaction in post-barrier eye tunics the level of IL-I in the aqueous humor did not increase (Kulkarni P.S., 1991). It is not excluded that PgE_2 serve as a factor preventing the increase of IL-I and IL-II production in immunocompetent cells.

5. The role of transforming growth factor in pathogenesis of cataracts and glaucomas

Nowadays rather informative evidence is available on the role of $TGF_{\beta\text{-}2}$ in the mechanisms of immunological tolerance activation at senile and complicated cataracts. High regional immunological tolerance in eye tunics is ensured through the enhanced $TGF_{\beta\text{-}2}$ synthesis by the cells of eye tunics: ciliary body, cornea, and retina (Stefan C. et al., 2008; Dawes L. et al., 2009; Hindman H. et al., 2010; Pattabiraman P., Rao P., 2010).

It is established that the active immunological tolerance at senile non-complicated cataracts is targeted at activation of T-helper and T-suppressor subpopulations in immune competent cells of the eye; these latter play an important role in prevention of autoimmune reactions aimed to produce antibodies against the lens tissues (Streilein J. et al., 1992; Wilbanks G. et al., 1992).

In the most relief mode the entire cascade of immunological shifts is presented in the aqueous humor of patients with senile and complicated cataracts, as a result of which currently the aqueous humor is considered as a rather informative bio-object characterizing the course of immunological reactions responsible for anterior chamber associated immune deviation (ACAID) formation.

In the specified aspect there are rather informative scientific publications, according to which at senile non-complicated cataracts during the post-surgery period is engaged the similar $TGF_{\beta\text{-}2}$-dependent mechanism that underlies the suppresson of local humoral immunity reactions through *in situ* activation of cytotoxic lymphocytes (Fleenor D. et al., 2006; Streilein J. et al., 1992).

At the same time our own investigation (Zilfyan A., 2009) allowed establishing that unlike senile non-complicated cataracts occurring on the background of glaucoma and pseudoexfoliative syndrome already in the pre-surgery period in eye tunics there originated immunopathological disorders manifested as activation of reactions responsible for antibody formation (high level of CD_4 and IgG in the aqueous humor – on the background of a marked decrease in CD_8 level).

Data obtained signify in favour of the fact, according to which $TGF_{\beta\text{-}2}$-dependent mechanism engaged in ACAID formation is actually not the single one at complicated cataracts (Zilfyan A.A., Zilfyan A.V., 2013).

Thus, our studies revealed that at complicated cataracts in the aqueous humor there is a marked increase of cortisol, prolactin and PgE_2 (Zilfyan A., 2009; 2012). Moreover, high concentrations

http://dx.doi.org/10.5772/58229

of mentioned hormones and PgE_2 are conditioned by their "non-arrival" from the periphery (as a result of increase in hematoophthalmic barrier permeability), or most likely, as a result of the enhanced synthesis in the eye tunics.

According to the proposed concept, relatively high concentrations of the above-mentioned biologically active compounds might act as endogenous factors activating *in situ* reactions of humoral immunity, because their selective influence towards the immune competent cells T-helpers and B-cellular populations is considered to be established (Goodwin J., Ceuppens J., 1983; McMurray R. et al., 1991; Lahat N. et al., 1993;).

Thus, in cases of complicated cataracts we revealed earlier unknown mediatory mechanisms engaged in launching the humoral immunity reactions, which apart the surgery-related trauma produce rather unfavourable impacts to the course of the regional pathological process.

In the light of data thus obtained, the role of $TGF_{\beta\text{-}2}$ in glaucomatous pathogenesis should be considered from the alternative standpoint. In particular, $TGF_{\beta\text{-}2}$ produced in the cornea and the ciliary body stimulates *in situ* synthesis of insulin-like growth factor-1 (IGF-1) and fibronectin, i.e. precisely those cytokines the excessive concentrations of which are considered as *provoking* factors hindering the normal outflow of the aqueous humor; this latter is fraught with the increase of aqueous humor in glaucoma.

Our previous studies also signify to the existence / presence of the similar $TGF_{\beta\text{-}2}$-dependent mechanism (Zilfyan A., 2013); it was demonstrated that at complicated cataracts on the background of glaucoma and pseudoexfoliative syndrome high concentrations of fibronectin and IGF-1 are determined in the aqueous humor (compared to those recorded in the aqueous humor of patients with senile non-complicated cataract).

Hence, the role of $TGF_{\beta\text{-}2}$ in pathogenesis of cataracts and glaucomas is far from being unambiguous. In particular, on the one hand, in senile non-complicated cataract $TGF_{\beta\text{-}2}$ modulates in the eye tunics processes of active immune tolerance aimed at prevention of autoimmune aggression against the antigenic determinants of the lens; on the other hand,-the same cytokine produced a rather unfavourable impact to the course and duration of glaucomas through its direct and/or indirect impact to the processes of fibronectin and IGF-1 enhanced synthesis in the trabecular meshwork of the eye. The excessive accumulation of both cytokines brings to impaired function of the eye anterior chamber trabecular meshwork, thus eventually accompanied by the increase of intraocular pressure.

On the basis of studies performed, within the entire context of available published data, from the qualitatively new positions we should consider the established, earlier unknown, $TGF_{\beta\text{-}2}$-independent hormonal mediatory mechanisms underlying the abolition of reactions responsible for ACAID formation and the increase of intraocular pressure at complicated cataracts.

6. Conclusion

Currently existing term "immune privilege of an eye" is mostly associated with evolutionary secured mechanisms, which ensure the regional immune homeostasis in eye tunics and in the eye liquid media both at norm and pathology. In particular, at cataracts in some eye tunics there are engaged mechanisms promoting the "active immunological tolerance" that is selectively targeted against the "bared" (revealed) antigenic determinants of the lens tissues. In modern ophthalmology the symptom complex of immune reactions occurring in eye tunics is defined as "anterior chamber associated immune deviation – ACAID".

Hence, it is considered to be proved that at senile non-complicated cataracts in the post-surgery period there are *in situ* activated immune processes, which manifest as activation of cytotoxic lymphocytes (T-suppressors and T-killers) due to which the "active immunological tolerance" is formed averting the processes of autoimmune aggression against the bared antigenic tissues of the lens.

Based on the evidence of available modern literature and our own research findings new earlier unknown hormonal mediatory mechanisms appear to the proscenium of the stage; those mechanisms at complicated cataracts are responsible for abolition of reactions promoting the ACAID function.

Thereupon, from qualitatively new positions should be considered the role of cortisol, prolactin fibronectin, $TGF_{\beta\text{-}2}$ and PgE_2, which are produced in specific eye tunics, in mechanisms of *in situ* realization of the immune reactions responsible for ACAID formation and abolition. It should be emphasized that all the above-mentioned biologically active substances in case of complicated cataracts (cataracts on the background of anterior open-angle glaucoma and pseudoexfoliative glaucoma) act as "provoking" factors, which take an active part in both impairment of the eye trabecular meshwork drainage function and the increase of intraocular pressure.

At the same time, in complicated cataracts the specified factors might take an active part in abolishing the reactions providing the "active immunological tolerance" through *in situ* activity of cytotoxic lymphocytes and activation of autoimmune processes targeted against the antigenic determinants of the eye tissues and tunics.

Based on the analysis of the available literature and the presented own studies we consider it purposeful to present to the attention of the readers the main regional immune and hormonal-mediatory mechanisms responsible for ACAID formation and abolition in senile and complicated cataracts also depicting them in detail as summary Schemes 1 and 2.

Immune and hormonal-mediatory factors engaged in ACAID formation at non-complicated cataracts are presented as Scheme 1.

During the surgery intervention for phacoemulsification of cataract (PhEC) there occurs baring of antigenic determinants of the lens tissues (BADLT). According to available evidence of scientific publications, 3 mechanisms are engaged in ACAID formation.

The first mechanism is associated with the activation of $TGF_{\beta\text{-}2}$ synthesis in the eye cornea, ciliary body and retina as a result of which there occurs stimulation of cytotoxic lymphocytes (T-ct).

http://dx.doi.org/10.5772/58229

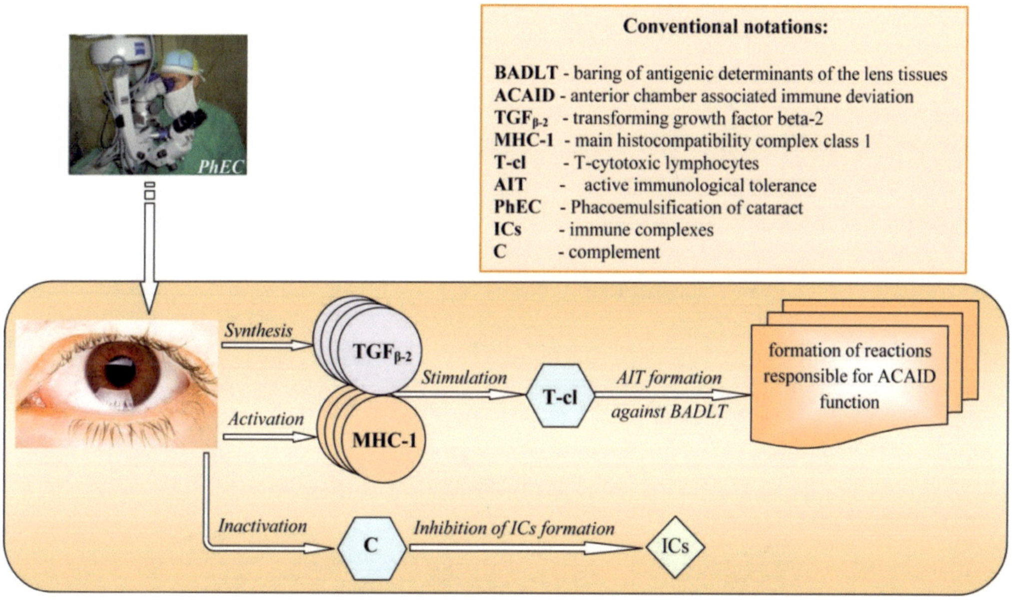

Scheme 1. Regional immune andmediatory mechanisms responsible for ACAID function.

As a result of the targeted stimulation of T-suppressor and T-killer subpopulations there occurs an active immunological tolerance (AIT) against the bared antigenic determinants of lens tissues, in particular through inhibition of activity in T-helper subpopulation of lymphocytes.

The second mechanism is associated with *in situ* activation of the main histocompatibility complex class 1 (MHC-1) with the subsequent activation of T-killer subpopulations.

The third mechanism is associated with *in situ* inactivation of the complement (C); therefore, the formation of immune complexes (IC) does not occur.

As a result, one of the possible mechanisms of autoaggression is excluded through deposition of the immune complexes on the lens tissues followed by their subsequent impairment.

According to the bulk of scientific data, similar mechanism is engaged in the post-surgery period at senile non-complicated cataracts.

From the result of our investigations we do not exclude that ACAID function is also engaged in cataracts occurring on the background of diabetes mellitus and arterial hypertension, because in both cases the recovery process was without complications, even without the aseptic autoimmune iridocyclitis.

Thus performed, our studies allowed establishing that at specific types of complicated cataracts (cataract on the background of primary open-angle and pseudoexfoliative glaucoma) regional immune mechanisms responsible for ACAID function were impaired (Scheme 2).

Thus, in both cases after the performed phacoemulsification of cataract (PhEC) and baring of antigenic determinants of the lens tissues (BADLT) the aqueous humor levels of cortisol (Cor)

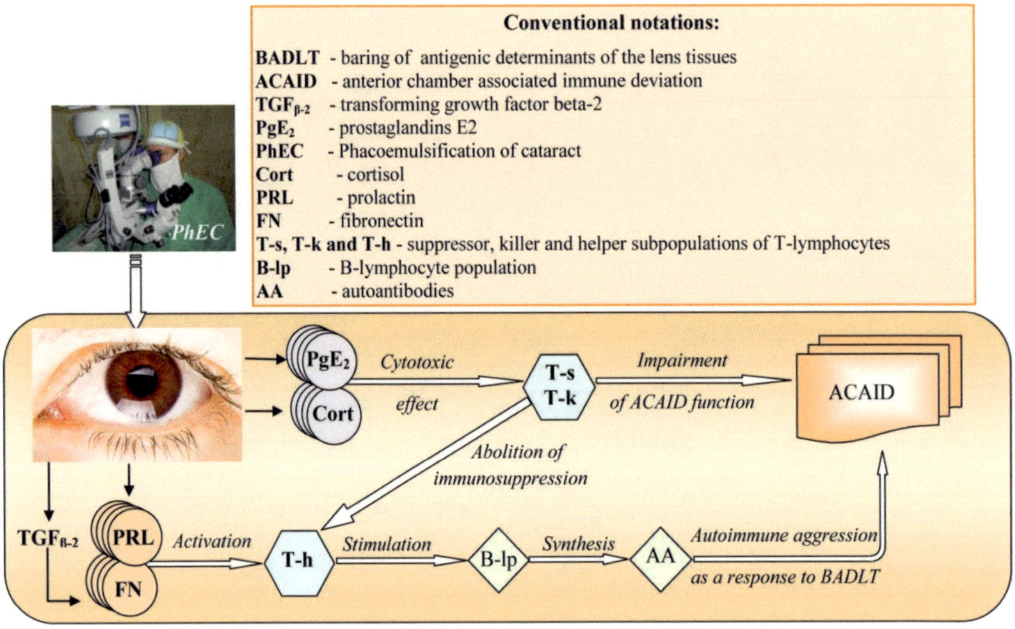

Scheme 2. Regional immune and hormonal mediatory mechanisms responsible for abolishing the ACAID function at complicated cataracts.

and PgE_2 increased. Both factors had unidirectional cytotoxic action towards the specific lymphocytic subpopulations – T-suppressors and T-killers (T-s, T-k). Hence, there occurred the abolition of the immunosuppressive action of those latter to the T-helper subpopulation of lymphocytes (T-h). Against this background we recorded high concentrations of prolactin (PRL) and fibronectin (FN) in the aqueous humor. The FN high level was conditioned by the stimulant influence of transforming growth factor beta-2 ($TGF_{\beta\text{-}2}$) towards the eye cornea cells and the trabecular meshwork. Both factors, prolactin (PRL) and fibronectin (FN), activate T-helper subpopulation of lymphocytes (T-h). As a result of surgery-related impairment of the lens tissues on the background of cytotoxic lymphocytes-abolished suppression there occurs stimulation of T-helper subpopulation that is fraught with formation of autoantibodies (AA) against the impaired tissues of lens followed with their autoimmunoaggrression towards both impaired and "structurally" preserved tissues of lens.

As a rule, such a complication as aseptic autoimmune iridocyclitis developed in the specified contingent of patients during the post-surgery period.

Undoubtedly, the presented Schemes 1 and 2 are not ultimate; moreover, they are not comprehensive. These Schemes should be supplemented (enriched) with new evidence on the role of earlier unknown biologically active substances of immune, hormonal, mediatory genesis, which are produced in eye tunics, in formation of in situ reactions responsible for formation and abolition of the ACAID function.

http://dx.doi.org/10.5772/58229

Author details

Artashes A. Zilfyan[1] and Arto V. Zilfyan[2*]

*Address all correspondence to: namj@ysmu.am

1 Scientific-Research Center, Yerevan State Medical University, Yerevan, Armenia

2 "Shengavit" Medical Center, Yerevan, Armenia

References

[1] Abrahamian A., Xi M., Donnelly J., Rockey J. Effect of interferon-gamma on the expression of transforming growth factor-beta by human corneal fibroblasts: role in corneal immunoseclusion. J. Interferon Cytokine Res. 1995; 15(4): 323-330.

[2] Bakunowicz L., Lazarczyk A., Moniuszko T. et al. Levels of selected cytokines in aqueous humor of patients with cataract extraction. Klin. Oczna. 1997; 99(4): 235-237.

[3] Bell P., Munck A. Steroid-binding properties and stabilization of cytoplasmic glucocorticoid receptors from rat thymus cells. Biochem. J. 1973; 136(1): 97-107.

[4] Berczi I., Nagy E., Kovacs K., Horvath E. Regulation of humoral immunity in rats by pituitary hormones. Acta Endocrinol. Copenhagen. 1981: 98: 506-513.

[5] Camelo S., Kezic J., McMenamin P. Anterior chamber-associated immune deviation: a review of the anatomical evidence for the afferent arm of this unusual experimental model of ocular immune responses. Clin. Exper. Ophthalmol. 2005; 33(4): 426-432.

[6] Carr D., Blalock J. A molecular basis for intersystem communication between the immune and neuroendocrine systems. Int. Rev. Immunol. 1989; 4(3): 213-228.

[7] Chong A., Aw S. Postmortem endocrine levels in the vitreous humor. Ann. Acad. Med. Singapore. 1986; 15 (4): 606-609.

[8] Cinatl J., Blaheta R., Bittoova M., Scholz M., Margraf S., Vogel J., Cinatl J., Deorr H. Decreased neutrophil adhesion to human cytomegalovirus-infected retinal pigment epithelial cells is mediated by virus-induced up-regulation of Fas ligand independent of neutrophil apoptosis. J. Immunol. 2000; 165(8): 4405-4413.

[9] D'Orazio T., Niederkorn J. The nature of antigen in the eye has a profound effect on the cytoki milieu and resultant immune response. Eur. J. Immunnol. 1998; 28(5): 1544-1553.

[10] Dawes L.J., Sleeman M.A., Anderson I.K., Reddan J.R., Wormstone I.M. TGFbeta/Smad4-dependent and-independent regulation of human lens epithelial cells. Invest. Ophthalmol. Vis. Sci. 2009 Nov; 50(11): 5318-5327. Epub 2009 Jun 10.

[11] Duenas Z., Rivera J., Quiroz-Mercado H., Aranda J., Macotela Y., Montes de Oca P., Lopez-Barrera F., Nava G., Guerrero J., Suarez A., De Regil M., Martinez de la Escalera G., Clapp C. Prolactin in eyes of patients with retinopathy of prematurity: implications for vascular regression. Invest. Ophthalmol. Vis. Sci. 2004; 45(7): 2049-2055.

[12] Fleenor D., Shepard A., Hellberg P., Jacobson N., Pang I., Clark A. TGFbeta2-induced changes in human trabecular meshwork: implications for intraocular pressure. Invest. Ophthalmol. Vis. Sci. 2006: 47(1): 226-234.

[13] Fu T., Yang P., Huang X., Zhou H., Li F., Huang Q. Preventive effect of anterior chamber associated immune deviation on endotoxin-induced uveitis. Zhonghua Yi Xue Za Zhi. 2004; 84(18): 1562-1566.

[14] Goodwin J.S., Ceuppens J. Regulation of the immune response by prostaglandins. J. Clin. Immunol. 1983; 3(4): 295-315.

[15] Hindman H.B., Swanton J.N., Phipps R.P., Sime P.J., Huxlin K.R. Differences in the TGF-{beta}1-induced profibrotic response of anterior and posterior corneal keratocytes in vitro. Invest. Ophthalmol. Vis. Sci. 2010 Apr; 51(4): 1935-1942. Epub 2009 Nov 11.

[16] Jacob E., FitzSimon J., Brubaker R. Combined corticosteroid and catecholamine stimulation of aqueous humor flow. Ophthalmology. 1996; 103: 1303-1308.

[17] Kasavina B., Ukhina T., Churakova T. Distribution of labeled cortisol in the tissues and media of the eye. Bull. Exp. Biol. Med. 1977; 83: 401-402.

[18] Kawakami M., Nakata J., Ohguro N., Yoshihara S., Inoue T., Tatekawa T., Ikegame K., Oka Y., Kawase I., Ogawa H. A case of immune recovery vitritis induced by donor leukocyte infusion for the treatment of cytomegalovirus retinitis. Eur. J. Haematol. 2005; 75(4): 352-354.

[19] Kitaichi N., Namba K., Taylor A. Inducible immune regulation following autoimmune disease in the immune-privileged eye. J. Leukoc. Biol. 2005; 77(4): 496-502.

[20] Kulkarni P.S. The role of endogenous eicosanoids in rabbit-intraocular inflammation. J. Ocul. Pharmacol. 1991; 7(3): 227-241.

[21] Kuznik B., Vasiliev N., Zybikov N. [Immunogenesis, homeostasis and non-specific resistance of the organism][published in Russian]. Moscow. Medicina ("Medicine" Publishers). 1989. 320p.

[22] Lahat N., Shitler R., Zlotnik A.Y., Merin G. Early IL-2/sIL-2R surge following surgery leads to temporary immune refractoriness. Clinical and Experim. Immun. 1993 June; 92(3): 482-486.

[23] Lightman S., Towler H. Immunopathology and altered immunity in posterior uveitis in man: a review. Curr. Eye Res. 1992; 11(Suppl.): 11-15.

[24] Lindemann D., Racke K. Glucocorticoid inhibition of interleukin-4 (IL-4) and interleukin-13 (IL-13) induced up-regulation of arginase in rat airway fibroblasts. Naunyn Schmiedebergs Arch. Pharmacol. 2003; 368(6): 546-550.

[25] Martin W., Egan R., Stevens J., Woodward J.G. Lens-specific expression of a major histocompatibility complex class I molecule disrupts normal lens development and induces cataracts in transgenic mice. Invest. Ophthalmol. Vis. Sci. 1995; 36(6): 1144-1154.

[26] Matera L. Endocrine, paracrine and autocrine actions of prolactin on immune cells. Life Sci. 1986; 59(8): 593-614.

[27] McMurray R., Keisler D., Kanuckel K., Izui S., Walker S.E. Prolactin influences autoimmune disease activity in the female B/W mouse. J. Immunol. 1991; 147: 3780-3787.

[28] Muhaya M., Calder V., Towler H. et al. Characterization of phenotype and cytokine profiles of T-cell lines derived from vitreous humor in ocular inflammation in man. Clin. Exp. Immunol. 1999; 116(3): 410-414.

[29] Murray P., Hoekzema R., Luyendijk L., Konings S., Kijlstra A. Analysis of aqueous humor immunoglobulin G in uveitis by enzyme-linked immunosorbent assay, isoelectric focusing, and immunoblotting. Invest. Ophthalmol. Vis. Sci. 1990: 31(10): 2129-2135.

[30] Nelson E.L. Prostaglandins and inflammation in the eye. Review. Mod. Probl Ophthalmol. 1976; 16: 125-130.

[31] Nishi O., Nishi K., Imanishi M. Synthesis of interleukin-1 and prostaglandin E2 by lens epithelial cells of human cataracts. Br. J. Ophthalmol. 1982; 76: 338-341.

[32] Orge Y., Gungor S. Immunological etiopathogenesis of senile and complicated cataract. Microbiol Bul. 1984; 18(3): 145-153.

[33] Patel J.I., Hykin P.G., Cree I.A. Diabetic cataract removal: postoperative progression of maculopathy – growth factor and clinical analysis. Br. J. Ophthalmol. 2006; Jun; 90(6) 697-701. Epub 2006 Mar 15

[34] Pattabiraman P.P., Rao P.V. Mechanistic basis of Rho GTPase-induced extracellular matrix synthesis in trabecular meshwork cells. Am. J. Phys. Cell Phys. 2010 Mar; 298(3): 749-763. Epub 2009 Nov 25.

[35] Pazirandeh A., Xue Y., Prestegaard T., Jondal M., Okret S. Effects of altered glucocorticoid sensitivity in the T cell lineage on thymocyte and T cell homeostasis. FASEB J. 2002; 16(7): 727-729.

[36] Pleyer U., Gupta D., Weidle E., Lisch W., Zierhut M., Thiel H. Elevated prolactin levels in human aqueous humor of patients with anterior uveitis. Graefes. Arch. Clin. Exp. Ophthalmol. 1991; 229(5): 447-451.

[37] Pleyer U., Yang J., Knapp S., Schacke H., Schemes N., Orlic N., Otasevic L., De Ruijter M., Ritter T., Keipert S. Effects of a selective glucocorticoid receptor agonist on experimental keratoplasty. Graefes. Arch. Clin. Exp. Ophthalmol. 2005; 243(5): 450-455.

[38] Podos S.M., Jaffe B.M., Becker B. Prostaglandinsand glaucoma. Br. Med. J. 1972 Oct 28; 4(5834): 232.

[39] Rauz S., Cheung C., Wood P., Coca-Prados M., Walker E., Murray P., Stewart P. Inhibition of 11β-hydroxysteroid dehydrogenase type 1 lowers intraocular pressure in patients with ocular hypertension. QJM. 2003; 96(7): 481-490.

[40] Rauz S., Walker E., Shackleton C., Hewison M., Murray P., Stewart P. Expression and putative role of 11 beta-hydroxysteroid dehydrogenase isozymes within the human eye. Invest. Ophthalmol. Vis. Sci. 2001; 42(9): 2037-2042.

[41] Robinson M., Reed G., Csaky K., Polis M., Whitcup S. Immune-recovery uveitis in patients with cytomegalovirus retinitis taking highly active antiretroviral therapy. Am. J. Ophthalmol. 2000: 130(1): 103-106.

[42] Sawada H., Fukuchi T., Tanaka T. Abe H. Tumor necrosis factor-alpha concentrations in the aqueous humor of patients with glaucoma. Invest. Ophthalmol. Vis. Sci. 2010 Feb; 51(2): 903-906.

[43] Slepova O.S., Gerasimenko V.A. Makarov V.P., Kushnir V.N., Zakharov G.Iu., Bykovskaia G.N., Vartanian I.R., Sadrislamova L.F. [Comparative study of the role of cytokines in different forms of eye diseases. 1. Tumor necrosis factor-alpha][Article in Russian]. Vestn. Ophthalmol. 1998 May-Jun; 114(3): 28-32.

[44] Sonoda A., Sonoda Y., Muramatu R., Streilein J., Usui M. ACAID induced by allogeneic corneal tissue promotes subsequent survival of orthotopic corneal grafts. Invest. Ophthalmol. Vis. Sci. 2000; 41(3): 790-798.

[45] Southren A., Gordon G., Yeh H., Dunn M., Weinstein B. Nuclear translocation of the cytoplasmic glucocorticoid receptor in the iris-ciliary body of the rabbit. Invest. Ophthalmol. Vis. Sci. 1979; 18(5): 517-521.

[46] Stambuk N., Curkovic T., Trbojevic-Cepe M., Dujmov I. Interleukin-4, IgG and oligoclonal IgG in aqueous humor of cataract patients. Graefes Arch. Clin. Exp. Ophthalmol. 1994; 232(2): 103-106.

[47] Stefan C., Dragomir L., Dumitrică D.M., Ursaciuc C., Dobre M., Surcel M. [TGF-beta-2 involvements in open angle glaucoma][published in Romanian]. Oftalmologia. 2008; 52: 110-112.

[48] Streilein J., Stein-Streilein J. Does innate immune privilege exist? J. Leukoc. Biol. 2000; 67(4): 479-487.

[49] Streilein J., Wilbanks G., Taylor A., Cousins S. Eye-derived cytokines and the immunosuppressive intraocular microenvironment: a review. Curr. Eye Res. 1992: 11(Suppl.): 41-47.

[50] Toris C.B., Gabelt B.T., Kaufman P.L. Update on the mechanism of action of topical prostaglandins for intraocular pressure reduction. Surv. Ophthalmol. 2008; 53: 107-120.

[51] Tripathi B.J., Tripathi R.C., Chen J., Gotsis S., Li J. Trabecular cell expression of fibronectin and MMP-3 is modulated by aqueous humor growth factors. Exp. Eye Res. 2004; 78: 653-660.

[52] Uenoyama K., Kanagawa R., Tamura M., Matoba M., Enomoto Y., Ohmi S. Experimental intraocular lens implantation in the rabbit eye and in the mouse peritoneal space. Part IV: Cell adhesion, fibroblast-like cell, and lymphocytic cluster observed on the implanted lens surface. J. Cataract. Refract. Surg. 1989; 15(5): 559-566.

[53] Visser J. Sparing interleukin-10 receptor expression by glucocorticoids is a prerequisite for the synergistic immunosuppressive effects of interleukin-10 and glucocorticoids. Transplantation 2003; 76(10): 1534-1535.

[54] Wilbanks G., Mammolenti M., Streilein J. Studies on the induction of anterior chamber-associated immune deviation (ACAID). III. Induction of ACAID depends upon intraocular transforming growth factor-beta. Eur. J. Immunol. 1992; 22(1): 165-173.

[55] Wilbanks G., Streilein J. Characterization of suppressor cells in anterior chamber-associated immune deviation (ACAID) induced by soluble antigen. Evidence of two functionally and phenotypically distinct T-suppressor cell populations. Immunol. 1990; 71(3): 383-389.

[56] Wordinger R.J., Fleenor D.L., Hellberg P.E., Pang I.H., Tovar T.O., Zode G.S., Fuller J.A., Clark A.F. Effects of TGF-beta2, BMP-4, and gremlin in the trabecular meshwork: implications for glaucoma. Invest. Ophthalmol. Vis. Sci. 2007 Mar; 48(3): 1191-1200.

[57] Yarilin A., Belyakov I. [Thymus as an organ of endocrine system][Article in Russian]. Immunologiya. 1996. P. 4-10.

[58] Zhou Z., He S., Liang Y. An experimental study of pathomorphology in the iris and ciliary body after intraocular lens implantation. Zhonghua Yan Ke Za Zhi. 1996; 32(6): 421-423.

[59] Zilfyan A.A. Modern Aspects of Glaucoma Pathogenesis Local Factors for Development of Primary Open-Angle Glaucoma Associated with Impairment of Secretory Functions of the Eye Membranes. Chapter 5 in: "Glaucoma – Basic and Clinical Aspects". Edited by Shimon Rumelt. INTECH. Croatia. 2013. P. 75-102.

[60] Zilfyan A.A. Shifts in content of fibronectin, insulin-like growth factor-1 and E_2 prostaglandins in aqueous humor in case of senile and complicated cataracts. The New Armenian Medical Journal. 2012; 6(3): 34-41.

[61] Zilfyan A.A. The role of cortisol, prolactin, CD_4 and CD_8 in induction of anterior chamber associated immune deviation (ACAID) in case of cataracts. The New Armenian Medical Journal. 2009; 3(1): 59-67.

[62] Zilfyan A.A., Zilfyan A.V. Hormonal-Mediatory Mechanisms in the Process of Anterior Chamber Associated Immune Deviation. The New Armenian Medical Journal. 2013; 7(3): 85-88.

Chapter 23

Paranasal Sinus Mucoceles – Opthalmic Manifestations, Radiological Imaging, Endoscopic Endonasal Marsupilization and Outcome

Balwant Singh Gendeh

Additional information is available at the end of the chapter

http://dx.doi.org/10.5772/58331

1. Introduction

Langeback first described paranasal sinus mucoceles in 1820. It was only in the early 1900s that mucoceles were given their name by Rollet and popularized by Gerber, who published 178 cases. In 1995, Lambert attributed frontal or ethmoid mucoceles as the most common nasal condition to produce proptosis [1]

A mucocele is an epithelial-lined mucus containing sac that fills a paranasal sinus and is able to expand by alternative bone resorption and bone formation. A mucocele occurs when a sinus ostium or a compartment of a septated sinus becomes obstructed, thus causing the sinus cavity to become filled with mucus or to become airless. Paranasal sinus mucoceles may result from inflammation, tumor, trauma or surgical manipulation [2].Because of the anatomic proximity of the orbit, the pathologic process of paranasal sinus mucocele will easily affect the orbit [3,4]. Anatomically, the frontal, ethmoid, sphenoid and maxillary sinuses all interface with the orbit. The maxillary sinus shares the floor of the orbit, the frontal sinus is part of the orbital roof, the ethmoid extends along most of the medial wall of orbit and the sphenoid almost completely surrounds the orbital apex [3, 4]. Thus, mucoceles of the paranasal sinuses can easily affect the orbit and cause ophthalmic symptoms such as proptosis, blurred vision and displacement of globe [4,5]. Patients with paranasal mucoceles with orbital symptoms are often seen by the ophthalmologist first and then referred to otorhinolaryngologist [5].Occasionally they can present with intracranial complications.

It is essential to differentiate a mucocele from a mucus retention cyst. A mucus retention cyst is just a fluid filled sac along the sinus lining which does not expand and push into the eye socket, nose or brain and does not cause problems in the vast majority of cases. Notably, mucus retention cysts in the sinuses are more common than expected. Infact, about 30-40% of the population with absolutely no complaints of sinus problems will have cysts of the paranasal sinuses when they have CT scans performed. Most retention cysts of sinuses spontaneously shrink or do not change in size over the long term [6]. In the absence of associated complaints "wait and see" may be the appropriate management strategy for these retention cysts.

2. Material and methods

From 2005 to 2012, 13 patients with paranasal sinus mucoceles were treated with wide endoscopic endonasal marsupilization at the UKM Medical Center in Kuala Lumpur, Malaysia. Review of the patients' complete medical records, including out-patient clinical records, operative notes and reports of imaging and histopathology were performed. The radiological imaging (CT/MRI) on preoperative coronal and axial views were reviewed.

3. Results

The demographic data on the 13 patients includes the age, sex, race, clinical presentation, type of radiological imaging performed, the surgical details and the post-operative follow-up are listed in Table 1. The most common sinus involved was the frontal, followed by the ethmoid, maxillary and sphenoid (Table 2). The most common clinical presentation was headache followed by eye and nasal symptoms (Table 3). Figure 1 shows a radiological image of a right ethmoidal mucocele in an adult patient with diplopia and headache. Figure 2 shows a radiological image of a gross right frontal mucocele in an adult patient with headache, reduced vision and proptosis. Figure 3 shows a radiological image of a sphenoid mucocele in a child with headache and vomiting. Figure 4 shows a radiological image of left maxillary mucocele in an adult patient with nasal blockage and foul smelling discharge.

Patient / Age/sex/ race	Presentation	Sinus involvement on endoscopy	Imaging	Surgery	Follow-up
1. 40/M/C	supra orbital swelling, no diplopia or nasal symptoms	Left frontal and ethmoid sinuses involvement	CT: Expansile cystic mass Lt fronto ethmoid region	Endoscopic marsupialization of fronto-ethmoidal mucocele	Symptom free at 1 year follow up with no sign of recurrence
2. 59/M/C	Right frontal swelling with diplopia	Right frontal sinus involvement	CT: Expansile cystic lesion pushing interfrontal sinus septum with	Bicoronal flap cranialization with endoscopic endonasal frontal sinusotomy and marsupilization	Symptom free at 1 year follow up with no evidence of recurrence

http://dx.doi.org/10.5772/58331

Patient / Age/sex/ race	Presentation	Sinus involvement on endoscopy	Imaging	Surgery	Follow-up
			orbital roof involvement		
3. 40/M/M	Nasal block, rhinorrhoea with anosmia	Right frontal sinus involvement with bilateral nasal polyposis	CR & MRI: Right frontal expansile cystic mass with intracranial extension, no evidence of mass effect or ring enhancement	Endoscopic right frontal sinusotomy and bilateral ethmoidectomy with marsupilization	Symptoms improvement with no evidence of recurrence of nasal polyps at 6 month follow-up
4. 55/F/M	Headaches with, right diplopia	Right ethmoid sinuses involvement	CT & MRI: Expansile right ethmoidal mass with thinning of lamina papyracea	Endoscopic anterior and posterior ethmoidectomy with marsupilization	Symptom free at 6 month follow up with no evidence of recurrence
5. 59/M/Bengali	Headaches, proptosis with reduced left eye movement	Bilateral frontal sinus involvement	CT: Expansile mass involving bilateral frontal sinuses	Endoscopic drainage of bilateral frontal mucopyocele with marsupilization	Symptom free at 6 month follow up with no evidence of recurrence
6. 73/M/C	Reduced vision, eye pain, headaches with nasal blockage	Sphenoid sinus involvement	CT: Expansile mass within sphenoid sinus compressing on optic nerves	Endoscopic sphenoethmoidectom y and marsupialization	Symptom free at 1 year follow up with no evidence of recurrence
7. 75/F/C	Left epiphora with swelling at medial cantus	Left Fronto-Ethmoid sinuses involvement	CT: Opacification of left frontal and ethmoidal sinuses	Endoscopic left frontal sinustomy with anterior and posterior ethmoidectomy with marsupialization	Symptom free at 1 year follow up with no evidence of recurrence
8. 71/F/C	Right nasal blockage, rhinorrhea, sneezing with epiphora	Right maxillary sinus involvement	CT: Hypodense mass in right maxillary sinus with remodeling of maxillary wall and hard plate	Endoscopic right MMA with Marsupialization	Symptom free at 6 months follow up with no evidence of recurrence

Patient / Age/sex/ race	Presentation	Sinus involvement on endoscopy	Imaging	Surgery	Follow-up
9. 63/F/C	Pain left eye with reduced vision and headaches	Left spheno-Ethmmoid sinuses involvement	CT & MRI: Bilateral opacity of ethmoid and sphenoid sinuses with evidence of compression of optic nerve and cavernous sinus	Endoscopic ethmosphenoidectomy with marsupialization	Symptom free at 1 year follow up with no evidence of recurrence
10. 39/M/I	Headaches with right protosis, and diplopia	Right frontal sinus involvement	MRI: Opacity within right frontal sinus with mass effect on right superior and medial wall	Endoscopic right frontal sinusotomy with marsupialization	Symptoms improvement with no evidence of recurrence at 1 year follow up
11. 8/M/I	Headaches with vomitting	Sphenoid sinus involvement	MRI: Expansile mass within sphenoid sinus involving the sphenoethmoidal recess	Endoscopic sphenoethmoidectomy with marsupialization	Symptoms improved with no recurrence at 3 months
12. 62/M/C	Lt nasal blockage with foul smelling nasal discharge	Left maxillary sinus involvement	CT: Expansile left maxillary mass	Endoscopic wide left MMA with marsupilization	Post DXT NPC with no recurrence at 3 months
13. 58/M/M	Rt nasal blockage with foul smelling nasal discharge	Right maxillary sinus involvement	CT: Expansile right maxillary mass	Endoscopic wide right MMA with marsupilization	Symptoms improved with no recurrence at 6 months

M – Male

F – Female

Race-M (Malay), C (Chinese), I (Indian)

Rt– Right

Lt – Left

MMA – Middle meatal antrostomy

Table 1. Dermographic presentation of 13 patients with paranasal sinus mucocele

	Frontal	Ethmoid	Maxillary	Sphenoid
Number of cases	6	4	3	3

Table 2. Sites of involvement of paranasal sinuses

	Headache	Diplopia	Proptosis	Reduced vision	Reduced eye movement	Nasal symptoms	Vomiting
Number of cases	7	2	5	3	2	5	1

Table 3. Clinical presentation of head and eye symptoms

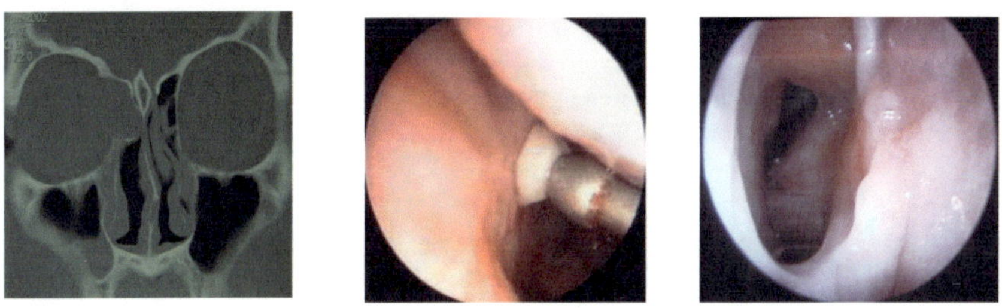

Figure 1. Coronal CT imaging of patient number 4 showing a right iatrogenic frontoethmoid mucocele with intraoperative endoscopic drainage and follow up at 3 months post surgery showing a patent frontal sinustomy

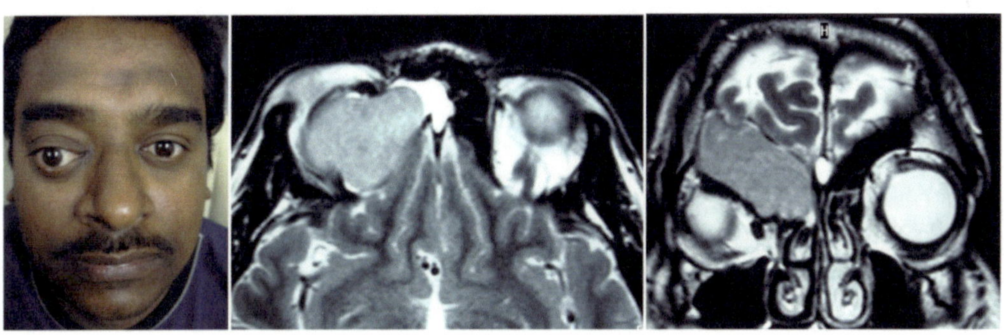

Figure 2. Picture of patient number 10 showing gross right protosis and the respective axial and coronal MRI sections revealing expansile frontal sinus lesion with loss of scalloping suggestive of a mucocele

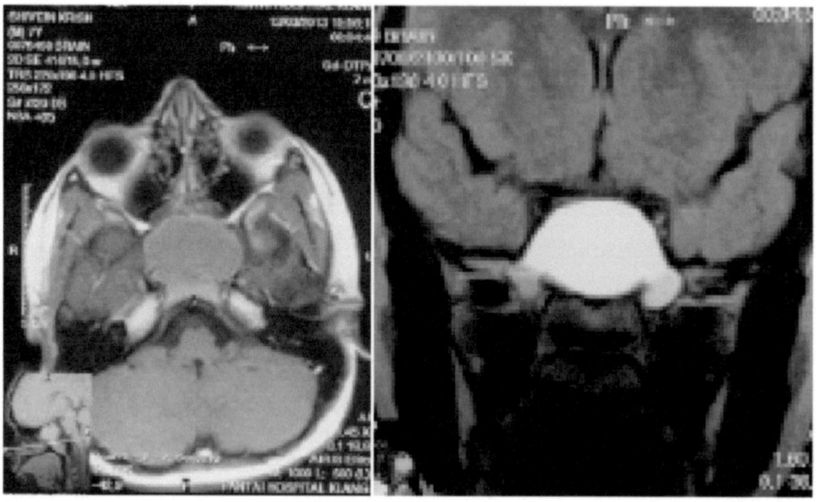

Figure 3. Axial views and coronal sections of T1 and T2 weighted MRI images of patient number 11 showing an expansile sphenoid lesion suggestive of mucocele in a 8-year Indian male.

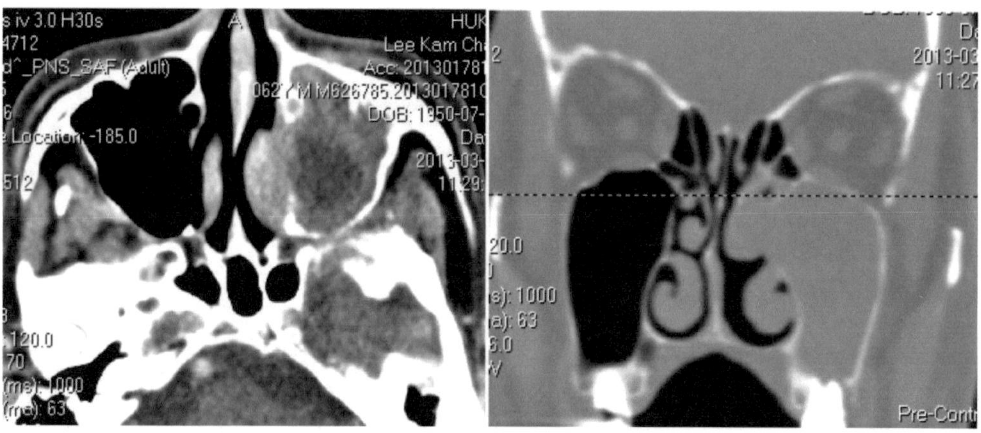

Figure 4. Axial views and coronal sections of CT images of patient number 12 showing a left expansile mass in the maxillary sinus suggestive of a mucocele in a 62 year male Chinese.

3.1. Surgical technique

All patients were operated under general aneasthesia. The patient is placed in supine position with head slightly elevated. Packing that has been soaked in a 4% cocaine solution is placed in the nasal cavity to initiate mucosal vasoconstriction. Both eyes are exposed in the surgical field. Under endoscopic visualization, submucosal injections of 1% lidocaine with epinephrine are administred along the lateral nasal wall and middle turbinate. Briefly the endoscopic endonasal marsupilization is as follows: wide middle meatal antrostomy and marsupilization for maxillary mucocele; initially complete ethmoidectomy followed by removal of antero-inferior wall of the sphenoid mucocele and marsupilizing the cavity for ethmoid and sphenoid mucocele;uncinectomy, anterior ethmoidectomy and widening of the frontal recess (Draf type 2 procedure) and marsupilization for fronto-ethmoid mucocele.Patients' are observed at weekly follow-up with secretion aspirated and sinonasal washing with saline solution upto one month post-surgery. Patients are checked upon at follow-ups every three months for first year than once a year.

4. Discussion

Paranasal sinus mucoceles are rare in children but relatively common in adults. In the literature, the etiologies of pediatric mucoceles have focused on impaired secretion process such as cystic fibrosis, pathological pneumatization processus, atopy and trauma, [7,8].

Mucoceles are commonly caused by post-operative ostial obstruction or secondary to trauma but can also present as primary disease. Paranasal sinus mucoceles predorminently occur in the fronto-ethmoid region (64%), followed by the maxillary sinus (18.6%), the sphenoid sinus (8.4%) and the posterior ethmoid sinus (6.7%) [9] which was similar to that in our study. Another common site for occurrence of mucocele is within the supraorbital ethmoid region. Primary sphenoid mucoceles can be found in association with chronic ethmoid sinusitis and/or nasal polyposis and are uncommon in isolation [10].

In the literature review, proptosis, periorbital pain and impairment of ocular mobility were the most common manifestations of mucoceles in the anterior paranasal sinuses while blurred vision and impairment of ocular mobility [11] were frequently seen in mucoceles in the posterior sinuses. Mucoceles of the anterior paranasal sinuses may expand the anterior and medial sinus walls, pushing the globe outward and downward and restrict movement of the extraocular muscles, thus causing proptosis and impairment of ocular mobility [4, 12, 13].

The natural development of sinus mucoceles consists of gradual expansion. This slow growing expansion can result in bone remodeling, bulging and erosion and reaches adjacent structures such as other sinuses, orbit, clivus, skull base or brain. In case of an intracranial complication, infection may even lead to conditions such as meningitis, subdural or brain abcess [14]. By extension into adjacent structures, the mucocele gives rise to a variety of clinical manifestations. The most common symptoms reported are headaches, facial pain, anosmia, ocular displacement, ocular palsy and visual failure. Visual symptoms in patients with sphenoid mucocele include diplopia, ocular muscle paresis, exopthalmus and complete visual loss [15, 16, 17, 18]. One should also be aware of unusual presentation including hypopituitarism [19, 20, 21].

The anatomical proximity and fragility of the orbital structures explains the high occurrence of ocular complications in sinusopathy. As the optic nerve enters the orbital apex from the intracranial portion, the nerve is encompassed by the narrow bony canal and is in close proximity to the posterior ethmoid and/or sphenoid sinus. In majority of cases the bony wall between the nerve and the sinuses is as thin as 40-60um [22, 23]. Intracranially the optic nerve is covered by the pia mater, arachnoid and CSF. As the nerve enters the canal, it is surrounded by two layers of nerve sheath, the outer which is continuous with the periorbita and the inner which en sheaths the nerve to the eyeball. The optic nerve canal can be identified as a semi-circular tube when viewed from the inside of the posterior ethmoid or sphenoid sinus. Since the optic nerve canal contains the nerve and two layers of nerve sheath without any soft tissues such as fat, pressure due to expansion of the mucocele may easily impact the nerve if the thin protecting bony wall is resorbed or if it is dehiscent congenitally.

Blurred vision is more often associated with mucoceles in the posterior than anterior paranasal sinuses and can affect the optic or other cranial nerves via two pathways. Firstly, expansion of the paranasal sinus wall may compress the optic nerve or compromise its blood supply with subsequent optic atrophy [12, 24, 25]. Secondly, optic neuritis may result from direct spread of suppuration from adjacent paranasal sinuses via bone loss or bone fissure [12, 26]. Both optic nerve compression and neuritis can cause deterioration of visual acuity [12, 26]. Besides the optic nerve, other cranial nerves (abducent or oculomotor) passing through the orbital apex or superior orbital fissure may be involved, thus resulting in impairment of ocular mobility [12, 25, 26, 27].

In a review of 47 patients suffering from ethmoid or sphenoid mucoceles, Moriyama et al [28] highlighted 70 per cent of patients first sought help from the ophthalmology department. The mucocele may compress the optic canal and cause visual disturbances, leading to loss of eye sight in severe cases. Further to direct pressure, ischemia or venous congestion around the optic nerve subsequently occurs [28]. Besides compression and its local effects, inflammation due to infection of the mucocele can spread to the nerve through zones of bony erosion. Therefore, the visual loss may be due to a local inflammatory response which responds to steroid therapy [29] but further diagnosis and immediate surgical drainage are imperative.

Preoperative diagnosis is usually based on CT and MRI. On CT scan, mucoceles usually fill a sinus structure and bulge against adjacent anatomical structures, but without infiltration and usually the bony margins of the lesion are well defined. MRI of mucoceles in both T1 and T2 weighted images show variable signal intensities as depicted in Fig 3. CT scans are preferable for definitive evaluation, assessment of bony involvement and presurgical planning. MRI scans are helpful in the evaluation of orbital or intracranial extension and in ruling out a neoplasm or fungus disease [30]. Therefore, CT and MRI imaging are complementary for the diagnostic evaluation of an expansile mass around the posterior ethmoid and sphenoid sinus. In the differential diagnosis, one should rule out a mucopyocele, sinus malignancy, hypophyseal tumor, craniopharyngioma, meningioma or optic nerve glioma, intracranial chordoma,cholesteatoma and neoplastic lesions of nasopharynx.

An urgent surgical intervention is advocated in a paranasal sinus mucocele with vision loss. The endoscopic endonasal approach is the most convenient for the treatment of mucocele in view of easy access, lower morbidity and a reduction in potential complications compared to intracranial route [31]. Several recent literatures have reported successful results in the management of mucoceles with endoscopic marsupilization as the main choice of treatment [32]. It has the advantage of magnification of the operative field, is minimally invasive, preserves the sinus architecture and produces good long-term results with adequate post-operative care. Some conditions are not suitable for endoscopic surgery alone including a far laterally placed frontal mucocele, hypertrophic bone occluding the area of the fronto-nasal recess and a mucocele arising secondarily from a malignancy [33]. With respect to patient number 2, the extensive mucocele with intraorbital extension was removed using both an endoscopic and an external approach through bicoronal flap and cranialization [34].

The paranasal sinus mucocele is widely opened and a sufficient part of the wall or outflow pathway is resected for adequate drainage and ventilation. With exposure of the dura or peri-orbital wall, the wall of the mucocele acts as a cover and no attempts are made to remove this mucosal lining to protect the orbit, optic nerve, dura and carotid artery. On adequate marsu-pilization of the mucocele, one should expect a rapid improvement of visual acuity but in cases with complete loss of vision prior to surgery, the prognosis may be much poorer. The micro-debrider is used in endonasal surgery with great easiness and good surgical outcome. The degree of improvement of the visual acuity after mucocele marsupilization depends on the severity of the initial loss prior to surgery, the mode of development and the location of the mucocele and the time from onset of the opthalmological disorder until the surgical marsu-pilization [9]. Prompt surgical treatment is necessary in order to avoid permanent visual impairment and other sequel [3, 18]. If vision is seriously impaired, immediate surgery should be performed, preferably within 24 hours after the onset of visual disturbances [35].

5. Differential diagnosis

5.1. Paranasal sinus tumors

The differential diagnosis of mucocele includes paranasal sinus tumors as shown in Table 4.

Non-neoplastic	Neoplastic
Mucosal cyst	Papillomas
Antrochonal polyp	Mesenchymal tumors (fibroma, lipoma, myxoma)
Fungal disease	Vasiform tumors (hemangioma, aneurysmal bone cyst, hemangiopericytoma)
Cholesterol granuloma	Tumors of muscle origin (leiomyoma, rhabdomyoma)
Hematoma	Odontogenic tumors
Antrolithiasis	Fibroosseous lesions (osteoma, ossifying fibroma, fibrous dysplasia, osteoblastoma)
Eosinophilic angiocentric fibrosis	Neuroectodermal tumors (schwannoma, neurofibroma)

Table 4. Classification of benign lesions of the paranasal sinus tumors

6. Non-neoplastic

6.1. Mucosal cyst

Mucosal cyct of the paranasal sinuses are common with and incidence between 12 and 36% detected on radiography [36, 37, 38]. They are broadly classified into secretory and non-secretary cysts [39]. Obstruction of mucosal gland leads to formation of secretory cysts which are less common. The more common non secretory cysts are presumably caused by an accumulation of exudates in the sinus mucosa lifting the epithelial lining. The aetiologic factors behind cyst formation remain unknown. They are mostly unilateral but can be bilateral in 10 to 20% cases [40], [41]. They are usually seen as homogenous, dome-shaped opacities on CT scanning and are usually a chance diagnosis on sinus radiography.

6.2. Antrochoanalpolyp (ACP)

ACP is a benign lesion that originates from the mucosa of the maxillary sinus and grows into the nasal cavity to reach the choana (Fig 5). ACPs account for 4 to 6% of all nasal polyps with increased incidence of 33% in children [42], [43]. ACPs are usually unilateral with only a small number of reported cases with bilateral polyps [16]. It has been suggested that most ACPs originate from the posterior-medial wall [44]. Mean age of presentation is 17 years and it is reported to be twice as common in males than females [44].

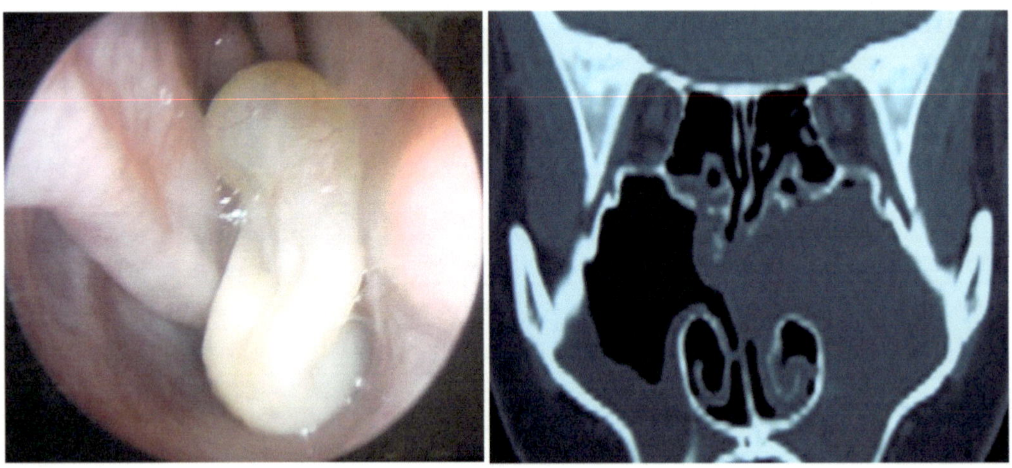

Figure 5. (A) A zero degree endoscope view of a left antrochoanal polyp in an adult male and (B) a coronal CT section of same patient showing a homogenous opaque mass in the maxillary sinus with opasification of the middle meatus and extension into choana.

Clinical manifestations usually start with unilateral nasal obstruction but other symptoms have been reported such as epistaxis, purulent rhinorrhea, post-nasal drip, snoring, obstructive sleep apnea, dysphonia and dysphagia [42, 44].

http://dx.doi.org/10.5772/58331

6.3. Fungal disease

Most sinus fungal infections are caused by Aspergillus species. Aspergilus flavus is the most common cause of sinus fungal ball. Infections by dematiaceous fungi such as Bipolaris, Curvularia or Alternaria are commonly seen in patients with allergic fungal sinusitis. Zygomycetes, such as Mucorales or Rhizopus are well-described aggressive organisms implicated in many cases of invasive fungal sinusitis [45, 46, 47].Fungal rhinosinusitis can be classified as invasive or non-invasive (Table 5). The prognosis of the fungal sinus infections is more dependent on the manifestation of the disease than on the specific causative species.

Noninvasive	Invasive
Saprophytic	Acute invasive fungal sinusitis
Allergic fungal sinusitis	Chronic granulomatous invasive sinusitis
Fungal ball	Chronic invasive fungal sinusitis

Table 5. Classification of fungal sinusitis

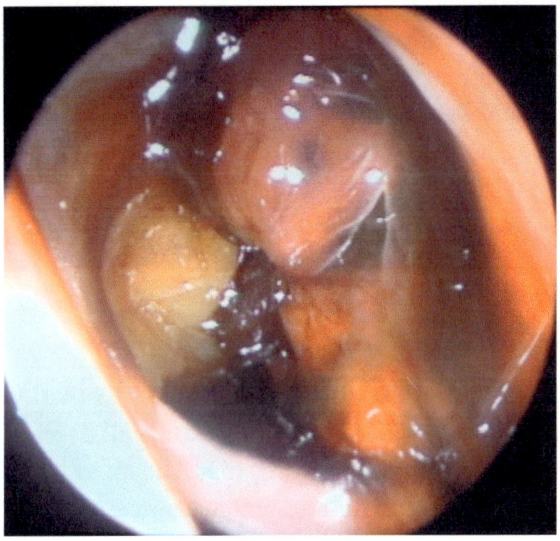

Figure 6. A zero degree endoscopic view of right nasal cavity showing evidence of allergic mucin in an adult male presenting with chronic rhinosinusitis

Associated nasal polyposis is seen in up to 10% due to the chronic inflammatory response. Maxillary sinus fungal ball often presents with unilateral sinus disease and unrelenting symptoms of rhinosinusitis. Allergic fungal sinusitis is characterized by the presence of allergic mucin in patients with symptoms of chronic rhinosinusitis, polyposis and an IgE-mediated hypersensitivity reaction to fungal elements resulting in a self-perpetuating inflammatory cascade (Fig 6). A high index of suspicion for invasive fungal sinusitis is necessary in patients with immunodeficiency, fever and symptoms referable to the paranasal sinuses. CT of paranasal sinuses is often ordered to evaluate refractory symptoms. Complete or subtotal opacification of the involved sinus is not uncommon. Up to 41% demonstrated heterogenous opacification with calcifications (Fig 7). Bony erosion or sclerosis from mass effect can be identified in 17 to 36% [48, 49, 50].

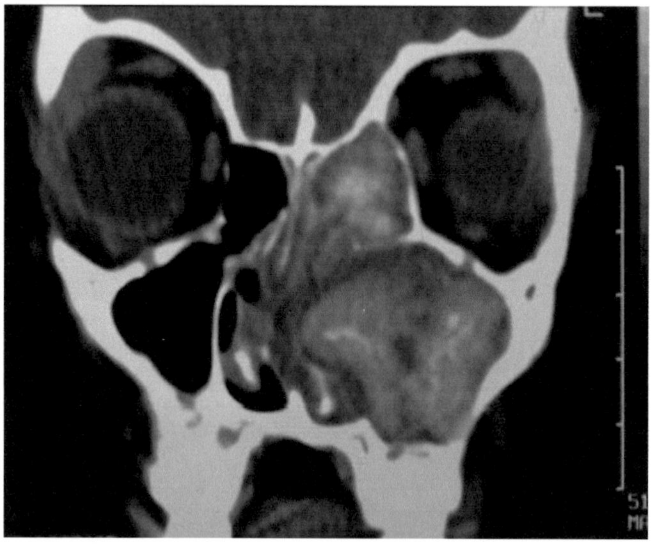

Figure 7. A CT scan coronal section showing heterogenous opacification of the left nasal cavity with calcification in an adult female with fungal sinusitis

6.4. Cholesterol granuloma (CG)

CG is a histologic term used to describe the coexistence of granulation tissue with cholesterol crystals and foreign body giant cells [51].The condition is well described in the temporal bone but is rarely encountered in the paranasal sinuses [52]. The maxillary sinus is most commonly involved [52, 53]. Only one case of bilateral maxillary sinus involvement has been reported [53]. CG has been observed more in men with 3:1 male to female ratio and an average age of 41 years.Only a small number of patients had a history of previous trauma or surgery [52, 53].

The factors contributing to the formation of CG includes disturbed ventilation in a bony cavity, impaired drainage and hemorrhage [52, 53, 54, 55]. Impaired drainage would result in obstruction to venous and lymphatic circulation thus predisposing to mucosal hemorrhage. The insufficient lymphatic drainage would fail to eliminate lipid components in red blood cells and contribute to accumulation of cholesterol crystals. These act as foreign material that stimulates the granulomatous reaction in the sinus cavity [52, 53, 56].

Patients with CG present with symptoms and signs resembling chronic sinusitis [52, 53]. Most of the patients present with nasal obstruction, post-nasal drip, rhinorrhea, facial pain or headaches (Fig 8 A). CT shows a cyst-like opacity which does not enhance with contrast (Fig 8B). Bony erosion or expansion has been reported in a small number of cases [53, 56].

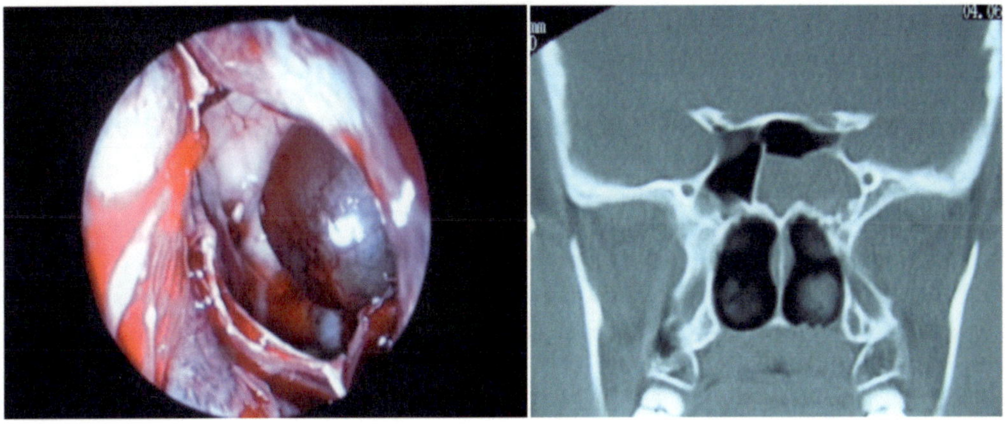

Figure 8. (A) Intraoperative view with 45 degree endoscope showing a polypoid left sphenoid sinus cholesterol granuloma in a young adult female presenting with persistent vertax headaches and (B) a CT scan coronal section showing a homogenous partial opacification of the affected sphenoid sinus

6.5. Hematoma

Hematoma of the maxillary sinus is also known as organized hematoma or hemorrhagic pseudotumor [57, 58, 59]. It is an uncommon cause of maxillary sinus mass with only a small number of reported cases from Korea and Japan [58]. Some of the hematoma have been reported in patients with bleeding diathesis such as Von Willebrand disease but there are several patients who present with what appears to be a spontaneous etiology [58, 59, 60]. Initially, a blood clot accumulates in the maxillary sinus secondary to facial trauma, operative bleeding, recurrent epistaxis or bleeding diathesis. Subsequently the hematoma develops and due to poor ventilation and obstruction of drainage it transforms into an organized hematoma by means of neovascularization and fibrosis [58, 59]. Encapsulation of the blood clot by fibrous tissue prevents reabsorption of the hematoma. Further bleeding causes increasing pressure and progressive expansion which leads to erosion of adjacent structures [59], [60].

The most common symptom at presentation is epistaxis followed by unilateral obstruction and facial swelling [57, 58]. Symptoms due to pressure on adjacent structures such as proptosis and infraorbital hypoaesthesia have been reported [61, 62]. CT scanning shows the hematoma as a nonenhancing soft tissue mass which can be heterogeneous or homogenous. Histologically the hematoma has a peripheral wall that consists of dense fibrous tissue with a spindle-shaped myofibroblast cells. The center of the hematoma consist of loose fibrous tissue which is relatively acellular and contains some intact erythrocytes [57, 58, 62].

6.6. Antrolithiasis

Antrolithiasis are calcified bodies that are formed from mineral salt deposition around a nucleus within the maxillary sinus cavity [63]. These are synonymous with rhinoliths which are reported within the nasal cavity. Anthroliths result from either endogenous (blood clot, mucus or pus) or exogenous factors (teeth and roots or other foreign material. The majority of cases reported had tooth extraction prior to presentation. The patients can be asymptomatic and may present with symptoms of unilateral chronic maxillary sinusitis. CT scan shows antroliths as radiopaque masses of varying sizes and shapes with irregular borders.

6.7. Eosinophilic Angiocentric Fibrosis (EAF)

EAF is an uncommon inflammatory fibrotic lesion that affects the submucosa of the nose, larynx and orbit [64, 65]. The pathologic process is manifested by predorminently eosinophilic perivascular inflammation and gradual replacement with progressive fibrosis [64, 67]. EAF is found with slightly higher incidence in young to middle-aged women than men [64]. The etiology of EAF is unknown but it has been closely linked to granuloma faciale [64, 68]. Majority of the lesions involve the nasal septum and lateral nasal wall with only few cases involving the maxillary sinus.

EAF is slow growing and can take many years to manifest [64, 65]. Symptoms are non specific and can initially include nasal obstruction, rhinorrhea,epistaxis and facial pain [64, 67, 68]. Due to mass expansion the patients will present later with facial swelling [64, 65]. Involvement of the orbit can lead to periorbital edema and proptosis [64]. Nasal endoscopy reveals thickening of the nasal septum with an intranasal mass [64, 65].

7. Neoplastic

7.1. Papillomas

Papillomas are the most common benign epithelial tumor found in the sinonasal area accounting for 10% of all neoplasms in this region [66].Histologically they are divided into inverted,cylindrical and everted [67]. Everted papilloma more often arises on the nasal septum whereas both inverted and cylindrical papillomas mostly arise on the lateral nasal wall within the middle meatus (Fig 9). The age of presentation is from 35 to 60 years with a male preponderance of 3.5: 1 [66, 68]. It is more common in Caucasions compared with other racial groups. A viral aetiology has been suggested with a link to papilloma viral subtypes 6, 11,16 and 18 [68].

Patients generally present with obstructive nasal symptoms, rhinorrhea and chronic rhinosinusitis [66, 68]. CT scans shows a mass in lateral nasal wall with areas of apparent calcification and there may be sclerosis of the walls of the sinus [81] (Fig 10). Both a high recurrence rate and malignant transformation have been documented. A recent review of the literature of over 200 cases calculated 7.1% synchronous carcinoma and 3.6% metachronous carcinoma [70].

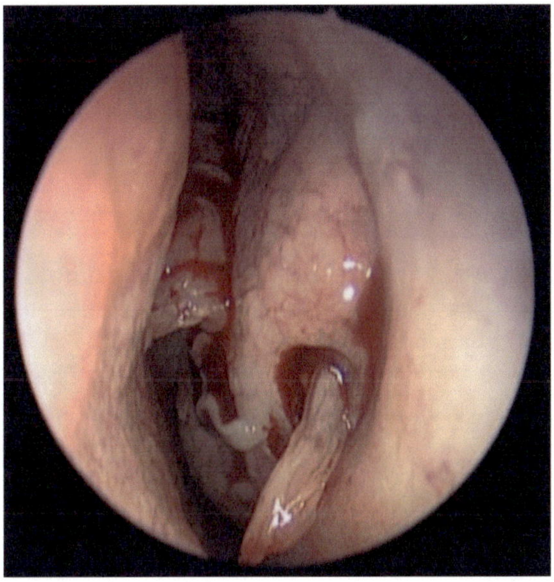

Figure 9. A zero degree endoscopic view of a left inverted papilloma arising from the lateral nasal wall in an elderly male

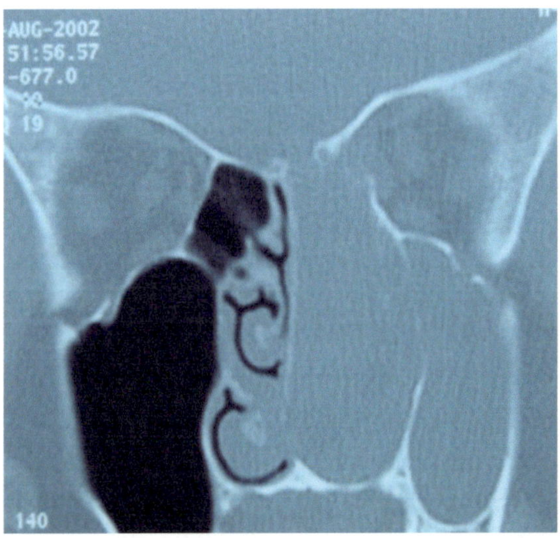

Figure 10. A coronal CT scan section showing an aggressive inverted papilloma (hybrid tumor) arising from the left nasal cavity with evidence of anterior skull base erosion in an elderly Chinese male presenting with CSF rhinorrhea

7.2. Mesenchymal tumors: Fibroma, lipoma and myxoma

These rare tumors may be encountered in the nose and sinuses and generally present prior to adulthood. Isolated tumors within maxillary sinus are very rare.

7.2.1. Fibromas

Fibromas result from progressive inflammation or fibroblastic proliferation of the nasal mucosa [71]. They present as slow-growing, grey-white, smooth surfaced masses producing obstructive nasal symptoms.

7.2.2. Lipoma

Lipoma is the most common soft tissue tumor in adulthood in contrast to intraosseouslipoma which is a rare condition.The etiology of intraosseous lipoma is unknown but infaction, ischaemia, trauma and irradiation may be contributing factors [72]. Cases have been reported within the nasal cavity and very rarely in the maxillary sinus. The presentation is of nasal swelling and possible nasal obstruction.

7.2.3. Myxoma

Myxoma of the maxillary sinus is very rare but more frequent than fibromas and lipomas [73]. The age of presentation is between 2 and 15 years and may be related to dental malformations or missing teeth.

7.3. Vasiform Tumors: Hemangioma, Aneurysmal Bone Cyst and Hemangiopericytoma

These benign lesions arise from vascular tissue within the mucosa or bone of the nose and sinuses.

7.3.1. Hemangiomas

Hemangiomas represent about 20% of benign non-epithelial tumors of nasal cavity and paranasal sinuses [74]. Mean age of diagnosis is 40 years and the most frequent presenting symptoms are nasal obstruction and epistaxis. Invovement of maxillary sinus have been reported less frequently [91]. Both cavernous and capillary hemangiomas have been reported.

7.3.2. Aneurysmal bone cyst (ABCs)

ABCs are expansile lesions of unknown etiology that involves long bones and vertebrae of patients younger than 20 years. About 2% of ABCs are encountered in the head and neck region with jaw being the most frequently involved site. The present with facial swelling and obstructive nasal symptoms in the age group between 5 and 23 years. ABCs consist of multiple cavities filled with blood and serous fluids which are separated by septa and surrounded by rim of bone [75]. ABCs have a "honeycomb"appearance on gadolinium-enhanced MRI studies [75].

7.3.3. Hemangiopericytoma (HPC)

HPC is a rare benign vascular tumor derived from extracapillary cells (pericytes). Less than one-third of HPC occur in the head and neck and 5% are located in the nasal cavity and

http://dx.doi.org/10.5772/58331

paranasal sinuses [76, 77]. Sphenoid and ethmoid sinuses are involved more frequently than the maxillary sinus. Both sexes are equally affected and can occur at any age but often develop after the second decade. The patients usually present with epistaxis and nasal obstruction with reddish submucosal nasal mass (Fig 11).

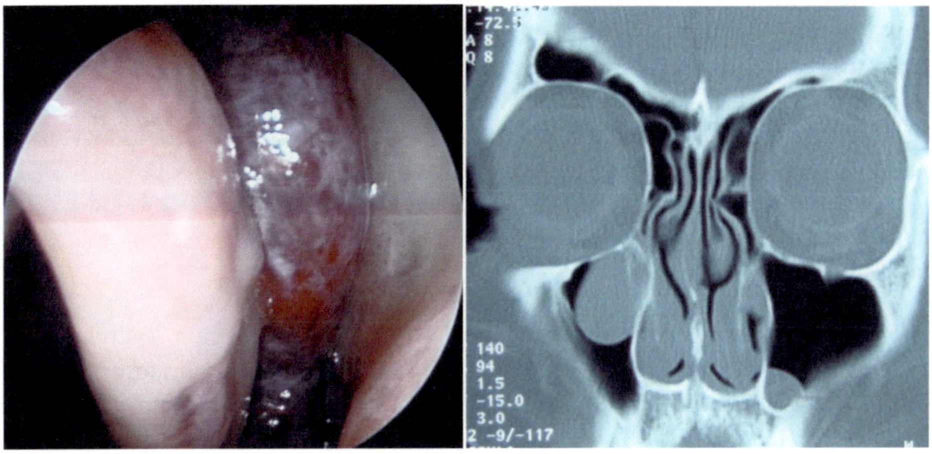

Figure 11. (A) View with 30 degree endoscope in an adult Chinese female presenting with right nasal obstruction and maxillary sinus discomfort and (B) CT scan coronal section showing a polypoidal mass arising from the right maxillary sinus and histopathology report consistent with hemangiopericytoma

7.4. Tumors of muscle origin: Leiomyoma and rhabdomyoma

7.4.1. Leiomyoma

Leiomyoma is a smooth muscle tumor that originates in areas of abundance of muscle like the uterus.

It is extremely rare for these tumors to present in the sinonasal tract because of the paucity of smooth muscle. And only a handful of cases have been reported in the maxillary sinus [78]. The tumor seem to be slow-growing and non-aggressive and presenting with obstructive nasal symptoms.

7.4.2. Rhabdomyoma

Rhabdomyomais a skeletal muscle tumor and is extremely rare in the paranasal sinus.,which has a benign behavior and low recurrence rate [79, 80].

7.5. Odontogenic tumors

Odontogenic tumors originate either within the maxillofacial skeleton (intraosseous) or within the gingival or alveolar mucosa overlying the tooth bearing areas (extraosseous). They are usually slow growing and have been associated with non-eruption of the teeth. Patients usually present with swelling of alveolar process along with nasal obstruction and epistaxis. Superior displacement of globe has been reported with large odontogenic tumors.

7.5.1. Ameloblastoma

Ameloblastomais the most common odontogenic tumor. It is slow growing, locally invasive and has a high rate of recurrence if not treated effectively. Patients between the ages of 16 and 60 years are generally affected with the region of canine tooth and maxilla being the most common sites. They are often asymptomatic but can present with a painless swelling of the cheek, gingival and palate that may reach a large size. Ameloblastoma presents as a unilocular or multilocular radiolucency that may be associated with an impacted tooth.

7.6. Fibro-osseous lesions: Osteoma, ossifying fibroma, fibrous dysplasia and osteoblastoma

Fibro-osseous lesions represent a class of bony abnormalities: osteoma, ossifying fibroma, fibrous dysplasia and osteoblastoma. They are distinct but lie along a continuum from the most to the least content. They have some similarities in appearance but their clinical implications differ.

7.6.1. Osteomas

Osteomas are frequent incidental finding in up to 3% of CT scans of the paranasal sinuses [81] (Fig 12). Eighty percent occur in the frontal sinuses followed by the ethmoids and least in the maxillary sinuses. The etiology is either embryologic or secondary to trauma or an infective process. There is an association with Gardner syndrome which is an autosomal dominant condition characterized by intestinal polyposis and pigmented skin lesions in addition to osteomas [82]. Maxillary sinus osteomas are slow growing and usually asymptomatic but they may become symptomatic depending on the location and onset [83].

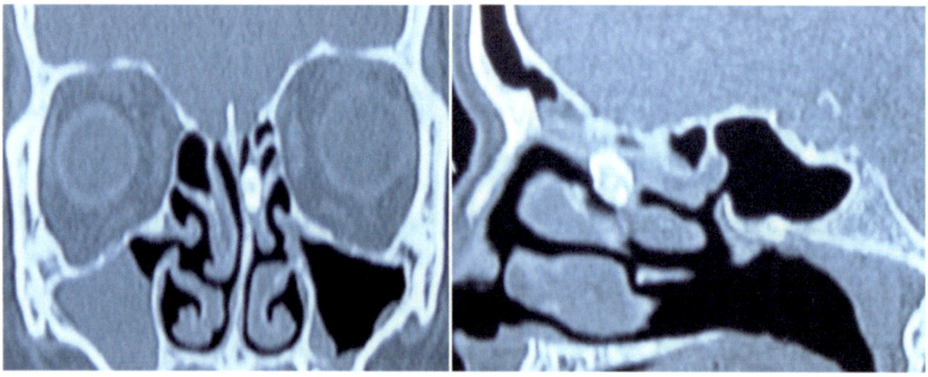

Figure 12. (A) A CT scan coronal and (B) sagittal section showing osteoma arising from the anterior ethmoid sinuses in an adult female presenting with frequent headaches

http://dx.doi.org/10.5772/58331

7.6.2. Ossifying fibroma (OF)

OF is a well-circumscribed lesion that continues to grow after sexual maturity and can attain dramatic proportions [81, 84]. The vast majority is located in the posterior region of the mandible; those involving the maxillary sinus are uncommon [85]. Patient usually present between the third and forth decades and the lesion is more common in women [85]. The most common presentation is of painless cheek swelling but involvement of the orbit or nasal cavity may be signified by proptosis, loss of visual acuity, epiphora, nasal obstruction and epistaxis [81, 85]. Radiologically, the lesion is sharply circumscribed with an egg shell rim and central radiolucency which differentiates it from fibrous dysplasia with its indistinguishable borders.

7.6.3. Fibrous dysplasia (FD)

FD is a slow, progressive disorder where normal bone is replaced by fibrous tissue and immature woven bone [81, 84]. There are two main forms of FD: monostatic (70-85%) that involves only one bone and polystatic (15-30%) where multiple bones can be involved (Fig 13). The maxilla and mandible are the most commonly involved bones generally in the monostatic form. FD is a disease of the young where patients present in their first or second decade and is assumed to be "burnt out" as the patients reach skeletal maturity. The usual symptom is of painless facial deformity although other complaints such as loosening of teeth, nasal obstruction or epistaxis have been encountered [86]. CT scans shows lesions with indistinct borders and a homogenous "ground glass" appearance.

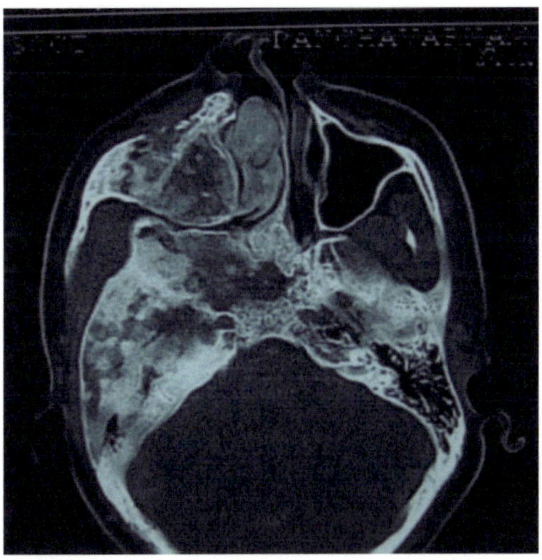

Figure 13. An axial CT section showing a polystatic fibrous dysplasia in an adult female

7.6.4. Osteoblastoma

Osteoblastoma is an uncommon neoplasm characterized by proliferation of osteoblasts forming bone trabeculae set in a vascularized fibrous connective tissue stroma [87]. The tumor occur predorminantly in vertebrae and long bones and can affect craniofacial bones with the mandible being the most commonly involved. It is reported less in the maxillary bone and rarely in the maxillary sinus [88]. The majority of the patients are under 30 years and present with a facial swelling and is often painful [87]. CT scan features range from radiolucent to radiopaque lesions and are often mistaken for other fibro-osseous lesions.

7.7. Neuroectodermal tumors: Schwannoma and neurofibroma

7.7.1. Schwannomas

Schwannomas are benign nerve sheath tumors of which 50% occur in the head and neck region. They are very uncommon in the paranasal sinuses (only 4%) and a very small number involve the maxillary sinus [84]. The lesion slowly expands in the sinus cavity resulting in swelling, pressure symptoms and bony necrosis. The patients mostly present with nasal obstruction but other symptoms such as proptosis, epiphora, headaches, facial anesthesia and epistaxis have been reported [90]. CT scan shows a homogenous radio-opaque mass with evidence of bone remodeling (Fig 14).

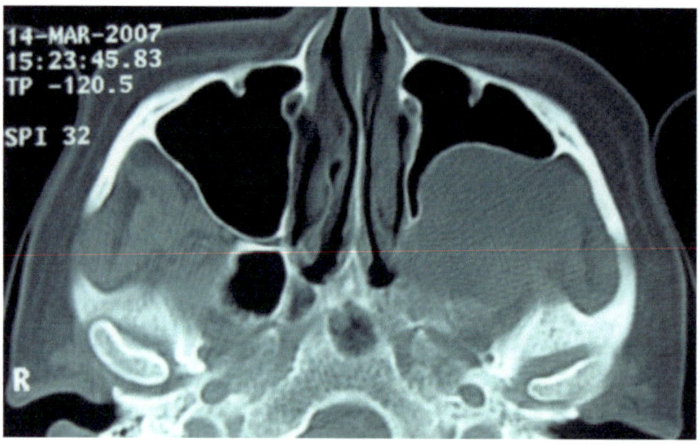

Figure 14. An axial CT section showing a left homogenous radio-opaque mass involving the maxillary sinus and infratemporal region in an adult female

7.7.2. Neurofibromas

Neurofibromas are heterogenous peripheral nerve tumors that arise from the connective tissue of the nerves especially the endoneurium [91]. They may occur as sporadic lesions but are much more common in association with neurofibromatosis type 1 (NF 1). Neurofibromas of the maxillary sinus are exceedingly rare.As with schwannomas, they slowly grow and expand within the sinus cavity causing swelling, pressure symptoms and bone necrosis. Presentation is similar to other expanding masses in the maxillary sinus. CT scan shows a well-circumscribed mass with some bony erosion.

8. Conclusion

Mucocele of the paranasal sinuses are well described complication of chronic sinusitis in adults but they rarely occur in the pediatric population. Mucocele can be associated with ophthalmic complications or intracranial complications. Radiological imaging includes CT-scan and sometimes MRI when intracranial complications are suspected. The differential diagnosis of mucocele includes paranasal sinus tumors. Usually a wide endoscopic endonasal marsupilization of paranasal sinus mucocele is a safe and less invasive than external approaches. Thus, a good understanding of paranasal sinus mucoceles by ophthalmologists and otorhinolaryngologists is essential for early diagnosis and rapid surgical intervention.

Author details

Balwant Singh Gendeh*

Address all correspondence to: bsgendeh@gmail.com

Department of Otorhinolaryngology-Head Neck Surgery, UKM Medical Center, Jalan Yaacob Latif, Bandar Tun Razak, Kuala Lumpur, Malaysia

References

[1] Alberti PW, Marshall HF, Black JI. 1968. Fronto-ethmoidalmucocele as a cause of unilateral proptosis. Br J Ophthalmol52: 833-838

[2] Johnson JT, Ferguson BJ. 1998. Infection in: Cummings CW, Fredrickson JM, Harker LA, Krause CJ, Schuller DE, Rhicharson MA, eds Otolaryngology Head Neck Surgery, 3rd edition. St Louis: Mosby1115-1116

[3] Maniglia AJ, Kronberg FG, Culbertson W. 1984. Visual loss associated with orbital and sinus disease. Laryngoscope 94(8): 1050-1059

[4] Curtin HD, Rabinov JD. 1998. Extension to the orbit from paraorbital disease. Radiol Clin North Am 36: 1201-1213

[5] Moriyama H, Hesaka H, Tachibana T, Honda Y. 1992. Mucoceles of ethmoid and sphenoid sinus with visual disturbance. Arch Otolaryngol Head Neck Surg 118: 141-146

[6] Wang JW, JangYT, Lee BJ. 2007. Natural course of retention cysts of the maxillary sinus: long term follow-up results. Laryngoscope 117(2):341-344

[7] Olze H, Matthias C, Degenhardt P. 2006. Pediatr ic paranasal sinus mucoceles. Eur J Pediatr ic Surg 16: 192-196

[8] Timon CL, O'Dwyer TP. 1989. Ethmoidal mucoceles in children. J Laryngol Otol 103: 284-246

[9] Rombaux Ph, Bertrand B, Eloy Ph, Collet S, Daela J, Bachert C, Claes J. 2000. Endoscopic endonasal surgery for paranasal sinus mucoceles. Acta Oto-Rhinol-Laryngologica Belg 54:115-122

[10] Daniilidis J, Nikolaou A, Kondopoulos V. 1992. An unusual case of sphenoid sinus mucocele with severe intracranial extension. Rhinology 31:135-137

[11] Tseng CC, Ho CY, Kao SC. 2005. Ophthalmic manifestation of paranasal sinus mucocele. J Chin Med Ass 68(6): 260-264

[12] Shimo-Oku M, Miyazaki S, Shiraki K, Sugimoto T, Sotani H. 1989. Optic nerve involvement in posterior paranasal sinus diseases. Neuroophthalmology 9:145-155

[13] Lund VJ, Rolfe ME. 1989. Ophthalmic considerations in fronto-ethmoid mucoceles. J Laryngol Otol 103:667-669

[14] Nugert GR, Sprinkle P, Bloor BM. 1970. Sphenoid sinus mucocele. J Neurosurg 32:443-451

[15] McCarthy WL, Frenkel M. 1972. Visual loss as the only symptom of sphenoid sinus mucocele. Am J Ophthalmol 74: 1140-1143

[16] Casteels F, De Loof E, Brock P, Jorissen M, Dralands L, Missotten L, Wilms G. 1992. Sudden blindness in a child: Presenting symptoms of sphenoid sinus mucocele. Br J Opthalmol 76: 502-504

[17] Hao SP. 1994. Mucocele of sphenoid sinus with acute blindness: report of a case. J Formosan Med Ass 93: 519-521

[18] Munee A, Jones NS. 1997. Unilateral abducens nerve palsy: a presenting sign of sphenoid mucoceles. J Laryngol Otol 111: 644-646

[19] Valvassoori G, Putterman AM. 1973. Ophthalmological and radiological findings in sphenoid mucoceles. Arch Ophthal 90:416-419

[20] Rosselet PO. Gomez F, Mange B, Savery M, Grigorin D. 1984. Sphenoid sinusitis and panhypopituitarism. Schweiz Med Wonchenschr 114: 1340-1342

[21] Pitkaranta A, Atula T, Lindokl P, Saxen H, Malmberg H. 2000. Unilateral blindness in a child with acute sinusitis. Rhinology 38:43-44

[22] Slavin ML, Glacer JS. 1987. Acute severe irreversible visual loss with sphenoethmoiditis – "Posterior" orbital cellulitis. Arch Ophthal 105: 345-348

[23] Kainz J, Stammberger H. 1992. Danger areas of the posterior rhinobasis. Acta Otolaryngol 112:852-861

[24] McCrary JA. 1997. Spheno-ethmoidal mucocele, chondrosarcoma and unilateral visual loss. In: Smith JL, ed. Neuroophthalmology Update. New York: Masson Publishing, 105-109

[25] Weille FL, Vang RR. 1953. Sinusitis as focus of infection in uveitis, keratitis and retrobulbar neuritis. Arch Ophthalmol, 58:154-165

[26] Rothstein J, Maisel RH, berlinger NT, Writschaffer JD. 1984. Relationship of optic neuritis to disease of the paranasal sinuses. Laryngoscope 94:1501-1508

[27] Lundgren A, Olin T. 1961. Mucopyocele of sphenoidal sinus or posterior ethmoidal cells with special reference to apex orbital syndrome. Acta Otolaryngol 53:61-79

[28] Moriyama H, Nakajima T, Honda Y. 1992. Studies on mucoceles of the ethmoid and sphenoid sinuses. Analysis of 47 cases. J Laryngol Otol 106:23-27

[29] Fujitani T, Takahashi T, Asai T. 1984. Optic nerve disturbance caused by frontal and fronto-ethmoidal mucopyoceles. Arch otolaryngol 110:257-269

[30] Kennedy DW, Josephson JS, Zinreich SJ, Mattox DE, Goldsmith MW. 1989. Endoscopic sinus surgery for mucoceles: A viable alternative. Laryngoscope 99:885-895

[31] Bheasley NTP, Jones NS. 1995. Paranasal sinus mucoceles: modern management. Am J Rhinol 9: 251-256

[32] Kennedy DW, Keogh B, Senior B, Lanza DC. 1996. Endoscopic approach to tumors of anterior skull base and orbit. Oper Tech Otolaryngol Head Neck Surg 7:257-263

[33] Conboy PJ, Jones NS. 2003. The place of endoscopic sinus surgery in the treatment of paranasal sinus mucoceles. Clin Otolaryngol Allied Sci 28;207-210

[34] Namavar E, loh JCN, Gendeh BS. 2012. Paranasal sinus mucocele:Endoscopicmarsupilization and surgical outcome, Egyptian J Otolaryngol 28(2): 95-97

[35] Yomoto E, Hyodo M, Kawatika S, Aibara R. 1997. Effect of sinus surgery on visual disturbances caused by Sphenoethmoidal mucoceles. Am j Rhinol 11: 337-343

[36] Bhattacharyya N. 2000. Do maxillary sinus retention cysts reflect obstructive sinus phenomena? Arch Otolaryngol Head Neck Surg 126(11):1369-1371

[37] Harar RPS, Chadha NK, Rogers G. 2007. Are maxillary sinus mucosal cysts a manifestation of inflammatory sinus disease? J Laryngol Otol 121(8):751-754

[38] Kanagalingham J, Bhatia K, Georgalas C, Fokkens W, Miszkiel K, Lund VJ. 2009. Maxillary mucosal cyst is not a manifestation of rhinosinusitis: results of prospective three-dimentional CT study of ophthalmic patients. Laryngoscope 119(1):8-12

[39] Gardner DG. Pseudocysts and retention cysts of the maxillary sinus. 1984. Oral Surg Oral Med Oral Pathol 58(5):561-567

[40] Casamassimo PS, lilly GE. 1980. Mucosal cysts of the maxillary sinus: a clinical and radiographic study. Oral Surg Oral Med Oral Pathol 50(3):282-286

[41] Fisher EW, Whittet HB, Croft CB. 1989. Symptomatic mucosal cysts of the maxillary sinus:antroscopic treatment. J Laryngol Otol 103(12):1184-1186

[42] Maldonado M, Martinez A, Alobid I, Mullol J. 2004. The antrochoanal polyp. Rhinology 42(4):178-182

[43] Mahfouz ME, Elsheikh MN, Ghoname NF. 2006. Molecular profile of the antrochoanalpolyp:up-regulation of basic fibroblast growth factor and transforming growth factor beta in maxillary sinusmucosa. Am J Rhinol 20(4):178-182

[44] Aydin O, Keskin G, Ustundag E, Iseri M, Ozkarakas H. 2007. Choanal polyps:an evaluation of 53cases. Am j Rhinol 21(2):164-168

[45] Deshazo RD, 2009. Syndromes of invasive fungal sinusitis. Med Mycol 47(Suppl 1):S309-S314

[46] Michael RC, Michael JS, Ashbee RH, Matthews MS. 2008. Mucological profile of fungal sinusitis:an audit of specimens over a 7-year period in a tertiary care hospital in Tamil Nadu. Indian J PatholMicrobiol 51(4): 493-496 Abstract

[47] Plszewski J, Milonski J. 2008. The analysis of the bacterial and fungal flora in maxillary sinuses in patients operated due to FESS method. Otolaryngol Pol 62(4):458-461

[48] Ferguson BJ. 2000. Fungal balls of the paranasal sinuses. Otolaryngol Clin North Am 33(2):389-398

[49] Ferreiro JA, Carlson BA, Cody DT. 1997. Paranasal sinus fungal balls. Head Neck 19(6):481-486

[50] Klossek JM, Serrano E, Peloquin L, Percodi J, Fontanel JP, Pessey JJ. 1997. Functional endoscopic sinus surgery and 109 mycetomas of paranasal sinuses. Laryngoscope 107(1):112-117

[51] Friedmann I, Osborn DA. 1982. Pathology of granulomas and neoplasms of the nose and paranasal sinuses. In: WStCSymmers, ed. Systemic Pathology. Edinburgh/London/New York:Churchill Livingston:1920235

[52] Astarci HM, Sungu N, Samim EE, Ustun H. 2008. Presence of cholesterol granuloma in the maxillary and ethmoid sinuses. Oral Maxillofac Surg 12(2):101-103

[53] Chao TK. 2006. Cholesterol granuloma of the maxillary sinus. Eur Arch Otorhinolaryngol 263(6):592-597

[54] Graham J, Michaels L. 1978. Cholesterol, granuloma of the maxillary antrum. Clin Otolaryngol Allied Sci 3(@):155-160

[55] Niho M. 1986. Cholesterol crystals in the temporal bone and the paranasal sinuses. Int J Pediatr Otorhinolaryngol 11(1):79-95

[56] Kunt T, Ozturkan S, Egilmez R. 1998. Cholesterol granuloma of the maxillary sinus: six cases from the same region. J Laryngol Otol 112(1):65-68

[57] Lim M, Lew-Ghor S, Beale T, Ramsay A, Lund VJ. 2008. Maxillary sinus haematoma. J Laryngol Otol 122(2): 210-212

[58] Song HM, Jang YJ, Chung YS, Lee BJ. 2007. Organizing hematoma of the maxillary sinus. Otolaryngol Head Neck Surg 136(4):616-620

[59] LeePK, Wu JK, Ludemann JP. 2004. Hemorrhagic pseudotumor of the maxillary sinus. J Otolaryngol 33(3):206-208

[60] Ozhan S, Arac M, Isik S, Oznur 11, Atilla S, Kemaloglu Y. 1996. Pseudotumor of the maxillary sinus in a patient with von Willebrand's disease. Am J Roentgenol 166(4): 950-951

[61] Lee BJ, Park HJ, Hoe SC. 2003. Organized hematoma of the maxillary sinus, Acta Otolaryngol 123(7): 869-872

[62] Tabaee A, Kacker A. 2002. Hematoma of the maxillary sinus presenting as a mass- a case report and review of literature. Int J Pediatr Otorhinolaryngol 65(2):153-157

[63] Guneri P, Kaya A, Caliskan MK. 2005. Antroliths:survey of the literature and report of a case. Oral Surg Oral Med Oral Pathol Oral Radiol Endod 99(4):517-521

[64] Kosarac O, Luna MA, RoJ Y, Ayala AG. 2008. Eosinophilic angiocentric fibrosis of the sinonasal tract. Ann Diagn Pathol 12(4):267-270

[65] Paun S, Lund VJ, Gallimore A. 2005. Nasal fibrosis:long-term follow-up of four cases of Eosinophilic angiocentric fibrosis. J Laryngol Otol 119(2):119-124

[66] Lund VJ. 2000. Optimum management of inverted papilloma. J Laryngol Otol 114(3): 194-197

[67] Michaels L. 1996. Benign mucosal tumors of the nose and paranasal sinuses. Semi-n Diagn Pathol 13(2):113-117

[68] Minovi A, Kollert M, Draf W, Bockmuhl U. 2006. Inverted papilloma: feasibility of endonasal surgery and long-term results of 87 cases. Rhinology 44(3):205-210

[69] Savy L, Lloyd G, Lund VJ, Howard D. Optimum imaging for inverted papilloma. J Laryngol Otol 114(11):891-893

[70] Mirza S, Bradley PJ, Acharya A, Stacey M, Jones NS. 2007. Sinonasal inverted papillomas:recurrence and synchoronous and metachronous malignancy. J Laryngol Otol 121(9):857-864

[71] Lin HL, Huang CC, Lee TJ. 2004. Endoscopic sinus surgery treatment for a huge sinonasal fibroma. Chang Gung Med J 27(3):233-237

[72] Uysal A, Kayiran O, Cuzdan SS, Bektas CI, Aslan G, Caydere M. 2007. Maxillary sinus lipoma:an unanticipated diagnosis. J Craniofac Surg 18(5):1153-1155

[73] Gregor RT, Loftus-Coll B. 1994. Myxoma of the paranasal sinuses. J Laryngol Otol 108(8):679-681

[74] Rabaso E, Rosell A, Plaza G, Martinez-Vidal A. Haemangioma of the maxillary sinus. J Laryngol Otol 111(7):638-640

[75] Fyrmpas G, Constantinidis J, Televantou D, Konstantinidis I, Daniilidis J. 2006. Primary aneurismal bone cyst of the maxillary sinus in a child: case report and review of the literature. Eur Arch Otorhinolaryngol 263(7):695-698

[76] Herve S, AbdAlsamad I, Beautru R, et al. 1993. Management of sinonasal hemangiopericytomas. Rhinology 37(4):153-158

[77] Stomeo F, Fois V, Cossu A, Meloni F, Pastore A, Bozzo C. 2004. Sinonasal hemangiopericytoma: a case report. Eur Arch Otorhinolaryngol 261(10): 555-557

[78] LaBruna A, Reagan B, Papageorge A, 1995. Leiomyoma of the maxillary sinus; a diagnostic dilemma. Otolaryngol Head Neck Surg 112(4): 595-598

[79] Fu YS, Perkin KH. 1976. Nonepithelial tumors of the nasal cavity, paranasal sinuses and nasopharynx: a clinicopathologic study of skeletal muscle tumors(rhabdomyoma and rhabdosarcoma). Cancer 37(1):364-376

[80] Reitter GS. 1921. Rhabdomyosarcoma of the nose: report of case. JAMA 76:22-23

[81] Eller R, Sillers M. 2006. Common fibro-osseous lesions of the paranasal sinuses. Otolaryngol Clin North Am 39(3): 585-600

[82] Alexander AA, Patel AA, Odland R. 2007. Paranasal sinus osteomas and Gardner's syndrome. Ann OtolRhinolLaryngol 116(6):658-662

[83] Park W, Kim HS. 2006. Osteoma of maxillary sinus: a case report. Oral Surg Oral Med Oral Pathol Oral Radiol Endod 102(6):e26-e27

[84] Harrison DF. 1984. Osseous and fibro-osseous conditions affecting the craniofacial bones. Ann OtolRhinolLaryngol 93(3 Pt 1):199-203

[85] Chong VF, Tan LH. 1997. Maxillary sinus ossifying fibroma. Am J Otolaryngol 18(6): 419-424

[86] Muraoka H, Ishihara A, Kumagai J. 2001. Fibrous dysplasia with cystic appearance in maxillary sinus. Auris Nasus Larynx 28(1):103-105

[87] Jones AC, Prihoda TJ, Kacher JE, Odingo NA, Freedman PD. 2006. Osteoblastoma of the maxilla and mandible: A report of 24 cases and review of literature and discus-

sion of its relationship to osteodosteoma of the jaw. Oral Surg Oral Med Oral Pathol Oral Radiol Endod 102(5):639-650

[88] Osguthorpe JD, Hungerford GD. 1983. Benign osteoblastoma of the maxillary sinus. Head Neck Surg 6(1): 605-609

[89] Sarioglu S, Ozkal S, Guneri A, et al 2002. Cystic schwannoma of the maxillary sinus. Auris Nasus Larynx 29(3):297-300

[90] Sheikh HY, Chakravathy RP, Slevin NJ, Sykes AJ, Banerjee SS. 208. Benign schwannoma in paranasl sinuses: a clinic-patological study of five cases emphasizing diagnostic difficulties. J Laryngol Otol 122(6):598-602

[91] Boedeker CC, Ridder GJ, Kayser G, Schipper J, Maier W. 2005. Solitary neurofibroma of the maxillary sinus and pterygopalatine fossa. Otolaryngol Head Neck Surg 133(3): 458-459